Improving Outcomes in Heart Failure

An Interdisciplinary Approach

Edited by

Debra K. Moser, DNSc, RN
Associate Professor
The Ohio State University
CHF Community Case Manager
Mount Carmel Health System
Columbus, Ohio

Barbara Riegel, DNSc, RN, CS, FAAN
Professor
School of Nursing
San Diego State University
Clinical Researcher
Sharp HealthCare
San Diego, California

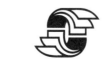

AN ASPEN PUBLICATION®
Aspen Publishers, Inc.
Gaithersburg, Maryland
2001

The authors have made every effort to ensure the accuracy of the information herein. However, appropriate information sources should be consulted, especially for new or unfamiliar procedures. It is the responsibility of every practitioner to evaluate the appropriateness of a particular opinion in the context of actual clinical situations and with due considerations to new developments. The authors, editors, and the publisher cannot be held responsible for any typographical or other errors found in this book.

Library of Congress Cataloging-in-Publication Data

Improving outcomes in heart failure: an interdisciplinary approach/
editors, Debra K. Moser, Barbara Riegel.
p. ; cm.
Includes bibliographical references and index.
ISBN 0-8342-1644-2 (alk. paper)
1. Congestive heart failure.   2. Outcome assessment (Medical care).
I. Moser, Debra K.   II. Riegel, Barbara, 1950–
WG 370I34 2000
616.1'2906—dc21
00-063958

Orders: (800) 638-8437
Customer Service: (800) 234-1660

About Aspen Publishers • For more than 40 years, Aspen has been a leading professional publisher in a variety of disciplines. Aspen's vast information resources are available in both print and electronic formats. We are committed to providing the highest quality information available in the most appropriate format for our customers. Visit Aspen's Internet site for more information resources, directories, articles, and a searchable version of Aspen's full catalog, including the most recent publications: **www.aspenpublishers.com**
Aspen Publishers, Inc. • The hallmark of quality in publishing
Member of the worldwide Wolters Kluwer group.

Editorial Services: Timothy Sniffin
Library of Congress Catalog Card Number: 00-063958
ISBN: 0-8342-1644-2

Printed in the United States of America

1 2 3 4 5

Contents

Contributors ix

Foreword xiii

Preface xv

PART I—THE SYNDROME OF HEART FAILURE:
      PERSONAL AND SOCIETAL IMPACT 1

Chapter 1— **Epidemiology of Heart Failure** 3
Marjorie Funk, Kerry A. Milner, and Harlan M. Krumholz

    Causes and Risk Factors 4
    Incidence 7
    Prevalence 8
    Morbidity 12
    Prognosis and Morality 12
    Conclusion 15

Chapter 2— **Health-Related Quality of Life Outcomes in Heart Failure:**
      A Conceptual Model 18
Martha Shively and Ira B. Wilson

    What Is Health-Related Quality of Life? 18
    A Conceptual Model of HRQL for Clinicians 20
    Understanding the HRQL Model in Heart Failure: Empirical Data ... 25
    Conclusion and Implications 27

Chapter 3— **Managing Heart Failure: Economic Impact and Outcomes** 31
Kathleen M. McCauley and Mary D. Naylor

    Introduction 31
    Economics of Heart Failure: Overview of Key Concepts 31
    Incidence and Economic Impact 32
    Cost-Effectiveness of Pharmacologic Therapy 33

Economic Outcomes Associated with Alternative Models of Care 35
Conclusion and Recommendations for Further Study 38

PART II—IMPROVING OUTCOMES BY INFLUENCING THE PERSONAL IMPACT OF HEART FAILURE **41**

Chapter 4— Impact of Pharmacologic Therapy on Health-Related Quality of Life in Heart Failure: Findings from Clinical Trials 43
Derek V. Exner and Eleanor B. Schron

Pathophysiology 43
Pharmacologic Therapy: Impact on Physiologic Parameters,
   Morbidity, and Morality 43
Pharmacologic Therapy: Impact on Quality of Life 44
Trials Evaluating Quality of Life in Heart Failure 44
Conclusion 49

Chapter 5— Impact of Surgical Therapy on Quality of Life in Heart Failure 52
Kathleen L. Grady, William Piccione, Jr., and Rick J. Marcantonio

Introduction 52
Methodologic Issues in Quality of Life Research 52
Surgical Revascularization in Heart Failure Patients 54
Mitral Valve Repair in Heart Failure Patients 56
Quality of Life after Surgical Revascularization and/or Mitral
   Valve Repair 58
Implantable Left Ventricular Assist Devices 60
Quality of Life after Ventricular Assist Device Implantation 63
Cardiac Transplantation 65
Quality of Life after Heart Transplantation 67
Recommendations for Future Research 71

Chapter 6— Impact of Nonpharmacologic Therapy on Quality of Life in Heart Failure 77
Debra K. Moser and Kathleen Dracup

Association between Quality of Life and Morbidity and
   Morality Outcomes 77
Interventions To Improve Quality of Life in Patients with
   Heart Failure 78
Biobehavioral Therapy 85
Exercise Training 86
An Integrated Theory To Explain Mechanism 92
Conclusion and Recommendations for Research and Practice 92

**PART III—IMPROVING OUTCOMES WITH NONPHARMACOLOGIC
        MANAGEMENT** **97**

Chapter 7— Nutritional Management of the Patient with Heart Failure **99**
            Susan J. Bennett, Laurie Hackward, and Sara A. Blackburn

        Nutrition Assessment   99
        Management of Malnutrition/Cachexia   112
        Management of Symptoms..   117
        Management of Sodium Retention and Hypervolemia   118
        Management of Hypovolemia and Dehydration   119
        Compliance with Medical Nutrition Recommendations   120
        Recommendations for Future Research   121

Chapter 8— Exercise in Heart Failure **124**
            John R. Wilson, Don B. Chomsky, and Karen Dahle

        Pathophysiology of Exercise Intolerance in Heart Failure   124
        Exercise Training and Heart Failure   128
        Exercise Prescriptions in Clinical Practice...   131
        Conclusion   133

Chapter 9— Risk Factor Modification in Heart Failure **136**
            *Lynn V. Doering, Susan J. Bennett, Laurie Hackward, Sara A. Blackburn,
            and Karol E. Watson*

        Introduction   136
        Behavioral Health Assessment in Heart Failure   136
        Hypertension   138
        Hyperlipidemia   142
        Diabetes Mellitus and Insulin Resistance   143
        Obesity   143
        Smoking   144
        Alcohol   146
        Inactivity..   146
        Conclusion   148

**Chapter 10—Biobehavioral Therapy in the Management of Patients with
            Heart Failure** **152**
            Debra K. Moser and Lynne W. Stevenson

        Biobehavioral Therapy: Biofeedback and Relaxation in Patients with
            Cardiovascular Disease   153
        Biobehavioral Therapy: Biofeedback and Relaxation in Patients with
            Heart Failure   155
        Conclusion   159

PART IV—IMPROVING OUTCOMES BY ENHANCING TREATMENT COMPLIANCE **163**

Chapter 11—Extent of the Problem of Noncompliance in Patients with Heart Failure **165**
Martha N. Hill

The Compliance Challenge 165
Impact of Noncompliance 165
Patient and Family Factors Contributing to Noncompliance 168
Provider Factors Contributing to Noncompliance 171
System Factors Contributing to Noncompliance 172
Research Recommendations To Enhance Compliance 173
Conclusion 175

Chapter 12—Heart Failure Patient and Family Education **178**
Deborah Knox, Lisa Mischke, and Randall E. Williams

Traditional Heart Failure Education 179
Conclusion 189
Appendix 12–A: Monitoring and Educating Using Disease Management
    To Improve Compliance Instrument (MEDICI) 192
Appendix 12–B: Consumer Information 197

PART V—THE ROLE OF FAMILY IN HEART MANAGEMENT **199**

Chapter 13—Supportive Resources for the Patient with Heart Failure **201**
Linda S. Baas, Robin Trupp, and William T. Abraham

Overview of Supportive Resources 201
A Theoretical Approach To Facilitating Supportive Resources 202
Supportive External Resources 205
Supportive Internal Resources 212
The Role of Health Care Providers in Enhancing Supportive Resources 214
Aims of Intervention 215
Conclusion 216

Chapter 14—Transitioning Heart Failure Care to the Family **219**
Peggy M. O'Connor

Introduction 219
Family Theory 219
Caring for the Caregiver 222
Conclusion 229

**PART VI—IMPROVING PERSONAL AND SOCIETAL OUTCOMES
WITH NEW CARE DELIVERY MODELS** 233

Chapter 15—Outcomes Measurement in Heart Failure 235
*Christi Deaton, Derek V. Exner, Eleanor B. Schron, Barbara Riegel,
and Suzanne Prevost*

Initial Considerations in Outcomes Measurement 235
Selecting Appropriate Instruments for Outcomes Measurement 239
Measuring Health-Related Quality of Life 241
Measuring Financial Outcomes 251
Measuring Processes That Influence Outcomes 254
Suggestions for Future Outcomes Measurement in Heart Failure 258

Chapter 16—Heart Failure Disease Management Models 267
Barbara Riegel and Barbara LePetri

Definition 267
Evolution of Disease Management 268
Designing a Disease Management Program 275

Chapter 17—Community Case Management Models of Heart Failure Care 282
*Debra K. Moser, Marlene J. Macko, F. Kevin Hackett,
and Maggie Roush Hutchins*

Rationale for Heart Failure Community Case Management 282
Tested Heart Failure Community Case Management Programs 284
An In-Depth View and Outcomes of One Heart Failure Community Case
Management Program 290
Conclusion 298

Chapter 18—The Clinic Model of Heart Failure Care 301
Gregg C. Fonarow, Julie Walden Creaser, and Nancy Livingston

Components of a Heart Failure Clinic 302
Heart Failure Patient Evaluation 307
Heart Failure Patient Management 307
The UCLA Heart Failure Program Experience 308
Patient Teaching 310
Evaluation of Outcomes 312
Analysis of Variables That May Influence Outcomes 313
Outcomes Measurement 314
Conclusion 315

Chapter 19—Telephonic Case Management Models of Heart Failure Care **318**
Nancy Houston Miller and Jeffrey A. West

An Overview of Case Management Models 318
The Stanford Cardiac Rehabilitation Program Experience 322
Conclusion 326
Appendix 19–A: Kaiser/Stanford Heart Failure Program Sodium
      Progress Report #2 329

**Chapter 20—Multidisciplinary Disease Management Models of Heart
      Failure Care** **331**
Barbara Riegel and Michael W. Rich

An In-Depth Analysis of Existing Programs 331
Analysis and Directions for Future Research 337

PART VII—SUMMARY AND THE FUTURE **341**

Chapter 21—Summary and the Future of Heart Failure Care **343**
Debra K. Moser and Barbara Riegel

Improving Outcomes 344
Are We Focusing on the Best Outcomes? 347
What Does the Future Hold? 350

List of Sources **355**

Index **359**

Contributors

William T. Abraham, MD, FACP, FACC
Professor of Medicine
Chief, Division of Cardiology
University of Kentucky College of Medicine
Lexington, Kentucky

Linda S. Baas, PhD, RN, CS, ACNP
Associate Professor
University of Cincinnati College of Nursing
Nurse Practitioner
University Hospital Community Heart Failure
    Program
Cincinnati, Ohio

Susan J. Bennett, DNS, RN
Professor
Indiana University School of Nursing
Clarian Health Partners, Inc.
Bloomington, Indiana

Sara A. Blackburn, RD, DSc
Clinical Associate Professor
Nutrition and Dietetics Program
School of Allied Health Sciences
Indiana University School of Medicine
Indianapolis, Indiana

Don B. Chomsky, MD
Assistant Professor of Medicine
Cardiology Division
Vanderbilt University
Nashville, Tennessee

Julie Walden Creaser, MN, RN
Clinical Nurse Specialist
Ahmanson-UCLA Cardiomyopathy Center
Los Angeles, California

Karen Dahle, RNC, MSN, ACNP
Nurse Practitioner
Department of Cardiovascular Sciences at
    St. Thomas Heart Institute
St. Thomas Health Services
Nashville, Tennessee

Christi Deaton, PhD, RN
Assistant Professor
Nell Hodgson Woodruff School of Nursing
Emory University
Atlanta, Georgia

Lynn V. Doering, DNSc, RN
Assistant Professor
UCLA School of Nursing
Los Angeles, California

Kathleen Dracup, DNSc, RN
Dean and Professor
University of California, San Francisco,
    School of Nursing
San Francisco, California

Derek V. Exner, MD, MPH, FRCPC
Clinician Scientist
Medical Research Council of Canada
Assistant Professor of Medicine and
    Community Health Sciences
University of Calgary
Calgary, Canada

Gregg C. Fonarow, MD, FACC
Associate Professor of Medicine
Director, Ahmanson-UCLA Cardiomyopathy
    Center
University of California, Los Angeles
Los Angeles, California

Marjorie Funk, PhD, RN
Professor
Yale University School of Nursing
New Haven, Connecticut

Kathleen L. Grady, PhD, RN, FAAN
Professor, College of Nursing
Associate Professor, College of Medicine
Rush-Presbyterian-St. Luke's Medical Center
Rush University
Chicago, Illinois

F. Kevin Hackett, MD
Cardiologist
Columbus Cardiology Consultants
Clinical Assistant Professor of Medicine
The Ohio State University College of Medicine
    and Public Health
Columbus, Ohio

Laurie Hackward, MS, RD
Nutrition Manager
Indiana University General Clinical Research
    Center
Bloomington, Indiana

Martha N. Hill, PhD, RN, FAAN
Professor
Johns Hopkins University School of Nursing
Baltimore, Maryland

Maggie Roush Hutchins, ACSW/LISW
Case Manager
Mount Carmel Health System
Columbus, Ohio

Deborah Knox, MS, RN, CCRN
Congestive Heart Failure Coordinator
Evanston Northwestern Healthcare
Evanston, Illinois

Harlan M. Krumholz, MD, MSc
Associate Professor
Codirector, Robert Wood Johnson Clinical
    Scholars Program
Yale University School of Medicine
Director
Center for Outcomes Research and Evaluation
Yale-New Haven Hospital
New Haven, Connecticut

Barbara LePetri, MD, FACC
Medical Director
Cardiovascular Risk Factors Group
Pfizer Pharmaceuticals, Inc.
New York, New York

Nancy Livingston, MN, RN, NP
Advanced Practice Nurse
Ahmanson-UCLA Cardiomyopathy Center
Los Angeles, California

Marlene J. Macko, MS, RN
CHF Community Case Manager
Mount Carmel Health System
Columbus, Ohio

Rick J. Marcantonio, PhD
Master Analyst
SPSS, Inc.
Chicago, Illinois

Kathleen M. McCauley, PhD, RN, CS, FAAN
Associate Professor of Cardiovascular Nursing
Cardiovascular Clinical Specialist
University of Pennsylvania School of Nursing
Philadelphia, Pennsylvania

Nancy Houston Miller, RN, BSN
Associate Director
Stanford Cardiac Rehabilitation Program
Stanford University School of Medicine
Stanford, California

Kerry A. Milner, DNSc, RN
Research Scientist
Yale University School of Nursing
New Haven, Connecticut

Lisa Mischke, MS, RN
Congestive Heart Failure Coordinator
Evanston Northwestern Healthcare
Evanston, Illinois

Debra K. Moser, DNSc, RN
Associate Professor
Ohio State University
CHF Community Case Manager
Mount Carmel Health System
Columbus, Ohio

Mary D. Naylor, PhD, RN, FAAN
Ralston Endowed Term Chair and Professor
University of Pennsylvania School of Nursing
Philadelphia, Pennsylvania

Peggy M. O'Connor, MSN, RN
Home Health and Hospice Case Manager
Sharp HealthCare
San Diego, California

William Piccione, Jr., MD, FACS
Associate Professor of Surgery
Rush-Presbyterian-St. Luke's Medical Center
Chicago, Illinois

Suzanne Prevost, PhD, RN, CNAA
Professor and National HealthCare Chairholder
Middle Tennessee State University
Murfreesboro, Tennessee

Michael W. Rich, MD, FACC
Associate Professor of Medicine
Washington University School of Medicine
St. Louis, Missouri

Barbara Riegel, DNSc, RN, CS, FAAN
Professor
School of Nursing
San Diego State University
Clinical Researcher
Sharp HealthCare
San Diego, California

Eleanor B. Schron, MS, RN, FAAN
Nurse Director
Division of Epidemiology and Clinical
　Applications
National Heart, Lung and Blood Institute
Bethesda, Maryland

Martha Shively, PhD, RN
Professor
San Diego State University School of Nursing
Associate Chief Nursing Service/Research
Veterans Affairs San Diego Healthcare System
San Diego, California

Lynne W. Stevenson, MD
Associate Professor
Harvard Medical School
Brigham and Women's Hospital
Boston, Massachusetts

Robin Trupp, RN, MSN, CS-ACNP, CCRN
Nurse Practitioner and Heart Failure
　Program Manager
University of Kentucky
Lexington, Kentucky

Karol E. Watson, MD
Cardiologist and Assistant Professor of
　Medicine
UCLA School of Medicine, Division of
　Cardiology
Los Angeles, California

Jeffrey A. West, MD
Clinical Assistant Professor of Medicine
　(Cardiovascular Medicine)
Stanford University School of Medicine
Medical Director
CareThere, Inc.
Stanford, California

Randall E. Williams, MD
Director
Congestive Heart Failure Program
Evanston Northwestern Healthcare
Evanston, Illinois

Ira B. Wilson, MD, MSc
Assistant Professor of Medicine
New England Medical Center
Tufts University School of Medicine
Boston, Massachusetts

John R. Wilson, MD, BA
Professor of Cardiology
Director, Vanderbilt Heart Failure Program
Vanderbilt University
Nashville, Tennessee

Foreword

The medical literature first described the syndrome of heart failure over two centuries ago. Yet in the year 2000, it remains a disease of epidemic proportions in the industrialized world. Both the human and economic toll associated with heart failure are enormous. The majority of patients with heart failure have symptoms—including fatigue, edema, and breathlessness—that dramatically affect the quality of their lives, while heart muscle disease also is responsible for markedly shortening life expectancy. In addition, the cost of caring for patients with heart failure in the inpatient and outpatient settings is nearly $50 billion each year. Since the risk of developing heart failure increases substantially with age, the graying of baby boomers in the United States and the increased longevity of the population are expected to result in a marked increase in the more than 5 million patients who presently have this syndrome. Recent advances in medical therapy have resulted in improved survival and decreased hospitalizations for patients with heart failure; however, these therapies are not curative and thus the overall burden of the syndrome remains unchanged.

Heart failure has often been described as the "cancer" of heart disease. However, this comparison belies the large differences between how we care for patients with malignancies and patients with heart failure. Patients with cancer often receive care from multispecialty centers of excellence where social workers, pharmacists, nutritionists, and nurses work collaboratively. Local support groups provide counseling to both patients and their family members, while sophisticated educational programs allow patients to have an understanding of both their disease and their treatment options. By contrast, our care of patients with heart failure has historically has focused largely on pharmacologic therapy and transplantation. However, over the past few years the paradigms for heart failure care have begun to change. Quality of life has become an increasingly important endpoint in both clinical trials and assessment of quality of care; the role of diet and nutrition has proven important; the importance of exercise has been recognized; and risk factor modification has become an increasingly important therapeutic target. Furthermore, it has been recognized that treatment compliance can only be fully attained when the patient's family members become stakeholders in the patient's care. Indeed, the family has been shown to have a role of great importance in improving a patient's outcome and quality of life.

Recent studies have demonstrated clearly that patients with heart failure are best cared for in multidisciplinary settings where multiple specialties can interact collaboratively in the management of individual patients. Whether such multidisciplinary care is most effectively provided in a nurse-managed heart failure clinic, through community case management, or in the context of a disease management program remains to be defined. However, it remains clear that the paradigm of heart failure care is changing dramatically.

In *Improving Outcomes in Heart Failure: An Interdisciplinary Approach*, the editors have focused attention for the first time on the personal impact of heart failures as well as its effect on the sociology of the family by providing a thorough and broad review of the impact of important nonpharmacologic therapies on outcomes, including quality of life. This discussion is timely as a large number of studies have recently demonstrated the overwhelming benefits of care that involves physicians, nurses, social workers, dietitians, and pharmacists. These studies have led to the development of multiple algorithms for comprehensive and multidisciplinary care which now must meet the test of time. Such discussions are also important in order to eradicate the misconception that heart muscle disease is a terminal and unrelenting disease. In addition, this work personifies the need to teach patients about "living" with heart failure and thus will be a text that will hopefully be read by both caregivers and patients alike.

Arthur M. Feldman, MD, PhD
Past President, 1998–2000
Heart Failure Society of America
Director
Cardiovascular Institute of the
UPMC Health System
University of Pittsburgh Medical Center
Pittsburgh, Pennsylvania

Preface

Heart failure is thought by many clinicians and researchers to have the classic characteristics of an epidemic. Unfortunately, heart failure is an epidemic on the rise—its incidence and prevalence are increasing, it is not easily treated, and its presence is associated with high morbidity and mortality. As a consequence, heart failure is now the single largest health care expenditure in the United States, and heart failure is being recognized as an enormous health care problem worldwide that produces substantial personal and societal burden. A disproportionate amount of the economic cost associated with heart failure care is attributable to hospitalizations. By several estimates many, if not most, of these hospitalizations might be prevented or delayed significantly with better health care delivery and improved patient participation in their own care.

Most of the emphasis in heart failure research has been placed on elucidating its complex pathophysiology and discovering optimal pharmacologic management that influences morbidity and mortality outcomes. This emphasis has produced remarkable advances in the treatment of heart failure, yet even the best pharmacologic therapy produces only a modest improvement in survival and sometimes no improvement in patients' quality of life. Currently most heart failure reference texts reflect this emphasis on pathophysiology and pharmacology and devote little attention to the concerns of patients and families, which can interfere with their ability to take advantage of optimal therapy, or to the failure of clinicians to prescribe optimal therapy. Moreover, texts to date have not fully recognized the power of interdisciplinary collaboration to improving outcomes in patients with heart failure.

The concerns of patients and their families are many and relate both to the manifestations of heart failure and to the management regimen imposed by health care providers. For patients with heart failure and their families, morbidity and mortality are, of course, important concerns, but for most, quality of life is an equally important outcome. Quality of life can be affected adversely by heart failure and prescribed treatment. For example, patients have difficulty contending with symptoms because the chronic heart failure symptoms of dyspnea and fatigue disturb every aspect of their daily lives. On the other hand, in this background of chronic symptoms, most patients have difficulty identifying acutely increasing symptoms that could warn them of impending exacerbation. These symptoms often are subtle and difficult for patients to interpret. To compound the problem, patients often are "blamed" by clinicians for their failure to properly interpret and respond to changing symptom status in a timely manner. Moreover, for many patients, clinicians' directions for daily management of heart failure are overwhelming as patients try to cope with complex, unfamiliar regimens and unwelcome life-style changes. Patients can become confused as they try to contend with sometimes mixed messages regarding diet, activity, and medication management.

Contributing to difficulty in managing heart failure are the many physical, psychologic, and social challenges that patients face as they attempt to manage their condition. Most heart failure patients are elderly and have one or more comorbidities or functional impairments that confound their care. Confusion and sensory abnormalities compound difficulties in self-management. Many elderly individuals or those with multiple chronic health problems live in poverty with all its attendant problems that contribute to difficulty with the successful management of heart failure. Anxiety and depression are relatively common in elderly chronically ill patients and are associated with poor compliance, risk for higher morbidity, and poor quality of life. Social isolation, also common in elders, is particularly troublesome because support from family or other caregivers is fundamental to improved patient outcomes. Low literacy level or inability to speak the majority language also can increase problems.

What patients and families need to assist them in managing their condition is a number of things that clinicians may not be trained to provide. Patients and their families need more open, honest communication and less paternalism from clinicians. They need concrete, consistent answers to their questions and problems that are based on applicable research and published evidence-based consensus guidelines. They need to know that there is hope for a better quality of life despite having heart failure. They need attention to the individual challenges that each of them face, such as social isolation and functional impairment. Finally, they need vigorous follow-up with continuing care and mentoring about heart failure self-management after an acute event.

Improving Outcomes in Heart Failure: An Interdisciplinary Approach takes a different tack in the management of patients with heart failure than most current references. We discuss, in depth, quality of life as an outcome of equal importance with the traditional outcomes of morbidity and mortality. We provide an overview of the current state of knowledge regarding the impact of different innovative health care delivery models and other nonpharmacologic/noninvasive approaches to management on patient outcomes. We provide discussions about how to address heart failure management issues facing patients and their families in the context of the daily challenges they face, as well as methods of incorporating current research findings into clinical practice. The vital role of interdisciplinary collaboration is threaded throughout the book.

Our hope is that the information in this book will help us all look at this epidemic through the eyes of our patients and their loved ones and to truly understand the personal burden of heart failure as well as we have come to understand the economic burden. An adequate body of knowledge is now available to assist clinicians to provide optimal care that addresses not only the physiologic changes associated with heart failure, but also the social and psychologic changes, and that improves outcomes in each of these areas. By using this scientific knowledge in practice, we believe that the care we provide will grow in excellence, and our patients will benefit by improved outcomes in all of the areas important to them and to society.

Debra K. Moser
Barbara Riegel

PART I

The Syndrome of Heart Failure: Personal and Societal Impact

CHAPTER 1

Epidemiology of Heart Failure

Marjorie Funk, Kerry A. Milner, and Harlan M. Krumholz

As a major public health problem, heart failure is responsible for substantial health care expenditures and disability. Over the past several decades, mortality from the most common cause of heart failure, coronary heart disease, has declined.[1] However, the incidence and prevalence of heart failure, and resulting morbidity and mortality, seem to have dramatically increased. Indeed, the declining mortality rates for coronary disease may in part be responsible for the apparent rise in heart failure rates, because prolonged survival with coronary heart disease is likely to result in more heart failure cases.[2] Other factors responsible for the "epidemic" of heart failure include the aging of the population and growing prevalence of diabetes mellitus among older individuals, especially women.[2]

Understanding how heart failure has been defined is crucial to an accurate interpretation of studies that report epidemiologic characteristics of this condition. A liberal definition may include many individuals with borderline heart failure and thus inflate the incidence and prevalence rates and indicate a better prognosis. A very strict definition that depends on clinically apparent symptoms may make the condition appear to be less common but have a worse prognosis. Unfortunately, there is little agreement about the definition of heart failure. Traditionally, it has been defined as a syndrome that develops as a consequence of cardiac disease and is recognized clinically by a constellation of symptoms and signs produced by complex circulatory and neurohormonal responses to cardiac dysfunction.[3] The cardinal clinical manifestations of heart failure are shortness of breath and exercise intolerance.[4] The presence and severity of heart failure can be assessed by questionnaires, physical and radiographic examination, and by measures of ventricular performance and exercise capacity. All these methods, however, have major limitations when used independently.[3] Many investigators have used the set of clinical criteria for the diagnosis of heart failure developed for the Framingham Heart Study.[5] See Exhibit 1–1. The Framingham Heart Study is an ongoing population-based prospective study that initially enrolled more than 5,000 men and women free of cardiovascular diseases in the late 1940s. The original cohort and their offspring have been examined every 2 years.

In any overview of the epidemiology of heart failure, methodological limitations of reported research must be considered. Epidemiologic studies have been carried out in different types of settings, using various definitions of heart failure, groups of patients, and methods of case ascertainment. Studies have also been conducted across long time periods in which the etiology and treatment of heart failure have changed.

Most hospital-based studies depend solely on the principal discharge diagnosis to determine the presence of heart failure. This definition is adequate to estimate hospitalizations for heart failure but not to understand the entire burden of this condition on the population. It is also important to consider the group of patients studied. In many cases, small select groups of patients have

Exhibit 1–1 Criteria for Diagnosis of Heart Failure Used in the Framingham Study[5]

Major criteria
Paroxysmal nocturnal dyspnea or orthopnea
Neck vein distention
Rales
Cardiomegaly
Acute pulmonary edema
S_3 gallop
Increased venous pressure >16 cm of water
Circulation time   25 seconds
Hepatojugular reflux

Minor criteria
Ankle edema
Night cough
Dyspnea on exertion
Hepatomegaly
Pleural effusion
Vital capacity ↓ 1/3 from maximum
Tachycardia (rate of 120/minute)

Major or minor criterion
Weight loss 4.5 kg in 5 days in response to treatment

For establishing a definite diagnosis of heart failure, two major or one major and two minor criteria have to be present concurrently.

---

been surveyed, and the incidence and prevalence of heart failure may not be generalizable to the entire population. In particular, some studies have excluded women and older adults.[6–9] The sampling time frame is also important to consider because the etiology of heart failure has changed dramatically over the past 40 years. Studies that include large numbers of individuals across a long time period may be mixing distinct subpopulations.[10] Although hypertension and valvular disease were the most common causes of heart failure 40 to 50 years ago, coronary heart disease is currently the most common etiology. In addition, recent changes in recommended therapy may have modified the prognosis of heart failure reported in populations more than a decade ago. Because there are limited recent population-based data available regarding

the epidemiology of heart failure, it is difficult to assess temporal trends in the incidence, prevalence, and prognosis associated with this condition.[11,12]

This chapter will review the epidemiology of heart failure in terms of causes and risk factors, incidence, prevalence, morbidity, and prognosis and mortality. Definitions of commonly used epidemiologic terms are presented in Exhibit 1–2.

CAUSES AND RISK FACTORS

The terms "cause" and "risk factor" are both used in discussions of the etiology of heart failure. To be considered a *cause* of a disease, a characteristic must meet certain criteria, such as a strong association, biologic credibility, consistency across investigations, appropriate temporal sequence, and a dose–response relationship. On the other hand, a *risk factor* is a characteristic that is suspected to be related to the occurrence of a particular disease, but it is neither a necessary nor sufficient cause of the disease.

Exhibit 1–2 Definitions of Commonly Used Epidemiologic Terms

Incidence—the number of new cases of a disease in a given period of time.

Prevalence—the number of existing cases of a disease at a particular point in time. Prevalence is influenced by factors that affect the occurrence of the disease (incidence) and by factors that affect the severity or duration of the disease (mortality).

Relative Risk or Risk Ratio—the ratio of the risk in the group with the characteristic (exposed) to the risk in the group without the characteristic (unexposed).

Attributable Risk—the proportion of the total risk for a particular outcome attributable to a particular exposure. It is obtained by subtracting the incidence rate for the group without the characteristic from the rate for the group with the characteristic.

Heart failure occurs as the final common pathway in a variety of cardiovascular disorders. Causes of heart failure have changed considerably over time. Early data from the Framingham study revealed that hypertension was the most common precipitating factor of heart failure in 37% of men and 33% of women. Hypertension was a cofactor in another 38% of men and 41% of women.[5]

In subsequent analyses that evaluated both the original cohort and their offspring, substantial changes in the etiology of heart failure were observed.[10,13] Coronary heart disease seems to be increasingly responsible for heart failure in recent years, whereas hypertension is a diminishing determinant. In a 1993 report of the Framingham cohort,[10] coronary heart disease was the attributable cause of heart failure in 59% of men and 48% of women, whereas hypertension alone was the attributable cause in only 21% of men and 26% of women.

Ho et al[14] report that heart failure was more commonly attributable to coronary heart disease in later decades in the Framingham cohort (22% of patients in the 1950s, 36% in the 1960s, 53% in the 1970s, and 67% in the 1980s), whereas valve disease was a less frequent cause in later decades (16% in the 1950s, 15% in the 1960s, 13% in the 1970s, and 10% in the 1980s). Preceding hypertension and left ventricular hypertrophy also became less frequent as isolated causes of heart failure over time. Although it is not certain to what extent this evolution away from hypertension to coronary heart disease as the primary cause of heart failure reflects a true change or improved diagnosis of coronary heart disease, major advances in the detection and treatment of hypertension and the decreasing prevalence of left ventricular hypertrophy argue for a declining role of hypertension.[2] Congenital heart disease and acquired valve disease are powerful risks for heart failure, but also carry a lower attributable risk because they are less prevalent,[13] and both surgical and medical treatment for these conditions have improved.

Others have confirmed the increasing importance of coronary heart disease as a primary etiology of heart failure. A retrospective review of hospital records in western Sweden used standard clinical criteria for the diagnosis of heart failure, coronary heart disease, and hypertension. Coronary heart disease was found to be the cause of heart failure in 40% of patients, and hypertension was a primary factor in 17%.[15] In addition, a recent review of 13 randomized multicenter heart failure treatment trials involving >20,000 patients published in the *New England Journal of Medicine* from 1986 to 1997 revealed that coronary heart disease was present in 68% of patients with heart failure.[16]

The etiology of heart failure varies according to geographic location, socioeconomic status, and economic standard of the region. Although coronary heart disease and hypertension account for most cases of heart failure in developed countries, rheumatic valve disease and nutritional cardiac disease are much more common in the developing world.[3,17]

In addition to the identified causes for heart failure, other conditions also predispose individuals to heart failure. Advancing age is clearly associated with heart failure. Changes in the cardiovascular system that occur with aging include (1) reduced responsiveness to β-adrenergic stimulation, (2) increased vascular stiffness, (3) increased stiffness of the heart itself, and (4) altered myocardial energy metabolism. The combination of age-related changes in the cardiovascular system in conjunction with a high prevalence of age-related cardiovascular diseases conspire to produce an exponential rise in heart failure prevalence with advancing age.[18]

Many of the known risk factors for coronary heart disease have also been found to be independent predictors of heart failure. Table 1–1 shows the impact of coronary heart disease risk factors (hypertension, left ventricular hypertrophy, diabetes, smoking, and elevated cholesterol) on the risk of heart failure based on data from the Framingham Heart Study.

Although hypertension has declined in importance as the primary cause of heart failure, it is still a major contributor to the occurrence of heart failure.[6,13,19] Despite improvements in the detection and treatment of hypertension, it remains a common problem in the general popula-

Table 1–1 Risk Factors for Heart Failure: 36-Year Follow-up of Framingham Study[13]

| | Age-Adjusted Risk Ratio Age 35–64 | | Age-Adjusted Risk Ratio Age 65–94 | |
	Males	Females	Males	Females
Hypertension	4.0	3.0	1.9	1.9
Left ventricular hypertrophy (by ECG)	15.0	12.8	4.9	5.4
Diabetes	4.4	7.7	2.0	3.6
Smoking	1.5	1.1*	1.0*	1.3
Serum cholesterol >240 mg/dL	1.2*	0.7*	0.9*	0.8*

All but * significant at $P < .0001$

tion. Framingham data[19] indicate that hypertension increases the risk of heart failure by about twofold in men and threefold in women. In this cohort, hypertension antedated the development of heart failure in 91% of cases. Levy et al[19] examined population-attributable risk, which represents the percentage of heart failure cases that can be attributed to a risk factor given its prevalence and hazard ratio. Hypertension carried the greatest population-attributable risk for heart failure of all risk factors considered: 39% in men and 59% in women. In contrast, the population-attributable risk for heart failure for myocardial infarction was 34% for men and 13% for women. The population-attributable risk for heart failure carried by coronary heart disease was not reported.

Framingham data[13] also revealed that the risk of heart failure increases progressively with the severity of the hypertension, and systolic and diastolic values equally predict risk. Risk is even substantial in patients with isolated systolic hypertension—a condition common in the elderly. In women, systolic pressure is most predictive, whereas in men pulse pressure confers the highest risk. Recently, elevated pulse pressure was found to be a strong independent predictor of risk of heart failure in the Established Populations for Epidemiologic Studies of the Elderly cohort.[20,21]

A common consequence of longstanding, poorly controlled hypertension is left ventricular hypertrophy (LVH). The Framingham data indicate that LVH (per electrocardiogram) is strongly associated with an increased incidence of heart failure, independent of hypertension.[10] As shown in Table 1–1, LVH carried a 15-fold increase in relative risk of heart failure in younger men and a 13-fold increase in younger women. Although the relative risk associated with LVH declines in older men and women, the absolute risk remains very high. A small relative risk that applies to a large number of people may produce many excess cases of the disease. Because LVH is more common in older people, a small relative risk results in a high incidence of heart failure.

Diabetes predisposes patients to heart failure because of its association with accelerated coronary atherosclerosis, hypertension, and obesity, and it also appears to damage the myocardium directly. Functional, structural, and metabolic aberrations demonstrated in the hearts of patients with diabetes suggest the existence of diabetic cardiomyopathy. Thus, it seems to be a microangiopathy similar to that seen in the skin, retina, and kidneys, not the simple acceleration of atherosclerosis, that increases the risk of heart failure. Diabetes predisposes patients to heart failure whether there is concomitant coronary heart disease or hypertension or not. In addition, diabetes is more likely to be a predisposing factor for heart failure in women than in men.[22,23]

Other conditions have been found to be significantly associated with heart failure, although the relationships are weaker than for hypertension, LVH, and diabetes. Cigarette smoking moderately increases the risk of heart failure in younger men and older women[13] and was a major independent risk factor in Swedish men born in 1913.[6] Although the serum total cholesterol is only weakly related to occurrence of heart failure, dyslipidemia characterized by a high total-to-high density lipoprotein cholesterol ratio is powerfully associated with heart failure in both sexes.[13]

Although risk ratios for obesity were not reported by Framingham investigators, obesity is an important contributor to heart failure, particularly in women. Its effect is both direct and indirect—by its promotion of hypertension, LVH, diabetes, and dyslipidemia.[13] In the study of Swedish men born in 1913, indices of obesity were associated with the development of heart failure, and the relationship tended to be stronger with increasing age. In particular, body weight was an independent predictor of heart failure when hypertension and smoking were taken into account. Eriksson et al[6] hypothesized that salt and water retention or increased left ventricular load may explain the independent association of obesity and heart failure.

Several other factors, such as increased heart volume on chest radiograph, T-wave abnormalities on electrocardiogram, intraventricular conduction abnormalities, heart rate variability, proteinuria, abnormal hematocrit values, reduced peak expiratory flow rate, psychologic stress, and a possible genetic marker—Fy-antigen, have been found to be independently associated with heart failure. It is unclear, however, whether these factors are indicators of reduced myocardial function rather than risk factors for the development of heart failure.[6,10,22,24]

The presence of multiple risk factors in the same individual dramatically and disproportionately increases the risk of heart failure. Therefore, any strategy directed toward early identification and subsequent risk factor modification for prevention of heart failure must address all these factors and promote particularly aggressive approaches in individuals with multiple risk factors.[6,24]

INCIDENCE

Incidence refers to the number of new cases of a disease in a given period of time. Incidence can be determined by two approaches: (1) re-examining individuals within a cohort at intervals to identify those who have developed heart failure; or (2) by a population-based surveillance system in which subjects who develop heart failure for the first time are identified. The Framingham Heart Study and the Gothenburg, Sweden, study are good examples of the first approach. The Eastern Finland and the Rochester, Minnesota, studies are examples of the second approach, which has the advantage that incident cases of heart failure presenting to the health care system are identified prospectively and may, therefore, be fully characterized at the time of diagnosis rather than retrospectively.[3]

A summary of studies evaluating incidence rates of heart failure is shown in Table 1–2. In the Framingham study, which followed cohorts of individuals for approximately 40 years, the incidence of heart failure increased dramatically with advancing age and was higher in men than in women. The annual incidence was 2.0 per 1000 patient-years for men aged 45 to 54 years and rose to 14.0 per 1000 in men aged 75 to 84 years. Similarly, in women, the annual incidence increased from 1.0 per 1000 in the youngest group to 13.0 per 1000 in the oldest group. The overall age-adjusted annual incidence of heart failure was 2.3 cases per 1000 in men and 1.4 cases per 1000 in women.[10] In the Framingham cohort, the diagnosis of heart failure was based on clinical factors (see Exhibit 1–1). It did not include persons with impaired subclinical function now detectable by the newer noninvasive technology. Thus, the incidence rates were probably underestimated.

Using diagnostic criteria similar to those in the Framingham study, Senni et al[12] evaluated 107 patients in 1981 and 141 patients in 1991 with a new diagnosis of heart failure living in Rochester, Minnesota. They also found that incidence rates were higher among men than women and increased with advancing age. The total incidence rate of heart failure, after adjustment for

Table 1–2 Incidence of Heart Failure (per 1,000 patient-years)

Study Age Groups	Men	Women
Framingham, MA[10]		
45–54	2.0	1.0
55–64	4.0	3.0
65–74	8.0	5.0
75–84	14.0	13.0
Rochester, MN[12]*		
<50	<1	1
50–59	2	2
60–69	10	3
70–79	34	20
>79	61	57
Eastern Finland[8]†		
45–54	1.9	0
55–64	3.1	1.5
65–74	8.2	2.0
Gothenburg, Sweden[6]		
50–54	1.5	
55–60	4.3	
61–67	10.2	

*Extrapolated from 1991 cohort data in Figure 3 in Senni M, et al., 1999[12]
†per Boston criteria for heart failure.

age and sex, did not differ in the 1981 and 1991 cohorts.

Incidence rates in two Scandinavian studies, Eastern Finland[8] and Gothenburg, Sweden,[6] were similar to those of the United States cohorts. In the Eastern Finland study, investigators evaluated the incidence of heart failure in 45- to 74-year-old inhabitants of four rural communities. General physicians referred all their patients with suspected heart failure during a 2-year period to the study. The Boston criteria, which includes history, physical examination, and chest radiographic criteria, were used to verify the diagnosis of heart failure. The Gothenburg study followed a cohort of men born in 1913 for 17 years from 1963 to 1980. A diagnosis of heart failure was based on medical interview and physical examination.

All of these studies reveal an increase in the incidence of heart failure with advancing age

and a higher incidence in men, presumably because of higher rates of coronary heart disease in older individuals and in men. Results of these studies can be used to estimate the number of individuals who develop heart failure each year. An extrapolation of the Framingham data to the age-adjusted population of the United States reveals that approximately 550,000 new cases of heart failure occur each year in the United States.[2,25]

Although it is widely stated that the incidence of heart failure is increasing over time, national secular trends in measures of incidence for the United States are not available. Recent data from the Framingham and Rochester studies, with uniform criteria and case ascertainment over the decades of follow-up, do not suggest an increase in the incidence of heart failure.[12,13]

Although recent data do not support an increase in the incidence of heart failure, there is a pervasive belief that the number of new cases is increasing. Several factors may explain this presumed increase in incidence of heart failure. Improved therapies for coronary heart disease and hypertension are allowing patients with these disorders to survive or avoid other clinical manifestations of these diseases, only to have heart failure develop at a later time. Thus, patients who might have died from acute myocardial infarction 20 years ago are now surviving, but with residual left ventricular dysfunction that may contribute to heart failure months or years later. Similarly, improved treatment of hypertension has led to a 60% decline in stroke mortality, yet these same patients remain at risk for heart failure developing.[18]

PREVALENCE

Prevalence is the number of existing cases of a disease at a particular point in time. It is determined both by factors that affect the occurrence of disease (incidence) and those that affect the severity or duration of disease (mortality). For example, as mortality from coronary heart disease decreases and more people are saved from premature death, the prevalence of heart failure increases. Three possible causes for an increase in prevalence include (1) reduction in mortality from myocardial infarction, (2) improved management of hypertension, and (3) the aging of the population.

Prevalence rates vary widely depending on diagnostic criteria, geographic region and population demographics, and the source of data. For example, data obtained from population-based studies, such as Framingham, National Health and Nutrition Examination Survey (NHANES), and Helsinki, are likely to differ from data obtained from medical records, such as Rochester and the Cardiovascular Health Study. When medical records are the primary source of data, only those people whose condition is severe enough to require hospitalization will be included. Prevalence rates based on population-based studies will generally be higher because these figures include those with milder heart failure not necessitating hospitalization.

An overview of the prevalence of heart failure by age and sex in various studies is presented in Table 1–3. In this table, studies are presented in chronological order of publication and the method of case ascertainment is included.

The population-based prospective Framingham study indicated that the prevalence of heart failure increases progressively with age and is highest in women 80 to 89 years of age.[10]

The NHANES study[9] included an initial cohort of 14,407 noninstitutionalized adults 25 to 74 years old. The prevalence of heart failure was determined by self-report in the entire cohort and by clinical criteria, including symptoms, physical examination, and chest X-ray, in a subset of 6913 individuals. Prevalence rates were lower when identification was solely by self-report, presumably because individuals may have been unaware of having heart failure or unwilling to report their condition. Prevalence rates for combined age and sex groups were 1.1% by self-report and 2.0% by clinical definition. Similar to that found in the Framingham study, prevalence rates increased with advancing age and were similar in men and women.

The NHANES data are limited by the exclusion of individuals older than 74 years of age, whereas the Helsinki Ageing Study, a population-based clinical and echocardiographic study, included only those 75 to 86 years.[26] As expected, prevalence rates were considerably higher than rates found in other population-based studies evaluating younger cohorts. Although the difference was not statistically significant, a trend toward higher prevalence rates in women was noted.

Case ascertainment based on review of medical records was the primary method of determining the prevalence of heart failure in the Rochester study.[27] In the Cardiovascular Health Study,[28] case ascertainment was based on a combination of interview, physical examination, and medical record review. As expected, the prevalence of heart failure is lower in these two studies compared with rates reported in cohorts in which the identification of heart failure was based on self-report and/or clinical criteria. An unexpected finding in the Cardiovascular Health Study is the decline in prevalence rates in individuals 85 and older.

The Evans County study,[7] an early population-based series that used interviews and physical examinations, is the only study in which racial groups were compared. There were no statistically significant differences in prevalence rates for the race-sex groups. As with other cohorts, prevalence appeared to increase with advancing age, but the data suggested that the peak prevalence rate for African-Americans may be in the middle-age group of 55 to 64 years (4.2%, vs 1.2% in the oldest age group of 65 to 74 years).

Because it is a broad-based community survey, NHANES[9] may provide the best estimate of the prevalence of heart failure in the United States.[2] The prevalence of heart failure from 1971 to 1975 ranged from 1.1% to 2.0% of the noninstitutionalized adult population < 75 years old. Extrapolating these rates to include institutionalized and older individuals, as well as accounting for current demographic characteristics of the population, provides the basis for the recent estimate of 4.6 million Americans currently living with heart failure.[25] A strong argument can be made for collecting new data because this figure is based on crude methods and data col-

Table 1–3 Prevalence of Heart Failure

Study Age Groups	Case Ascertainment	Men (%)	Women (%)	Total (%)
Tecumseh, MI[56]	Physical examination			
0–39		0	.3	.1
40–49		.9	.6	.7
50–59		1.2	1.2	1.2
60–69		5.0	6.5	5.3
70–79		4.0	10.9	7.7
80+		15.2	14.0	14.5
Evans County, GA[7]	Interview; physical examination			
45–54		.9	1.0	1.0
55–64		3.4	2.3	2.8
65–74		4.6	2.5	3.5
Montgomery County, NC[57]	Physician surveillance of own practice			
<45		.1	<.1	.1
45–64		1.0	1.5	1.2
65–74		4.7	4.5	4.6
75+		12.4	9.5	10.8
Caledonia County, VT[57]	Physician surveillance of own practice			
<45		0	<.1	<.1
45–64		1.0	.9	.9
65–74		4.3	4.5	4.4
75+		8.2	10.5	9.5
Gothenburg, Sweden[6]	Physical examination			
50		2.1		
54		2.4		
60		4.3		
67		13.0		
NHANES—I (1971–1975; self-report)[9]	Questionnaire			
25–54		.4	.3	.4
55–64		2.2	2.0	2.1
65–74		3.7	3.2	3.4
NHANES—I (1971–1975; clinical score)[9]	Physical examination			
25–54		.8	1.3	1.1
55–64		4.5	3.0	3.7
65–74		4.8	4.3	4.5
Framingham, MA[10]	Physical examination			
50–59		.8	.8	.8
60–69		2.2	2.2	2.2
70–79		5.1	4.3	4.7
80–89		6.6	7.9	7.3
Rochester, MN[27]	Medical record review			
45–54		<.1	.2	.1
55–64		1.0	.5	.7
65–74		2.7	1.9	2.3

continues

Table 1–3 continued

Study Age Groups	Case Ascertainment	Men (%)	Women (%)	Total (%)
Cardiovascular Health Study[28]	Interview; physical examination; medical record review			
65–69		2.2	1.2	1.6
70–74		1.9	1.5	1.7
75–79		3.2	2.4	2.7
80–84		3.2	2.5	2.8
85+		2.9	2.2	2.6
Helsinki Ageing Study[26]	Physical examination			
75–86		5.2	9.3	8.2

lected more than two decades ago. An accurate estimate of the prevalence of heart failure is important when developing new strategies for managing this condition.[2]

Data from NHANES reveal that the prevalence of heart failure increased substantially between 1976 and 1991 and then leveled off between 1991 and 1994. This pattern is consistent for whites and African-Americans and for men and women[29] (see Figure 1–1). The increase in numbers of persons with heart failure is primarily driven by the aging population, but this trend persists even after adjustment for age. The likely explanation for this pattern, which is unique among cardiovascular diagnoses, is the improved survival of patients with other chronic cardiovascular conditions, particularly coronary heart disease, hypertension, and diabetes.[2]

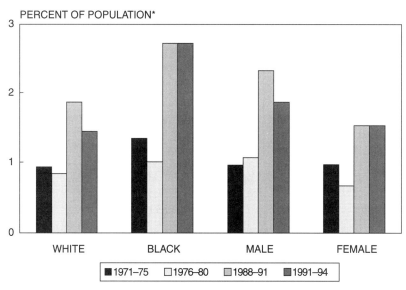

PERCENT OF POPULATION*

Legend: ■1971–75 □1976–80 ▨1988–91 ▨1991–94

Between 1976–80 and 1988–91, the prevalence of CHF increased substantially in each group: male and female, African-American and white, and remained at about those levels in 1991–94.

* Age-adjusted to the 2000 standard

Figure 1–1 Prevalence of heart failure in the United States from 1971 to 1994, by race and sex, age 25–74.[29]

MORBIDITY

Hospitalizations for heart failure are perhaps the best marker of morbidity,[2] although these data relate only to those individuals who require hospital treatment. Most data using hospitalizations are based on heart failure as the primary diagnosis; however, morbidity is better reflected when both primary and secondary diagnoses of heart failure are considered.

Hospitalizations for heart failure rise sharply with age, from 12 per 10,000 persons <65 years old to 328 per 10,000 >74 years old, making heart failure the most frequent cause of hospitalization in the Medicare population.[2,3,30] Hospitalizations are approximately 15% more frequent in women and in African-Americans.[2] On average, nonwhite men experienced annual hospitalization rates 33% higher than white men, whereas for women the corresponding nonwhite rates were 50% higher.[31]

Hospitalizations for heart failure are also rising over time, from 377,000 in 1979 to 957,000 in 1997.[25] A review of Medicare hospital claims records for patients hospitalized with heart failure in 1986 (n = 631,306) and 1993 (n = 803,506) showed that rates of initial hospitalization for heart failure were higher in 1993 than in 1986 among men and women, and especially among African Americans.[32] Although hospitalization for heart failure is rising, the total number of hospital days for this diagnosis has leveled off since 1988, probably because of a substantial decline in length of stay.[2]

One possible consequence of decreasing length of stay is an increase in hospital readmission. A number of studies have documented that elderly patients who survive hospitalization for heart failure are particularly vulnerable to readmission.[33–36] Three-month readmission rates ranged from 29% to 47%,[35,36] and 6-month rates ranged from 36% to 44%.[33,34] In the largest of these studies, Krumholz and colleagues[34] reported that 44% of 17,448 Medicare beneficiaries in Connecticut were readmitted within 6 months after hospitalization for heart failure. Significant independent predictors of readmission included male sex, at least one prior admission within 6 months of the index hospitaliza-

tion, Deyo comorbidity score of >1, and length of stay in the index hospitalization of >7 days. These high readmission rates emphasize the vulnerability of these patients to recurrent illness.

PROGNOSIS AND MORTALITY

Once heart failure is recognized, it has a very high mortality rate. In fact, heart failure is associated with a shorter life expectancy than that of many types of cancer.[10] One-year mortality rates for newly diagnosed cases average between 35% and 45%.[10,27]

Data regarding prognosis and mortality are derived from various types of sources, such as national mortality statistics, population-based studies (eg, Framingham, Rochester), hospital discharge data, and drug trials. National mortality statistics are compiled from death certificates filed in state vital statistics offices. These statistics are based on the underlying cause of death recorded on the death certificate by the attending physician, medical examiner, or coroner.[37] The fact that heart failure is more commonly a contributing cause of death rather than an underlying cause of death must be considered when interpreting national mortality statistics. Mortality rates in population-based studies reflect deaths from heart failure in the particular community under study and may not be generalizable to areas with different demographic characteristics. Hospital series tend to reflect the patient population of specialist referral centers, and drug trials are composed of a highly select group of patients.[3]

Mortality caused by heart failure increases with advancing age. In 1995, age-specific rates were 633.5 per 100,000 for persons 85 years, 130.8 for persons 75 to 84 years, and 32.2 for persons 65 to 74 years.[37] Framingham data also revealed that survival is adversely affected by age, with a 27% increase in mortality per decade of advancing age in men and a 61% increase in women.[13]

In general, mortality rates are higher in men than women and higher in African-Americans compared with whites. In 1990, heart failure death rates were higher in African-Americans than whites, with the greatest racial differences found in the younger age groups. At ages 45 through 49, rates in African-American men and women were about four times those in whites.[1] Among persons 65 years, age-adjusted rates for 1995 were 126.1 per 100,000 for African-American men, 117.0 for white men, 107.6 for African-American women, and 101.2 for white women.[37]

Survival time after the diagnosis of heart failure is poor. In the Framingham study, 37% of men and 38% of women died within 2 years of diagnosis. The median survival time after the diagnosis of heart failure was 1.7 years for men and 3.2 years for women. For men, 1-, 2-, 5-, and 10-year survival rates were 57%, 46%, 25%, and 11%, respectively. For women, corresponding survival rates were better: 64%, 56%, 38%, and 21%.[14,22,38] In the Rochester study, only 79% and 85% of persons remained alive 6 months after diagnosis, 72% and 77% at 1 year, and 34% and 33% at 5 years in the 1981 and 1991 cohorts, respectively.[12] In addition, the 8-year survival of persons diagnosed in 1981 was 30%.[27]

Sudden death (usually defined as death within 1 hour of the onset of symptoms) is a typical feature of mortality in persons with heart failure. In those with heart failure, sudden cardiac death occurs at six to nine times the rate of the general population.[25] In the Framingham cohort, 25% of men and 13% of women experienced sudden death within 6 years of initial diagnosis of heart failure,[22] and 40% to 50% of all heart failure deaths were sudden.[38] Most of the remainder of deaths were due to progressive pump failure. In a review of 27 published studies of patients with heart failure, Narang et al[39] reported that 39% of deaths were due to circulatory failure, whereas sudden death accounted for only 32% to 34% of deaths. The precise mechanisms implicated in sudden death in patients with heart failure remain to be explained, but antiarrhythmic therapy (with the possible exception of amiodarone in severe heart failure) has not been shown to prevent such deaths.[3]

A number of factors have been associated with a poorer prognosis in persons with heart failure. In both the Framingham and Rochester cohorts, advanced age was the most powerful predictor of long-term survival[12,14] In the Framingham study, once the diagnosis of heart failure was established, the hazard ratio was 1.27 per decade in men (ie, a 27% higher mortality rate) and 1.61 in women.[2,14]

Data regarding the association between the type of underlying heart disease and the prognosis with heart failure conflict. Data from early hospital-based studies revealed significantly shorter survival in persons with severe heart failure and evidence of coronary heart disease.[40,41] On the other hand, data from community-based studies such as Framingham and Rochester revealed that coronary heart disease was not an independent predictor of mortality.[12,14] Among men in the Framingham cohort, heart failure attributed to valvular heart disease carried a particularly poor prognosis compared with heart failure secondary to coronary heart disease.[14] Recent data from Rochester revealed that valvular heart disease was not an independent predictor of survival.[12]

Evidence exists that functional classification, as determined by New York Heart Association classification or the 6-minute walk test, predicts survival in persons with heart failure.[2,3] In general, the more severe the functional impairment, the worse the prognosis.[3] One-year mortality rates in drug treatment trials exclusively enrolling New York Heart Association Class IV patients[42] or Class III or IV with ejection fractions near 20%[43,44] were substantially higher than rates in trials enrolling only Class II and III patients.[40,45,46] In the Studies of Left Ventricular Dysfunction (SOLVD) Registry Substudy, distance walked in 6 minutes was a strong independent predictor of mortality.[47]

Other factors have also been found to predict outcome in patients with heart failure. These include diabetes (in women only),[14] LVH (in women only),[14] left ventricular ejection fraction,[47,48] left ventricular filling pressure,[41] peak exercise oxygen consumption,[45,48] cardiothoracic ratio > 0.55,[48] ventricular arrhythmias,[48] and plasma norepinephrine.[48] The latest report of the Rochester data[12] indicated that creatinine concentration >115 μmol/L was an independent negative predictor of long-term survival (relative risk of death = 1.649; 95% confidence interval = 1.07–2.54), and hypertension tended to be an independent positive predictor of survival (relative risk of death = 0.682; 95% confidence interval = 0.45–1.04).

Although unadjusted mortality rates in persons with heart failure have increased dramatically since the 1970s, trends after adjustment for age and other factors do not show the same striking increase. In fact, during the 40-year period of observation of the Framingham cohort, there was no significant temporal change in age-adjusted survival after the onset of heart failure.[14]

More recently, national data showed similar trends. Age-adjusted mortality rates in persons 65 years with heart failure increased from 1980 to 1988, declined from 1988 to 1990, and then remained fairly constant through 1995[37] (see Figure 1–2). Age-adjusted rates for the United States population aged 65 years declined from 116.9 per 100,000 standard population in 1988 to 107.6 in 1995 (an average annual decline of 1.1% compared with 1988 rates). The largest average annual percentage decline compared with

1988 rates occurred among African-American men (3.0% per year), followed by African-American women (2.2%), white men (1.7%), and white women (0.5%). Because of greater declines in death rates for heart failure among African-American adults, from 1980 to 1995 the African-American/white ratio for men narrowed from 1.3:1 to 1.1:1 and for women from 1.4:1 to 1.1:1.[37] Narrowing of the African-American/white ratio for heart failure mortality may reflect improved control of hypertension and access to medical care among older African-American adults.[37]

A recent report of the Rochester cohort, which is predominantly white, compared survival rates of 107 patients presenting with new-onset heart failure in 1981 with survival rates of 141 patients with new onset failure in 1991. Survival adjusted for age, sex, and New York Heart Association functional class was not significantly different in patients with heart failure in 1981 and 1991.[12]

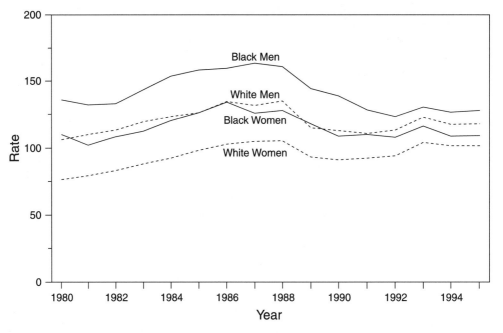

*Per 100,000 population, standardized to the 1970 Bureau of the Census population aged >65 years.
†*International Classification of Diseases, Ninth Revision,* code 428.
§Data for racial/ethnic groups other than blacks and whites were too small for meaningful analysis.

Figure 1–2 Age-adjusted death rate* for heart failure† for persons 65 years, by race, § sex, and year—United States, 1980–1995.

It has been shown that angiotensin-converting enzyme (ACE) inhibitors[42,46,49,50] and β-blockers[51] improve prognosis in patients with heart failure. Despite the use of ACE inhibitors in more than 40% of patients in the 1991 Rochester cohort, there were no changes in survival rates. The lack of an impact of ACE inhibitor therapy on survival may be related to the low percentage of patients treated, as well as to inadequate dosing and duration of therapy.[12] In a study of quality of care for elderly patients hospitalized with heart failure, it was found that although 86% of patients were eligible for ACE inhibitor therapy, only 14% received what the investigators considered to be sufficient doses.[52]

In contrast to the relative lack of change in mortality rates derived from national data and population-based studies, a progressive decline in mortality from heart failure over time has been observed in hospital-based studies. Hospital mortality rates decreased from 10.7 per 100 discharges in 1983 to 7.2 per 100 discharges in 1993.[53,54] Although it is possible that the decline in mortality may reflect improvement in heart failure therapy, it may also result from differences in admission and discharge practices and, in particular, a tendency of early discharge to extended care facilities.[2]

CONCLUSION

Heart failure is the final common pathway in a variety of cardiovascular disorders. In recent years, coronary heart disease has become the leading cause of heart failure. Many risk factors for coronary heart disease are also independent predictors of heart failure. Advanced age, hypertension, left ventricular hypertrophy, and diabetes are the strongest predictors of heart failure. Approximately 550,000 new cases of heart failure are diagnosed in the United States each year.

Incidence increases with age and is higher in men than women. Approximately 4.9 million Americans are currently living with heart failure. Prevalence increases with age and is similar in men and women. Heart failure is the most common cause of hospitalization in people 65 years of age and older. Hospitalizations for heart failure increase with age and are more frequent in women and African-Americans.

Heart failure is associated with very high mortality rates. Mortality increases with age and is higher in men. The median survival time from diagnosis is 1.7 years for men and 3.2 years for women. Major factors associated with a poorer prognosis include advanced age and functional impairment. Although unadjusted mortality rates are increasing over time, age-adjusted rates have remained constant or are even declining slightly in some groups.

Although some[12,55] have pointed out that limitation of infarct size by thrombolysis or revascularization and the widespread use of antihypertensive therapy should result in a reduction in the incidence of heart failure, this has not yet been observed. Goldberg and Konstam[11] propose that new population-based registries of heart failure in a number of communities throughout the United States are needed to characterize the present population burden from heart failure.

Clearly, heart failure has reached epidemic proportions. As with any epidemic, the focus needs to shift from the treatment of already affected individuals, whose prognosis is limited, to prevention and early intervention.[2] Continued efforts toward decreasing the occurrence of coronary heart disease by modifying risk factors, as well as limiting infarct size through early initiation of drug therapies and revascularization, should result in improvements in the incidence and prognosis of heart failure in the future.[23,55]

REFERENCES

1. Gillum RF. Trends in acute myocardial infarction and coronary heart disease death in the United States. *J Am Coll Cardiol.* 1994;23:1273–1277.

2. Massie BM, Shah NB. Evolving trends in the epidemiologic factors of heart failure: Rationale for prevention strategies and comprehensive disease management. *Am*

Heart J. 1997;133:703–712.

3. Cowie MR, Mosterd A, Wood DA, et al. The epidemiology of heart failure. *Eur Heart J.* 1997;18:208–225.

4. Lenfant C. Report of the Task Force on Research in Heart Failure. *Circulation.* 1994;90:1118–1123.

5. McKee PA, Castelli WP, McNamara PM, Kannel WB. The natural history of congestive heart failure: The Framingham Study. *N Engl J Med.* 1971;285:1441–1446.

6. Eriksson H, Svärdsudd K, Larsson B, et al. Risk factors for heart failure in the general population: The study of men born in 1913. *Eur Heart J.* 1989;10:647–656.

7. Garrison GE, McDonough JR, Hames CG, Stulb SC. Prevalence of chronic congestive heart failure in the population of Evans County, Georgia. *Am J Epidemiol.* 1966;83:338–344.

8. Remes J, Reunanen A, Aromaa A, Pyörälä K. Incidence of heart failure in eastern Finland: A population-based surveillance study. *Eur Heart J.* 1992;13:588–593.

9. Schocken DD, Arrieta MI, Leaverton PE, Ross EA. Prevalence and mortality rate of congestive heart failure in the United States. *J Am Coll Cardiol.* 1992;20:301–306.

10. Ho KKL, Pinsky JL, Kannel WB, Levy D. The epidemiology of heart failure: The Framingham Study. *J Am Coll Cardiol.* 1993;22:6A–13A.

11. Goldberg RJ, Konstam MA. Assessing the population burden from heart failure: Need for sentinel population-based surveillance systems. *Arch Intern Med.* 1999;159:15–17.

12. Senni M, Tribouilloy CM, Rodeheffer RJ, et al. Congestive heart failure in the community: Trends in incidence and survival in a 10-year period. *Arch Intern Med.* 1999;159:29–34.

13. Kannel WB, Ho K, Thom T. Changing epidemiological features of cardiac failure. *Br Heart J.* 1994;72:S3–S9.

14. Ho KKL, Anderson KM, Kannel WB, Grossman W, Levy D. Survival after the onset of congestive heart failure in Framingham Heart Study subjects. *Circulation.* 1993;88:107–115.

15. Andersson B, Waagstein F. Spectrum and outcome of congestive heart failure in a hospitalized population. *Am Heart J.* 1993;126:632–640.

16. Gheorghiade M, Bonow RO. Chronic heart failure in United States: A manifestation of coronary artery disease. *Circulation.* 1998;97:282–289.

17. Killip T. Epidemiology of congestive heart failure. *Am J Cardiol.* 1985;56:2A–6A.

18. Rich MW. Epidemiology, pathophysiology, and etiology of congestive heart failure in older adults. *J Am Geriatr Soc.* 1997;45:968–974.

19. Levy D, Larson MG, Vasan RS, Kannel WB, Ho KKL. The progression from hypertension to congestive heart failure. *JAMA.* 1996;275:1557–1562.

20. Chae CU, Pfeffer MA, Glynn RJ, Mitchell GF, Taylor JO, Hennekens CH. Increased pulse pressure and risk of heart failure in the elderly. *JAMA.* 1999;281:634–639.

21. Chen Y, Vaccarino V, Williams CS, Butler J, Berkman LF, Krumholz HM. Risk factors for heart failure in the elderly: A prospective community-based study. *Am J Med.* 1999;106:605–612.

22. Kannel WB, Belanger AJ. Epidemiology of heart failure. *Am Heart J.* 1991;121:951–957.

23. Funk M, Krumholz HM. Epidemiologic and economic impact of advanced heart failure. *J Cardiovasc Nurs.* 1996;10(2):1–10.

24. Deedwania PC. Prevalence and prognosis of heart failure. *Cardiol Clin.* 1994;12(1):1–8.

25. American Heart Association. *2000 Heart and Stroke Statistical Update.* Dallas, TX: Author; 1999.

26. Kupari M, Lindroos M, Iivanainen AM, Heikkilä J, Tilvis R. Congestive heart failure in old age: Prevalence, mechanism and 4-year prognosis in the Helsinki Ageing Study. *J Intern Med.* 1997;241:387–394.

27. Rodeheffer RJ, Jacobsen SJ, Gersh BJ, et al. The incidence and prevalence of congestive heart failure in Rochester, Minnesota. *Mayo Clin Proc.* 1993;68:1143–1150.

28. Mittelmark MB, Psaty BM, Rautaharju PM, et al. for the Cardiovascular Health Study Collaborative Research Group. Prevalence of cardiovascular diseases among older adults: The Cardiovascular Health Study. *Am J Epidemiol.* 1993;137:311–317.

29. National Heart, Lung, and Blood Institute. *Morbidity & Mortality: 1998 Chartbook on Cardiovascular, Lung, and Blood Diseases.* Bethesda, MD: Author; 1998.

30. Hennen J, Krumholz HM, Radford MJ. Twenty most frequent DRG groups among Medicare inpatients age 65 or older in Connecticut hospitals, fiscal years 1991, 1992, and 1993. *Conn Med.* 1995;59(1):11–15.

31. Ghali JK, Cooper R, Ford E. Trends in hospitalization rates for heart failure in the United States. *Arch Intern Med.* 1990150:769–773.

32. Croft JB, Giles WH, Pollard RA, Casper ML, Anda RF, Livengood JR. National trends in initial hospitalization for heart failure. *J Am Geriatr Soc.* 1997;45:270–275.

33. Gooding J, Jette AM. Hospital readmissions among the elderly. *J Am Geriatr Soc.* 1985;33:595–601.

34. Krumholz HM, Parent EM, Tu N, et al. Readmission after hospitalization for congestive heart failure among Medicare beneficiaries. *Arch Intern Med.* 1997;157:99–104.

35. Rich MW, Freeland KE. Effect of DRGs on three-month readmission rate of geriatric patients with congestive heart failure. *Am J Public Health.* 1988;78:680–682.

36. Vinson JM, Rich MW, Sperry JC, Shah AS, McNamara T. Early readmission of elderly patients with congestive heart failure. *J Am Geriatr Soc.* 1990;38:1290–1295.

37. Centers for Disease Control and Prevention. Changes in mortality from heart failure—United States, 1980–1995. *MMWR.* 1998;47:633–637.

38. Kannel WB, Plehn JF, Cupples LA. Cardiac failure and sudden death in the Framingham Study. *Am Heart J.* 1988;115:869–875.

39. Narang R, Cleland GF, Erhardt L, et al. Mode of death in chronic heart failure: A request and proposition for more accurate classification. *Eur Heart J.* 1996;17:1390–1403.

40. Cohn JN, Archibald DG, Ziesche S, et al. Effect of vasodilator therapy on mortality in chronic congestive heart failure: Results of a Veterans Administration Cooperative Study. *N Engl J Med.* 1986;314:1547–1552.

41. Franciosa JA, Wilen M, Ziesche S, Cohn JN. Survival in men with severe chronic left ventricular failure due to either coronary heart disease or idiopathic dilated cardiomyopathy. *Am J Cardiol.* 1983;51:831–836.

42. The Consensus Trial Study Group. Effects of enalapril on mortality in severe congestive heart failure: Results of the Cooperative North Scandinavian Enalapril Survival Study (CONSENSUS). *N Engl J Med.* 1987;316:1429–1435.

43. Packer M, Carver JR, Rodeheffer RJ, et al. for the PROMISE Study Research Group. Effect of oral milrinone on mortality in severe chronic heart failure. *N Engl J Med.* 1991;325:1468–1475.

44. Packer M, O'Connor CM, Ghali JK, et al. for the Prospective Randomization Amlodipine Survival Evaluation Study Group. Effect of amlodipine on morbidity and mortality in severe chronic heart failure. *N Engl J Med.* 1996;335:1107–1114.

45. Roul G, Moulichon M-E, Bareiss P, et al. Prognostic factors of chronic heart failure in NYHA class II or III: Value of invasive exercise haemodynamic data. *Eur Heart J.* 1995;16:1387–1398.

46. The SOLVD Investigators. Effect of enalapril on survival in patients with reduced left ventricular ejection fractions and congestive heart failure. *N Engl J Med.* 1991;325:293–302.

47. Bittner V, Weiner DH, Yusuf S, et al. for the SOLVD Investigators. Prediction of mortality and morbidity with a 6-minute walk test in patients with left ventricular dysfunction. *JAMA.* 1993;270:1702–1707.

48. Cohn JN, Johnson GR, Shabetai R, et al. for the V-HeFT Cooperative Studies Group. Ejection fraction, peak exercise oxygen consumption, cardiothoracic ratio, ventricular arrhythmias, and plasma norepinephrine as determinants of prognosis in heart failure. *Circulation.* 1993;87:VI5–VI16.

49. Pfeffer MA, Braunwald E, Moyé LA, et al. on behalf of the SAVE Investigators. Effect of captopril on mortality and morbidity in patients with left ventricular dysfunction after myocardial infarction: Results of the Survival and Ventricular Enlargement Trial. *N Engl J Med.* 1992;327:669–677.

50. Pitt B, Cohn JN, Francis GS, et al. The effect of treatment on survival in congestive heart failure. *Clin Cardiol.* 1992;15:323–329.

51. CIBIS-II Investigators and Committees. The Cardiac Insufficiency Bisoprolol Study II (CIBIS-II): A randomised trial. *Lancet.* 1999;353:9–13.

52. Krumholz HM, Wang Y, Parent EM, Mockalis J, Petrillo M, Radford MJ. Quality of care for elderly patients hospitalized with heart failure. *Arch Intern Med.* 1997;157:2242–2247.

53. Graves EJ. National Hospital Discharge Survey: Annual summary, 1988. *Vital and Health Statistics.* (Series 13: Data from the National Health Survey, No. 106), 1991;1–55.

54. Graves EJ. National Hospital Discharge Survey: Annual summary, 1993. *Vital and Health Statistics.* (Series 13: Data from the National Health Survey, No. 106), 1995;1–63.

55. Yamani M, Massie BM. Congestive heart failure: Insights from epidemiology, implications for treatment. *Mayo Clin Proc.* 1993;68:1214–1218.

56. Epstein FH, Ostrander Jr, LD, Johnson BC, et al. Epidemiological studies of cardiovascular disease in a total community—Tecumseh, Michigan. *Ann Intern Med.* 1965;62:1170–1187.

57. Gibson TC, White KL, Klaine LM. The prevalence of congestive heart failure in two rural communities. *J Chron Dis.* 1966;19:141–152.

CHAPTER 2

Health-Related Quality of Life Outcomes in Heart Failure: A Conceptual Model

Martha Shively and Ira B. Wilson

Heart failure affects about 4.6 million Americans and results in high mortality, reduced quality of life, and significant economic burden on society.[1,2] Historically, the care of these patients has been episodic and aimed at delaying death. Because of advances in therapy, the focus of care has shifted from episodic, inpatient care to outpatient care. The goals of care today are to prevent costly hospital readmissions, prevent unnecessary outpatient visits, and maintain or improve health-related quality of life (HRQL).

Interest in HRQL as an outcome in clinical care and research comes from several sources. One, as noted previously, is that mortality, fortunately, is less common and therefore less useful as an end point. A second is that state-of-the-art heart failure therapy now involves multiple medications, each of which carries some risk of side effects. Understanding the net effects of pharmacologic therapies requires the use of outcomes that aggregate the beneficial and adverse effects of therapeutic regimens, and HRQL measures are ideal for this purpose.[3–5] A third reason for interest in HRQL is that new therapies are inevitably relatively expensive, and payers are increasingly demanding that therapies be not only effective but also cost-effective.[6] HRQL measures can be used as the denominator for cost-effectiveness ratios. Finally, more and more patients want to know how the illness of heart failure and needed drug therapies are going to affect their lives, and clinicians need HRQL data to respond to these reasonable questions.

This chapter explores HRQL as it pertains to patients with heart failure. The goals of this chapter are to (1) provide a brief overview of the construct of HRQL, (2) demonstrate how a previously published conceptual model of HRQL can be applied to heart failure, and (3) discuss empirical data that support the relationships specified in the conceptual model. Cost outcomes are addressed elsewhere in this book. This chapter does not propose to review all of the conceptual and practical factors that need to be considered in designing and carrying out studies of HRQL in patients with heart failure (see Chapter 15). Interested readers can find thorough HRQL reviews in other places.[7–10]

WHAT IS HEALTH-RELATED QUALITY OF LIFE?

The terms "quality of life" and "health-related quality of life" are prevalent in the health care literature. Often, the terms are interchanged. Quality of life has been defined as the "excellence of one's life as a whole"; the meaning of the term quality of life varies among individuals and groups.[11] Ferrans and Powers[12] defined quality of life as "a person's sense of well-being that stems from satisfaction or dissatisfaction with the areas of life that are important to him/her."

HRQL is a distinct construct, different but related to quality of life. HRQL is a multidimensional construct with no simple definition. In the medical literature HRQL has been used to describe the quality of changes that occur as a result of medical interventions. However, some authors use a broader conceptualization to examine the reciprocal relationships between health and general well-being.[11] The term HRQL has also been used synonymously with health status and functional status. Patrick and Erickson define health-related quality of life as "the value assigned to duration of life as modified by the impairments, functional states, perceptions, and social opportunities that are influenced by disease, injury, treatment, or policy."[7(p22)] Perhaps the most concise definition is that offered by Gill and Feinstein, who define HRQL as "the uniquely personal perception of one's own health status."[13(p624)] In the context of health care, the term HRQL is preferred over quality of life because the focus is on health rather than the more global aspects of quality of life. Health professionals typically do not address the broad environmental, economic, and social aspects of quality of life. HRQL is also preferred because it is less restrictive than the terms health status or functional status, terms that are often thought to mean only clinical outcomes or physical functioning. Just as there are many definitions for HRQL there are many conceptual models of this construct.

Conceptual Models of HRQL

Many authors have proposed conceptual models of quality of life or HRQL to examine or measure relationships among the concepts or variables embedded within health and quality of life. A brief description of a few models is provided here to show the reader the diversity in conceptualization of HRQL. Thorough discussions can be found in references by Patrick and Erickson,[7] Haas,[10] Renwick et al,[11] Guyatt et al,[14] Padilla,[15] Patrick and Bergner,[16] Spilker,[17] and Stewart.[18]

Ware[19] proposed a model of HRQL that shows disease at the center of a series of concentric boxes. The concepts of personal functioning, psychological distress/well-being, general health perceptions, and social/role functioning move outward from disease. The concepts are also shown to be influenced by characteristics

intrinsic to an individual and to the larger social environment.

Patrick and Bergner[16] proposed a causal model in which a sequence of events occurs from disease to opportunity for health. HRQL concepts in the model are disease and injury, impairments, functioning, health perceptions, and opportunity or capacity for health. They propose that the environment and prognosis influence the other concepts. Disease influences duration of life.

Raeburn and Rootman[20] proposed a "Comprehensive Health, Well-Being, and Quality of Life Framework" to examine the integrated relationships among quality of life, health, and health promotion. They state the model is useful for understanding issues related to health promotion and rehabilitation. Health is shown as encompassing three of the nine domains of quality of life—physical being, psychologic being, and social belonging. The authors show clear boundaries that distinguish health from the other domains of life. Health promotion interventions can have an impact on quality of life determinants and health domains.

George and Bearon[21] proposed four dimensions of quality of life for older persons. The subjective dimensions are life satisfaction and self-esteem. The objective dimensions are general health and functional status and socioeconomic status. Ferrans and Powers[12] adapted the quality of life conceptual framework from George and Bearon[21] and used the framework to develop an instrument that would measure specific life domains and allow health care professionals to plan interventions to improve quality of life. The instrument (*Quality of Life Index*) measures the importance of the domains to subjects and subjective satisfaction with the domains.

Cowan et al[22] presented a conceptual model for examining quality of life during chronic illness. Perceived quality of life was the outcome variable. Antecedent variables were severity of disease, treatment aggressiveness, and socioeconomic status. Mediating variables were symptom distress, functional alterations, and cognitive adaptation. The authors pilot tested their model in patients with myocardial infarction and melanoma. Results indicated that the proposed relationships in the model were generic, not disease specific.

Most of the models briefly described here were developed by social scientists in an attempt to comprehensively describe quality of life. Comprehensive models of quality of life can be extremely valuable when the goal of measurement is to compare two different populations of patients or to assess the impact of an intervention. However, such models are not necessarily useful in clinical care. Clinicians are trained to think of disease in terms of biology and physiology. They assess symptoms by means of a careful history and signs by the physical examination. To be useful to clinicians caring for patients, the concepts in a theoretical model of HRQL should have some logical and intuitive relationship to the clinical variables that clinicians are familiar with and make use of in clinical decision making. Further, it is not only clinicians who are interested in these relationships. Patients want to know how much a treatment is going to improve their dyspnea, whether they will sleep better, and whether they will be less tired. A model of HRQL described by Wilson and Cleary[23] explicitly attempts to link clinical variables and clinical concepts with concepts such as physical functioning, social functioning, and general health perceptions. Because of this clinical focus, we believe that this model has particular salience for patients with heart failure. In the section that follows, we will describe this model in detail.

A CONCEPTUAL MODEL OF HRQL FOR CLINICIANS

The principal goal of clinical care is improvement of patients' health outcomes. To achieve this goal, clinicians need to craft interventions for their patients that they know are causally related to specific outcomes that patients value. For example, if a patient with systolic dysfunction has pedal edema, dyspnea with exertion, and paroxysmal nocturnal dyspnea, both the clinician and the patient will want to know that treatment with diuretics, digoxin, an angio-tensin-converting enzyme (ACE) inhibitor, or spironolactone (Aldactone) therapy will improve those symptoms. But this is not all they might want to know. They might want to know how much the dyspnea with exertion will improve, whether the patient will be well enough to return to work as a construction worker or an accountant, and whether the patient will be less anxious and depressed. The relationships between clinical variables such as pedal edema, jugular venous distention, and an ejection fraction of 20% and concepts such as social functioning and general health perceptions have not been adequately conceptualized to date, either in heart failure or in other conditions. Wilson and Cleary[23] have developed a model of HRQL that facilitates a better understanding of these relationships and may be useful in the formulation of strategies to improve patients' functioning and HRQL. Although the model has not been previously used in heart failure, empirical testing of the model in patients with human immunodeficiency virus supports the models' underlying assumptions.[24,25]

This model, shown in Figure 2–1, classifies the types of concepts that are usually used in understanding HRQL into five distinct groups or levels: biologic/physiologic factors, symptoms, functioning, general health perceptions, and overall quality of life. The model also proposes that there are causal relationships between adjacent levels in the model and that the dominant direction of causation is from left to right in the diagram (as shown by arrows). Clinicians are intimately familiar with the first three levels in the model, biologic/physiologic factors, symptoms, and functioning, but may be less familiar with the concepts or measures of general health perceptions and overall quality of life. One goal in developing this model was to describe the causal relationships between traditional clinical measures and less familiar measures of HRQL. Another goal was to stimulate efforts to quantify these relationships in a variety of different conditions, such as heart failure. Characteristics of both the individual and the environment potentially influence each of these levels. Wilson and Cleary emphasize that the relationships between

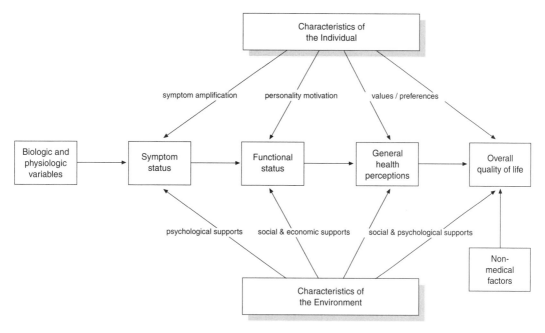

Figure 2–1 Health-Related Quality of Life Conceptual Model.

adjacent levels of the model may be reciprocal and that nonadjacent levels may also be related. That is, the levels are not necessarily linear or unidirectional. For example, functional status may influence or be associated with symptom status or physiologic variables.

Model Levels

The five major model levels will be discussed in the context of heart failure. Biologic and physiologic factors—the first major level in the model and the most basic determinants of health—focus on genetic, cellular, organ, and organ system function. Examples of biologic and physiologic variables related to heart failure include genetic evidence of hypertrophic cardiomyopathy, coronary artery anatomy, evidence of ventricular systolic and/or diastolic dysfunction, S_3 gallop, rales, and elevated jugular venous pressure. Such biologic and physiologic variables are usually assessed by instruments of one kind or another (eg, electro-

physiology test results, pulmonary artery catheter readings, echocardiograph, physical examination), or by trained observers.

Symptoms, the second model level, are the "patient's perception of an abnormal physical, emotional, or cognitive state"[23(p61)]; they are by definition subjective. That is, symptoms are self-reports of problems. The relationships between symptoms and other levels of the model are complex. Symptoms prompt persons to seek health care and may be influenced by characteristics of the individual (eg, mood) and environment (eg, access to care, insurance). Symptom status is a major component of HRQL and may also affect health services use because people who have more symptoms may use health care services more than people without symptoms. Examples of common symptoms in heart failure are dyspnea on exertion, fatigue, paroxysmal nocturnal dyspnea, and orthopnea.

Functioning, the third level in the model, refers to assessments of ability to perform specific tasks or functions. There are different kinds of functioning, such as physical functioning, social functioning, emotional functioning, and role functioning. Cognitive functioning may also be important because cognitive impairment is prevalent in patients with heart failure.[26] Functioning is usually assessed by asking patients to answer questions about what they can and cannot do, but functioning can also be observed and reported by others. For example, family members may be able to describe the functioning of the patient. Wilson and Cleary[23] review the relationships among physiologic variables, symptoms, and functional status. They suggest that symptoms, as well as biologic and physiologic variables, are important determinants of functioning. For example, symptoms such as dyspnea on exertion and fatigue limit physical functioning in patients with heart failure.

General health perceptions, the fourth level, are patients' global perceptions about their health and take into account the weights or values that patients attach to different symptoms or functional impairments. Like symptoms, general health perceptions can only be assessed by self-report. Self-report questions that assess general health perceptions typically ask, "Overall, how would you rate your health?" or "Is your health: excellent, very good, fair, poor?" Patients may consider their symptoms and functional status, as well as the importance of health or satisfaction with health status, when they answer such questions. Health perceptions are thought to integrate the physiologic factors, symptoms, and functioning levels of the model. General health perceptions have been used as a single measure of HRQL.

Quality of life is the fifth and most complex level of the model. As previously noted, quality of life is described as a person's subjective sense of well-being, happiness, and satisfaction with life overall.[23] Others have referred to quality of life as "the adequacy of people's material circumstances and to their feelings about those circumstances."[8(p381)] Quality of life is a global construct with many objective and subjective dimensions: cultural, social, psychologic, interpersonal, spiritual, economic, political, temporal, and philosophical.[7] Because health is only one aspect of overall quality of life, quality of life may be only weakly related to health. Overall quality of life, the last concept in the model, therefore, may not be a useful outcome in clinical studies.

The levels or concepts addressed thus far provide most of the structure of Wilson and Cleary's model of HRQL. However, additional factors are acknowledged as important determinants of the overall construct. Characteristics of the individual and the environment potentially influence all levels of the model. For example, a person's coping and problem-solving skills, motivation and self-efficacy, and social support may be related to symptom status, functioning, and general health perceptions. Self-efficacy, or confidence in one's own ability to perform certain tasks, could influence attempts to exercise. Self-efficacy is an important determinant of health behavior change in the face of chronic illness,[27] and such self-management behaviors have been shown to influence general quality of life health outcomes.[28,29]

The quality of the patient–provider interaction and organizational characteristics of the health care delivery system may also have an impact on HRQL.[30] For example, Greenfield et al studied patients with peptic ulcer disease,[31] hypertension,[32] and diabetes[33] and showed that interventions designed to improve interpersonal care can improve patients' health outcomes.

Other factors such as patient preferences or values may influence general health perceptions and overall quality of life. Utility assessment elicits patients' values for particular states of health and is often used as an overall measure of HRQL.[23] The term "utility" has been defined as "the value of a particular health state or improvement in health status."[7(p53)] Individuals are asked to rank or order their preferences or values for specific health states or outcomes. The health state being evaluated may be a current or past health state or a hypothetical state. However, measures of utility may reflect factors other than health status, such as the value patients place on life, their risk aversion, or their attitudes toward medical interventions.[9,23]

Measuring Variables in the HRQL Model

The previous section defined and described the levels of the model. This section reviews selected generic and condition-specific measures to facilitate applying the model to clinical practice or research related to heart failure studies. Table 2–1 shows where some of these measures may fit in the HRQL model. Note that some measures described in this section may not necessarily map directly onto the Wilson and Cleary conceptual model. For example, the physical and emotional dimension scores from the Minnesota Living with Heart Failure (MLHF) questionnaire do not directly correspond to any level in the Wilson and Cleary model. On the other hand, the dyspnea and fatigue that are dimensions of the Chronic Heart Failure Questionnaire (CHFQ) are symptoms and would fit nicely into the model, as would emotional function.

Generic measures can be used with many populations and allow for comparisons across interventions, populations, and conditions. A limitation of generic measures is that they may not be as responsive to changes over time in specific conditions as condition-specific measures.[14,34,35] Conversely, although condition-specific measures may be more sensitive to changes over time for a certain condition, they do not allow for comparisons across conditions or populations. Many studies include both generic and condition-specific measures to avoid these significant potential tradeoffs.

Other factors to consider in selecting HRQL measures include the purpose of the research or clinical evaluation, the HRQL domains to be evaluated, the psychometric properties of the measure(s), the planned target audience and dissemination of results, and respondent burden. Stuifbergen and Rogers[36] suggest that measuring the importance of life domains and satisfaction with those domains should be considered in persons living with chronic illness.

Three different instruments to measure generic health status have emerged from the Medical Outcomes Study (MOS). The first was the 20-item Short Form-20 (SF-20).[37] The SF-20 was one of the first comprehensive and generic short-form health surveys. The SF-20 was used to profile functioning and well-being in chronically ill patients. Domains measured in the SF-20 were physical, role, and social functioning; mental health; health perceptions; and bodily pain.

The Short Form-36 (SF-36) Health Survey is the best-known generic measure for monitoring outcomes in patients with chronic conditions[38,39] and followed the SF-20. Like the SF-20, it is useful in understanding population differences in physical and mental health, the health burden of chronic illness, and the effects of interventions on general health status. The SF-36 has eight dimensions: physical functioning, role limitations caused by physical health problems, bodily pain, general health, vitality (energy/fatigue), social functioning, role limitations caused by emotional problems, and mental

Table 2–1 Selected Outcome Measures for Patients with Heart Failure and Fit with the *Wilson and Cleary Health-Related Quality of Life* Model

Biologic and Physiologic Factors	Symptom Status	Functional Status	General Health Perceptions	Quality of Life
• Ejection fraction	• Chronic Heart	• NYHA classification	• SF-36/SF-12	
• Peak oxygen	Failure	• Specific Activity		
consumption	Questionnaire	Scale		
• Tumor necrosis		• SF-36/SF-12		
factor-α		• 6-minute walk		

NYHA = New York Heart Association; SF = short form.

health (psychologic distress and psychologic well-being). Extensive psychometric testing has been done with the SF-36 and is described in the *SF-36 Health Survey Manual and Interpretation Guide*.[39]

Norm-based data from the MOS (SF-36) are available for patients with heart failure.[39] Patients with heart failure ($n = 216$) had a mean age of 67, and 52% were women. The lowest mean scores were on the "role limitations due to physical problems" scale, and the highest mean scores were on the mental health scale. Forty-four percent of respondents scored at the lowest possible level (floor effect) on the "role limitations due to physical problems" scale; 53% scored at the highest possible level on the "role limitations due to emotional problems" scale. The authors caution that the norms were not adjusted for sociodemographic characteristics and other comorbidities that could affect the scale scores.

The Short Form-12 (SF-12) Health Survey is the third instrument to be released. It is a shorter version of the SF-36 and has good psychometric properties.[40] The SF-12 has been used in surveys of general and specific populations and longitudinal studies of health outcomes. Ware et al[40] state that the SF-12 gives less precise estimates of individual health scores but should be similar to the SF-36 in detecting changes in health status over time.[41]

Performance-based measures are generic measures of functioning. Performance-based measures generally require that participants be observed while performing specific activities rather than having patients report on what they can and cannot do. One type of performance-based measure tests specific muscle groups[42,43] such as measures of isometric knee extension strength. Another type of performance-based measure assesses several different muscle groups. For example, in the chair rise test a participant is timed trying to rise from a level stool 0.42 meters from the floor.[44,45] A third strategy is to assess maximal aerobic performance.[46] A fourth strategy, the Physical Performance Test,[47,48] assesses global performance. A disadvantage of performance-based testing compared with survey methods is that it is more time-consuming and more expen-

sive.[49] However, for some research hypotheses performance-based tests are clearly preferable. For example, a measure of activities of daily living may not be relevant for an intervention designed to improve exercise capacity. In the course of daily living, subjects may do no exercise, so questionnaire items directed at improved exercise capacity may not be answerable. In such a case performance-based measurement would be a necessity. In one of the few studies that directly compared performance-based and self-report measures, performance-based measures had no greater predictive ability than self-report measures.[48] Others have recommended that performance-based measures be used with caution until more is understood about their relationship to self-report measures.[49]

The 6-minute walk test is a commonly used generic and performance-based measure of exercise capacity or functional ability. Patients are instructed to walk as far as they can in 6 minutes. They may sit or rest during that time. The distance walked in 6 minutes is the variable measured. This test has been widely used in patients with heart failure.[50-58] It is user-friendly to the clinician, time efficient, and safe for patients with heart failure.[52] Concurrent validity and reproducibility are good.[57] The procedure for the walk test should be standardized by using the same physical area for the test, giving the same directions to patients, and by having the same researcher or clinician supervise all the tests. The 6-minute walk relies heavily on lower extremity functioning and may be difficult to interpret in an elderly population with different types and severity of lower extremity problems. In the presence of limiting hip arthritis, for example, the test might be insensitive to clinically important improvements in aerobic capacity.

Several different condition-specific health outcome scales have been developed for use with persons with heart failure.[34,59] Outcome measures used in heart failure studies have varied widely and prohibit cross-study comparisons.

Of the condition-specific measures, the MLHF has been used the most, and data about its performance characteristics are ample. The MLHF is a patient self-assessment of therapeutic response to interventions for heart failure. The MLHF is a 21-item Likert-type questionnaire that focuses on physical and emotional impairments that patients attribute to heart failure and that are amenable to therapy. Items are rated from 0 (no impairment) to 5 (very much impaired) to "quantitate the degree of disability related to each item."[60(p1018)] A total score, physical dimension score (sum of eight questions), and emotional dimension score (sum of five questions) are calculated. This questionnaire has been used as the primary efficacy measure in multicenter, randomized, clinical drug trials.[60,61] Rector et al[62] addressed validity of the MLHF with patients enrolled in the Studies of Left Ventricular Dysfunction. Patients without overt heart failure had significantly lower MLHF scores (less impairment) than patients with overt heart failure treated with medication. Improvements in the total and physical dimension scores of the enalapril group were significantly better than scores of the placebo group. Reliability has been evaluated in a sample of 198 patients diagnosed with heart failure and rated primarily as New York Heart Association (NYHA) Class III; Cronbach's alphas were 0.94 for the total score, 0.94 for the physical dimension, and 0.90 for the emotional dimension.[60]

The CHQ is another condition-specific measure for heart failure that was developed by Guyatt et al.[63] This 16-item questionnaire measures three domains: dyspnea (five items), fatigue (four items), and emotional function (seven items). The CHQ is intended to measure longitudinal change over time within persons. Items for each domain are presented as 7-point scales. In the dyspnea domain patients are asked to identify five activities and rate the extent of their dyspnea in those activities. The fatigue and emotional function questions are the same for all respondents. The CHQ is administered by means of an interview.

The most common clinical measure of functional status in cardiac patients is presently the NYHA classification. Clinicians and researchers commonly use the NYHA classification. Historically, this has been a subjective measure of the clinician's assessment of a patient's func-

tional capacity, and it has been criticized for its interrater reliability and validity problems. The most recent version of the NYHA classification includes the subjective functional capacity classes (I–IV) and an objective assessment section.[64] The Specific Activity Scale (SAS) is a 5-item scale that can be used to assess cardiac functional class.[65] The SAS is similar to the NYHA classification system but is used to assign cardiac functional class (I–IV) on the basis of the metabolic equivalents (METs) or work associated with each class. These and other measures of HRQL are discussed further in Chapter 15.

UNDERSTANDING THE HRQL MODEL IN HEART FAILURE: EMPIRICAL DATA

In this section we examine examples from the literature of studies that assess relationships between different levels in the model. The HRQL model is at the early stages of its evolution to a theoretical framework in that hypotheses about the relationships between and among concepts can be articulated and some have been tested. This section of the chapter presents empirical data that support the links between the HRQL model levels. Variables that may not be explicitly shown in the model but important to conceptualizing HRQL are also discussed.

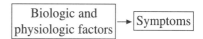

The most basic links in the HRQL model between biologic/physiologic factors and symptoms are perhaps the most familiar to clinicians and researchers. However, relationships between biologic/physiologic factors and symptoms, when studied, can be surprisingly weak. For example, patients with heart failure may have abnormal biologic or physiologic parameters but few symptoms. Marantz et al[66] reported that 20% of patients with an ejection fraction less than 40% met no clinical criteria for heart failure. Mattleman et al[67] found that only 42% of patients with left ventricular ejection fractions less than 30% had dyspnea on exertion. Many patients with moderate-to-severe left ventricular systolic dysfunction or early symptoms have no physical signs of heart failure.[2] These studies emphasize something that experienced clinicians intuitively understand: the presence of abnormal symptoms should prompt a search for abnormal biology and physiology, but the absence of symptoms in no way rules out the presence of abnormal biology and physiology.

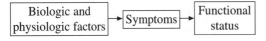

The next and more complex level of the model is functional status. The relationships between physiologic factors, symptoms, and functional status represent an active area of research. Examples of these studies include the role of neurohormonal activation and cytokine levels in heart failure, the relationship between systolic dysfunction and exercise capacity, the relationship between exertional symptoms and hemodynamic dysfunction, and the effect of an ACE inhibitor on ventilatory function and exercise capacity. These research examples are described below.

One interesting area of research examines the links between cytokine levels (a physiologic factor), symptoms, and functional status, as well as the relationship between neurohormonal activation and cytokine levels (two physiologic factors). One cytokine, tumor necrosis factor-α (TNF-α), has been shown to produce negative inotropic effects in cardiac tissue. Recent data indicate that there is a link between the presence of TNF-α and symptoms of fatigue, weight loss, and shortness of breath.[68] Torre-Amione et al[68] found that blood levels of TNF-α were 10 times higher in study patients with failing hearts compared with normal volunteers and hypothesized that TNF-α may be one of several mechanisms responsible for advanced heart failure decompensation (deterioration of heart function, increase in symptoms, and decline in functioning).

In another study Torre-Amione et al[69] assessed the relationship of proinflammatory cytokine levels (TNF-α and interleukin-6) to neurohormonal levels and NYHA functional class. There was no significant relationship between neurohormonal and cytokine levels, except for a weak correlation between TNF-α and atrial natriuretic factor. TNF-α levels were significantly ($P < .001$) elevated compared with age-matched controls and were progressively elevated in relation to decreasing functional status (NYHA class). However, there is disagreement about whether TNF-α contributes to the primary progression of heart failure or is simply a marker of disease severity.

Another area of research focuses on the relationship between systolic dysfunction (physiologic factors) and exercise capacity (functional status). Smith et al[70] examined the relationships between ejection fraction at rest, exercise capacity (oxygen consumption at peak exercise), and patient (heart condition assessment) and physician assessments (NYHA classification) of clinical severity in 804 patients with moderate heart failure. There were weak correlations between patient and physician assessments of clinical severity and exercise capacity. The investigators concluded that neither the NYHA class nor the patient quality of life scores was a useful assessment of peak exercise capacity because of wide individual patient variation. Investigators have also shown that low ejection fraction was only weakly related to exercise capacity.[70,71] These authors concluded that LV systolic function was not a key determinant of peak exercise capacity.

Wilson et al[72] examined the relationship between exertional symptoms, ventilatory and skeletal muscle dysfunction, and circulatory function in 52 ambulatory patients with heart failure. Patients underwent pulmonary artery catheterization and maximal symptom-limited treadmill testing. Patients demonstrated varied hemodynamic responses (mild, moderate, or severe dysfunction) to exercise. Peak oxygen consumption ($\dot{V}O_2$) was not significantly different in patients classified as having mild, moderate, or severe hemodynamic dysfunction. Perceived dyspnea was not related to the pulmonary artery wedge pressure and minimally related to the level of excessive ventilation. The level of perceived fatigue was moderately correlated with the blood lactate level ($r = .55$, $P < .01$). There was no correlation between peak $\dot{V}O_2$ and the total, physical, and emotional scores of the MLHF questionnaire. There was a moderate correlation between the peak $\dot{V}O_2$ and the dyspnea-fatigue index ($r = .48$, $P < .05$). The authors concluded that the level of exertional symptoms reported by patients does not reflect the level of hemodynamic dysfunction and that multiple factors other than cardiac function may influence symptoms, such as skeletal muscle deconditioning, body composition, motivation, and tolerance of discomfort.

McConnell et al[73] studied the effect of the ACE inhibitor captopril on the minute ventilation/carbon dioxide output ($\dot{V}E/\dot{V}CO_2$) ratio at submaximal exercise in 135 patients with reduced left ventricular function after myocardial infarction. Patients had cycle ergometer exercise tests three times over a 24-month period. The investigators concluded that captopril therapy resulted in reduced $\dot{V}E/\dot{V}CO_2$ ratio during submaximal exercise and that ACE inhibitors may be more effective at improving exercise tolerance at submaximal levels rather than maximal or peak levels. They hypothesized that the reduced ventilation may allow patients to perform normal activities at a lower perception of difficulty, reduce symptoms, and improve quality of life. However, they did not measure symptoms and quality of life.

The studies described previously demonstrate the need to explain the relationships among the pathophysiology of heart failure (physiologic factors), symptoms, and patient functioning. More studies are needed that quantitatively assess linkages so that symptoms, functioning, and HRQL can be improved through effective clinical interventions. These linkages will become clearer as new knowledge develops about the pathophysiology and management of heart failure.

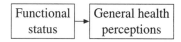

The more complex relationships between functioning and general health perceptions also need more investigation. Only one study has been found that links functional status and general health perceptions in patients with heart failure. Survivors of an acute exacerbation of heart failure have been shown to retain good functional status and health perceptions.[74] Jaagosild et al[74] studied 1390 patients with an acute exacerbation of severe heart failure to determine HRQL, mortality, and resource use. Health perceptions improved at 60 and 180 days after the acute episode, and functional status remained the same. This research shows that functioning may be maintained and health perceptions may improve even with severe illness.

CONCLUSION AND IMPLICATIONS

In this chapter we defined HRQL in relation to the more general construct of quality of life. We described a model of the relationships between different measures of HRQL and reviewed empirical studies in heart failure patients that relate to the model. Biologic and physiologic variables are easier to influence than functioning or health perceptions variables. It is not surprising, therefore, to find that there is more empirical evidence describing relationships among biologic variables, physiologic variables, and symptoms than there is for relationships at higher levels of the models (eg, health perceptions and overall quality of life).

The HRQL model described in this chapter should be useful to clinicians and researchers. The model can guide clinicians in conceptualizing and evaluating functioning and HRQL. Clinicians may also find the model helpful in evaluating the effect of interventions on HRQL outcomes. The HRQL model can guide investigators to conceptualize and define the domains of HRQL relevant for specific research questions and provide a framework for data analysis and interpretation. The model is appropriate for pharmacologic and behavioral intervention research with heart failure patients because it includes the multiple domains of HRQL. The model can be refined as empirical data emerge.

The strengths of this model are the clear and logical conceptual relationships proposed and the dominant causal associations and clinical applicability. The model needs to be further tested in research applications to provide empirical data for the conceptual links and reciprocal relationships and to identify any weaknesses in conceptualization or proposed relationships. As diagrammed, the model is very specific with regard to the first four levels of the model (physi-ologic variables, symptom status, functional status, and general health perceptions); however, the connections between general health perceptions and overall quality of life are not as clearly delineated. These connections will become clearer with future research.

REFERENCES

1. American Heart Association. 1999 heart and stroke statistical update. Retrieved October 1, 1999 from the World Wide Web: http://www.americanheart.org/statistics/index.html.

2. Konstam M, Dracup K, Baker D, et al. Heart failure, evaluation and care of patients with left-ventricular systolic dysfunction. Clinical Practice Guideline No. 11. AHCPR Publication No. 94–0612. Rockville, MD, Agency for Health Care Policy and Research, Public Health Service, U.S. Department of Health and Human Services; June 1994.

3. Croog SH, Levine S, Testa MA, et al. The effects of antihypertensive therapy on the quality of life. N Engl J Med. 1986;314:1657–1664.

4. Bombardier C, Ware J, Russell IJ, Larson M, Chalmers A, Read JL. Auranofin therapy and quality of life in patients with rheumatoid arthritis. Results of a multicenter trial. Am J Med. 1986;81:565–578.

5. Bozzette SA, Kanouse DE, Berry S, Duan N. Health status and function with zidovudine or zalcitabine as initial therapy for AIDS. JAMA. 1995;273:295–301.

6. Gold MR, Siegel JE, Russell LB, Wienstein MC. Cost-Effectiveness in Health and Medicine. Oxford, England: Oxford University Press; 1996.

7. Patrick DL, Erickson P. Health Status and Health Policy: Quality of Life in Health Care Evaluation and Resource Allocation. New York: Oxford University Press; 1993.

8. McDowell I, Newell C, eds. Measuring Health: A Guide to Rating Scales and Questionnaires. 2nd ed. New York: Oxford University Press; 1996.

9. Fowler FJ, ed. The proceedings of the conference of measuring the effects of medical treatment [entire issue]. Med Care. 1995;33(4 suppl):AS1-AS306.

10. Haas BK. Clarification and integration of similar quality of life concepts. Image: J Nurs Scholarship. 1999;31(3): 215–220.

11. Renwick R, Brown I, Nagler, M. Quality of Life in Health Promotion and Rehabilitation, Conceptual Approaches, Issues, and Applications. Thousand Oaks, CA: Sage; 1996.

12. Ferrans CE, Powers MJ. Psychometric assessment of the Quality of Life Index. Res Nurs Health. 1992;15:29–36.

13. Gill TM, Feinstein AR. A critical appraisal of the quality of quality-of-life measurements. JAMA. 1994;272:619–626.

14. Guyatt GH, Feeny DH, Patrick DL. Measuring health-related quality of life. Ann Intern Med. 1993;118:622–629.

15. Padilla GV. State of the art in quality of life research. Communicating Nurs Res. 1993;26:71–80.

16. Patrick DL, Bergner M. Measurement of health status in the 1990s. Ann Rev Public Health. 1990;11:165–183.

17. Spilker B, ed. Quality of Life Assessments in Clinical Trials. New York: Raven; 1990:7.

18. Stewart AL. Conceptual and methodological issues in defining quality of life: State of the art. Prog Cardiovasc Nurs. 1992;7:3–11.

19. Ware JE. Conceptualizing disease impact and treatment outcomes. Cancer. 1984;53(suppl):2316–2323.

20. Raeburn JM, Rootman I. Quality of life and health promotion. In: Renwick R, Brown I, Nagler M, eds. Quality of Life in Health Promotion and Rehabilitation, Conceptual Approaches, Issues, and Applications. Thousand Oaks, CA: Sage; 1996.

21. George LK, Bearon LB. Quality of Life in Older Persons: Meaning and Measurement. New York: Human Sciences Press; 1980.

22. Cowan MJ, Graham KY, Cochrane BL. Comparison of a theory of quality of life between myocardial infarction and malignant melanoma: A pilot study. Prog Cardiovasc Nurs. 1992; 7(1):18–28.

23. Wilson IB, Cleary PD. Linking clinical variables with health-related quality of life. A conceptual model of patient outcomes. JAMA. 1995;273:59–65.

24. Wilson IB, Cleary PD. Clinical predictors of physical function in persons with acquired immune deficiency syndrome. Med Care. 1996;34:610–623.

25. Wilson IB, Cleary PD. Clinical predictors of declines in physical functioning in persons with AIDS: Results of a longitudinal study. J Acquir Immune Defic Syndr Hum Retrovirol. 1997;16:343–349.

26. Cacciatore F, Abete P, Ferrara N, et al for the Osservatorio Geriatrico Campano Study Group. Congestive heart failure and cognitive impairment in an older population. J Am Geriatr Soc. 1998;46:1343–1348.

27. Lorig K, Stewart A, Ritter P, Gonzalez V, Laurent D, Lynch J. *Outcome Measures for Health Education and Other Health Care Interventions*. Thousand Oaks, CA: Sage Publications, Inc.; 1996.

28. Glasgow RE, Toobert DJ, Hampson SE, Wilson W. Behavioral research on diabetes at the Oregon Research Institute. *Ann Behav Med.* 1995;17(1):32–40.

29. Lorig KR, Sobel DS, Stewart AL, et al. Evidence suggesting that a chronic disease self-management program can improve health status while reducing hospitalization: A randomized trial. *Med Care.* 1999;37(1):5–14.

30. Landon BE, Wilson IB, Cleary PD. A conceptual model of the effects of health care organizations on the quality of medical care. *JAMA.* 1998;279:1377–1382.

31. Greenfield S, Kaplan SH, Ware JE. Expanding patient involvement in care: effects on patient outcomes. *Ann Intern Med.* 1985;102:520–528.

32. Kaplan SH, Greenfield S, Ware JE. Impact of the doctor–patient relationship on the outcomes of chronic disease. In: Stewart M, Roter D, eds. *Communicating with Medical Patients*. Newbury Park: Sage Publications; 1989:228–245.

33. Greenfield S, Kaplan SH, Ware JE, Yano EM, Frank HJL. Patients' participation in medical care: Effects on blood sugar control and quality of life in diabetes. *J Gen Intern Med.* 1988;3:448–457.

34. Guyatt GH. Measuring health-related quality of life in heart failure. *J Am Coll Cardiol.* 1993;22(Suppl A):185A–191A.

35. Patrick DL, Deyo RA. Generic and disease-specific measures in assessing health status and quality of life. *Med Care.* 1989;27(3 suppl):S217–S232.

36. Stuifbergen AK, Rogers S. Health promotion: An essential component of rehabilitation for persons with chronic disabling conditions. *Adv Nurs Sci.* 1997;19(4):1–20.

37. Stewart AL, Greenfield S, Hays RD, et al. Functional status and well-being of patients with chronic conditions—results from the Medical Outcomes Study. *JAMA.* 1989;262:907–913.

38. Ware JE, Sherbourne CD. The MOS 36-item short-form health survey (SF-36). I. Conceptual framework and item selection. *Med Care.* 1992;30:473–483.

39. Ware JE, Snow KK, Kosinski M, Gandek B. *SF-36 Health Survey Manual and Interpretation Guide*. Boston: The Health Institute, New England Medical Center; 1993.

40. Ware JE, Kosinski M, Keller SD. *SF-12: How To Score The SF-12 Physical and Mental Health Summary Scales*. 2nd ed. Boston: The Health Institute, New England Medical Center; 1995.

41. Ware JE, Kosinski M, Keller SD. A 12-item short-form health survey. Construction of scales and preliminary tests of reliability and validity. *Med Care.* 1996;34:220–233.

42. Edwards RHT, Young A, Hosking GP, Jones DA. Human skeletal muscle function: Description of tests and normal values. *Clin Sci Mol Med.* 1977;52:283–290.

43. Hook O, Tornvall G. Apparatus and method for determination of isometric muscle strength in man. *Scand J Rehabil Med.* 1969;1:139–142.

44. Skelton DA, Greig CA, Davies JM, Young A. Strength, power and related functional ability of healthy people aged 65–89 years. *Age Aging.* 1994;23:371–377.

45. Fiatarone MA, Marks EC, Ryan ND, Meredith CN, Lipsitz LA, Evans WJ. High-intensity strength training in nonagenarians. Effects on skeletal muscle. *JAMA.* 1990;263:3029–3034.

46. Schambelan M, Mulligan K, Grunfeld C, et al. Recombinant human growth hormone in patients with HIV-associated wasting. A randomized, placebo-controlled trial. Serostim Study Group. *Ann Intern Med.* 1996;125:873–882.

47. Reuben DB, Siu AL. An objective measure of physical function of elderly outpatients. The Physical Performance Test. *J Am Geriatr Soc.* 1990;38:1105–1112.

48. Reuben DB, Siu AL, Kimpau S. The predictive validity of self-report and performance-based measures of function and health. *J Gerontol.* 1992;47:M106–M110.

49. Manandhar MC. Functional ability and nutritional status of free-living elderly people. *Proc Nutr Soc.* 1996;54:677–691.

50. Dracup K, Walden JA, Stevenson LW, Brecht M-L. Quality of life in patients with advanced heart failure. *J Heart Lung Transplant.* 1992;11:273–279.

51. Kostis JB, Rosen RC, Cosgrove NM, Shindler DM, Wilson AC. Nonpharmacologic therapy improves functional and emotional status in congestive heart failure. *Chest.* 1994;106:996–1001.

52. Bittner V, Weiner DH, Yusuf S, et al, for the SOLVD Investigators. Prediction of mortality and morbidity with a 6-minute walk test in patients with left ventricular dysfunction. *JAMA.* 1993;1702–1707.

53. Cahalin LP, Mathier MA, Semigran MJ, Dec GW, DiSalvo TG. The six-minute walk test predicts peak oxygen uptake and survival in patients with advanced heart failure. *Chest.* 1996;110:325–332.

54. Woo MA, Moser DK, Stevenson LW, Stevenson WG. Six-minute walk test and heart rate variability: Lack of association in advanced stages of heart failure. *Am J Crit Care.* 1997;6:348–354.

55. Gorkin L, Norvell NK, Rosen RC, et al, for the SOLVD Investigators. Assessment of quality of life as observed from the baseline data of the Studies of Left Ventricular Dysfunction (SOLVD) Trial quality-of-life substudy. *Am J Cardiol.* 1993;71:1069–1073.

56. Walden JA, Stevenson LW, Dracup K, Wilmarth J, Kobashigawa J, Moriguchi J. Heart transplantation may not improve quality of life for patients with stable heart failure. *Heart Lung.* 1989;18:497–506.

57. Lipkin DP, Scriver AJ, Crake T, Poole-Wilson PA. Six minute walking test for assessing exercise capacity in chronic heart failure. *Br Med J.* 1986;292:653–655.

58. Guyatt G. Use of the six-minute walk test as an outcome measure in clinical trials in chronic heart failure. *Heart Failure.* 1987;3:211–217.

59. Bulpitt CJ. Quality of life with ACE inhibitors in chronic heart failure. *J Cardiovasc Pharmacol.* 1996;27(Suppl 2):S31–S35.

60. Rector TS, Cohn JN. Assessment of patient outcome with the Minnesota Living with Heart Failure questionnaire, reliability and validity during a randomized, double-blind, placebo-controlled trial of pimobendan. *Am Heart J.* 1992;124:1017–1025.

61. Rector TS, Johnson G, Dunkman B, et al, for the V-HeFT VA Cooperative Studies Group. Evaluation by patients with heart failure of the effects of enalapril compared with hydralazine plus isosorbide dinitrate on quality of life, V-HeFT II. *Circulation.* 1993;87(suppl VI):VI-71–VI-77.

62. Rector TS, Kubo SH, Cohn JN. Validity of the Minnesota Living with Heart Failure questionnaire as a measure of therapeutic response to enalapril or placebo. *Am J Cardiol.* 1993;71:1106–1107.

63. Guyatt GH, Nogradi S, Halcrow S, Singer J, Sullivan MJJ, Fallen EL. Development and testing of a new measure of health status for clinical trials in heart failure. *J Gen Intern Med.* 1989; 4:101–107.

64. American Heart Association Medical/Scientific Statement: 1994 revisions to classification of functional capacity and objective assessment of patients with diseases of the heart. Retrieved November 12, 1999 from the World Wide Web: http://www.americanheart.org/Scientific/statements/1994/079401.html

65. Goldman L, Hashimoto B, Cook EF, Loscalzo A. Comparative reproducibility and validity of systems for assessing cardiovascular functional class: Advantages of a new specific activity scale. *Circulation.* 1981;64(6):1227–1234.

66. Marantz PR, Tobin JN, Wassertheil-Smoller S, et al. The relationship between left-ventricular systolic function and congestive heart failure diagnosed by clinical criteria. *Circulation.* 1988;77:607–612.

67. Mattleman SJ, Hakki A, Iskandrian AS, Segal BL, Kane SA. Reliability of bedside evaluation in determining left-ventricular function: Correlation with left-ventricular ejection fraction determined by radionuclide ventriculography. *J Am Coll Cardiol.* 1983;1:417–420.

68. Torre-Amione G, Kapadia S, Lee J, et al. Tumor necrosis factor-alpha and tumor necrosis factor receptors in the failing human heart. *Circulation.* 1996;93(4):704–711.

69. Torre-Amione G, Kapadia S, Benedict C, Oral H, Young JB, Mann DL. Proinflammatory cytokine levels in patients with depressed left ventricular ejection fraction: A report from the Studies of Left Ventricular Dysfunction (SOLVD). *J Am Coll Cardiol.* 1996;27(5):1201–1206.

70. Smith RF, Johnson G, Ziesche S, Bhat G, Blankenship K, Cohn JN, for the V-HeFT VA Cooperative Studies Group. Functional capacity in heart failure. Comparison of methods for assessment and their relation to other indexes of heart failure. *Circulation.* 1993;87(suppl VI):VI-88–VI-93.

71. Cohn JN, Johnson GR, Shabetai R, et al. Ejection fraction, peak exercise oxygen consumption. Cardiothoracic ratio, ventricular arrhythmias, and plasma norepinephrine as determinants of prognosis in heart failure. *Circulation.* 1993;87(suppl VI):VI-5–VI-16.

72. Wilson JR, Rayos G, Yeoh TK, Gothard P, Bak K. Dissociation between exertional symptoms and circulatory function in patients with heart failure. *Circulation.* 1995;92:47–53.

73. McConnell TR, Menapace FJ, Hartley LH, Pfeffer MA. Captopril reduces the VE/VCO_2 ratio in myocardial infarction patients with low ejection fraction. *Chest.* 1998;114:1289–1294.

74. Jaagosild P, Dawson NV, Thomas C, et al, for the SUPPORT Investigators. Outcomes of acute exacerbation of severe congestive heart failure. *Arch Intern Med.* 1998;158:1081–1089.

CHAPTER 3

Managing Heart Failure: Economic Impact and Outcomes

Kathleen M. McCauley and Mary D. Naylor

INTRODUCTION

Currently, there are nearly 5 million patients in the United States with heart failure. Of these, 1.4 million are classified as New York Heart Association (NYHA) Class III or IV.[1] The incidence and prevalence of heart failure are expected to grow primarily because of recent declines in mortality from coronary heart disease and the aging of the population. Because of its high prevalence and associated medical resource consumption, heart failure is now the single most costly cardiovascular illness in the United States.[1] The cost of caring for heart failure patients is anticipated to escalate well into the twenty-first century.

The current model of heart failure care relies heavily on frequent hospitalizations to manage either deterioration in the underlying condition or escalating symptoms related to inadequate outpatient management. At least 75% of the nonhotel costs of hospitalization occur within the first 48 hours of admission, and half of heart failure readmissions may be preventable. Thus, cost containment strategies must address improved management of the underlying disease and more effective outpatient and home management.[1]

For these reasons, there has been enormous interest in identifying costs associated with heart failure and its management, as well as tremendous growth in heart failure research aimed at identifying the therapies and interventions that will improve both clinical and economic out-comes for this patient group. This chapter will examine the economics of heart failure associated with existing models of care and explore the potential of alternative modes of therapy and innovative models of care for improving patient and economic outcomes. We will attempt to identify what is known about the economics of heart failure from the perspective of society and will identify issues relevant to the cost of heart failure for the individual and her or his family.

ECONOMICS OF HEART FAILURE: OVERVIEW OF KEY CONCEPTS

In health care economics, the concept of cost as applied to an illness such as heart failure has at least three dimensions. It includes the direct cost of the illness, indirect costs, and intangible costs.[2,3] Direct costs include the actual costs of services such as hospitalizations, medications, and home care. Indirect costs include loss of income for the individual patient and/or family caregiver and travel expenses to health care settings. Perhaps the most difficult to measure are intangible costs, the costs associated with physical and emotional pain and suffering.

Most heart failure studies are focused on direct costs and usually attention is limited to hospital costs. These findings help us to understand the cost of health care from a societal perspective, albeit a limited one. This relatively narrow approach to cost assessment contributes little to our appreciation of the two other important dimensions of cost, indirect and intangible.

Direct costs may be assessed using charges, payment, or the actual cost of the treatment. The actual costs of providing a service are difficult to determine, because they include such diverse resources as personnel, space, equipment, and depreciation. For this reason, charges or reimbursements are often substituted as a proxy. Both of these substitutes have limitations. Charges may be unreliable because of cost shifting, and reimbursements may be unreliable because the basis for payment varies with the payer.[2] Cost analyses may be conducted in a variety of ways. Cost alone may be calculated or it may be related to effectiveness (measured as years of life saved), benefit (measured in dollars), or usefulness (measured in quality-adjusted life years, QALYs).[3]

INCIDENCE AND ECONOMIC IMPACT

Heart failure is estimated to afflict more than 1.3% of the population and accounts for 5% of the population of Medicare HMO patients.[2,4] With more than 2 million annual heart failure admissions, it has been estimated that the cost approaches $23.1 billion dollars or about 8.6% of the 1991 total costs for nonfederal hospitals.[5]

More recent data from 1995 indicate that heart failure as a primary or secondary diagnosis accounts for about 2,672,000 admissions.[6] Assuming that each patient has about 3.4 outpatient visits per year, the yearly cost per patient would be about $4238 or $14.7 billion nationally.[5] The overall pattern of outpatient visits has increased so that as of 1993, they numbered about 2.9 million visits annually.[2] The combined cost of inpatient and outpatient care, including the cost of heart transplant ($270 million), is approximately $37.8 billion. This represents about 5.4% of 1991 federal health care expenditures of about $700 billion.[5] A new estimation of the costs of heart failure care that recognizes the increased cost of each heart failure hospitalization and the increased number of hospitalizations indicates that estimated costs for 1999 were $56 billion.[1]

The magnitude of heart failure as a worldwide health problem is reflected in incidence data reported from multiple countries. In Northern Europe, it is estimated that there are 15,000 cases of symptomatic heart failure per million adults. An estimated additional 15,000 cases per million of asymptomatic patients, coupled with an estimate of 3,000 per million new patients each year, warrant concern both from a disease management and an economic perspective. Hospitalizations for heart failure have doubled in the past 15 years, and it is estimated that about 8,000 heart failure patients per million of the population of Northern Europe will be hospitalized each year. Considering expenditures in terms of 1998 US dollars, heart failure management costs range from a low of 1% of the total health care budget in The Netherlands to 2% in the United States. Expenditures in other European countries such as the United Kingdom and France fall between these extremes.[7]

Little evidence exists regarding the incidence and impact of heart failure in developing nations. Recent data from Malaysia, however, indicate that heart failure is a frequent cause of hospital admissions and accounts for 9% of medical admissions to an urban teaching hospital in Kuala Lumpur.[8]

Severity of heart failure has an effect on costs associated with treatment. Patients with severe heart failure may incur greater costs of treatment over a short-term analysis (6 to 12 months) because of frequent hospitalizations.[7] Most treatment costs occur in patients' final 6 to 12 months of life.[4] The mild to moderately ill heart failure patient, however, may incur greater expenses over time because of longer life resulting in more outpatient visits and more expensive pharmacologic therapy, despite fewer hospitalizations.[7] Recent innovations in pharmacologic management, while providing longer and higher quality lives, place significant financial burdens on patients who may not have the resources to pay for these therapies. Consequently, the beneficial goal of prolonging life for patients with heart failure will have economic consequences when the cost of drug therapy and clinical management programs are considered. Some analyses have been done of the cost impact of both components of heart failure management.

COST-EFFECTIVENESS OF PHARMACOLOGIC THERAPY

Several investigators have examined the economic impact of digoxin therapy for patients in heart failure. Data from the RADIANCE and the PROVED trials suggest that for patients in sinus rhythm, savings of $400 million per year would result from widespread use of digoxin. Although the number of hospitalizations in these studies was small, the data suggested that a 50% to 75% reduction in hospitalization was possible.[7,9-11] The larger Digitalis Investigation Group (DIG) study demonstrated a more modest reduction in risk of hospitalization (risk ratio, 0.72; 95% confidence interval, 0.66 to 0.79; $P < .001$).[12] This corresponds to a reduction in hospitalization of about 28% with potential savings of about $100 million.[7] Digoxin had a significant impact in reducing all cause hospitalizations and those caused by general cardiovascular causes.[12]

Early investigations of the use of vasodilators in heart failure demonstrated that a combination of hydralazine and isosorbide dinitrate reduced risk of dying by 36% over 3 years while improving left ventricular ejection fraction compared with either placebo or prazosin.[13] Later, the SOLVD investigators found that enalapril significantly reduced total mortality (39.7% vs 35.2%) and death caused by progressive heart failure or related arrhythmia (19.5% vs 16.3%) compared with placebo. This corresponds to a 16% reduction in the risk of death. The risk of either death or hospitalization for worsening heart failure was reduced by 26%. The investigators estimated that for every 1,000 heart failure patients treated with an angiotensin-converting enzyme (ACE) inhibitor for 3 years, about 50 premature deaths would be prevented and about 350 hospitalizations averted.[14] Consequently, the V-HeFT II trial compared enalapril with isosorbide dinitrate and hydralazine in patients already receiving digoxin and diuretics. The enalapril group had significant reductions in 2-year mortality (28.2%), but the difference diminished to a 10.3% reduction by 4 years. There were no significant differences between groups in numbers of hospitalizations.[15]

More extensive analyses of the economic impact of ACE inhibitor therapy in patients with mild-to-moderate or severe heart failure caused by significant left ventricular dysfunction have been done. Although ACE inhibitors are more expensive than older agents such as isosorbide dinitrate and hydralazine, their improved effect on mortality rates warrants consideration for use despite cost differences. If the cost of enalapril were reduced so that it is about 1.6 times as expensive as the isosorbide dinitrate and hydralazine combination, the ACE inhibitors would be considered the drug of choice for economic and clinical reasons.[16]

Cost analysis from the SAVE data was used to calculate a cost-effectiveness ratio that incorporates the cost of the drug and an adjustment for quality of life on the basis of a time tradeoff utility, or QALY. This analysis attempts to provide cost estimates for improved quality of life rather than simple survival years gained. If a patient with a given condition were asked to estimate hypothetically how many total years lived they would trade for years in better health, the resulting estimate is termed a QALY. This analysis found that treatment with captopril has a cost-effectiveness ratio of $3,600 to $60,800 per QALY when a conservative estimation of a limited benefit assumption is made. The disparity of savings estimates correlates with the age of the patient. Older patients (80 years of age) are expected to incur lower costs of treatment and younger patients (50 year of age) are at risk for most expensive treatment costs if the effectiveness of captopril exceeds the benefits of placebo for only 4 years. When a persistent benefit assumption is used (benefits exceed 4 years), the incremental cost-effectiveness ratio would range from $3,700 for older patients to $10,400 for younger patients per QALY in 1991 dollars. Compared with other accepted therapies for secondary prevention of heart disease such as aspirin or β-blocker therapy, ACE inhibitor treatment to improve ventricular remodeling is competitive.[17]

Increased sympathetic activity and resulting potentiation of the renin angiotensin system in patients with heart failure have been associated with poor outcomes such as hemodynamic dysfunction, poor exercise tolerance, and increased mortality. Consequently, the use of β-adrenergic blocking agents such as carvedilol and metoprolol has received clinical and scientific attention, and they are now added to standard therapy for heart failure.[18]

For a sample of patients with dilated cardiomyopathy and low ejection fraction, metoprolol was found to significantly reduce the need for heart transplant, improve quality of life, exercise capacity at 12 months, ejection fraction, and New York Heart Association class. The primary end point of death or need for heart transplant approached significance for improved outcome in the metoprolol group ($P = .058$). Hospital readmissions for all patients and the mean number of readmissions per patient were significantly less with metoprolol treatment.[19]

In a study terminated early because of a pronounced beneficial treatment effect, carvedilol was associated with a 65% reduction in risk of death for patients with heart failure. The overall reduction in the risk of hospitalization was 27%, and a combined reduction of 38% in the risk of death or hospitalization for cardiovascular reasons was seen.[20]

Delea and colleagues[21] examined the cost-effectiveness of carvedilol therapy in a hypothetical cohort of chronic heart failure patients. A Markov model was used to project life expectancy and the cost of medical care over the lifetime of treatment with conventional therapy alone (ACE inhibitors, digoxin, and diuretics) or this treatment plus carvedilol. Given the findings of the US Carvedilol Heart Failure Trials Program,[20] a reduced risk of death and hospitalization was assumed for the carvedilol treatment group. Because this clinical trial was ended early, long-term follow-up data are not available. Delea and colleagues[21] therefore projected outcomes beyond 6 months using a limited benefits and extended benefits approach. They assumed that if the drug were to have short-term benefits, patients in the carvedilol treatment group would revert to outcomes similar to standard treatment after 6 months. The extended benefits approach assumed that the probabilities

of either death or hospitalization for heart failure would increase in a linear fashion over time for carvedilol-treated patients and revert to the outcomes seen with conventional therapy after 3 years. Costs of drug therapy, outpatient care, and hospitalization were estimated using wholesale drug prices plus dispensing fees, Medicare data, and Health Care Cost and Utilization project data. Adding carvedilol to conventional therapy is expected to cost $6,745 over the patient's lifetime under a limited benefits assumption or $7,718 if extended benefits are assumed. This corresponds to an incremental cost per year of life saved of $29,477 (limited benefits) or $12,911 (extended benefits).

A new treatment strategy is likely to be associated with extra benefits and the added cost of adopting that treatment. Cost-effectiveness is the economic analysis that describes this relationship. Once this analysis is done, the treatment can then be compared with already accepted treatments for the target disease and other well-recognized diseases and treatments. The threshold can then be established to compare therapies. Currently, the accepted threshold is $50,000 per life-year added. Treatments that greatly exceed this threshold, such as costs of $100,000 per life-year added, may be considered less desirable from a cost-effectiveness perspective.[7,22]

Cleland[7] noted that both ACE inhibitors and β-blockers reduce heart failure hospitalizations, improve longevity, and are economical compared with other accepted therapies. These therapies have been estimated to either actually reduce the overall cost of care or add an estimated $2,500 cost over 5 years per year of life gained. Aspirin for myocardial infarction has been associated with a cost of $3,100 per life-year gained over 2 years. Coronary artery bypass graft surgery for multivessel disease costs $50,000 per life-year gained over 5 years, and cholesterol management with 3-hydroxy-3-methylglutaryl coenzyme A (HMG CoA) reductase inhibitors incurs a cost of $30,000 to $40,000 per life-year gained over 5 years.

When a new treatment strategy is found to improve outcomes at an equal or lower cost compared with standard treatment, the new treatment is termed a dominant strategy by economists. This type of analysis is termed cost minimization and is helpful in guiding clinicians and payers in treatment decisions. For example, data on clinical effectiveness and cost from the recent trials evaluating digoxin in heart failure suggest that use of digoxin in heart failure may reduce cost and may be therefore considered dominant.[9–11] These analyses serve to inform clinicians and payers about the greater societal impact of new and traditional pharmacologic therapies. Compared with other accepted therapies for heart disease, these agents are competitive, predominantly because of their effect in reducing hospitalizations. However, while providing important economic data to supplement clinical effectiveness findings, this type of analysis fails to describe the impact on the patient who must pay for these often expensive agents. The reality for many patients without medication insurance coverage is that the therapies that hold such clinical promise force economic choices that are difficult or impossible.

Current experience in our ongoing randomized clinical trial (RCT) in heart failure indicates that patients adjust dosages, skip doses, or stop drugs altogether because of these difficult financial dilemmas. In this trial, advanced practice nurses follow elders with heart failure from hospitalization to home for a 3-month intervention designed to improve symptom management, enhance function, and reduce hospitalizations and costs. In the process of helping patients and families manage the complexity of heart failure, we have learned that patient nonadherence to drug therapy is multifactorial. The cost of drug therapy, however, is a significant barrier for many patients. Although the societal benefit of a new drug therapy may be economically competitive, the cost may be prohibitive for many patients and families.

ECONOMIC OUTCOMES ASSOCIATED WITH ALTERNATIVE MODELS OF CARE

In the United States, two-thirds of heart failure patients return home or to self-care after discharge. Because more than 80% of heart failure patients are 65 years of age or older,[5] the burden of managing heart failure is further complicated by the diminished physical, social, and economic resources of aging. In recent years, nonpharmacologic therapies alone or in combination with pharmacologic treatments have received increased attention in the management of heart failure patients.[23–28] The recognition that multiple factors influence outcomes for this patient group has led to great interest in such approaches. These factors include multiple coexisting health problems; behavioral, social, and economic issues; and problems with the management of heart failure (eg, poor continuity of care).[29] Studies of more comprehensive approaches to care have generally been led by research teams made up of more than one discipline who have tested multidisciplinary interventions. Although only a few of these studies have explicitly examined cost outcomes, many have investigated the interventions' effects on health resources utilization, often a very good proxy for costs.[23–28]

Relatively few investigators have used RCTs to examine the effects of multimodal interventions on outcomes for heart failure patients. In an RCT exclusively targeting heart failure patients, Rich and colleagues[23] tested the effects of conventional care supplemented by a nurse-directed interdisciplinary team with those achieved by conventional, physician-directed care alone. The sample included 282 elders hospitalized with heart failure. The intervention was made up of intensive patient education, dietary consultation, social service evaluation, medication review, and close follow-up by telephone and home visits by a home health specialist and study nurse. At 90 days after hospital discharge, the following outcomes were demonstrated for the intervention compared with the control group: all-cause readmissions were reduced by 44%, heart failure readmissions were reduced by 56%, and the number of patients experiencing multiple readmissions was reduced by 61%. Patients in the intervention group also experienced an improved quality of life and greater compliance with medications and diet than patients in the usual care group.

Cost data were collected only for a subgroup of patients enrolled in this study ($n = 57$) and analyzed in the following four domains: readmission costs (based on allowable diagnosis-related group reimbursement); other direct medical costs (eg, medications); caregiver costs (ie, time spent by family caring for patient, prorated at $6/hour); and, the costs of the intervention (based on direct time spent by clinicians, social work, and home care team at an hourly rate of $20). Overall costs were calculated using mean readmission costs for all patients plus average costs of nonhospital services and costs of treatment for intervention group only. The cost analysis revealed net cost savings per patient of $460.

Stewart and associates[24] examined the long-term effects of a home-based intervention on the frequency of unplanned readmissions and out-of-hospital deaths among a subgroup of heart failure patients ($n = 97$) with a mean age of 75 years, who participated in a larger scale RCT. In addition to usual care, the intervention group in the larger study received predischarge teaching by a study nurse and a single home visit by a nurse and a pharmacist 1 week after discharge. The patient's clinical status and compliance with therapies were assessed at the home visit. In addition, the study nurse reviewed each patient's status with the primary care physician.

At 18 months after discharge, the intervention group experienced 50% fewer readmissions. Mean hospital costs per patients were 52% lower in the intervention compared with the control group ($P = .02$). Outpatient clinic costs were found to be comparable between groups. Other community-based costs were not reported. The cost of the original intervention was estimated to be approximately $190 per patient. The measurement of health resource utilization and the methods used to calculate costs for this study are not described in this report.[24]

More recently, the effects of a multidisciplinary home-based intervention similar to that just described was the focus of a second RCT conducted by Stewart and his team.[25] Once again, the intervention supplemented usual care. Patients in the intervention group received a structured home visit by a cardiac nurse 7 to 14 days after discharge. In addition to assessment of patients' health status and adherence to therapies, teaching and counseling were provided. If needed, referrals for emergency care were initiated, and flexible diuretic regimens were arranged. Findings from this visit were reported to the patient's cardiologist and primary care physician.

Compared with the usual care group ($n = 100$), the intervention group ($n = 100$) had fewer unplanned readmissions at 6 months ($P = .03$). At this end point, more intervention patients than usual care patients remained event-free, defined as unplanned readmission plus all-cause out of hospital deaths. Although the intervention group had lower total and mean hospital-based costs (ie, inpatient, outpatient, and emergency care) than the usual care group, the differences were not statistically significant. The mean per patient cost of the intervention was approximately $350. Other community-based costs, assessed for only a subset of patients ($n = 66$), were similar for both groups. Once again, limited information was provided about the measurement of resource utilization and calculation of costs.

Elders hospitalized with heart failure have been a targeted patient group in three RCTs conducted by Naylor and colleagues and funded by the National Institute of Nursing Research, National Institutes of Health.[26–28] In their most recently completed study, the effects of a comprehensive discharge planning and home follow-up protocol for patients hospitalized with heart failure and other common medical and surgical reasons for admissions of Medicare beneficiaries were examined.[27] The intervention group received a comprehensive discharge planning and home follow-up protocol designed specifically for elders at risk for poor outcomes and implemented by master's prepared nurses. The intervention substituted for traditional care and extended from hospital admission through 1 month after discharge. A total of 363 patients was enrolled in the study; 60 of these patients had been hospitalized for heart failure (diagnosis-related group 127). By 24 weeks after discharge, fewer intervention group patients had been rehospitalized ($P < .001$), had multiple readmissions ($P = .01$), and had fewer hospital days per patient ($P <$

.001). Time to first readmission was increased in the intervention group ($P < .001$). The intervention also resulted in a decrease in the number of patients readmitted for prolonged hospital stays (ie, more than 10 days).[28]

Group differences in actual Medicare reimbursements were reported. The index hospital reimbursement included the costs of discharge planning services for both groups. Data on hospital readmissions; unscheduled acute care visits; and home visits by nurses, allied health professionals, and assistive personnel were obtained from patient records and validated, and standardized Medicare reimbursements were applied. Costs of pharmaceuticals, over-the-counter drugs, assistive devices, and indirect costs (eg, productivity costs) were not calculated. The cost of advanced practice nurse (APN) services after discharge was estimated by assessing APN intervention-related effort (from logs) and applying Medicare reimbursements. At 6 months after index posthospital discharge, the estimated savings in Medicare reimbursements for intervention versus control groups revealed a mean per patient savings of almost $3000. Thus, the intervention was dominant from an economic perspective—improved outcomes were achieved at reduced cost.[27]

With the exception of elders hospitalized with heart failure, the intervention was effective in achieving the outcomes noted for all medical and surgical problems studied. Although statistical evidence was weak that the relative efficacy of the intervention differed between patients with and without congestive heart failure ($P = .11$), in clinical terms, the intervention's relative efficacy was significantly greater for patients without congestive heart failure compared with patients with congestive heart failure (rate ratio, 1.6 vs 2.7). Significant reductions in rehospitalizations for this patient group were demonstrated for a shorter period of time after the completion of the intervention.[27]

An analysis of logs maintained by the master's-prepared nurses who implemented this intervention revealed two possible reasons for the lack of longer term effects.[29] Relative to other patient subgroups, elders with heart failure

had many more unresolved issues at the end of the intervention linked to (1) the complexity of health problems and associated therapies and (2) long-standing poor general health behaviors.

Building directly on these findings, we are examining, in an ongoing RCT, the effects of a comprehensive clinical intervention designed to increase the ability of elder patients to manage their heart failure and improve their general health behaviors. The intervention extends from hospital admission through 3 months after discharge and incorporates plans of care developed, implemented, and coordinated by master's-prepared nurses in collaboration with a team of heart failure experts; educational and behavioral strategies to increase each patient's ability to manage heart failure and improve general health behaviors; and a strong patient–provider relationship. The intervention's effect on patient and cost outcomes is being assessed at multiple data points through 1-year postindex hospital discharge.

The study population for the RCTs completed to date has been older adults. Research is needed to determine whether younger patients would benefit from such comprehensive interventions. In general, studies are needed to help identify which of the subgroups of heart failure patients will benefit most from comprehensive interventions. Compared with traditional care, the few RCTs that have targeted heart failure have consistently resulted in decreased acute care resource utilization, specifically reduced hospital readmissions. It is, however, difficult to understand the relationship between the nature and intensity of the interventions studied and health resource outcomes. For example, the long-term reduction in hospital readmissions demonstrated by Stewart and colleagues[24,25] for a relatively low-intensity intervention is similar to that achieved by Rich and his team[23] for a much higher intensity intervention assessed in a much shorter time period. It is also difficult to interpret why studies with similar reductions in readmissions and intervention costs did not consistently demonstrate differences in associated costs.

Replication of these studies with a more diverse group of heart failure patients is desirable. In addition, research is needed to identify the best interventions from both a clinical and economic perspective for a growing group of heart failure patients. Enhanced reporting of the exact nature of the intervention and the processes used to measure resource use and calculate costs is essential to facilitate such efforts.

Multiple studies using a pre–post intervention design have evaluated the effects of a multidisciplinary approach to the management of heart failure patients on health resource utilization. The interventions tested have included specialized clinics,[30-32] disease management protocols,[33,34] intensive home follow-up,[35] use of a home-based computer-assisted telemonitoring system supplemented by patient education,[36] and the combined use of a pharmacologic and nonpharmacologic therapy.[37,38] These efforts have consistently demonstrated reductions in costly hospital readmissions compared with the preintervention care, suggesting their potential to improve economic outcomes for this patient group. Unfortunately, substantial differences exist among these studies in the nature and intensity of the intervention, the study population, and the follow-up evaluation period. In addition, little information is provided about the measurement of resource use and associated costs. Rigorous testing of such innovations is the next logical step.

On the basis of available data, it cannot be concluded definitively that multidimensional interventions are the most cost-effective methods of delivering care. Clear and compelling cost data are lacking. However, study findings suggest that the potential exists for this type of intervention to improve clinical and economic outcomes for the individual, family, and society. On that basis, more widespread adoption of these innovations seems warranted.[2] At the same time, continued study of such approaches to care should be a high priority.

CONCLUSION AND RECOMMENDATIONS FOR FURTHER STUDY

Heart failure is a chronic, debilitating illness. Despite recent advances in pharmacologic therapy and management strategies that promise to prolong life and reduce rehospitalizations, patients and families must deal with the physical, emotional, and economic consequences of this progressive condition. Although economic analyses of the cost-effectiveness of pharmacologic therapies, as presented here, point to tremendous benefit at a cost that is often comparable to therapies for other conditions, the cost to the individual patient may be prohibitive. Inadequate insurance coverage forces many patients to choose between the drugs that are needed to manage symptoms and prolong life and life's necessities.

These patients frequently have multiple and complex comorbid conditions requiring coordinated and often expensive therapy. Poor general health behaviors, knowledge deficits, and inadequate tangible and emotional support systems often complicate attainment of an optimal state of health. Patients and families face the challenge of negotiating a health care system composed of multiple general and specialist providers. Management programs that bridge the transition from hospital to home and that enhance the patient and family's ability to manage heart failure and the complexities of aging are needed.

Greater attention is needed to define the economic impact of heart failure and its treatment for patients and families. It has been estimated that adherence to the drug therapy for patients with heart failure varies from 30% to 60%, depending on the complexity of the treatment plan.[4] The economic component of this nonadherence deserves analysis and creative attention. Patients who are willing and able to take their medications should not be excluded from this therapy for cost reasons.

Future multidisciplinary intervention trials designed to identify best practices in overall management of heart failure should also begin to include more comprehensive data on the range of costs. These include lost time from work while family members care for patients with failure, transportation costs for outpatient visits, and the cost of interventions to reduce social isolation. The evidence is clear that heart failure is a huge health problem with enormous societal and individual costs. The promise of extended life with new drug therapies will bring additional economic consequences that must be addressed.

REFERENCES

1. O'Connell JB. The economic burden of heart failure. *Clin Cardiol*. 2000;23 (suppl III):III-6–III-10.

2. Rich M, Nease R. Cost-effectiveness analysis in clinical practice. The case of heart failure. *Arch Intern Med*. 1999;159:1690–1700.

3. Willens H, Chakko S, Simmons J, Kessler K. Cost-effectiveness in clinical cardiology: Part 1: Coronary artery disease and congestive heart failure. *Chest*. 1996;109:1359–1369.

4. Mackowiak J. Cost of heart failure to the healthcare system. *Am J Man Care*. 1998;4 Suppl:S338–S342.

5. O'Connell J, Bristow M. Economic impact of heart failure in the United States: time for a different approach. *J Heart Lung Transplant*. 1993;3:S107–S112.

6. American Heart Association. *Heart and Stroke Statistical Update*. Dallas, TX: American Heart Association; 1998.

7. Cleland JG. Health economic consequences of the pharmacologic treatment of heart failure. *Eur Heart J*. 1998;19(suppl P):P32–P39.

8. Teh B, Lim M, Robiah W, et al. Heart failure hospitalizations in Malaysia [abstract]. *J Card Fail*. 1999;5(3) Suppl 1:64.

9. Packer M, Gheorghiade M, Young J, et al. Withdrawal of digoxin from patients with chronic heart failure treated with angiotensin converting enzyme inhibitors. *N Engl J Med*. 1993;329:1–7.

10. Uretsky B, Young J, Shahidi F, Yellen L, Harrison M, Jolly M. on behalf of the PROVED Investigative Group. Randomized study assessing the effect of digoxin withdrawal in patients with mild to moderate chronic congestive heart failure: results of the PROVED trial. *J Am Coll Cardiol*. 1993;22:955–962.

11. Ward R, Gheorghiade M, Young J, Uretsky B. Economic outcomes of withdrawal of digoxin therapy in adult patients with stable congestive heart failure. *J Am Coll Cardiol*. 26:93–101.

12. The Digitalis Investigation Group. The effect of digoxin on mortality and morbidity in patients with heart failure. *N Engl J Med*. 1997;336:525–533.

13. Cohn J, Archibald D, Ziesche S, et al. Effect of vasodilator therapy on mortality in chronic congestive heart failure: the results of a Veterans Administration cooperative study. *N Engl J Med*. 1986;314:1547–1552.

14. The SOLVD Investigators. Effect of enalapril on survival in patients with reduced left ventricular ejection fractions and congestive heart failure. *N Engl J Med*. 1991;325:293–302.

15. Cohn J, Johnson G, Ziesche S, et al. A comparison of enalapril with hydralazine – isosorbide dinitrate in the treatment of chronic congestive heart failure. *N Engl J Med*. 991;325:303–310.

16. Paul S, Kuntz K, Eagle K, et al. Costs and effectiveness of angiotensin converting enzyme inhibition in patients with congestive heart failure. *Arch Intern Med*. 1994;154:1143–1149.

17. Tsevat J, Duke D, Goldman L, et al. Cost effectiveness of captopril therapy after myocardial infarction. *J Am Coll Cardiol*. 1995;26:914–919.

18. Frishman W. Drug therapy: carvedilol. *N Engl J Med*. 1998;339:1759–1765.

19. Waagstein F, Bristow M, Swedberg K. Beneficial effects of metoprolol in idiopathic dilated cardiomyopathy. *Lancet*. 1993;342:1441–1446.

20. Packer M, Bristow M, Cohn J, et al. The effect of carvedilol on morbidity and mortality in patients with chronic heart failure. *N Engl J Med*. 1996;334:1349–1355.

21. Delea T, Vera-Llonch M, Richner R, Fowler M, Oster G. Cost effectiveness of carvedilol for heart failure. *Am J Cardiol*. 1999;83:890–896.

22. Mark D. Economics of treating heart failure. *Am J Cardiol*. 1997;80:33H–38H.

23. Rich MW, Beckham V, Wittenberg C, Leven CL, Freedland KE, Carney RM. A multidisciplinary intervention to prevent the readmission of elderly patients with congestive heart failure. *N Engl J Med*. 1995;333:1190–1195.

24. Stewart S, Vandenbroek AJ, Peason S, Horowitz JD. Prolonged beneficial effects of a home-based intervention on unplanned readmissions and mortality among patients with congestive heart failure. *Arch Intern Med*. 1999;159:257–261.

25. Stewart S, Marley JE, Horowitz JD. Effects of a multidisciplinary, home-based intervention on unplanned readmissions and survival among patients with chronic congestive heart failure: a randomised controlled study. *Lancet*. 1999;354:1077–1083.

26. Naylor M, Brooten D, Jones R, Lavizzo-Mourey R, Mezey M, Pauly M. Comprehensive discharge planning for the hospitalized elderly: A randomized clinical trial. *Ann Intern Med*. 1994;120:999–1006.

27. Naylor M, Brooten D, Campbell R, et al. Comprehensive discharge planning and home follow-up intervention on elders hospitalized with common medical and surgical cardiac conditions. *JAMA*. 1999;281:613–620.

28. Naylor M, McCauley K. The effects of a discharge planning and home follow-up intervention on elders hospitalized with common medical and surgical cardiac conditions. *J Cardiovasc Nurs*. 1999;14:44–54.

29. Happ M, Naylor M, Roe-Prior P, Campbell R, Jacobsen B. Factors contributing to rehospitalization of elderly patients with heart failure. *J Cardiovasc Nurs*. 1997;11:75–84.

30. Lasater M. The effect of a nurse-managed CHF clinic on patient readmission and length of stay. *Home Healthcare Nurse.* 1996;14:351–356.

31. Roglieri JL, Futterman R, McDonough KL, et al. Disease management interventions to improve outcomes in congestive heart failure. *Am J Managed Care.* 1997;3:1831–1839.

32. Smith LE, Farbri SA, Pai R, et al. Symptomatic improvement and reduced hospitalization for patients attending a cardiomyopathy clinic. *Clin Cardiol.* 1997;20:949–954.

33. Hanumanthu S, Butler J, Chomsky D, Davis S, Wilson JR. Effect of a heart failure program on hospitalization frequency and exercise tolerance. *Circulation.* 1997;96:2842–2848.

34. Riegel B, Thomason T, Carlson B, et al. Implementation of a multidisciplinary disease management program for heart failure patients. *Congestive Heart Failure.* 1999;5:164–170.

35. Kornowski R, Zeeli D, Averbuch M, et al. Intensive home-care surveillance prevents hospitalization and improves morbidity rates among elderly patients with severe congestive heart failure. *Am Heart J.* 1995;129:762–766.

36. Roglieri J, Futterman B, McDonough K, et al. Disease management interventions to improve outcomes in congestive heart failure. *Am J Man Care.* 1997;3:1831–1839.

37. West JA, Miller NH, Parker KM, et al. A comprehensive management system for heart failure improves clinical outcomes and reduces medical resource utilization. *Am J Cardiol.* 1997;79:58–63.

38. Fonarow GC, Stevenson LW, Walden JA, et al. Impact of a comprehensive heart failure management program on hospital readmission and functional status of patients with advanced heart failure. *J Am Coll Cardiol.* 1997;30:725–732.

PART II

Improving Outcomes by Influencing the Personal Impact of Heart Failure

Impact of Pharmacologic Therapy on Health-Related Quality of Life in Heart Failure: Findings from Clinical Trials

Derek V. Exner and Eleanor B. Schron

Heart failure is the most important public health problem in cardiovascular medicine,[1] affecting more than 5 million persons in North America alone.[1,2] In addition to causing excess mortality, heart failure has a tremendous impact on the lives of patients and their families. Because of the increasing age of the population,[2,3] the prevalence of heart failure will continue to increase, as will its impact on individuals and society. Thus, an intense search for therapies to improve outcomes in heart failure has been, and continues to be, an important goal in clinical research. This chapter reviews the outcomes achieved in the major clinical trials, with an emphasis on the effectiveness of pharmacologic therapy on health-related quality of life (HRQL) in individuals with heart failure.

PATHOPHYSIOLOGY

During the initial stages of heart failure, activation of the sympathetic nervous system increases heart rate, myocardial contractility, and peripheral vasoconstriction, resulting in the maintenance of blood pressure. Concurrently, activation of the renin-angiotensin-aldosterone system leads to further vasoconstriction and increased intravascular volume. However, sustained activation of these systems is counterproductive, leading to progressive left ventricular systolic dysfunction.[4,5] This pathophysiology drives the choice of pharmacologic agents tested in clinical trials.

PHARMACOLOGIC THERAPY: IMPACT ON PHYSIOLOGIC PARAMETERS, MORBIDITY, AND MORTALITY

Angiotensin-converting enzyme (ACE) inhibitors reduce the production of renin and angiotensin, improve hemodynamic parameters and exercise performance, and alter the progression of ventricular dysfunction in patients with heart failure. Further, controlled trials have demonstrated the efficacy of ACE inhibitors in a variety of patient groups. ACE inhibitors reduce mortality and hospitalizations in patients with symptomatic left ventricular systolic dysfunction, reduce hospitalizations in patients with asymptomatic left ventricular systolic dysfunction, and reduce mortality and hospitalizations in patients with heart failure after myocardial infarction.[6–15] Recently, the addition of the aldosterone antagonist, spironolactone, to ACE inhibitor therapy has been shown to further reduce mortality in patients with advanced heart failure.[16] β-Adrenoceptor blockers have also been shown to favorably alter ventricular function, improve exercise performance, and reduce mortality and hospitalizations in patients with moderately symptomatic left ventricular systolic dysfunction.[17–19] Digoxin therapy has also been shown to improve ventricular function, enhance exercise performance, and reduce morbidity in patients with heart failure.[20] Finally, a number of inotropic agents (eg, milrinone, flosequinan, vesnarinone) have been demonstrated to have favorable effects on hemodynamic function, exercise performance, and overall quality of life in patients with heart failure but lead to an increased risk of death in these patients.[21–23]

PHARMACOLOGIC THERAPY: IMPACT ON QUALITY OF LIFE

In addition to the ability of pharmacologic agents to favorably alter surrogate outcomes (eg, hemodynamic parameters, exercise performance) and hard end points (eg, mortality, hospitalization), clinical investigators have been interested in the effect of treatment on self-reported HRQL.[24] This interest is primarily related to the recognized importance of HRQL assessment in providing insight into the influence of therapies on the lives of patients. In addition to biologic and physiologic factors, individual characteristics and environmental factors importantly modify self-perceived HRQL[25] (see Chapter 2). Thus, poor correlation between self-perceived HRQL and surrogate markers or hard end points would not be unexpected in some individuals. For example, a patient with heart failure who receives a β-blocker is likely to have an improvement in their left ventricular function and be at lower risk of dying. However, this individual may experience adverse effects, such as dizziness and fatigue, or suffer financial stress related to the cost of the therapy. Thus, their self-perceived HRQL may either not change or even decline. Some studies have found an inverse relationship between mortality and HRQL,[23] whereas other trials have shown positive correlation between self-perceived HRQL and both surrogate outcomes (eg, 6-minute walk distance)[26,27] and mortality.[28,29] In this chapter, we discuss several large clinical trials that illustrate many of these issues. A discussion of the specific instruments, the importance and methods of collecting high-quality HRQL data, the influence of missing data on the interpretation of HRQL results, and recent advances in longitudinal data analysis are discussed elsewhere in this book (see Chapter 15).

TRIALS EVALUATING QUALITY OF LIFE IN HEART FAILURE

Six major pharmacologic clinical studies that included assessments of HRQL are discussed in the following sections. In addition to the studies discussed here, a large number of other heart failure trials have also assessed functional status and quality of life. The studies reviewed here were chosen because they illustrate the important issues in the evaluation of the effect of pharmacologic therapy on HRQL. Summaries of the other studies and their results can be found elsewhere.[30,31]

Veterans Administration Heart Failure Trials

The Veterans Administration Heart Failure Trials (V-HeFT) evaluated the efficacy of hydralazine-isosorbide dinitrate versus placebo (V-HeFT I) and hydralazine-isosorbide dinitrate versus enalapril (V-HeFT II) in 1,446 men with New York Heart Association (NYHA) Class II to III symptoms of heart failure[6,8] (Table 4–1). V-HeFT II demonstrated that enalapril increased survival compared with hydralazine-isosorbide dinitrate. Both the Heart Condition Assessment (HCA) and the Living with Heart Failure (LIhFE) questionnaire were self-administered at baseline, 3 months, 6 months, and thereafter every 6 months after randomization. Neither active study regimen was associated with significantly improved HRQL. In fact, progressive declines in self-perceived well-being and in serial measures of physiologic parameters (ejection fraction, peak oxygen consumption) were observed.

The reasons for the observed discrepancies between improved survival but declines in self-reported HRQL and physiologic parameters are unclear. It is plausible that the HCA and LIhFE questionnaires were not responsive to changes in physical functioning and mental well-being.[32] Alternatively, these questionnaires may provide a responsive measure of HRQL, but mortality and HRQL may be poorly correlated. Because HRQL is a multidimensional construct, it is not

Table 4–1 Trials Assessing Quality of Life

Trial (Year)	Population/ Comparison	QoL Components	Results
Veterans Affairs Heart Failure Trials (V-HeFT) (1986, 1991)[6,8,32]	• NYHA II–IV • EF < 0.40 or ↓ exercise • n = 1446 (both) • *V-HeFT I—* isosorbide dinitrate vs placebo • *V-HeFT II—* enalapril vs isosorbide dinitrate	• Perceived health • Symptoms • Physical function • Emotional function • Sexual function • Employment	• Reduced mortality with isosorbide dinitrate (V-HeFT I) • Further reduction in mortality with enalapril (V-HeFT II) • No improvement in QoL with isosorbide dinitrate or enalapril
Studies of Left Ventricular Dysfunction (SOLVD) (1991, 1992)[11,12,26–28]	• *Treatment*—NYHA II–IV • *Prevention*—NYHA I–II • EF < 0.35 (both) • n = 6797 (both) • Enalapril vs placebo	• Life satisfaction • Perceived health • Symptoms • Physical function • Emotional function • Sexual function • Employment	• Reduced mortality with enalapril (treatment trial) • Reduced risk of death or hospitalization with enalapril (both trials) • Improved QoL with enalapril (both) • Increased 6-minute walk distance with enalapril (both)
Digoxin Investigation Group (DIG) (1997)[20,34]	• NYHA class I–IV • n = 7788 • Digoxin vs placebo	• Perceived health • Symptoms • Physical function • Emotional function • Sexual function • Socioeconomic	• No alteration in mortality with digoxin • Reduced hospitalizations with digoxin • No alteration in QoL with digoxin
Prospective Randomized Evaluation of Carvedilol on Symptoms and Exercise (PRECISE) (1996)[33]	• EF 0.35 • Six-minute walk distance 150–425 m (492–1394 ft) • n = 278 • Carvedilol vs placebo	• Perceived health • Symptoms • Physical function • Emotional function • Sexual function • Socioeconomic	• Reduced risk of death or hospitalization with carvedilol • Improved NYHA functional class and increased 6-minute walk distance with carvedilol • Improved generic QoL, but no alteration in heart failure-specific QoL with carvedilol
Vesnarinone Trial (1998)[23]	• NYHA Class III/IV • EF 0.30 • n = 3883 • Vesnarinone vs placebo	• Perceived health • Symptoms • Physical function • Emotional function • Sexual function • Socioeconomic	• Higher mortality with vesnarinone • Improved QoL with vesnarinone
Metoprolol Randomised Intervention Trial in Heart Failure (MERIT-HF) (2000)[19,29]	• NYHA Class II–IV • EF 0.40 • n = 3991 • Metoprolol CR/XL vs placebo	• Perceived health • Symptoms • Physical function • Emotional function	• Reduced mortality with metoprolol • Improved generic QoL, but no alteration in heart failure–specific QoL, with metoprolol

surprising that poor correlation between changes in self-perceived HRQL with either physiologic surrogates or hard outcomes was observed. Measurement of self-perceived HRQL incorporates factors such as social status, health perceptions, and emotional factors, which may not be significantly altered by drug or device therapy. Thus, although alteration in certain aspects of self-perceived HRQL may be observed with specific interventions (eg, improved physical functioning), significant alterations in other aspects (eg, social status) would not be anticipated. Finally, problems related to incomplete data may, in part, account for these observations (see Chapter 15).

Studies of Left Ventricular Dysfunction

The Studies of Left Ventricular Dysfunction (SOLVD) evaluated HRQL of patients with left ventricular dysfunction, defined by an ejection fraction 0.35. Patients were enrolled in either the Treatment ($n = 2569$)[11] or Prevention trial ($n = 4228$),[12] depending on the presence or absence of heart failure symptoms, respectively. Of the 6797 participants in the SOLVD trials, 5025 (74%) completed one or more HRQL assessments (treatment trial $n = 2465$; prevention trial $n = 2560$). Patients in both trials were randomly assigned to enalapril or placebo. A brief, self-administered set of HRQL questionnaires was completed at baseline, 6 weeks, 12 months, and 24 months of follow-up (Table 4–1).[26–28] These questionnaires contained 14 scales that addressed seven components of HRQL. They included physical functioning (vigor, activities of daily living), emotional distress (anxiety, depression), social health (social functioning, social life), intimacy, life satisfaction, perceived health, general health perception, and productivity or job performance. Questions were drawn from the LIhFE, RAND Physical Limitations, Psychological Distress, and Health Perceptions instruments. An additional question on shortness of breath was adapted from the Dyspnea Scale. Cognitive functioning (vocabulary, digit span) was also assessed.

In the Treatment trial (symptomatic patients), enalapril therapy was associated with a modest, but significantly improved level of HRQL at 6 weeks and 1 year compared with placebo. Specifically, enhanced social functioning, reduced dyspnea and improvements in scales measuring activities of daily living, life satisfaction, and general health perception were observed among symptomatic patients receiving enalapril versus placebo. In the Prevention trial (asymptomatic patients) enalapril therapy was associated with enhanced social functioning compared with placebo. In both trials, the observed alterations in HRQL were not significantly related to improved functional status, as assessed with a 6-minute walk test. In addition to this brief assessment, a trained psychologist conducted a more detailed assessment of psychosocial, physical, and intellectual functioning in 308 patients. The results obtained from this substudy were consistent with the results observed in the overall population (L. Gorkin, personal communication, 1999).

Similar to the V-HeFT trials, the modest alteration in HRQL observed in the SOLVD trials may relate to the anticipated incongruity between altered survival and changes in self-perceived HRQL. However, the significant amount of missing or incomplete data in the SOLVD HRQL substudy likely had a significant influence on the results observed, demonstrating the importance of attending to consistent and careful data collection on the HRQL variables.

PRECISE

The Prospective Randomized Evaluation of Carvedilol in Symptoms and Exercise (PRECISE) trial enrolled 278 patients who were assigned to placebo ($n = 145$) or carvedilol ($n = 133$) for the 6-month study period.[17,33] The primary study end point was exercise tolerance. Carvedilol produced symptomatic improvement, as assessed by NYHA functional class ($P = 0.01$), had marginal effects on exercise tolerance ($P < .05$), but had a significant impact on global health perceptions (81% improvement with carvedilol vs 53% with placebo; $P < 0.01$). However, carvedilol had no significant influence on disease-specific HRQL, as assessed using the LIhFE questionnaire. Patients randomly assigned to carvedilol had a significant increase in ejection fraction ($P < 0.001$) and a significant reduction in the combined risk of death or hospitalization ($P < 0.03$) compared with patients randomized to placebo. Thus, this relatively small study showed positive correlation between both surrogate and hard end points and global HRQL. However, no significant alteration in heart failure–specific HRQL was observed.

The reasons why generic HRQL improved in these patients but disease-specific HRQL did not are unclear, but probably relate to the components of the assessment tools. For example, the LIhFE questionnaire assesses a variety of physical and psychologic parameters, including adverse symptoms. In PRECISE, adverse symptoms (eg, dizziness and fatigue) were more common in carvedilol-treated patients and may have offset any beneficial effects of carvedilol on self-perceived HRQL measured using the LIhFE questionnaire. In contrast, adverse symptoms are not incorporated in global health and NYHA functional class assessments. Thus, poor correlation between changes in LIhFE scores versus NYHA functional class or global health scores is not surprising.

DIG

The Digoxin Investigators Group (DIG) trial randomized 6800 patients with left ventricular ejection fraction values 0.45 to digoxin ($n = 3397$) or placebo ($n = 3403$) in addition to diuretics and ACE inhibitors. An additional 988 patients with ejection fraction values >0.45 were separately assigned to digoxin ($n = 492$) or placebo ($n = 496$).[20] Mortality was unaffected by digoxin therapy (risk ratio 0.99; 95% confidence interval, 0.91 to 1.07; $P = 0.8$), but a reduction in hospitalizations for worsening heart failure was observed (risk ratio, 0.72; 95% confidence interval, 0.66 to 0.79; $P < 0.001$). Although exercise performance (6-minute walk distance) and self-perceived HRQL (global depression or LIhFE scores) improved over time in participants overall, no differences between the digoxin and placebo groups were observed.[34] Interestingly, older patients had more substantial functional limitation on 6-

minute walk testing (358 m for age < 65 vs 334 m for ages 65–74 vs 247 m for age >74 years at baseline), but reported similar levels of functional limitation (mean physical functioning values of 20, 21, and 20, respectively). Mean LIhFE scores (39, 27, and 25, respectively) corresponded more closely to 6-minute walk distances than to physical functioning scores.

The DIG investigators attributed the differences in self-perceived versus objective physical functioning to reduced expectations. These findings may simply reflect differences in the instruments used, but previous research has indicated that as heart failure progresses, the expectations of the patient may diminish and *usual* activities become progressively less demanding.[35] This possibility has important implications for the measurement of physical functioning in heart failure patients.

Vesnarinone Trial

The Vesnarinone study evaluated the capacity of the inotropic agent vesnarinone to reduce mortality and improve HRQL in 3833 patients with moderately severe heart failure (Table 4–1). In contrast to the V-HeFT and SOLVD trials, this study demonstrated a marked improvement in HRQL with the active therapy as assessed using the LIhFE questionnaire.[23] However, patients receiving active therapy had an increased risk of death.[23] These results raise several important issues, not the least of which is: What is the most appropriate means of assessing treatment efficacy in patients with heart failure—quality of life, longevity, or their combination? Although vesnarinone led to a 21.2% (relative) increased risk of death, it was associated with a strikingly similar 21.4% (relative) improvement in HRQL. The implications of these findings remain unclear. One potential explanation for these results is that vesnarinone led to the demise of patients with the worst HRQL. Thus, the population who survived would have, on average, higher HRQL scores than those treated with vesnarinone (patients who died plus those who survived). Undoubtedly, the reason for this observation is likely far more complex.

The Vesnarinone trial results highlight the ongoing controversy over the relative importance of balancing HRQL and longevity. Several points are worth mentioning with respect to this controversy. First, it is difficult to apply the results of this trial, obtained in a group of patients, to an individual patient with heart failure. Clearly, the desires of individual patients must enter the decision-making process surrounding treatment choices. It is worth noting that previous research has demonstrated that patients generally express either a strong preference for improved survival or for improved HRQL.[36,37] Second, under what circumstances is HRQL assessment necessary in a clinical trial? For instance, when evaluating a potentially curative treatment that is free of adverse effects, is the assessment of HRQL necessary? This may be a mute point, however, because we rarely have highly effective treatments that are free of significant adverse effects. Thus, HRQL assessment should be an integral part of most studies. Third, HRQL may be a more relevant end point than longevity in certain situations. For example, the influence of a therapy on HRQL is likely to be of more relevance than longevity in a group of seriously ill patients with an incurable disease. Likewise, when comparing treatments with similar effects on mortality, but different side effect profiles, or treatments that improve survival but have significant adverse effects, HRQL may be a more relevant outcome than longevity.[38,39]

As mentioned at the outset of this chapter, survival has traditionally been the primary end point evaluated in cardiovascular clinical trials. The main reason for this is that determining whether someone is alive or dead is far simpler, and less prone to error, than determining an individual's HRQL. Because of this simple fact, and other potential explanations for the results of the Vesnarinone trial, it seems prudent to not adopt a potentially harmful therapy based solely on a potential for improved HRQL. However, these results highlight the importance of additional research aimed at developing methods that incorporate survival and HRQL.[40,41]

MERIT-HF

The Metoprolol CR/XL Randomised Intervention Trial in Congestive Heart Failure was a randomized comparison of long-acting metoprolol versus placebo in 3991 patients with chronic heart failure, NYHA functional Class II to IV, and ejection fractions 0.40. [19,29] MERIT-HF clearly demonstrated that patients randomly assigned to metoprolol had a significantly lower risk of death (risk reduction, 19%; 95% confidence interval 27%; $P < 0.001$) and a lower number of days in the hospital for heart failure (3401 vs 5303 days; $P < 0.001$) compared with patients randomly assigned to placebo. Further, NYHA functional class, assessed by physicians, improved to a greater extent in patients randomly assigned to metoprolol (29% vs 26% for placebo; $P = 0.003$). Likewise, global self-perceived HRQL, assessed using the McMaster Overall Treatment Evaluation, improved to a greater extent in patients randomly assigned to metoprolol versus placebo ($P = 0.009$). However, no significant difference in heart-failure–specific HRQL, as assessed with the LIhFE, was observed between the groups (absolute difference in scores between the metoprolol and placebo group was –0.9; 95% confidence interval –3.4 to 1.6; $P = 0.2$).

These final two results (ie, improved global HRQL, but unchanged disease-specific HRQL) raise several important issues. First, is it possible that pharmacologic therapy is not sufficiently powerful to influence HRQL? It may be that HRQL depends primarily on emotions and social support—variables that are not typically influenced by pharmacologic therapies. Second, what set of instruments is required to detect meaningful changes in HRQL? Is a global assessment of HRQL preferable to a disease-specific one or vice versa? Should multiple measures be used that assess the full range of variables that make up the HRQL construct? Third, how does one interpret the results of a trial if one instrument shows no change, yet another indicates improvement or deterioration?

Although the specific answers to the preceding questions may vary, several basic tenets hold true. The combination of a generic or global and a disease-specific instrument are required in most clinical trials because they are designed to measure, and generally do assess, different aspects of self-perceived HRQL. Further, the choice of instruments depends on the research question being asked. If the researcher is interested in specific aspects of the patients' self-perceived health (eg, adverse symptoms from therapy, dyspnea), then the results of the disease-specific instrument would be most important. However, if general health status or outlook is of interest, then a generic instrument may provide the necessary information. The weighting of the results obtained with these instruments thus depends on the question(s) being asked. Finally, care must be taken to ensure accurate and complete HRQL data collection, because incomplete or inaccurate data greatly limit our ability to draw meaningful conclusions.

CONCLUSION

In this chapter we have discussed how the measurement of HRQL provides a means of assessing the impact of an illness or therapeutic strategy on an individual's well-being and the use of select instruments in large trials. Although we are able to accurately assess the impact of interventions on the prolongation of life and reduction in hospitalizations, evidence from randomized, controlled clinical trials suggest that we still have much to learn about how to measure changes caused by an intervention on self-perceived HRQL. Modest improvements in HRQL have been observed for participants with heart failure in several clinical trials. However, others have demonstrated a lack of correlation between survival and HRQL, and some have shown a decrease in HRQL with therapy.

Researchers are challenged to explore the HRQL construct conceptually and direct their attentions to interventions with potential to influence this important outcome. The main challenges in measurement of HRQL in heart failure involve issues of instrument choice, complete data collection, the use of analyses that can adjust for missing data over time, and the development of methods that incorporate both survival and HRQL.

REFERENCES

1. Garg R, Packer M, Pitt B, Yusuf S. Heart failure in the 1990s: evolution of a major public health problem in cardiovascular medicine. *J Am Coll Cardiol.* 1993; 22(Suppl):3A–5A.

2. Sharpe N, Doughty R. Epidemiology of heart failure and ventricular dysfunction. *Lancet.* 1998;352 (Suppl):SI3–S17.

3. Rich MW. Therapy for acute myocardial infarction in older persons. *J Am Geriatr Soc.* 1998;46:1302–1307.

4. Mann DL. Mechanisms and models in heart failure. A combinatorial approach. *Circulation.* 1999;100:999–1008.

5. Cohn JN. Structural basis for heart failure: ventricular remodeling and its pharmacological inhibition. *Circulation.* 1995;91:2504–2507.

6. Cohn JN, Archibald DG, Ziesche S, et al. Effect of vasodilator therapy on mortality in chronic congestive heart failure. Veterans Administration Cooperative Study. *N Engl J Med.* 1986; 314:1547–1552.

7. CONSENSUS Trial Study Group. Effects of enalapril on mortality in severe congestive heart failure. Results of the Cooperative North Scandinavian Enalapril Survival Study (CONSENSUS). *N Engl J Med.* 1987;316:1429–1435.

8. Cohn JN, Johnson G, Ziesche S, et al. Comparison of enalapril with hydralazine-isosorbide dinitrate in the treatment of chronic congestive heart failure. *N Engl J Med.* 1991;325:303–310.

9. Cohn JN. The Vasodilator-Heart Failure Trials (V-HeFT). Mechanistic data from the VA Cooperative Studies. Introduction. *Circulation.* 1993;87(Suppl):VI 1–VI 4.

10. Pfeffer MA, Braunwald E, Moye LA, et al. Effect of captopril on mortality and morbidity in patients with left ventricular dysfunction after myocardial infarction. Results of the survival and ventricular enlargement trial. *N Engl J Med.* 1992;327:669–677.

11. SOLVD Investigators. Effect of enalapril on survival in patients with reduced left ventricular ejection fractions and congestive heart failure. *N Engl J Med.* 1991;325:293–302.

12. SOLVD Investigators. Effect of enalapril on mortality and the development of heart failure in asymptomatic patients with reduced left ventricular ejection fractions. *N Engl J Med.* 1992;327:685–691.

13. Acute Infarction Ramipril Efficacy (AIRE) Study Investigators. Effect of ramipril on mortality and morbidity of survivors of acute myocardial infarction with clinical evidence of heart failure. *Lancet.* 1993;342:821–828.

14. Kober L, Torp-Pedersen C, Carlsen JE, et al. A clinical trial of the angiotensin-converting-enzyme inhibitor trandolapril in patients with left ventricular dysfunction after myocardial infarction. Trandolapril Cardiac Evaluation (TRACE) Study Group. *N Engl J Med.* 1995;333:1670–1676.

15. Ambrosioni E, Borghi C, Magnani B. The effect of the angiotensin-converting-enzyme inhibitor zofenopril on mortality and morbidity after anterior myocardial infarction. The Survival of Myocardial Infarction Long-Term Evaluation (SMILE) Study Investigators. *N Engl J Med.* 1995;332:80–85.

16. Pitt B, Zannad F, Remme WJ, et al. The effect of spironolactone on morbidity and mortality in patients with severe heart failure. Randomized Aldactone Evaluation Study Investigators. *N Engl J Med.* 1999;341:709–717.

17. Packer M, Bristow MR, Cohn JN, et al. The effect of carvedilol on morbidity and mortality in patients with chronic heart failure. *N Engl J Med.* 1996;334:1349–1355.

18. CIBIS-II Committees and Investigators. The Cardiac Insufficiency Bisoprolol Study II (CIBIS-II): a randomised trial. *Lancet.* 1999;353:9–13.

19. MERIT-HF Investigators. Effect of metoprolol CR/XL in chronic heart failure: Metoprolol CR/XL Randomised Intervention Trial in Congestive Heart Failure (MERIT-HF). *Lancet.* 1999;353:2001–2007.

20. Digitalis Investigation Group. The effect of digoxin on mortality and morbidity in patients with heart failure. *N Engl J Med.* 1997;336:525–533.

21. Packer M, Carver JR, Rodeheffer RJ, et al. Effect of oral milrinone on mortality in severe chronic heart failure. PROMISE Study Research Group. *N Engl J Med.* 1991;325:1468–1475.

22. Massie BM, Berk MR, Brozena SC, et al. Can further benefit be achieved by adding flosequinan to patients with congestive heart failure who remain symptomatic on diuretic, digoxin and an angiotensin converting enzyme inhibitor? *Circulation.* 1992;88:492–501.

23. Cohn JN, Goldstein SO, Greenberg BH, et al. A dose-dependent increase in mortality with vesnarinone among patients with severe heart failure. Vesnarinone

Trial Investigators. *N Engl J Med.* 1998;339:1810–1816.

24. Wenger NK, Mattson ME, Furberg CD, Elinson J. Assessment of quality of life in clinical trials of cardiovascular therapies. *Am J Cardiol.* 1984;54:908–913.

25. Wilson IB, Cleary PD. Linking clinical variables with health-related quality of life. A conceptual model of patient outcomes. *JAMA.* 1995;273:59–65.

26. Rogers WJ, Johnstone DE, Yusuf S, et al. for the SOLVD Investigators. Quality of life among 5,025 patients with left ventricular dysfunction randomized between placebo and enalapril: the studies of left ventricular dysfunction. *J Am Coll Cardiol.* 1994;23:393–400.

27. Gorkin L, Norvell NK, Rosen RC, et al. Assessment of quality of life as observed from the baseline data of the Studies of Left Ventricular Dysfunction (SOLVD) trial quality-of-life substudy. *Am J Cardiol.* 1993;71:1069–1073.

28. Konstam V, Salem D, Pouleur H, et al. Baseline quality of life as a predictor of mortality and hospitalization in 5,025 patients with congestive heart failure. SOLVD Investigations. Studies of Left Ventricular Dysfunction Investigators. *Am J Cardiol.* 1996;78:890–895.

29. Hjalmarson A, Goldstein S, Fagerberg B, et al. Effects of controlled-release metoprolol on total mortality, hospitalizations, and well-being in patients with heart failure: the Metoprolol CR/XL Randomized Intervention Trial in congestive heart failure (MERIT-HF). MERIT-HF Study Group. *JAMA.* 2000;283:1295–1302.

30. Berry C, McMurray J. A review of quality-of-life evaluations in patients with congestive heart failure. *Pharmacoeconomics.* 1999;16:247–271.

31. Leidy NK, Rentz AM, Zyczynski TM. Evaluating health-related quality-of-life outcomes in patients with congestive heart failure. A review of recent randomised controlled trials. *Pharmacoeconomics.* 1999;15:19–46.

32. Rector TS, Johnson G, Dunkman WB, et al. Evaluation by patients with heart failure of the effects of enalapril compared with hydralazine plus isosorbide dinitrate on quality of life. V-HeFT II. The V-HeFT VA Cooperative Studies Group. *Circulation.* 1993;87(Suppl):VI71–VI177.

33. Packer M, Colucci WS, Sackner-Bernstein JD, et al. for the PRECISE Study Group. Double blind, placebo-controlled study of the effects of carvedilol in patients with moderate to severe heart failure. *Circulation.* 1996;94:2793–2799.

34. Rich MW, McSherry F, Williford WO, et al. The DIG Study. Presented at the American Heart Association Meeting: *Do Existing Databases Hold the Answers to Clinical Questions in Geriatric Disease and Stroke?* Washington, DC, January 2000.

35. Waller DG. Effect of drug treatment on quality of life in mild to moderate heart failure. *Drug Safety.* 1991;6:241–246.

36. Rector TS, Tschumperlin LK, Kubo SH, et al. Use of the Living with Heart Failure questionnaire to ascertain patients' perspectives on improvement in quality of life versus risk of drug-induced death. *J Card Fail.* 1995;1:201–206.

37. Lewis EF, Johnson PA, Johnson W, et al. Heart failure patients express strong polarity of preference for either quality of life or survival [abstract]. *Circulation.* 1998;98:4544.

38. Quality of life and clinical trials. *Lancet.* 1995;346:1–2.

39. Gotay CC, Korn EL, McCabe MS, et al. Quality of life assessment in cancer treatment protocols: research issues in protocol development. *J Natl Cancer Inst.* 1992;84:575–579.

40. Glasziou PP, Simes RJ, Gelber RD. Quality adjusted survival analysis. *Stat Med.* 1990;9:1259–1276.

41. Feenstra J, Lubsen J, Grobbee DE, Stricker BHC. Heart failure treatments—Issues of safety versus issues of quality of life. *Drug Safety.* 1999;20:1–7.

CHAPTER 5

Impact of Surgical Therapy on Quality of Life in Heart Failure

Kathleen L. Grady, William Piccione, Jr., and Rick J. Marcantonio

INTRODUCTION

In addition to the more traditional outcomes of morbidity and mortality, quality of life increasingly has been recognized as a salient patient outcome to study, especially in patients with chronic illnesses. Furthermore, in the managed care environment, quality of life data provide important information for determining the benefits of costly new technologic interventions.[1] Heart failure is a chronic illness that has seen an increasing incidence and prevalence.[2] Several successful surgical interventions for New York Heart Association (NYHA) functional Class III and IV heart failure patients have been developed during the past 30 years. These include surgical revascularization and/or mitral valve repair, implantation of ventricular assist devices, and heart transplantation.

The impact of surgical revascularization and heart transplantation on heart failure patient outcomes has undergone extensive study. However, research on patient outcomes following implantation of ventricular assist devices is much less extensive. Furthermore, there are many methodologic issues related to the study of some patient outcomes, especially quality of life. The purposes of this chapter are to (1) describe methodologic challenges in the study of quality of life after surgical procedures and (2) describe surgical therapies for heart failure patients, including indications, surgical techniques, benefits, complications, outcomes, limitations, and quality of life and related methodologic issues.

METHODOLOGIC ISSUES IN QUALITY OF LIFE RESEARCH

Publication of research related to quality of life has flourished during the last two decades.[3] However, there is no consensus of opinion regarding a definition of quality of life, domains of quality of life, or a theoretical framework; although researchers agree that the concept of quality of life is multidimensional.[4] It has both subjective and objective components; it is also temporal and, therefore, changes over time. Researchers have used many different instruments to measure quality of life and often provide no definition on which to base instrument selection.[5] Research designs often are cross-sectional or pre- and posttreatment, such as before and after surgical procedures. Missing data are frequently not reported. In treatment trials, missing data on outcomes can result in underestimation of a treatment effect and overly optimistic statements about patient outcomes, especially when patients drop out of the study due to poor outcomes.[6] Although researchers have agreed on the multidimensional nature of quality of life, issues regarding type of design, handling of missing data, and related statistical tests have not been addressed as frequently and deserve further comment.

Longitudinal analysis is the recommended design for the study of quality of life. The statistical approach for longitudinal analysis is repeated measures analysis of variance. This method of statistical analysis is ideally suited for quality of life studies because its goal is the description and assessment of change occurring in experimental units that are measured over at least two (and possibly more) time intervals. Further, the assumptions that warrant its use are appropriate for the measure of quality of life. For example, subjects are considered independent and must be randomly drawn from the target population. In addition, responses for each individual must be related to some degree to prior responses. Lastly, at least one dependent variable (such as a satisfaction with life or health status) and the use of time as an independent variable must be included in the study design.

Often, however, a deeper look through the lens of applied research reveals that these same assumptions are either demonstrably false or inapplicable in many quasi-experimental or nonexperimental settings. First, it may be impossible, let alone impractical, to draw subjects independently and at random from some target population. Consider a study in which a number of heart transplant patients are to be assessed at various points after surgery. Although random assignment is plausible (if treatment and control groups are planned), random sampling is extremely difficult, if not impossible. Further, if several heart transplant programs contribute groups of patients to the study, the patients are naturally "clustered." In other words, the subjects treated by Program "A" form a group whose attributes on any number of dimensions may be more similar to each other than they are to a cluster belonging to Program "B." Such sampling and clustering problems clearly contribute to a violation of the assumption of independence in repeated measures analysis.

Secondly, repeated measures assumes *compound symmetry*, or constant covariance (ie, correlation) of the dependent variable from one time to the next.[7] However, other error structures may present a more realistic picture of quality of life changes. For example, in studies requiring subjects to recall prior events,[8] it is not at all unreasonable to observe that measures are more strongly correlated at adjacent time points than they are at time points further away. Such a structure indicates *autocorrelation*.[9,10] Further, responses may

show nonconstant variance over time; indeed, it may be hypothesized in many field settings that the variance of a certain outcome stabilizes over time and is by definition larger at the outset of a study than it is after an intervention.[11,12] As before, violation of the assumption of compound symmetry can weaken the power of repeated measures.

A third problem is that dependent variable(s) may not be distributed even reasonably close to normality in a given sample. A variety of variance-stabilizing or normality transformations can be investigated and applied to continuous measures such as age, weight, height, or income[13] when appropriate. However, many scales in behavioral research are at the ordinal level and are not strictly continuous. Attitude scales using the Likert scale of the "strongly agree" to "strongly disagree" variety seem particularly vulnerable to skewing. It is difficult to suggest a plausible transformation for such a scale when it is range-restricted or even a theoretical justification for doing so.

A related problem is that the dependent variable used in repeated measures analysis cannot be measured as an ordinal or nominal variable. Thus, repeated measures per se cannot be used to examine any research question that focuses on how proportions or probabilities change as a function of time.

Finally, only subjects who have completely responded to all the questions are included in the analysis. The requirement for the usual repeated measures analysis is that any subject who failed to respond at all time points is deleted, whatever the reason. In longitudinal research, attrition can be a serious issue.[11] Loss of subjects means not only an obvious waste of time, effort, and money; it also means a reduction of statistical power, or the probability of correctly rejecting the null hypothesis.[14,15]

Fortunately, statistical methods are being developed and refined to ameliorate these problems. One promising avenue of statistical research is mixed models,[16] also known as *random regression models*,[17] *hierarchical linear models*,[18] or *multilevel models*.[19]

Mixed models begin with the assumption that, regardless of the study design (cross-sectional or longitudinal), variation in obtained responses is due to at least two factors: the naturally occurring variation inherent in any measure (Level 1 variation), and the variation due to "nesting," or the "clustering" effect (Level 2 variation). In cross-sectional research, patients may be clustered, for example, within units, units within hospitals, or hospitals within counties. In longitudinal research, each individual is a cluster, the variation in responses then being partitioned into random variation within an individual over time (Level 1) and systematic variation due to individual differences (Level 2).

It is important to classify the variance of dependent measures into these components so that the explanatory power of all concomitant variables can be more precisely understood. For example, suppose that a longitudinal study has examined the health promotion behaviors of coronary artery bypass graft (CABG) patients with left ventricular dysfunction. Five different clinics were involved, all of which were administering the same medical regimen. Suppose that we discover in mixed modeling that 10% of the variance in the health-related measures is due not to between-patient differences but to between-clinic (ie, cluster) differences. Obviously, one's interpretation of the effectiveness of this medical regimen would be different and better informed than it would be if we had never known or thought about differences between clinics.

Important extensions to mixed models have been developed recently to overcome the limitation of need for continuous dependent variables in a repeated measures context. For dichotomous outcomes, Bock and Gibbons[20] have developed extensions to logit and probit analyses to multivariate cases. Ordinal multivariate analysis is also available, using mixed-effects proportional odds models.[10]

Finally, another advantage to mixed modeling is that all available observations are retained. Recall that, in repeated measures analysis of variance, only complete cases are used in the analysis. Because clusters in mixed models can have differing numbers of observations, missing data pose no particular structural limitation, in

and of themselves. Missing data points are estimated via an Expectation-Maximization (EM) algorithm.[15] Of course, whereas the nature of the missing data must be understood, methods are already under development for more effectively doing so,[21-23] providing even more advantage to the use of these models over traditional repeated measures analysis of variance. These techniques need to be tested in longitudinal studies of quality of life to determine the impact on reporting the results on heart failure patient outcomes after surgical therapies.

SURGICAL REVASCULARIZATION IN HEART FAILURE PATIENTS

Coronary artery disease (CAD) is currently the most common cause of heart failure in the adult population and is associated with a worse prognosis than with other causes.[24] Despite recent advances in medical therapy, the estimated 2-year survival rate for patients with severe left ventricular dysfunction of ischemic origin is only 30%.[25] Cardiac transplantation remains a highly effective therapy for these patients. However, the limited supply of donor hearts, high mortality of patients awaiting surgery, and progressive vasculopathy in the transplanted heart make it a less than optimal treatment modality.

Coronary artery bypass grafting in patients with ischemic cardiomyopathy and left ventricular dysfunction, with or without angina, is becoming an increasingly accepted alternative to transplantation. However, acceptance of this therapy has been hindered by clinicians' perceptions of an excessive surgical mortality in this group of patients. Historically, large randomized trials of CABG versus medical therapy intentionally excluded patients with left ventricular dysfunction (measured by left ventricular ejection fraction [LVEF] < 35%).[26] However, subsequent studies have shown that patients with severe left ventricular dysfunction can potentially benefit the most from revascularization, especially if angina is present.[27,28]

Previously, left ventricular dysfunction secondary to ischemic heart disease was thought to be largely irreversible, thus making revascularization difficult to justify, given the perceived excessive mortality rate. However, it is now understood that ischemic left ventricular dysfunction often is reversible with surgery, as evidenced by improvements in LVEF, exercise performance, and quality of life scores.[29,30] Therefore, a major challenge in this population is to identify accurately those patients with left ventricular dysfunction secondary to nonviable, irreversibly damaged myocardium versus those suffering from dysfunctional but viable myocardial segments, (ie, hibernating myocardium). The presence of hibernating or dysfunctional myocardium, which should improve following revascularization, can be predicted by techniques such as scintigraphy, positron emission tomography (PET), and dobutamine echocardiography.

Assessing Contractile Reserve

The most widely accepted physiologic test available to determine the presence of ischemic myocardium is perfusion scintigraphy, such as thallium 201 imaging.[28] Thallium is extracted from the blood and actively retained in the myocardial sarcolemmal process. Standard thallium imaging involving a 3- to 4-hour delayed image is not optimal for detecting all viable myocardium, due to a 40%–50% false-negative rate. Delayed thallium imaging for 8–24 hours reduces the false-negative rate to 15%–25%, and combining a rest study with redistribution imaging further reduces the false-negative rate to 5%–10%.[31] The finding of a "fixed defect" on thallium imaging implies nonviable myocardial scar.

However, a more sensitive means of demonstrating the presence and quantity of viable myocardium is PET. This test can identify metabolic patterns indicative of ischemic but viable myocardium versus nonviable myocardium by combining regional blood flow assessment and glucose metabolism. Increased myocardial uptake of F-fluorodeoxyglucose (FDG) in areas of decreased perfusion is diagnostic of viable myocardium with potentially reversible function. Decreased FDG uptake indicates scar tissue. Although PET scanning is much more sensitive than conventional scintigraphy, it has the disad-

vantage of being expensive and is not yet widely available.

Dobutamine stress echocardiography is another modality to assess contractile reserve indicative of potentially reversible ischemic myocardium. Although it is more widely available and less expensive than PET, dobutamine stress echocardiography appears to be less sensitive than PET.

The presence of angina is a clinical indication of ongoing ischemia but may not distinguish hibernating from nonfunctional myocardium. Several investigators have demonstrated a lack of correlation between the presence of angina and the degree of perfusion-metabolism mismatch (ie, hibernating myocardium) on PET scanning.[30,32] Conversely, the absence of angina in patients with left ventricular dysfunction does not exclude the possibility of extensive areas of dysfunctional but viable myocardium. Therefore, it is essential to consider the possibility of ischemic myocardium that is potentially reversible with revascularization when evaluating patients with left ventricular dysfunction, even in the absence of anginal symptoms.[28]

Revascularization

Prior to revascularization, patients should be optimized medically. In addition, invasive hemodynamic monitoring can be extremely helpful in guiding therapy for these patients. Preoperative placement of an intraaortic balloon pump (IABP) may be helpful in further optimizing the patient prior to surgery and in supporting the patient during the postoperative period.

During surgery, meticulous attention is given to protecting the myocardium from further ischemia or metabolic compromise. Cardioplegic solution is delivered, either antegrade alone or in combination with retrograde administration, depending on the degree of proximal coronary obstruction and the presence of previous bypass grafts. Cardioplegia is generally combined with moderate systemic hypothermia (28°–32° C) and topical cooling of the heart. Further precautions involve avoiding prolonged periods of aortic cross clamping. Additional operative time spent grafting very small or highly diseased vessels is generally counterproductive and may even compromise surgical outcomes. Extended coronary endarterectomies also prolong the operative time and are subject to a higher acute thrombosis rate and, therefore, should be avoided in this patient population. The use of arterial conduits, particularly the internal mammary artery, is encouraged if the conduit is of good caliber with acceptable flow. These vessels often are preferred over venous conduits because they are easier to reach and anastamose, and there is less stenosis than with use of saphenous veins. Small or marginal conduits should be avoided because they increase the risk of perioperative ischemia. Transesophageal echocardiography (TEE) is routinely used during surgery. Visualization of ventricular wall motion, in combination with simultaneous hemodynamic monitoring, allows the surgeon to assess more accurately the effectiveness of the procedure as well as the need for pharmacologic support.

Results of Surgical Revascularization

Results of surgical revascularization in patients with left ventricular dysfunction and demonstrable hibernating myocardium are encouraging. However, no controlled studies demonstrating that CABG improves survival in heart failure patients without angina are available. To date, CABG has been used to treat mostly those patients with left ventricular dysfunction and angina. However, several studies have provided substantial evidence that patients with left ventricular dysfunction and demonstrable areas of ischemic but viable myocardium benefit from CABG, even in the absence of angina.[32–34] Pagano and associates[29] recently studied 35 heart failure patients (NYHA functional Class III) with and without angina who underwent CABG. Patients were evaluated at baseline and at 6 months following CABG. Left ventricular function was assessed by transthoracic echocardiography and radionuclide ventriculography. Myocardial viability was assessed by PET. Overall, 30-day perioperative mortality

was 5.7%. The investigators found that, following CABG, LVEF improved significantly ($p < 0.0001$). Interestingly, the improvement in LVEF was greater in patients without angina. In addition, a linear correlation was found between the quantity of viable dysfunctional myocardium and the degree of improvement of LVEF following CABG. Quality of life scores improved significantly in both the angina and nonangina groups following CABG; however, no correlation was found between the amount of viable dysfunctional myocardium and changes in the quality of life score.

Limitations of CABG in heart failure patients include increased perioperative mortality. This can be reduced to an acceptable level with careful perioperative, intraoperative, and postoperative management. Demonstration of significant viable, yet dysfunctional myocardium is essential and is directly related to improvements in LVEF. Finally, the surgeon must be able to restore adequate blood flow to the affected ischemic area, which requires a suitable coronary artery to bypass. In carefully selected patients with left ventricular dysfunction, CABG can provide significant improvement and clearly has a role in the treatment of severe heart failure patients with coronary occlusive disease, even in the absence of angina.

MITRAL VALVE REPAIR IN HEART FAILURE PATIENTS

Mitral regurgitation of varying degree is a frequent finding in patients with both ischemic and idiopathic dilated cardiomyopathy. The mechanisms for regurgitation in this setting include dilatation of the mitral annulus and altered ventricular geometry, which affects the papillary–chordal complex or papillary dysfunction secondary to ischemia or infarction.[35,36] The resultant mitral regurgitation leads to progressive volume overload of the left ventricle, which in turn leads to greater annular dilatation and further regurgitation. This cycle leads to progressive left ventricular dysfunction and worsening symptoms of heart failure. Functional mitral regurgitation also is associated with substantial mortality; left ventricular dysfunction patients have a 1-year survival rate estimated as low as 30%.[37,38] Surgical intervention on the mitral valve in patients with severe left ventricular dysfunction has traditionally been avoided, due to the high operative mortality rates reported in patients undergoing mitral valve replacement. The worsening of left ventricular systolic function following mitral valve replacement is now known to be related to the loss of the normal annular–chordal–papillary continuity associated with traditional valve replacement.[39–41]

Surgical repair of the regurgitant mitral valve with preservation of the chordal attachments has been shown to result in improved preservation of systolic function and lower operative mortality, when compared with mitral valve replacement.[42–44] Subsequent studies have confirmed that valve reconstruction with chordal–papillary preservation results in maintenance of left ventricular geometry and valvular function, with better clinical outcomes.[45,46]

The potential benefit of surgical correction of mitral regurgitation in patients with left ventricular dysfunction was suggested by Hammermeister and associates.[47] In their study of 249 patients with mitral regurgitation, survival of the surgically treated group was superior to that of the medically treated group. Furthermore, the patient cohort with moderate left ventricular functional impairment demonstrated the greatest survival advantage, compared with the medically treated group. This observation, combined with the anticipated high mortality in patients with left ventricular dysfunction and severe mitral regurgitation, led investigators to consider mitral valve reconstructive surgery in this high-risk group of patients.

In 1995, Bach and Bolling[48] reported their initial experience with mitral valve repair in patients with severe left ventricular dysfunction. This initial group consisted of nine patients—eight with NYHA functional Class IV symptoms and one in Class III. All patients were receiving maximal medical therapy, and all had severe left ventricular dysfunction defined as an LVEF less than 25%. Patients were excluded from the study if they had evidence of mitral leaflet disease, if

the mitral regurgitation preceded the cardiomyopathy, or if bypass grafting also was required in the setting of ischemic cardiomyopathy.[48]

In the above study,[48] the surgical technique of mitral valve repair consisted of median sternotomy and cardiopulmonary bypass. The heart was arrested with standard cardioplegic techniques, and the mitral valve was visualized. All patients underwent implantation of a flexible ring annuloplasty. In addition, none of the patients required valve leaflet resection at the time of repair.

No perioperative deaths occurred in this series, and all patients reported subjective improvement in their functional status after surgery. NYHA functional class improved in all patients (Figure 5–1). Quantitative echocardiography confirmed mild or no residual regurgitation in all patients, with increases in ejection fraction and forward cardiac output.

A later study by the same group reported on 16 patients followed for a mean of 8 months. Similarly, no perioperative deaths were reported, and the 1-year actuarial survival was 75%.[49] All patients improved to NYHA functional Class I or II, and all experienced improve-

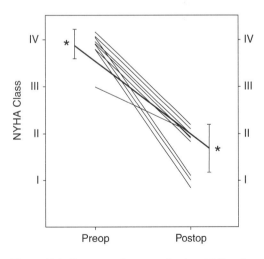

Figure 5–1 Symptomatic congestive heart failure before and after annuloplasty. Each patient noted subjective improvement in functional status at 17 ± 5 weeks of follow-up. Group NYHA Functional Class fell significantly, from 3.9 ± 0.3 to 1.7 ± 0.5. *$p < 0.001$.

ment in LVEF. Most recently, the follow-up of this cohort of patients has been expanded to 48 months, with a mean of 22 months (range 1–48 months).[50] Preoperatively, 40 patients were NYHA functional Class IV, and 8 were NYHA functional Class III. All patients were receiving maximal medical therapy consisting of digoxin, diuretics, and afterload reducers. Outcomes included one perioperative death, and one patient required IABP. All patients improved to NYHA functional Class I or II and had improvement in LVEF, from a mean of 17% preoperatively to 26% postoperatively ($p = 0.008$). Actuarial survival was 82% at 1 year and 72% at 2 years (Figure 5–2). Although the results have demonstrated positive clinical outcomes, limitations of the studies include the nonrandomized uncontrolled nature of the study design and lack of long-term follow-up. Nonetheless, these intermediate results remain extremely encouraging and deserve further investigation.

QUALITY OF LIFE AFTER SURGICAL REVASCULARIZATION AND/OR MITRAL VALVE REPAIR

The studies summarized in the preceding sections demonstrate that surgical revascularization and mitral valve repair are promising therapies for individuals with even severe heart failure. However, can these therapies improve quality of life in these patients? Several investigators have examined changes in quality of life from before to after open-heart surgical procedures and generally have found that it improved.[29,51–53] These improvements were found in both objective and subjective measures of quality of life. Improvement in the Canadian Cardiovascular Society angina class[54] and NYHA functional class[30,54] were noted by some authors (eg, improvement by one angina or functional class or more).

Several investigators examined change in quality of life over time, using self-report tools.

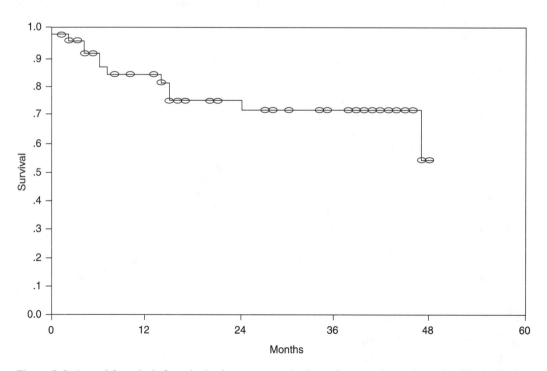

Figure 5–2 Actuarial survival after mitral valve reconstruction in cardiomyopathy, as determined by the Kaplan-Meier method.

Pagano et al[29] reported significantly improved quality of life in heart failure patients with angina ($n = 14$) and without angina ($n = 21$) prior to and 6 months after surgical revascularization in both physical and emotional functional status. Two researchers, who used similar instruments to measure quality of life, described improvements in the following dimensions: energy, sleep, physical mobility, social isolation, emotional reaction, and pain from pre- to 6 months post-CABG surgery and/or valve replacement.[51,52]

Quality of life is not uniformly improved after surgery, and certain subgroups are at higher risk for poorer quality of life. After surgery, Chocron et al[51] ($n = 199$) identified worse NYHA class as a predictor of less energy and less physical mobility, female gender as a predictor of more social isolation, and at least one comorbid disease as a predictor of worse emotional reaction. No differences in postoperative quality of life by type of procedure were found. Klersy et al[52] ($n = 259$) noted that males, younger patients, patients with NYHA functional Class I, patients with silent or stable angina, patients without additional cardiac surgical procedures, and patients without surgical complications had better perceived overall quality of life. Interestingly, in a smaller study of women ($n = 27$) who underwent cardiac surgical procedures, although NYHA class improved through 3 postoperative months, it was not associated with quality of life and life satisfaction.[55]

Complications and prolonged intensive care stay after cardiac surgery were found to affect quality of life as much as 1 year after surgery.[56,57] Of patients with a protracted recovery (ICU stay > 48 hours) after cardiac surgical procedures ($n = 162$, primarily CABG and/or valve replacement), 76 (47%) had significantly impaired quality of life at 1 postoperative year, compared with patients having a less complicated hospital course.[56] Similarly, 47 cardiac surgical patients (with multiple organ failure and requiring an ICU stay 5 days) who were matched with 47 uncomplicated cardiac surgical patients by gender and age had worse quality of life scores overall and in the following dimensions: energy, physical mobility, and emotional reactions at

1 year after surgery.[57] Cardiac surgical patients who experienced complications, when compared with the control group, also reported that their health status adversely affected three of six activities of daily living (ie, housework, sex life, and hobbies).

Several researchers examined change in quality of life in elderly patients undergoing cardiac surgical procedures. McHugh et al[58] reported improved NYHA class from 3 to 1.7 and less symptom severity in patients 75 years ($n = 80$) from before to after cardiac operation (revascularization, valvular surgery, or both) with no difference in postoperative quality of life between the old (75–79 years) and very old (80 years) patients. In another study, predictors of improved quality of life 6 months after CABG ($n = 97$ patients 70 years) were presence of angina and a worse NYHA class before surgery.[59] Two studies concluded that quality of life improved in octogenarians with cardiac dysfunction who underwent cardiac surgery.[60–62] Patients from these studies reported improved NYHA class,[60,61] improved angina class,[61] decreased frequency of cardiovascular symptoms,[61] increased activities of daily living,[60] less need for tangible support,[61] improved emotional status,[61] and more satisfaction with overall life.[61] No significant differences in life satisfaction and quality of life by age (< 70 years versus 70 years) were found in the study of 27 women who underwent cardiac surgical procedures.[55]

Quality of life data for cardiomyopathy patients who have undergone mitral valve repair are limited to the report of improvement in NYHA class and patient report of subjective improvement in functional status from the series of articles by the University of Michigan researchers, as previously described.[48–50]

Methodologic Issues and Gaps in the Literature

Issues in the assessment of quality of life in patients with cardiac dysfunction who undergo revascularization and/or valve replacement are related to sample, design, and measurement. Findings on women differed significantly from those of men in some studies. The small sample of women in most of these studies makes generalizations related to gender difficult at best. Also, racial and cultural differences in quality of life were not described, and the only age-related studies examined quality of life in patients who were > 70 years.

Although prospective, longitudinal designs were used by some researchers, sampling needs to be more frequent (only pre- and one postoperative time period were usually sampled). Also, studies were short-term and described changes in quality of life through only 6 months to 1 year after surgery. Future studies, therefore, need to be long-term and include assessment of quality of life beyond 1 postoperative year, perhaps through 5 postoperative years, with several sampling periods.

A final group of limitations are related to conceptualization and measurement of quality of life. Frequently, quality of life is not defined by investigators and is measured with a single instrument that only partially represents this multifactorial construct. Missing data were usually reported as missing due to loss of subjects during follow-up or death. Occasionally, return of incomplete instruments was cited as a reason for the missing data.

IMPLANTABLE LEFT VENTRICULAR ASSIST DEVICES

Early interest in mechanical circulatory support in the 1960s led to the development of the artificial heart program at the National Institutes of Health in 1964.[63] Initial interest was in the development of reliable devices for use in patients with postcardiotomy failure. Considerable interest also focused on the development of a permanent biventricular replacement device, the total artificial heart. The feasibility of developing mechanical left ventricular support alone in heart failure patients was soon realized, and in 1970, the National Heart, Lung and Blood Institute created a program for developing fully implantable left ventricular assist devices (LVADs).[64] In 1978, the first successful implantation of an LVAD as a bridge to transplantation

was undertaken in a 24-year-old man at the Texas Heart Institute.[65] Since that time, the efficacy and feasibility of long-term circulatory support with LVADs have been widely accepted.

In the United States, two implantable LVAD systems that provide pulsatile flow are currently available. These devices are the HeartMate LVAD system, available in both pneumatic and electrical configurations (Thermo Cardiosystems, Inc., Woburn, MA; Figure 5–3) and the Novacor electrically powered LVAD system (Baxter Healthcare, Oakland, CA; Figure 5–4). The Food and Drug Administration (FDA) has approved both systems as a bridge to transplantation.

Similarities and differences exist between the two LVAD systems. Both the HeartMate and Novacor systems are implanted through a median sternotomy and positioned below the diaphragm. The HeartMate was originally designed for intraperitoneal placement but can also be positioned in a subrectus properitoneal plane, which is typical of the Novacor device placement.[66,67] The left ventricle is drained through a large apical valve conduit, and blood is returned to the ascending aorta through a similarly valved outflow graft. The native heart with a functioning right ventricle remains in situ.

However, significant design differences exist between the HeartMate and Novacor devices. The Novacor device is electrically powered and utilizes a dual opposing pusher plate design. The pump has a maximum stroke volume of 70 mL and is capable of generating up to 10 L/minute of flow. Bovine pericardial tissue valves are used, and full anticoagulation therapy with warfarin and antiplatelet agents is recommended to reduce thromboembolic events.[68] In contrast, the HeartMate system utilizes a pusher plate design in both the pneumatic and electrical configurations. Maximum stroke volume is 85 mL, with a maximum pump output of 11 L/minute. Blood flow is directed by 25-mm porcine valves, and anticoagulation generally consists of antiplatelet agents alone.

Both the HeartMate and Novacor systems are generally operated in an automatic mode, rather than the optional "fixed rate" mode. In the automatic mode, the device will sense when it is 90%

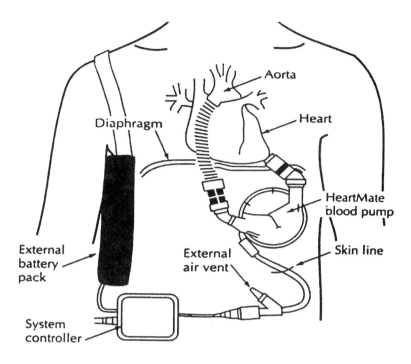

Figure 5–3 Vented electric model of the TCI HeartMate left ventricular assist device.

filled and, thus, will eject the blood. This feature, therefore, allows for greater physiologic compatibility with the cardiac output needs of the patient, in that pump flows will increase with exercise and diminish with rest. In a normally functioning system, the left ventricular pressures remain low because blood is immediately diverted to the pump. In a normal operating mode, the pump output, therefore, equals the patient's cardiac output.

Implantation of LVADs is generally performed via a median sternotomy. The incision is extended to just above the umbilicus. Both devices require a body surface area of at least 1.5 m² to incorporate the device comfortably. As previously mentioned, the HeartMate device can be placed either intraperitoneally or in a subrectus properitoneal pocket. Cardiopulmonary bypass is instituted, and the patient is cooled to moderate hypothermia (32° C). The aorta is cross-clamped, and the heart is arrested with cardioplegic solution. Following arrest, a core of left ventricular apex is removed, with care taken to not damage the ventricular septum. The Teflon sewing ring is then attached to the ventricular apex with a series of pledget sutures. The pump is then brought to the field and placed in the abdominal wall pocket. The valved inflow cannula is brought across an opening created in the diaphragm and secured in the apical sewing ring. The driveline is then tunneled and generally brought through the skin in the right subcostal area. Rewarming is then begun as the Dacron outflow graft is attached to the pump and trimmed to the appropriate length. This Dacron graft is then anastomosed in an end-to-side fashion to the proximal ascending aorta.

Several methods have been described regarding de-airing the system prior to initiation. However, whichever method the surgeon prefers, all intracardiac and intrapump air must be removed before initiation of the device. Transesophageal echocardiography is extremely helpful during this portion of the operation. Once totally de-

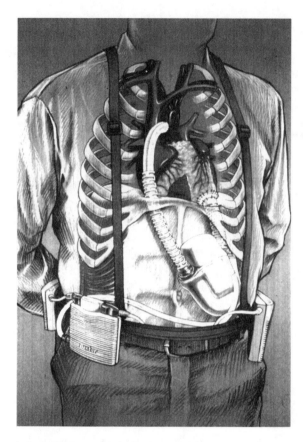

Figure 5–4 The Novacor left ventricular assist device.

aired, pump function is initiated, and the patient is gradually weaned from conventional cardiopulmonary bypass. Some degree of inotropic support is generally required to augment right ventricular flow because filling of the LVAD is dependent on adequate right ventricular function and blood crossing the pulmonary circuit.

Much has been written previously documenting the benefits of LVAD support in chronic heart failure patients awaiting transplantation. Following restoration of normal hemodynamics, end organ function typically improves with rehabilitation of the patient prior to transplantation.[69,70] The physiologic and rehabilitative capabilities of patients with LVADs awaiting transplantation are evidenced by the successful bridge to transplant rate in excess of 90% at Rush-Presbyterian-St. Luke's Medical Center in Chicago. Further, several investigators reported that improvements in physiologic and neurohumoral parameters experienced by LVAD patients resulted in improved patient survival and rehabilitation following cardiac transplantation.[71,72] Both the electric HeartMate and Novacor systems allow patients to be discharged from the hospital while awaiting transplantation.

Unfortunately, implantable LVAD systems, like other forms of mechanical support, are associated with significant complications. Early complications include hemorrhage, air embolism, and right ventricular failure. Beyond the perioperative period, late complications consist of infection, thromboembolism, and primary device failure. However, it is important to note that, with improved patient selection, pump design improvements, and increasing clinical experience, the incidence of LVAD-related complications should continue to decline.[73]

The favorable results obtained with use of implantable LVADs as a bridge to heart transplantation have provided an opportunity to study the efficacy of LVADs over extended bridging periods. Furthermore, this success has prompted investigators to develop protocols utilizing both the Novacor and the vented electric HeartMate devices as destination therapy, rather than as a bridge to transplant application.[74,75]

The Randomized Evaluation of Mechanical Assistance for the Treatment of Congestive Heart Failure (REMATCH) is one such study currently in progress that utilizes the HeartMate vented electric device. REMATCH is jointly sponsored by Thermo Cardiosystems, Inc. and the National Institutes of Health. REMATCH is a randomized, controlled, multisite clinical trial intended to evaluate the use of permanent implantable LVADs versus optimal medical therapy in NYHA functional Class IV heart failure patients who are ineligible for cardiac transplantation. In the current protocol, 140 patients will be enrolled and followed for 3 years. The primary end point of the study is patient survival. Additional outcomes, such as quality of life, morbidity, and economic issues, will also be studied. Upon completion, REMATCH should provide valuable information regarding the feasibility of chronic LVAD support and how well it compares with medical therapy. These results clearly will provide needed information about the possibility of using chronic LVAD support as an alternative to transplantation.

QUALITY OF LIFE AFTER VENTRICULAR ASSIST DEVICE IMPLANTATION

The study of quality of life in patients who receive ventricular assist devices is limited, and most of the studies conducted have had very small sample sizes. Moskowitz et al,[76] using a standard gamble approach, concluded that quality of life with a Thermo Cardiosystems, Inc.

HeartMate LVAD ($n = 6$) was better than before device implantation and not as good as after heart transplantation. Dew et al[77] compared the quality of life of 10 patients who received either a Novacor left ventricular assist system or a Thoratec ventricular assist device and were awaiting heart transplantation from before to after hospital discharge. The patients were compared with 55 other nonhospitalized heart transplant candidates and 97 posttransplant recipients. The investigators reported that the 10 patients discharged on LVADs improved in physical functioning and emotional well-being from before to after discharge, showed more improvement than did the nonhospitalized transplant candidates, and were most similar to the posttransplant recipients. Social interactions were most similar to those of nonhospitalized transplant candidates. In addition, the 10 patients no longer viewed themselves as burdens to their families.

In another small study, Catanese et al[74] also found a trend toward improved quality of life in discharged patients ($n = 4$) in the following dimensions: energy, pain, emotion, sleep, and physical mobility ($p = 0.06$) from before to 12 weeks after implantation of a vented electric HeartMate LVAD. Other very limited and often anecdotal comments about out-of-hospital experiences of heart assist device patients bridged to heart transplantation include improved physical[78,79] and emotional well-being;[78] increased involvement in home activities, recreational activities, and social life;[78-80] satisfactory sexual life;[79,80] successful airplane trips;[80] and return to work and school.[79-81]

In two reports, a 16-question survey[82] and a modified 12-question version of the same survey[83] were given to patients ($n = 12$ in both studies) after implantation of ventricular assist devices or extracorporeal membrane oxygenation. In the first study, seven of the patients had the device successfully removed, and five of the patients were bridged to heart transplantation, whereas in the second study, 11/12 patients were successfully bridged to transplant. In both studies, the majority of patients agreed that they had a brighter outlook on life since their illness, felt that they had returned to a normal lifestyle, would consent if they needed the device again, would recommend the device to someone who needed it, and believed that they had not suffered long-term effects while on the device. In addition, 92% of patients who received LVADs returned to work or stated that they were capable of doing so within 1 year of heart transplantation. In another report, patients receiving mechanical assistance reported increased independence in activities of daily living, increased exercise, and greater time in pursuit of hobbies.[84]

A small phenomenologic study was conducted with six patients who received a HeartMate pneumatic LVAD as a bridge to transplantation. Respondents answered questions about their experiences while the device was implanted.[85] Patients described physical concerns of discomfort (especially when trying to sleep), early postoperative pain, and early satiety. Psychosocial issues of being constantly reminded of their hearts, fear of the machine, and yet being comforted by the "whooshing" sounds were described. Patients believed that they had received a second chance in life and that a greater plan existed for them. Patients also reported positive coping experiences, including supportive relationships, use of humor, and diversional activities.

At Rush-Presbyterian-St. Luke's Medical Center, the authors have undertaken a multisite study of quality of life of patients who have received a heart assist device as a bridge to heart transplantation. Patients undergoing implantation of a HeartMate LVAD ($n = 150$) were studied before device implant, during the implant, and through 1 year after heart transplant. Twenty-eight patients (mean age = 53 years, 79% male, 79% married) were able to complete quality of life questionnaires immediately before and at 1–2 weeks after implantation of a HeartMate LVAD.[86] Patients who were unable to complete questionnaires were generally too sick to complete questionnaires at the preimplant time period. From immediately before to 1–2 weeks after HeartMate LVAD implantation, patients reported improved health status, improved quality of life, a trend toward

less stress, and similar coping ability.[86] Total symptom distress and cardiopulmonary distress decreased. Patients also reported decreased self-care ability at 1–2 weeks after LVAD implant versus before implant, probably due to the need to learn to care for themselves while on an LVAD. Regarding life satisfaction, although there was no difference in overall life satisfaction, patients reported significantly more satisfaction with health/functioning and significant others, and significantly less satisfaction with socioeconomic status from before, compared with after LVAD implantation.

In a second report from the same study,[87] 83 patients (89% male; 76% Caucasian, 21% African-American, and 3% other; mean age = 51 years, 74% married) were able to complete questionnaires at 1 month after HeartMate LVAD implantation. The majority of patients who did not complete questionnaires were too sick. Patients received either a pneumatic ($n = 38$) or vented electric ($n = 45$) LVAD. Ninety-two percent of the patients were still hospitalized at the time of questionnaire completion. Patients were very satisfied with the outcome of the assist device surgery, and 77% said that they would definitely have device surgery, knowing what they knew at 1-month postimplant. Predictors of better quality of life at 1 month after implantation of a HeartMate LVAD were having fewer psychologic symptoms and less overall stress, being African-American, and having a reoperation.[87] These four psychologic, demographic, and clinical variables explained 48% of variance in quality of life at 1 month after device implantation.

Methodologic Issues and Gaps in the Literature

Some of the same limitations pertaining to methodology in the revascularization and mitral valve replacement studies also exist in VAD studies. Issues related to sampling (ie, very small sample sizes and missing data due to morbidity and mortality[74,76–80,82–84,86,87]) can skew results because the data are reported by patients who have fewer complications and by survivors. Similarly, retrospective querying of patients[82,83] can also skew results because patients who reflect back on having had an assist device may report more positive perceptions than actually were experienced. Furthermore, issues related to instrumentation include the retrospective use of daily logs completed by patients[79] and use of instruments without report of preliminary psychometric testing for reliability and validity.[82,83] Other methodologic issues include use of cross-sectional designs[82–84] and report of quality of life for patients receiving many different types of assist devices[82] because there is no evidence regarding similarities in experiences of patients receiving different devices; and long-term follow-up of patients with short-term assist devices (mean length of support < 3 days)[84] because results may be confounded by many other intervening variables.

A strength of three of the studies was their description of quality of life in assist device patients from before to after assist device implantation[86] and from before to after discharge.[74,77] In addition, Grady et al[87] had a sufficient sample size to use multivariate statistical analyses. These data provide clinicians with the ability to generalize tentatively to patients with permanently implantable devices. Research on patients with heart assist devices as destination therapy is still in progress. Quality of life data in patients undergoing implantation of left ventricular assist devices as destination therapy will be invaluable as clinicians attempt to understand the impact of these technologic advancements on long-term patient outcomes. The results of studies (such as REMATCH) in which an LVAD is compared with medical therapy will be important to our understanding of the best ways to improve patients' quality of life.

CARDIAC TRANSPLANTATION

The first successful human-to-human heart transplant was performed on a 57-year-old man with ischemic heart disease at Groote Schuur Hospital in Cape Town, South Africa by Dr. Christian Barnard on December 3, 1967. Although the operation was a success, immunosuppression was crude by today's standards, and the patient died of pneumonia on the 18th post-operative day. Within weeks, the team at Stanford University, headed by Dr. Norman Shumway, performed the first successful heart transplant in the United States on January 6, 1968. Following these early successes, there was an enthusiastic response worldwide, and over the next 12 months, 102 heart transplants were performed in 17 countries, with more than one-half of those procedures performed in the United States. However, enthusiasm quickly waned, due to allograft rejection and infection, and by 1971, only 21 of the initial 165 patients transplanted were still alive, demonstrating a 10% survival rate at 2 years.[88] Following these less-than-favorable results, most programs abandoned clinical heart transplantation by the early 1970s. Fortunately, a few centers, most notably Stanford Medical School, persisted in promoting this as a therapeutic modality.

In the early days of transplantation, immunosuppression consisted generally of azathioprine and corticosteroids. The introduction of cyclosporine in 1980 marked the next major breakthrough in cardiac transplantation, with markedly improved clinical results. In 1986, the US government approved Medicare reimbursement for cardiac transplantation, which denoted the end of the experimental phase and identified transplantation as an accepted therapy in patients with severe heart failure. Since that time, results have continued to improve, and, currently, 1-year survival rates for heart transplantation are approximately 85% and 5-year survival rates are 70% (Figure 5–5).[89] Rejection of the transplanted heart and infection of the immunosuppressed recipient continue to remain the major sources of morbidity and mortality in the early postoperative period. Later in the recovery period, the development of vasculopathy in the transplanted heart is considered to be the major determinant of survival.

The basic technique of orthotopic heart transplantation was developed in the laboratory in the late 1950s and early 1960s and is still widely used today, with minor modifications. This standard biatrial approach proceeds as follows. The recipient is approached via a median sternotomy and placed on conventional cardiopulmonary

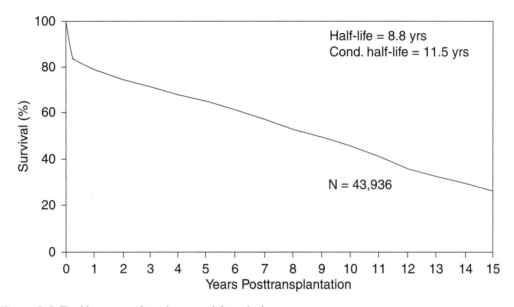

Figure 5–5 Total heart transplantation actuarial survival.

bypass. Moderate systemic hypothermia is achieved (28°–32° C). In coordination with the donor team, the recipient's diseased heart is removed by transecting the aorta and pulmonary artery just above the semilunar valves and excising the remainder of the heart, leaving cuffs of both the left and right atria. The donor heart is then brought to the operative field and inspected for patent foramen ovale. Corresponding cuffs of left and right atria are then fashioned, and anastomosis to the recipient proceeds, with the left atrial suture line first followed by a separate right atrial suture line. Separate end-to-end anastomoses of the pulmonary artery and aorta are accomplished, and the heart is de-aired. After rewarming, the patient is gradually weaned from cardiopulmonary bypass as the donor heart resumes support of the circulation.

Recent surgical modifications of this technique include both the bicaval approach as well as the so-called total orthotopic technique. In the bicaval approach, the entire recipient right atrium is removed. The left atrial cuff and anastomosis is then performed in the standard fashion, followed by individual anastomoses of both

the inferior and superior vena cavae. In the total orthotopic technique, the recipient's left atrium is also excised, leaving separate cuffs of both the right and left pulmonary veins. These separate pulmonary venous anastomoses are then performed to the donor heart, followed by bicaval anastomoses and completion of the aortic and pulmonary artery suture lines.

As previously stated, the results of cardiac transplantation have continued to improve over the ensuing 30 years since the first successful operation was performed. Although the surgical technique has changed little, major advances have been achieved in patient selection, perioperative management, and, most significantly, with improvements in immunosuppression.

A major limitation of cardiac transplantation as a therapy for heart failure remains the donor shortage. International registry data confirm that, following a peak in 1995, the total number of heart transplants performed worldwide has continued to decrease, despite the use of older donors (Figure 5–6).[89] This situation remains in sharp contrast to the number of patients who could potentially benefit from a transplant,

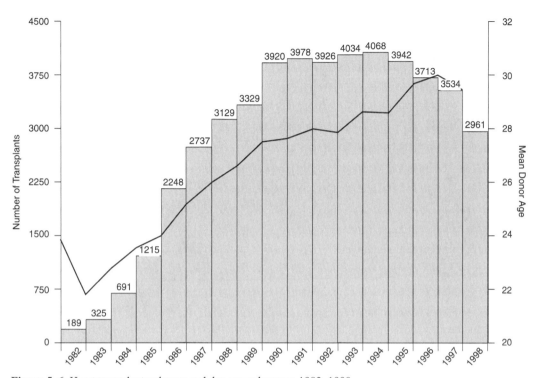

Figure 5–6 Heart transplant volumes and donor age by year, 1982–1998.

which is continuing to increase every year. Unfortunately, without extending the available donor pool, the number of heart transplants performed is likely to change little from the present levels. Despite this significant limitation, continued advances in perioperative management and in the development of more specific, less toxic immunosuppressive agents will most probably improve the survival and quality of life in patients who undergo cardiac transplantation.[90]

QUALITY OF LIFE AFTER HEART TRANSPLANTATION

Quality of life has been studied fairly extensively in patients after heart transplantation. Studies of quality of life in heart transplant patients have been primarily descriptive (short-term and long-term) and comparative (pre- versus posttransplant, comparisons to other patient groups and normative profiles, and comparisons by patient demographic and clinical characteristics). Most studies reported improvement in quality of life from before to after heart transplantation. Few studies effectively dealt with issues related to missing data.

Short-Term Studies on Outcomes after Heart Transplantation

Changes in outcomes have been compared in heart transplant patients from preoperatively to shortly after heart transplant and through 5 years after transplantation. Most studies, however, used short-term longitudinal designs. Generally, patients were found to experience an improvement in outcomes from before to up to 5 years after surgery. Patients reported less or no depression,[91–93] less anxiety,[91,92,94] less symptom distress,[94–96] greater well-being,[91,92,97] greater life satisfaction,[95] improved body image,[91] better health status,[95,98] better perceived quality of life,[95,99,100] better family relationships,[100] and improved functioning in the following areas: physical,[93–95,99,100] social,[93,99,101] emotional,[93,99–101] mental,[100] vocational,[101,102] domestic,[93,101] leisure activities,[93, 100] and sexuality.[95,100,101] Many of these changes were either maintained or further improved over the short term in several studies. No changes in the amount of stress or the use and effectiveness of coping were reported, but changes in the types of stressors experienced and types of coping strategies used were reported.[95] In some studies, patients stated that the following areas were worse: financial situation,[95,100] vocational functioning,[93] and sexual functioning.[103]

Outcomes within 5 years after heart transplant have been compared with other patient groups and with normative profiles. Comparative studies were conducted between heart transplant recipients and healthy individuals,[104] other cardiovascular patients (CABG[105,106] and heart failure patients[107]), and other transplant patients (kidney[108] and liver[109] recipients). Heart transplant recipients reported excellent or good overall quality of life and psychologic well-being comparable to healthy controls but were more bothered by symptoms.[104] The most positive life changes were in physical performance, health, and general quality of life; whereas the most negative life changes pertained to spouse/partner relationships, sexual activity/satisfaction, and return to work.[104]

When compared with CABG patients, heart transplant patients before surgery were significantly less healthy, and areas of their lives were more affected by health problems.[105] One year after surgery, however, both groups improved their health status, but the heart transplant patients tended to have more energy than did CABG patients.[105] In another study of heart transplant and CABG patients, researchers found that both groups were more satisfied with relationships but less satisfied with their sexual life, financial and work status, and health.[106] Comparisons between 6-month post-heart-transplant patients and heart failure patients with 6 months of sustained medical therapy revealed similar high levels of anxiety, depression, hostility, and poor adjustment to illness, yet better

physical and social functioning by heart transplant, as compared with heart failure patients.[107]

Researchers who studied differences in outcomes among organ transplant recipients reported that heart transplant recipients had worse outcomes than did kidney transplant recipients, with the exception of functional impairment.[108] Heart transplant candidates had more physical disability than did liver transplant candidates but improved their functional ability earlier after transplant.[109] These same heart and liver transplant recipients reported a similar, significant decrease in depression and anxiety up to 1 year after transplant.[109]

Additionally, differences in post-heart-transplant outcomes have been examined by pretransplant severity of illness indicators,[110] immunosuppression,[111,112] and work status.[113,114] Patients who were more severely ill before transplant (as defined by NYHA class and United Network for Organ Sharing [UNOS] status) were less satisfied with their overall quality of life, health functioning, psychologic status, socioeconomic status, and relationship with significant others 6 months after transplant than were less severely ill patients.[110] Patients receiving double immunosuppression (cyclosporine and azathioprine), as compared with triple immunosuppression (cyclosporine, azathioprine, and prednisone), experienced better perceived quality of life[111]; and patients on FK506 and prednisone versus cyclosporine, prednisone, and azathioprine also experienced better perceived quality of life.[112]

Regarding work status, patients who were employed after heart transplant versus patients who were not employed had a decreased length of medical disability before transplant, perceived themselves as being physically able to work, experienced a lower rate of loss of health insurance or disability income, and reported better self-esteem, identity stability (ie, not always questioning who you are), perceived quality of life, and body image.[113,114]

Functional capacity has also been studied through the use of objective measures of exercise capacity.[115–118] Exercise capacity has been found to improve after heart transplant, although it remained impaired, when compared to healthy subjects,[115–117] with the majority of improvement seen within the first posttransplant year.[115,118] Possible reasons for reduced patient exercise capacity include lack of functional cardiac reinnervation, cardiac dysfunction, poor conditioning, steroid use and skeletal muscle changes, increased pulmonary vascular resistance, female gender, older heart transplant recipient, and older donor age.[115–118] Researchers also revealed that heart transplant patients (with denervated hearts) demonstrated greater exercise capacity when using a gradual, individualized exercise protocol versus a standardized exercise protocol.[119]

Predictors of perceived quality of life at 1 year after heart transplantation were recently identified ($n = 232$) and included less stress, perception of more helpfulness of health-related information, better health perception, increased compliance with the transplant regimen, more effective coping, less functional disability, less symptom distress, older age, and fewer complications.[120] Another study identified life satisfaction, health status, and employment status as significant predictors of perceived quality of life at 6 months after heart transplant.[97] These findings help clinicians to identify those patients with better quality of life after heart transplantation and those who might be at risk for poorer quality of life or require psychosocial interventions.

Long-Term Studies of Outcomes after Heart Transplantation

Few long-term studies on outcomes of heart transplantation are reported in the literature. These studies were mostly cross-sectional (through 10–22 years' posttransplant), although a few were prospective, longitudinal (through 7–9 years' posttransplant). In two cross-sectional studies (on patients who were 6 months to 10–14 years' posttransplant), patients reported good to excellent outcomes, with positive life changes in physical condition (improved health and endurance), self-accomplishment, relationships, and social activities.[121] Negative life changes were reported in the areas of financial situation,[121] physical appearance,[122] sexual function,[121,122] endurance,[122] sleep patterns,[122] and domestic functioning.[122] The negative life changes were not associated with duration after heart transplant.[122]

A German study[123] of 77 patients between 9 and 13 years after heart transplantation revealed that, at follow-up, most recipients were now NYHA functional Class I or II (91%) and rated their overall health as good to excellent (79%). Health-related quality of life was inferior to that of a healthy population in physical function and role function; patients were limited by physical impairment, pain, and poor overall health. The most frequent complaints were bone and joint pain, back pain, oversensitivity to cold, and hirsutism. Overall quality of life was within the normal range, but work and recreational activities were hindered, due to disability. Although anxiety did not differ from healthy individuals, depression was significantly more prevalent in the study group.[123]

Another study of 27 patients who were followed up 11–22 years after heart transplant reported general well-being comparable to a normal male population, with a trend toward more distress in the areas of mobility, sleep, pain, and energy.[124] In addition, patient exercise capacity ($n = 14$) was 80%–90% of normal, 52% of patients were employed, 20% smoked, and 38% reported some sexual dysfunction.[124]

Prospective longitudinal studies demonstrated improvement in anxiety,[92] depression,[92,93] well-being,[92] social functioning,[98] emotional functioning,[98] sleep,[98] perceived quality of life,[93,97,125] and health status[98] from before to after heart transplant, which did not deteriorate through 4–6 years after transplant. Exercise capacity, which improved by 6 months after heart transplant, also did not change through 9 years of follow-up.[118] Only 53% of patients were working by 5 years' posttransplant.[93] A major limitation of these long-term studies is that many of the studies had very small sample sizes (6–27 patients) by 4–6 years after heart transplant.[92,93,97,98]

Differences in Heart Transplant Outcomes by Age, Gender, Racial/Ethnic Background, and Complications

Short- and long-term studies of differences in outcomes of heart transplant patients based on age, gender, racial/ethnic background, and complications are sparse. Patients > 65 years of age had more functional limitations than did patients < 65 years 6 months after heart transplant, but this difference was not significant at 1 year posttransplant.[126] Coffman et al[127] identified better overall quality of life and improved domestic environment, improved family relationships, and less psychologic distress in heart transplant recipients who were > 60 years, as compared with those < 60 years up to 4 years posttransplant. Likewise, Jones et al[91] reported less anxiety in older versus younger patients immediately after and 8 months after heart transplant. Rickenbacher et al[128] also found significantly improved overall quality of life, specifically in the areas of emotional reactions and sleep in heart transplant patients who were > 54 years of age. As stated previously, older age is a significant predictor of better perceived quality of life in patients at 1 year after heart transplant, although it did not account for a large amount of variance.[120]

Gender-specific issues after heart transplant often focus on (1) the effect of peripartum cardiomyopathy and previous pregnancy on posttransplant morbidity and mortality[129,130] and (2) pregnancy after heart transplant,[131,132] and not on other issues related to posttransplant outcomes. Lough et al[133] described frequent problems with menstruation in post-heart-transplant women and distress related to impotence in post-heart-transplant men. Women had a higher overall rate of symptom frequency, as compared with men.[133] A study examining differences in outcomes between men ($n = 80$) and women ($n = 22$) demonstrated differences in physical functional ability and psychosocial ability at 2 weeks after heart transplant but not at 1 year after surgery.[134] Another report of 145 patients (115 men and 30 women) at 3 months after heart transplant showed that female patients were more distressed by symptoms related to changes in appearance and coped more effectively, whereas men were more distressed by changes in sexual function and return to work.[135] No significant differences between the two groups were found in functional status, satisfaction with heart transplant, or overall life satisfaction.[135] Duitsman

and Cychosz[136] reported that women ($n = 29$) were more anxious and more dissatisfied with their body image than were men ($n = 102$) after heart transplant.

Racial/ethnic background was not examined in heart transplant studies of patient outcomes except to indicate racial background in the sample description.[96,101,108,109,114,137,138] Some heart transplant studies have been published by researchers from other countries, including Canada,[97] England,[98,102,105] Germany,[104,106,123] Austria,[100] and Australia,[91,92,111] but these studies also did not describe their patient sample by race and/or ethnic background.

The only reported evidence on the effect of postoperative complications on outcomes is from the study of predictors of quality of life at 1 year after heart transplant.[120] This study revealed a small but significant variance in perceived quality of life by number of posttransplant complications.[120] Strauss et al[106] generally did not find a relationship between psychosocial variables and medical complications after heart transplant, except between dissatisfaction with the relationship with children and postoperative complications. A weak relationship between postoperative medical variables and psychosocial variables was also reported by Jones et al.[91]

Methodologic Issues and Gaps in the Literature

Numerous short-term studies of quality of life after heart transplant (5 years' posttransplant) with acceptable designs and fairly adequate sample sizes provide evidence of positive outcomes after transplantation. These improvements were often sustained through 4–6 years after transplant. Researchers reported that physical functioning improved the most dramatically after heart transplantation, but patients continued to experience symptoms and stress, and to use coping strategies. However, the specific symptoms, stressors, and coping strategies used after transplantation were different from those used before transplantation. Equivocal findings regarding sexual and vocational function were found. Deterioration in financial situation was also demonstrated in some studies. Comparisons with other populations of patients revealed similar or better health status and improved functioning in some areas, with worse functioning in other areas. Further research in the short-term study of outcomes is recommended in the areas of sexual functioning, work, financial situation, and spirituality. Differences by age, gender, racial/ethnic background, and clinical variables, such as complications, need further exploration. In addition, only two studies examined predictors of perceived quality of life. More research is needed to identify the variables that predict quality of life. Further, most studies were descriptive or comparative in design. Trials of interventions which may alter quality of life after cardiac transplantation are needed.

Many gaps in the literature exist regarding the study of long-term outcomes of heart transplant patients in general and in differences by age, gender, racial/ethnic background, and complications. Cross-sectional, long-term studies[121–124] used a limited number of questionnaires (1–3 tools per study), which examined only a few outcomes. Sample sizes varied from 27 to 96 patients, with 42%–100% response rates. The range of participants' time since surgery was < 1 year to 14 years' posttransplant, making it difficult to compare findings. Long-term, longitudinal studies[92,93,97,98] of outcomes after heart transplant included only patients who were less than 6 years' posttransplant, had very small sample sizes (6–27 patients), and, after 1 year posttransplant, collected data no more frequently than annually. Most of the studies on differences in posttransplant outcomes by age, gender, and complications were short-term.[91,106,120,126–128,134,135] No studies regarding differences in outcomes after heart transplant by race or ethnicity were found in the literature. Some of the studies used no psychometric instruments or a limited number of instruments.[126–128,133] Research regarding the effect of medical complications on outcomes after transplant was equivocal.[91,106,120] Overall, studies of long-term outcomes after heart transplant were descriptive and comparative by design. Long-term studies of outcomes, including efforts to identify variables that predict the best outcomes, are still needed.

Finally, studies are needed that examine the effect of missing data on outcomes after heart transplantation. Many researchers have reported outcomes data without describing the number of patients who were unavailable for participation in the study or who were lost to follow-up subsequent to study enrollment. When missing data have been reported in the study of outcomes after heart transplantation, researchers have dealt with this problem by describing the number of patients in the total pool, the number/percent of patients who did not participate in the study and why (eg, exclusion criteria, refusal to participate, medical complications, or death) and the number/percent of patients who participated in the study.[92,95–97,100–102,104,106,110,111,113,123,124] Additionally, some researchers have acknowledged a marginal questionnaire response rate or stated that patient attrition may or may not have had an effect on study results.[114,122,136] A few researchers have indicated that patients were lost to follow-up after study enrollment, due to medical complications, noncompliance with the study protocol, or death.[97,109] More detail about missing data is essential if the medical community is ever to understand fully the impact of these therapies on quality of life outcomes.

RECOMMENDATIONS FOR FUTURE RESEARCH

The study of quality of life in heart failure patients who undergo surgical therapies is important. Studies must define quality of life and must include objective and subjective multidimensional measures of quality of life that are reliable, valid, and conceptually consistent with the definition. They must be adequately powered, include the use of prospective, longitudinal designs with appropriate statistical techniques and methods to handle missing data, identify predictors of quality of life, and test interventions to improve quality of life. Multisite studies by multidisciplinary teams of researchers will provide the basis from which to understand quality of life in patients who undergo advanced surgical procedures.

REFERENCES

1. Kane RL. *Understanding Health Care Outcomes Research.* Gaithersburg, MD: Aspen Publishers; 1997.
2. Starling RC. The heart failure pandemic: Changing patterns, costs, and treatment strategies. *Cleve Clin J Med.* 1998;65(7):351–358.
3. Haas BK. Clarification and integration of similar quality of life concepts. *Image: J Nurs Scholarship.* 1999;31(3):215–220.
4. Grady KL. Quality of life in patients with chronic heart failure. *Crit Care Nurs Clin North Am.* 1993;5(4):661–670.
5. Gill TM, Feinstein AR. A critical appraisal of the quality of quality-of-life measurements. *JAMA.* 1994;272(8):619–626.
6. Raboud JM, Singer J, Thorne A, Schechter MT, Shafran SD. Estimating the effect of treatment on quality of life in the presence of missing data due to dropout and death. *Quality of Life Res.* 1998;7:487–494.
7. Morrison DF. *Multivariate Statistical Methods, 2nd ed.* New York: McGraw-Hill; 1976.
8. Minnick A, Roberts M, Young WB, Kleinpell R, Marcantonio RJ. What influences patients' reports of three aspects of hospital services? *Med Care.* 1997;35(4):399–409.
9. Cryer J. *Time Series Analysis.* Boston: Duxbury Press; 1986.
10. Gibbons RD, Hedecker D. *Applications of Mixed-Effects Models in Biostatistics.* Sankhya; in press.
11. Cook TD, Campbell DT. *Quasi-experimentation: Design and Analysis Issues for Field Settings.* Boston: Houghton-Mifflin; 1979.
12. Marcantonio RJ, Cook TD. Convincing quasi-experiments: The interrupted time series and regression-discontinuity designs. In: Wholey J, Newcomer K, Hatry H, eds. *Handbook of Practical Program Evaluation,* San Francisco: Jossey-Bass Publishers; 1994.
13. Neter J, Wasserman W, Kutner MH. *Applied Linear Statistical Models,* 2nd ed. Homewood, IL: Richard D. Irwin; 1985.
14. Cohen J, Cohen P. *Applied Multiple Regression/Correlation Analysis for the Behavioral Sciences,* 2nd ed. Hillsdale, NJ: Erlbaum; 1983.
15. Little RJA, Rubin D. *Statistical Analysis with Missing Data.* New York: John Wiley & Sons; 1987.
16. Longford NT. A fast scoring algorithm for maximum likelihood estimation in unbalanced mixed models with nested effects. *Biometrika.* 1987;74:817–827.
17. Laird NM, Ware JH. Random effects models for longitudinal data. *Biometrics.* 1982;38:963–974.
18. Bryk AS, Raudenbush SW. *Hierarchical Linear Models. Applications and Data Analysis Methods.* Newbury Park, CA: Sage Publications; 1992.
19. Goldstein H. Multilevel mixed linear model analysis using iterative generalized least squares. *Biometrika.* 1986;73:43–56.
20. Bock RD, Gibbons RD. High dimensional multivariate probit analysis. *Biometrics.* 1996;52:1183–1194.
21. Hedeker D, Gibbons RD. Application of random-effects pattern-mixed models for missing data in longitudinal studies. *Psychol Methods.* 1997;2:64–78.
22. Little RJA. A class of pattern-mixture models for normal incomplete data. *Biometrika.* 1994;81:471–483.
23. Little RJA. Modeling the dropout mechanism in repeated-measures studies. *J Am Stat Assoc.* 1995;90:1112–1121.
24. Jessup-Likoff M, Chandler S, Kay H. Clinical determinants of mortality in chronic congestive heart failure secondary to idiopathic dilated or to ischemic cardiomyopathy. *Am J Cardiol.* 1987;59:634–638.
25. Franciosa JA, Wilen M, Ziesche S, Cohn JN. Survival in men with severe chronic left ventricular failure due to either coronary heart disease or idiopathic dilated cardiomyopathy. *Am J Cardiol.* 1983;51:831–836.
26. CASS Principal Investigators. Coronary Artery Surgery Study (CASS): A randomized trial of coronary artery bypass surgery. Survival data. *Circulation.* 1983;68:939–950.
27. Elefteriades JA, Kron IL. CABG in advanced left ventricular dysfunction. In: Elefteriades JA, Lee FA, Letsou GV, eds. *Cardiology Clinics: Advanced Treatment Options for the Failing Left Ventricle.* Philadelphia: WB Saunders Company; 1995;35–41.
28. Winkel E, Piccione W. Coronary artery bypass surgery in patients with left ventricular dysfunction: Candidate selection and perioperative care. *J Heart Lung Transplant.* 1997;16:S19–S24.
29. Pagano D, Townend JN, Littler WA, Horton R, Camici PG, Bonser RS. Coronary artery bypass surgery as treatment for ischemic heart failure: The predictive value of viability assessment with quantitative positron emission tomography for symptomatic and functional outcome. *J. Thorac Cardiovasc Surg.* 1998;115:791–799.
30. Dreyfus GD, Duboc D, Blasco A, et al. Myocardial viability assessment in ischemic cardiomyopathy: Benefits of coronary revascularization. *Ann Thorac Surg.* 1994;57:1402–1408.
31. Miller DD. Noninvasive diagnosis of myocardial viability. *J Myocard Ischemia.* 1994;6:22–30.
32. DiCarli MF, Davidson M, Little R, et al. Value of metabolic imaging with positron emission tomography for evaluating prognosis in patients with coronary artery disease and left ventricular dysfunction. *Am J Cardiol.* 1994;73:527–533.

33. DiCarli MF, Asgarzadie F, Schelbert HR, et al. Quantitative relation between myocardial viability and improvement in heart failure symptoms after revascularization in patients with ischemic cardiomyopathy. *Circulation.* 1995;92:3435–3444.

34. Eitzman D, Al-Aouar Z, Kanter HL, et al. Clinical outcome of patients with advanced coronary artery disease after viability studies with positron emission tomography. *J Am Coll Cardiol.* 1992;20:559–565.

35. Boltwood CM, Tei C, Wong M, Shah PM. Quantitative echocardiography of the mitral complex in dilated cardiomyopathy: The mechanism of functional mitral regurgitation. *Circulation.* 1983;68:498–508.

36. Kono T, Sabbah HN, Rosman H, Alam M, Jafri S, Goldstein S. Left ventricular shape is the primary determinant of functional mitral regurgitation in heart failure. *J Am Coll Cardiol.* 1992;20:1594–1598.

37. Blondheim DS, Jacobs LE, Kotler MN, Costacurta GA, Parry WR. Dilated cardiomyopathy with mitral regurgitation: Decreased survival despite a low frequency of left ventricular thrombus. *Am Heart J.* 1991;122(3 Pt 1):763–771.

38. Bach DS, Bolling SF. Improvement following correction of secondary mitral regurgitation in end-stage cardiomyopathy with mitral annuloplasty. *Am J Cardiol.* 1996;78:966–969.

39. Schuler G, Peterson KL, Johnson A, et al. Temporal response of left ventricular performance to mitral valve surgery. *Circulation.* 1979;59:1218–1231.

40. Pitarys CJ II, Forman MB, Panayiotou H, Hansen DE. Long-term effects of excision of the mitral apparatus on global and regional ventricular function in humans. *J Am Coll Cardiol.* 1990;15:557–563.

41. Sarris GE, Cahill PD, Hansen DE, Derby GC, Miller DC. Restoration of left ventricular systolic performance after reattachment of the mitral chordae tendineae. *J Thorac Cardiovasc Surg.* 1988;95:969–979.

42. Carpentier A, Deloche A, Dauptain J, et al. A new reconstructive operation for correction of mitral and tricuspid insufficiency. *J Thorac Cardiovasc Surg.* 1971;61:1–13.

43. Goldman ME, Mora F, Guarino T, Fuster V, Mindich BP. Mitral valvuloplasty is superior to valve replacement for preservation of left ventricular function: An intraoperative two-dimensional echocardiographic study. *J Am Coll Cardiol.* 1987;10:568–575.

44. Tischler MD, Cooper KA, Rowen M, LeWinter MM. Mitral valve replacement versus mitral valve repair: A Doppler and quantitative stress echocardiographic study. *Circulation.* 1994;89:132–137.

45. Rankin JS, Feneley MP, Hickey MstJ, et al. A clinical comparison of mitral valve repair versus replacement in ischemic mitral regurgitation. *J Thorac Cardiovasc Surg.* 1988;95:165–177.

46. Cohn LH, Kowalker W, Bhatia S, et al. Comparative morbidity of mitral valve repair versus replacement for mitral regurgitation with and without coronary artery disease. *Ann Thorac Surg.* 1988;45:284–290.

47. Hammermeister KE, Fisher L, Ward Kennedy J, Samuels S, Dodge HT. Prediction of late survival in patients with mitral valve disease from clinical, hemodynamic, and quantitative angiographic variables. *Circulation.* 1978;57:341–349.

48. Bach DS, Bolling SF. Early improvement in congestive heart failure after correction of secondary mitral regurgitation in end-stage cardiomyopathy. *Am Heart J.* 1995;129:1165–1170.

49. Bolling SF, Deeb GM, Brunsting LA, Bach DS. Surgery for acquired heart disease: Early outcome of mitral valve reconstruction in patients with end-stage cardiomyopathy. *J Thorac Cardiovasc Surg.* 1995;109:676–683.

50. Bolling SF, Pagani FD, Deeb GM, Bach DS. Intermediate-term outcome of mitral reconstruction in cardiomyopathy. *J Thorac Cardiovasc Surg.* 1998;115:381–388.

51. Chocron S, Etievent JP, Viel JF, et al. Prospective study of quality of life before and after open heart operations. *Soc Thorac Surg.* 1996;61:153–157.

52. Klersy C, Collarini L, Morellini MC, Cellino F. Heart surgery and quality of life: A prospective study on ischemic patients. *J Cardio-Thorac Surg.* 1997;12:602–609.

53. Kirkevold M, Gortner S, Berg K, Saltvold S. Patterns of recovery among Norwegian heart surgery patients. *J Adv Nurs.* 1996;24:943–951.

54. Elefteriades JA, Tolis G, Levi E, Mills LK, Zaret BL. Coronary artery bypass grafting in severe left ventricular dysfunction: Excellent survival with improved ejection fraction and functional state. *J Am Coll Cardiol.* 1993;22:1411–1417.

55. King KM, Gortner SR. Women's short-term recovery from cardiac surgery. *Prog Cardiovasc Nurs.* 1996;11(2):5–15.

56. Treasure T, Holmes L, Loughead K, Gallivan S. Survival and quality of life in patients with protracted recovery from cardiac surgery. *Eur J Cardiothorac Surg.* 1995;9:426–432.

57. Nielsen D, Sellgren J, Ricksten SE. Quality of life after cardiac surgery complicated by multiple organ failure. *Crit Care Med.* 1997;25(1):52–57.

58. McHugh GJ, Havill JH, Armistead SH, et al. Follow up of elderly patients after cardiac surgery and intensive care unit admission, 1991 to 1995. *N Z Med J.* 1997;110:432–435.

59. Gortner SR, Jaeger AA, Harr J, Miller T. Elders' expected and realized benefits from cardiac surgery. *Cardiovasc Nurs.* 1994;30(2):9–14.

60. Diegeler A, Autschbach R, Falk V, et al. Open heart surgery in the octogenarians: A study on long-term survival and quality of life. *Thorac-Cardiovasc Surg.* 1995;43:265–270.

61. Kumar P, Zehr KJ, Chang A, Cameron DE, Baumgartner WA. Quality of life in octogenarians after open heart surgery. *Chest.* 1995;108(4):919–926.

62. Kirsch M, Guesnier L, LeBesnerais P, et al. Cardiac operations in octogenarians: Perioperative risk factors for death and impaired autonomy. *Soc Thorac Surg.* 1998;60–67.

63. Frazier OH. The development of an implantable portable, electrically powered left ventricular assist device. *Semin Thorac Cardiovasc Surg.* 1994;6:181–187.

64. Frazier OH. Ventricular assistance: A perspective on the future. *Heart Failure.* December 1994/January 1995:259–264.

65. Norman JC, Cooley DA, Kalan BD, et al. Total support of the circulation of a patient with postcardiotomy stone heart syndrome by a partial artificial heart (ALVAD) for 5 days followed by heart and kidney transplantation. *Lancet.* 1978;1:1125–1127.

66. McCarthy PM, Wang N, Vargo R. Preperitoneal insertion of the HeartMate 1000 IP implantable left ventricular assist device. *Ann Thorac Surg.* 1994;57:634–638.

67. McCarthy PM, Sabik JF. Implantable circulatory support devices as a bridge to heart transplantation. *Semin Thorac Cardiovasc Surg.* 1994;6:174–178.

68. Wagner WR, Johnson PC, Kormos RL, Griffith BP. Evaluation of bioprosthetic valve-associated thrombus in ventricular assist device patients. *Circulation.* 1993;88:2023–2029.

69. McCarthy PM, Savage RM, Fraser CD, et al. Hemodynamic and physiologic changes during support with an implantable left ventricular assist device. *J Thorac Cardiovasc Surg.* 1995;109:409–417.

70. Burnett CM, Duncan JM, Frazier OH, et al. Improved multiorgan function after prolonged univentricular support. *Ann Thorac Surg.* 1993;55:65–71.

71. Frazier OH, Rose EA, McCarthy P, et al. Improved mortality and rehabilitation of transplant candidates treated with a long-term implantable left ventricular assist system. *Ann Surg.* 1995;222:327–338.

72. Kormos RL, Murali S, Dew MA, et al. Chronic mechanical circulatory support: Rehabilitation, low morbidity, and superior survival. *Ann Thorac Surg.* 1994;57:51–58.

73. Piccione W. Mechanical circulatory assistance: Changing indications and options. *J Heart Lung Transplant.* 1997;16:S25–S28.

74. Catanese KA, Goldstein DJ, Williams DL, et al. Outpatient left ventricular assist device support: A destination rather than a bridge. *Ann Thorac Surg.* 1996;62:646–653.

75. McCarthy PM, James KB, Savage RM, et al. Implantable left ventricular assist device: Approaching an alternative for end-stage heart failure. *Circulation.* 1994;90(II):83–86.

76. Moskowitz AJ, Weinberg AD, Oz MC, Williams DL. Quality of life with an implanted left ventricular assist device. *Soc Thorac Surg.* 1997;64:1764–1769.

77. Dew MA, Kormos RL, Winowich CJ, et al. Quality of life outcomes in left ventricular assist system inpatients and outpatients. *ASAIO J.* 1999;45:218–225.

78. Winowich S, Nastala CJ, Pristas JM, Griffith BP, Kormos RL. Discharging patients who are undergoing mechanical circulatory support. *Ann Thorac Surg.* 1996;61:478–479.

79. Myers TJ, Catanese KA, Vargo RL, Dressler DK. Extended cardiac support with a portable left ventricular assist system in the home. *ASAIO J.* 1996;42:M576–M579.

80. Vigano M, Scuri S, Cobelli F, et al. Staged discharge out of hospital of the Novacor left ventricular assist system (LVAS) recipients. *Eur J Cardio-Thorac Surg.* 1997;11:S45–S50.

81. Poirer VL. The HeartMate left ventricular assist system: Worldwide clinical results. *Eur J Cardio-Thorac Surg.* 1997;11:S39–S44.

82. Ruzevich SA, Swartz MT, Reedy JE, et al. Retrospective analysis of the psychologic effects of mechanical circulatory support. *J Heart Transplant.* 1990;9:209–212.

83. Abou-Awdi NL, Frazier OH. Quality of life of patients on LVAD support. In: *Quality of Life After Heart Surgery.* Dordrecht, the Netherlands: Kluwer Academic Publishers; 1992,397–401.

84. Baldwin RT, Radovancevic B, Duncan JM, et al. Quality of life in long-term survivors of the hemopump left ventricular assist device. *ASAIO Trans.* 1991;37:M422–M423.

85. Savage LS, Canody C. Life with a left ventricular assist device: The patient's perspective. *Am J Crit Care.* 1999;8(5):340–343.

86. Grady K, Mattea A, Meyer P, et al. Improvement in quality of life from before to after left ventricular assist device implantation. *J Heart Lung Transplant.* 2000;19(1):78.

87. Grady K, Meyer P, Mattea A, et al. Predictions of quality of life in patients at 1 month after left ventricular assist device implantation. *J Heart Lung Transplant.* 2000;19(1):59.

88. Young JB. The brouhaha surrounding cardiac transplantation: The need to place outcomes in perspective. *Curr Opin Organ Transplant.* 1998;3:1–5.

89. Hosenpud JD, Bennett LE, Keck BM, et al. The Registry of the International Society for Heart and Lung Transplantation: Sixteenth Official Report—1999. *J Heart Lung Transplant.* 1999;18:611–626.

90. Robbins RC, Barlow CW, Oyer PE, et al. Cardiothoracic transplantation: Thirty years of cardiac transplantation at Stanford University. *J Thorac Cardiovasc Surg.* 1999;117:939–950.

91. Jones BM, Chang VP, Esmore D, et al. Psychological adjustment after cardiac transplantation. *Med J Aust.* 1988;149:118–122.

92. Jones BM, Taylor F, Downs K, Spratt P. Longitudinal study of quality of life and psychological adjustment after cardiac transplantation. *Med J Aust.* 1992;157:24–26.

93. Fisher DC, Lake KD, Reutzel TJ, Emery RW. Changes in health-related quality of life and depression in heart transplant recipients. *J Heart Lung Transplant.* 1995;14:373–381.

94. Mai FM, McKenzie FN, Kostuk WJ. Psychosocial adjustment and quality of life following heart transplantation. *Can J Psychiatry.* 1990;35:223–227.

95. Grady KL, Jalowiec A, White-Williams C. Improvement in quality of life in patients with heart failure who undergo transplantation. *J Heart Lung Transplant.* 1996;15(8):749–757.

96. Jalowiec A, Grady KL, White-Williams C, et al. Symptom distress three months after heart transplantation. *J Heart Lung Transplant.* 1997;16:604–614.

97. Molzahn AE, Burton JR, McCormick P, Modry DL, Soetaert P, Taylor P. Quality of life of candidates for and recipients of heart transplants. *Can J Cardiol.* 1997;13(2):141–146.

98. Caine N, Sharples LD, English TAH, Wallwork J. Prospective study comparing quality of life before and after heart transplantation. *Transplant Proc.* 1990;22(4):1437–1439.

99. Packa D. Quality of life of adults after a heart transplant. *J Cardiovasc Nurs.* 1989;3(2):12–22.

100. Bunzel B, Grundbock A, Laczkovics A, Holzinger C, Teufelsbauer H. Quality of life after orthotopic heart transplantation. *J Heart Lung Transplant.* 1991;10(3):455–459.

101. Bohachick P, Anton BB, Wooldridge PJ, et al. Psychosocial outcome six months after heart transplant surgery: A preliminary report. *Res Nurs Health.* 1992;15:165–173.

102. Mulcahy D, Fitzgerald M, Wright C, et al. Long term follow-up of severely ill patients who underwent urgent cardiac transplantation. *Br Med J.* 1993;306:98–101.

103. Mulligan T, Sheehan H, Hanrahan J. Sexual function after heart transplantation. *J Heart Lung Transplant.* 1991;10:125–128.

104. Angermann CE, Bullinger M, Spes CF, Zellner M, Kemkes BM, Theiseu K. Quality of life in long-term survivors of orthotopic heart transplantation. *Kardiologie.* 1992;81:411–417.

105. Wallwork J, Caine N. A comparison of the quality of life of cardiac transplant patients and coronary artery bypass graft patients before and after surgery. *Quality Life Cardiovasc Care.* 1985;317–331.

106. Strauss B, Thormann T, Strenge H, et al. Psychosocial, neuropsychological and neurological status in a sample of heart transplant recipients. *Quality Life Res.* 1992;1:119–128.

107. Walden JA, Stevenson LW, Dracup K, Wilmarth J, Kobashigawa J, Moriguchi J. Heart transplantation may not improve quality of life for patients with stable heart failure. *Heart Lung.* 1989;18:497–506.

108. Evans RW, Manninen DL, Maier A, Garrison, Jr. LP, Hart LG. The quality of life of kidney and heart transplant recipients. *Transplant Proc.* 1985;XVII(1):1579–1582.

109. Riether AM, Smith SL, Lewison BJ, Cotsonis GA, Epstein CM. Quality of life changes and psychiatric and neurocognitive outcome after heart and liver transplantation. *Transplantation.* 1992;54:444–450.

110. Grady KL, Jalowiec A, White-Williams C. Quality of life 6 months after heart transplantation compared with indicators of illness severity before transplantation. *Am J Crit Care.* 1998;7(2):106–116.

111. Jones BM, Taylor FJ, Wright OM, et al. Quality of life after heart transplantation in patients assigned to double or triple drug therapy. *J Heart Transplant.* 1990;9:392–396.

112. Dew MA, Harris RC, Simmons RG, Roth LH, Armitage JM, Griffith BP. Quality of life advantages of FK 506 vs. conventional immunosuppressive drug therapy in cardiac transplantation. *Transplant Proc.* 1991;23(6):3061–3064.

113. Paris W, Woodbury A, Thompson S, et al. Social rehabilitation and return to work after cardiac transplantation—A multicenter survey. *Transplantation.* 1992;2(53):433–438.

114. Duitsman DM, Cychosz CM. Psychosocial similarities and differences among employed and unemployed heart transplant recipients. *J Heart Lung Transplant.* 1994;13:108–115.

115. Mandak JS, Aaronson KD, Mancini DM. Serial assessment of exercise capacity after heart transplantation. *J Heart Lung Transplant.* 1995;14:468–478.

116. Gullestad L, Haywood G, Ross H, et al. Exercise capacity of heart transplant recipients: The importance of chronotropic incompetence. *J Heart Lung Transplant.* 1996;15:1075–1083.

117. Renlund DG, Taylor DO, Ensley RD, et al. Exercise capacity after heart transplantation: Influence of donor and recipient characteristics. *J Heart Lung Transplant.* 1996;15:16–24.

118. Osada N, Chaitman BR, Donohue TJ, Wolford TL, Stelken AM, Miller LW. Long-term cardiopulmonary exercise performance after heart transplantation. *Am J Cardiol.* 1997;79:451–456.

119. Olivari MT, Yancy CW, Rosenblatt RL. An individualized protocol is more accurate than a standard protocol

for assessing exercise capacity after heart transplantation. *J Heart Lung Transplant*. 1996;15:1069–1074.

120. Grady KL, Jalowiec A, White-Williams C. Predictors of quality of life in patients at 1 year after heart transplantation. *J Heart Lung Transplant*. 1999;18:202–210.

121. Lough ME, Lindsey AM, Shinn JA, Stotts NA. Life satisfaction following heart transplantation. *J Heart Transplant*. 1985;IV:446–449.

122. Rosenblum DS, Rosen ML, Pine ZM, Rosen SH, Borg-Stein J. Health status and quality of life following cardiac transplantation. *Arch Phys Med Rehabil*. 1993;74:490–493.

123. Hetzer R, Albert W, Hummel M, et al. Status of patients presently living 9 to 13 years after orthotopic heart transplantation. *Ann Thorac Surg*. 1997;64:1661–1668.

124. DeCampli WM, Luikart H, Hunt S, Stinson EB. Characteristics of patients surviving more than ten years after cardiac transplantation. *J Thorac Cardiovasc Surg*. 1995;109:1103–1115.

125. Littlefield C, Abbey S, Fiducia D, et al. Quality of life following transplantation of the heart, liver, and lungs. *Gen Hosp Psychiatry*. 1996;18:36S–47S.

126. Heroux AL, Costanzo-Nordin MR, O'Sullivan JE, et al. Heart transplantation as a treatment option for end-stage heart disease in patients older than 65 years of age. *J Heart Lung Transplant*. 1993;12:573–579.

127. Coffman KL, Valenza M, Czer LSC, et al. An update on transplantation in the geriatric heart transplant patient. *Psychosomatics*. 1997;38:487–496.

128. Rickenbacher PR, Lewis NP, Valantine HA, Luikart H, Stinson EB, Hunt SA. Heart transplantation in patients over 54 years of age. *Eur Heart J*. 1997;18:870–878.

129. Johnson MR, Naftel DC, Hobbs RE, et al. The Cardiac Transplant Research Database Group. The incremental risk of female sex in heart transplantation: A multiinstitutional study of peripartum cardiomyopathy and pregnancy. *J Heart Lung Transplant*. 1997;16:801–812.

130. Keogh A, Macdonald P, Spratt P, Marshman D, Larbalester R, Kaan A. Outcome in peripartum cardiomyopathy after heart transplantation. *J Heart Lung Transplant*. 1994;13:202–207.

131. Wagoner LE, Taylor DO, Olsen SL, et al. Immunosuppressive therapy, management, and outcome of heart transplant recipients during pregnancy. *J Heart Lung Transplant*. 1994;13:993–1000.

132. Hunt SA. Pregnancy in heart transplant recipients: A good idea? *J Heart Lung Transplant*. 1991;10(4):499–503.

133. Lough ME, Lindsey AM, Shinn JA, Stotts NA. Impact of symptom frequency and symptom distress on self-reported quality of life in heart transplant recipients. *Heart Lung*. 1987;16(2):193–200.

134. Grady KL, Jalowiec A, Costanzo MR, et al. Differences in quality of life indicators based on UNOS status, age, and gender after heart transplantation. *J Heart Lung Transplant*. 1994;13:S45.

135. Grady KL, Jalowiec A,White-Williams C, et al. Gender differences in quality of life 3 months after heart transplantation. *Circulation*. 1994;90:(suppl 4):I–349.

136. Duitsman DM, Cychosz CM. Gender differences in psychosocial characteristics of heart transplant recipients. *J Transplant Coord*. 1995;5:137–143.

137. Grady KL, Jalowiec A, White-Williams C, Hetfleisch M, Penicook J, Blood M. Heart transplant candidates' perception of helpfulness of health care provider interventions. *Cardiovasc Nurs (AHA)*. 1993;29(5):33–37.

138. Grady KL, Jalowiec A, White-Williams C, et al. Predictors of quality of life in patients with advanced heart failure awaiting transplantation. *J Heart Lung Transplant*. 1995;14:2–10.

CHAPTER 6

Impact of Nonpharmacologic Therapy on Quality of Life in Heart Failure

Debra K. Moser and Kathleen Dracup

In a 1993 editorial aptly titled "From Shroud Waving to Quality of Life," Peter Mills exhorted clinicians who conduct clinical trials in cardiovascular medicine to include quality of life assessment as an equally important primary end point with mortality.[1] In another 1993 editorial, Redford Williams and Margaret Chesney wrote about patients with coronary heart disease (CHD) that "the clear demonstration that factors like depression and social isolation distinguish the CHD patients at highest risk means it would be unethical not to start trying to treat these factors with the goal of improving quality of life and minimizing the risks they engender."[2(pp.371)] Despite publication of subsequent research findings supporting these statements, quality of life still often is not included as an end point in cardiovascular clinical trials, nor are interventions systematically employed to improve quality of life in cardiovascular patients.

In heart failure specifically, the situation is no different. Quality of life is poor in patients with heart failure,[3–9] and relatively poorer quality of life is associated with higher mortality and more frequent heart failure hospitalizations.[10,11] Nonetheless, quality of life is not consistently measured as an end point in heart failure trials, and few investigators have examined the impact of interventions to alter quality of life. For example, since 1983, there have been at least 20 studies of the impact of heart failure disease management programs on patient outcomes.[12–32] Of these, less than 40% included quality of life as an outcome measure. In this chapter, we discuss the limited literature in which the effect on quality of life of specific nonpharmacologic interventions—heart failure disease management, biobehavioral therapy, and exercise training—was tested and will provide suggestions for clinical practice and future research.

ASSOCIATION BETWEEN QUALITY OF LIFE AND MORBIDITY AND MORTALITY OUTCOMES

There are two major reasons to develop and implement interventions to improve patients' quality of life. First, quality of life is impaired substantially in patients with heart failure.[3–9] In the Medical Outcomes Study, quality of life was found to be more negatively affected in heart failure than it was in several other common chronic diseases, such as hypertension, diabetes, arthritis, chronic lung disease, or angina.[5] Quality of life is impaired in a number of dimensions, and patients commonly report psychologic or emotional distress, severe limitation in ability to perform activities of daily living, disruption of work roles and family roles, impairment of social interactions at several levels, and reduced sexual activity and satisfaction.[3,6–9]

The second reason to develop and implement interventions to improve patients' quality of life is that poor quality of life has been linked to other adverse clinical outcomes (Table 6–1).[10,11,33] In a substudy of the Studies of Left Ventricular Dysfunction (SOLVD) trial, Konstam and colleagues[11] investigated the potential rela-

Table 6–1 Association between Quality of Life and Morbidity and Mortality in Patients with Heart Failure

Authors	Quality of Life	Outcomes
Konstam et al[11]	Quality of life* Depression Increased difficulty with activities of daily living Social functioning Patient's assessment of his or her health Vigor Patient's perception of his or her life	All-cause mortality
	Quality of life* Increased difficulty with activities of daily living Social functioning Patient's assessment of his or her health	Heart failure hospitalizations
	Quality of life* Increased heart failure symptoms Patient's assessment of his or her health	All-cause mortality and heart failure hospitalizations
Bennett et al[10]	Quality of life Total score on LHFQ Emotional subscale on LHFQ Alertness behavior scale of Sickness Impact Profile	Heart failure hospitalizations

*From univariate analyses and after controlling for age, ejection fraction, treatment, and NYHA multivariate analyses controlling for other medical and/or demographic factors.
LHFQ = Living with Heart Failure Questionnaire.

tionship of quality of life to mortality and heart failure rehospitalizations. These investigators followed 5,025 patients for an average of 3.5 years after they completed baseline measurements of quality of life. Even after controlling for patients' ejection fraction, age, treatment group, and New York Heart Association Functional Classification (NYHAFC), quality of life was predictive of all-cause mortality and rehospitalizations. Bennett and colleagues[10] used different quality of life instruments but similarly demonstrated that poorer quality of life was associated with higher rates of rehospitalization among patients with heart failure.

The clear demonstration of poor quality of life in many patients with heart failure and of the deleterious impact of poor quality of life on morbidity and mortality offers a compelling reason to design and test interventions or to implement already proven interventions that can positively influence quality of life. The failure of drug therapy alone to produce marked improvement in quality of life[34–37] further highlights the need to investigate interventions to improve heart failure patients' quality of life. Although few investigators have examined the impact of nonpharmacologic interventions on quality of life, there is evidence that heart failure disease management programs,[14,17,22–26,31,32,38] biobehavioral therapy,[39,40] and exercise[41–49] may improve quality of life in patients with heart failure.

INTERVENTIONS TO IMPROVE QUALITY OF LIFE IN PATIENTS WITH HEART FAILURE

Heart Failure Disease Management Programs

Quality of life has been included as an outcome in several types of heart failure disease management programs, including the multidisciplinary team approach,[14] heart failure clinic,[23,24,32] community case management,[17,25,26] and telephonic case management.[22,38] Although not a universal finding, most heart failure disease management programs in which quality of life was measured have had a positive impact on this outcome (Table 6–2). No program produced a deleterious effect on quality of life. Improvement in quality of life has been demonstrated with each of the four basic categories of heart failure disease management intervention.

Several trends are evident in this body of literature. First, quality of life improves as time from hospitalization increases, regardless of group assignment.[14,17,25,32] In most studies, baseline quality of life was measured during or soon after a hospitalization for heart failure and improved in both the intervention and control groups when measured again during follow-up. This finding highlights the second trend, that is, that the magnitude of change in quality of life may be overestimated in studies without a control group for comparison. This is because it is likely that the impact of intervention on quality of life is additive to the natural improvement that is seen as time from hospitalization increases. This explains why, in studies with a pre–post design, the degree of improvement seen in quality of life may be overestimated, compared with that seen in randomized controlled trials.[50]

A third trend seen is that quality of life improves to a greater degree, at least in the short term (ie, 30 days to 3–4 months), with intervention than with usual care.[14,17,25] Thus, although quality of life does improve across time since hospitalization in most patients, the degree of improvement seen is substantially greater in patients who receive intervention in some form of heart failure disease management program. For example, after receipt of an intervention from a multidisciplinary heart failure team,[14] the quality of life in the intervention group improved by 31%, compared with 15% in the usual care group. Patients who received home-based community case management demonstrated a 30% improvement in quality of life, whereas usual care patients demonstrated only a 2% improve-

ment.[17] In the randomized controlled trials conducted to date, regardless of which instrument or intervention was used, the magnitude of change was approximately 30%.[14,17,25]

As a group, these studies have been limited by three characteristics. First, all have had a relatively short length of follow-up (ie, 6 months). Long-term effects beyond 1 year have not been documented to date, so the ultimate effect of heart failure disease management on quality of life is unknown. Second, most studies compared an intensive intervention that involved heart failure nurse specialists, as well as other members of a multidisciplinary team, with care as usual. Patients clearly knew whether they had been assigned to the experimental group. The positive results on quality of life documented in the studies may have been the result of the increased attention that the patients received, rather than the specific intervention being tested. Third, the interventions were "bundled," in that close medical follow-up, an emphasis on patient self-care through increased education, involvement of family, and referral to specialists were often all included in the intervention. It is, therefore, impossible to identify which part of the intervention was effective and whether any could be deleted without a negative consequence on quality of life.

However, this group of studies also has multiple strengths that increase our confidence in the validity of the findings. A major strength is that some of the studies were conducted using randomized controlled trials, and their results are supported by those studies in which the less rigorous pre–post intervention comparison was used. Investigators across all studies used instruments to measure quality of life that had well-established reliability and validity in patients with heart failure. The two most commonly used instruments were the Medical Outcomes Study SF-36 and the Minnesota Living with Heart Failure Questionnaire.[51–56] Both have been used extensively in patients with heart failure and have demonstrated sensitivity to change. Use of the same instruments across studies is an added strength because it allows comparison among different studies with different interventions.

Table 6–2 Impact on Quality of Life of Heart Failure Disease Management Programs

Reference	Patients	Study Design	Intervention	Impact on Quality of Life	Quality of Life Measurement
Weinberger et al[31]	• n = 1,396 total, 504 with heart failure • NYHAFC I, 13%; II, 38%; III, 3%; IV, 16% • mean age 63 years • 98%–99% male	Randomized controlled trial (intervention compared with usual care) with follow-up for 6 months	Increased access to primary care • care directed by primary care physician and nurse teams • assessment by primary care nurse of postdischarge needs, provision of relevant education materials, assignment of primary care physicians • card given to patient with names and numbers of team • visit by primary care physician prior to discharge to discuss postdischarge regimen • phone call by primary care nurse within 2 days of discharge • clinic appointment within 1 week of discharge	No difference in quality of life at baseline or 1 and 6 months after the intervention between the control and intervention groups	Medical Outcomes Study SF-36 with 8 subscales: • physician functioning • physical role functioning • emotional role functioning • social functioning • bodily pain • mental health • vitality • general perceptions of health
Rich et al[14]	• n = 282 • mean NYHAFC 2.4 • median age 79 years • 37% male; 63% female	Randomized controlled trial (intervention compared with usual care) with follow-up of 90 days for intervention and 12 months for data collection	Nurse-directed multidisciplinary team with in-hospital education and home follow-up • comprehensive in-hospital education by geriatric cardiovascular nurse • individualized dietary instruction by registered dietician • detailed daily weighing instructions • simplification of medication regimen if possible • discharge planning by social worker and home care to manage economic, social, and transportation problems • intensive home follow-up visits and phone calls • increased access to study personnel	Quality of life improved in both groups across time, but to a greater extent in the treatment group overall and in all 4 subscales (P = 0.001) • For total score, 15% improvement over 90 days in control group versus 31% improvement over 90 days in intervention group	Chronic Heart Failure Questionnaire with 4 subscales • dyspnea • fatigue • emotional function • environmental mastery

continues

Table 6–2 continued

Reference	Patients	Study Design	Intervention	Impact on Quality of Life	Quality of Life Measurement
West et al[22]	• n = 51 • NYHAFC I, 22%; II, 38%; III, 28%; IV, 12% • mean age 66 ± 10 years • 71% male; 29% female	Within-subjects preintervention, postintervention comparison with follow-up of 138 ± 44 days for intervention and 12 months for data collection	Physician-supervised, nurse-managed telephonic case management • primary physician retained overall responsibility • nurse managed care; initial home visit followed by weekly phone calls for 6 weeks • cardiologist available for consultation in difficult cases • implementation of consensus heart failure guidelines • optimization of drug, specifically angiotensin-converting enzyme inhibitor or isosorbide dinitrate/hydralazine, therapy • comprehensive education	Improved quality of life, compared with baseline • significant improvement in physical function components (P = 0.04) • nonsignificant increase in mental component scores (P = 0.27)	Medical Outcomes Study SF-36
Hanumanthu et al[24]	• n = 134 (quality of life measured in a subset of 34 patients) • NYHAFC not indicated • mean age 52 ± 12 years • 71% male; 29% female	Within-subjects preintervention, postintervention comparison with follow-up of 12 months	Comprehensive outpatient heart failure clinic • heart failure/transplant physician-directed • nurse coordinators • team exclusively manages heart failure patients • optimization of medical therapy • other details not provided	Improved quality of life • 39% improvement, compared with baseline (P = 0.01)	Minnesota Living with Heart Failure Questionnaire
Smith et al[23]	• n = 21 • mean NYHAFC 2.6 ± 0.5 • mean age 61 years • 100% male	Within-subjects preintervention, postintervention comparison with follow-up of 6 months	Comprehensive heart failure clinic • care provided by physician or nurse practitioner • optimization of medical therapy • management of cause of heart failure • comprehensive patient education • practitioner available by phone • increased access to clinic without appointment	Improved quality of life • 36% improvement, compared with baseline (P = 0.001)	Minnesota Living with Heart Failure Questionnaire

continues

Table 6–2 continued

Reference	Patients	Study Design	Intervention	Impact on Quality of Life	Quality of Life Measurement
Cline et al[32]	• n = 190 • mean NYHAFC 2.6 ± 0.7 • mean age 75 ± 5 years • 52% male; 48% female	Randomized controlled trial (intervention vs usual care) with follow-up of 12 months	Nurse-directed outpatient clinic • comprehensive patient and family education prior to hospital discharge • medication organizer • patient diuretic self-management • 1-hour information visit for patient and family at home after discharge • easy access to a nurse-directed outpatient clinic with one prescheduled visit at 8 months • clinic nurses available by phone; can see patients at short notice • patients encouraged to contact clinic for any problems or questions	Quality of life improved at 1-year follow-up in both groups; no significant group differences	• Quality of Life in Heart Failure Questionnaire • Nottingham Health Profile (generic questionnaire) • Patients' global self-assessment
Stewart et al[17]	• n = 200 • NYHAFC II, 45%; III, 45%; IV, 10% • mean age 76 ± 8 years • 62% male; 38% female	Randomized controlled trial (intervention vs usual care) with follow-up of 6 months	Home-based education • intervention delivered by nurse • home visit 7–14 days after hospital discharge by nurse for assessment, comprehensive education, and counseling • consultation with primary care MD and cardiologist • flexible diuretic regimen • telephone follow-up at 3 and 6 months • Increased access to study nurse by phone	Improvement across time for both groups, but significantly greater improvement in the intervention group • At 3 months, 30% improvement in total score of Minnesota Living with Heart Failure Questionnaire for intervention group vs 2% improvement in usual care group ($P =$ 0.04 for Minnesota Living with Heart Failure Questionnaire; $P = 0.02$ for SF-36, physical function only) • no differences at 6 months	• Minnesota Living with Heart Failure Questionnaire • Medical Outcomes Study SF-36

continues

Table 6–2 continued

Reference	Patients	Study Design	Intervention	Impact on Quality of Life	Quality of Life Measurement
Heidenreich et al[38]	• n = 68 • NYHAFC II and III (% not indicated) • mean age 73 ± 13 years • 53% male; 47% female	Intervention patients compared with matched control group, preintervention period compared with postintervention period	Home education and monitoring • patient entry by phone of blood pressure, weights, symptoms • computer algorithm determines whether values in acceptable range set by MD, pages nurse if not • weekly for 1-year educational mailing and 10-minute phone calls from nurse	No change in quality of life in intervention group at 3 months' follow-up (no quality of life data available for control group)	Medical Outcomes Study SF-36
Jaarsma et al[26]	• n = 179 • NYHAFC III, 17%; III–IV, 22%; IV, 61% • mean age 72 ± 9 years • 58% male; 42% female	Randomized controlled trial (intervention vs usual care) with 9 months' follow-up	Hospital and home-based education and counseling • predischarge education, counseling, and support from nurse • One telephone call and one home visit after discharge	Quality of life improved after hospital discharge in both groups, with no differences between the groups across time	• Heart Failure Functional Status Inventory • Symptom occurrence, severity, and distress • Psychosocial Adjustment to Illness Scale • Cantril's Ladder of Life
Moser et al[25]	• n = 136 • NYHAFC II, 31%; III, 40%; IV, 29% • mean age 70 ± 13 years • 48% male; 52% female	Randomized controlled trial (intervention vs usual care) with 3 months' follow-up	Community case management • nurse home-based assessment, education, and counseling at first visit • frequent long-term follow-up by phone • comprehensive education and counseling about pharmacologic and nonpharmacologic therapy • behavioral strategies to improve compliance • patient access to nurse as needed • attention to social, environmental, financial, behavioral problems • coordination of social and health care services	Improved quality of life in both groups, but significantly greater improvement in intervention than control group	• Minnesota Living with Heart Failure Questionnaire

NYHAFC = New York Heart Association Functional Class.

Potential Mechanisms of Action

None of the studies described was designed to delineate the mechanism whereby quality of life improved as a result of participation in a heart failure disease management program. The task of trying to determine mechanisms is made more difficult by the fact that each of the programs consisted of several components. Nonetheless, a model of quality of life improvement based on changes in several dimensions can be postulated: decreased symptoms and associated distress, increased perception of control through education, improved emotional states through counseling, increased social support, and decreased exacerbations of heart failure and rehospitalizations. Heart failure disease management programs may exert a positive effect on quality of life for any one of these reasons or, more likely, for a combination of them, but each of them will be discussed individually.

A common effect of participation in a heart failure disease management program is improvement in the symptoms associated with heart failure and in their impact on patients' lives. Many patients report troubling disruptions in their abilities to perform their usual activities and roles, owing to the severity of heart failure symptoms.[4,57–60] These disruptions in ability to perform needed or desired activities contribute to declining quality of life in patients with heart failure. As symptoms decrease, patients are better able to perform their personal, work, and leisure activities and to participate in a variety of social interactive activities; subsequently, quality of life improves.[61,62] Symptom distress—the degree to which the symptoms a patient experiences cause discomfort or suffering—also is common in patients with heart failure and is associated with poor quality of life.[59,60] As symptoms improve, symptom distress decreases, and quality of life improves.

A second mechanism whereby heart failure disease management programs may result in improved quality of life is through an increase in patients' perception of control after they receive the comprehensive education common in most programs. By providing patients with informa-

tion and skills to adopt needed lifestyle changes, many of the uncertainties that distress patients with heart failure are relieved or reduced, and sense of control is increased.[63] Increased control has been associated with marked reductions in patients' anxiety, depression, and hostility.[64] Because negative emotions contribute to poorer quality of life, improved mood state results in enhanced quality of life.

A third, related mechanism is that of improved emotional states secondary to counseling. The counseling component of disease management programs is often hidden under the umbrella of comprehensive education and is sometimes difficult to recognize as an identifiable component. However, in most programs that include some element of frequent clinician contact, clinicians have the opportunity to perform a number of counseling activities. These counseling activities include assistance with problem-solving skills and behaviors; provision of support and assistance with management of anxiety and depression; identification of and assistance with management of financial, domestic, and social problems; and referral to appropriate social and psychologic services when needed. Each of these activities has the potential to improve coping with the many adverse manifestations of chronic heart failure and, thus, to enhance patients' quality of life.

A fourth potential mechanism involves social support derived from two sources: more frequent and effective contact with health care providers and, in the case of patients with family members, improved quality of social support provided by them as they receive information, problem-solving skills, and support from health care providers. Increased social support can improve quality of life by positively influencing psychologic state as quality and quantity of social interactions increase and sense of social isolation decreases.[65–67] It also may improve quality of life indirectly by promoting better adherence to the prescribed pharmacologic and nonpharmacologic regimen, thereby reducing symptoms and their negative impact.[65–67]

Finally, successful heart failure disease management reduces heart failure exacerbations,[12] and this may improve quality of life through a number of pathways. Fewer exacerbations result in less frequent visits to the physician or emergency department and, ultimately, fewer hospitalizations. One component of quality of life is the financial impact of illness. Therefore, the financial burden imposed by frequent exacerbations is lessened because even those patients with health care insurance assume greater financial costs as they use more health care resources. This is especially important for the many elderly patients who survive on very limited, fixed, poverty-level incomes. A decrease in the number of exacerbations also may improve quality of life by decreasing the negative impact of symptoms, as described previously. In addition, patients who experience fewer heart failure exacerbations have less disruption of their usual routine and ability to carry out their various social, domestic, and work roles, and must less often assume the sick role. As a consequence, patients who have fewer exacerbations experience better quality of life.

Lessons from Negative Studies

Attempts to determine mechanisms that explain how quality of life is improved with heart failure disease management are facilitated by examination of programs in which there was no impact on quality of life associated with the intervention.[26,31,32,38] Quality of life was either unchanged during follow-up or there were no differences across time between the intervention and control groups. In each of the negative studies, the investigator tested a less intense intervention that included limited contact with clinicians compared with the level of contact seen in successful programs. In less intensive interventions, when there are few contacts with clinicians, the social supportive and counseling aspects of heart failure disease management are limited, and there may be little opportunity to affect quality of life via these mechanisms. Resource utilization was also unaffected by the intervention in the studies with negative quality of life results, and these two outcomes may be related.

BIOBEHAVIORAL THERAPY

As described in Chapter 10, only two groups of researchers have investigated the role of biobehavioral therapy in the management of patients with heart failure.[39,40] Both have examined the impact of this therapy on quality of life and demonstrated improvement as a result of treatment. The findings of each of these groups are strengthened by use of randomized controlled study designs.

Kostis and associates[39] randomly assigned 20 patients with heart failure to one of three groups: (1) nonpharmacologic intervention; (2) digoxin therapy; or (3) placebo. Patients received standard background therapy with angiotensin-converting enzyme inhibitors and diuretics. Nonpharmacologic intervention consisted of biobehavioral therapy in the form of group-based cognitive-behavioral intervention that emphasized stress management using relaxation and coping with anxiety, anger, and depression. The nonpharmacologic intervention also had an exercise training component and a dietary intervention aimed at reducing dietary sodium intake, and weight reduction for moderately obese patients.

Although quality of life was not directly measured in this study, two emotional variables that contribute to quality of life—anxiety and depression—were measured. Anxiety and depression were significantly reduced only in the nonpharmacologic intervention group. Patients in the nonpharmacologic intervention group demonstrated a 52% reduction in depression and a 39% reduction in anxiety, versus a 15% increase in depression and a 24% increase in anxiety in the digoxin group, and a 25% increase in depression and a 45% increase in anxiety in the placebo group.

Moser and associates[40] examined the impact of biofeedback-relaxation training on a number of clinical variables (rehospitalizations, functional status, catecholamines, and heart rate variability), in addition to the psychosocial variables of perceived control, anxiety, depression, and quality of life. Patients with advanced heart failure ($n = 90$) were randomly assigned to 6 weeks of one-on-one biofeedback-relaxation training in addition to usual care or to usual care alone. Patients were followed for 6 months. Patients in the biofeedback-relaxation training group experienced a 66% increase in perceived control, a 45% decrease in anxiety, a 25% decrease in depression, and a 42% improvement in quality of life. In the control group, perceived control decreased, anxiety and depression increased, and quality of life decreased.

These studies demonstrate improved quality of life as a result of participation in biobehavioral therapy. Although these findings represent the work of only two groups and further research is needed to supplement this small body of work, the findings of these two groups are credible because both used randomized, controlled designs. Thus, it appears that gains in quality of life can be had with use of biobehavioral therapies. The magnitude of improvement is similar to that seen in heart failure disease management programs.

Potential Mechanisms of Action

Biobehavioral therapy may improve quality of life by three main mechanisms: improved coping with negative emotions, decreased symptoms and their negative impact, and increased perceived control that decreases emotional distress. Biobehavioral therapy that includes cognitive restructuring (as did the intervention tested by Kostis and associates[39]) assists patients to cope more effectively with negative emotions, such as anxiety, depression, and anger, that are common in patients with heart failure. Cognitive restructuring is a well-established method wherein an individual is first taught to assess systematically his or her negative emotions and expectations, then is taught skills for coping positively with these negative emotions and expectations.[39] Similarly, many biofeedback-relaxation programs contain a component that involves training patients to examine their negative emotional responses to acute or chronic stressors and to use the relaxation response to diminish or eliminate the negative response.[68] Thus, in biobehavioral therapy, quality of life may be improved as negative emotions are decreased.

Biobehavioral therapy may improve quality of life by decreasing symptoms and their impact. Theoretically, successful biobehavioral therapy in patients with heart failure results in improved symptom status through a reduction of sympathetic nervous system arousal and increased peripheral vasodilation, effects that may augment the impact of drug therapy and decrease symptoms.[69] Because symptoms and symptom distress are important contributors to quality of life, an improvement in symptom status can lead to improved quality of life.[61,62]

Another potential mechanism whereby quality of life is improved as a result of biobehavioral therapy is increased perceived control.[40] As previously described, increased perceived control is associated with a reduction in negative emotions, such as anxiety, depression, and anger, that can so adversely affect quality of life.[64]

EXERCISE TRAINING

As recently as the early 1990s, clinicians commonly were advised to recommend that patients with heart failure avoid exercise.[70] Although the role of exercise training in heart failure is still not completely understood and the impact of training on survival is unclear, many investigators have demonstrated that exercise training has several benefits for patients with heart failure (see Chapter 8).[71–83] These benefits include improved hemodynamics, improved muscle metabolism (ie, improved oxidative capacity), increased exercise capacity, and improved autonomic balance.[71–83] Fewer investigators have examined the impact of exercise training on quality of life, but those who have demonstrated benefit,[39,41–48] with one exception[49] (see Table 6–3). Although only a few investigators examined changes across more than two time points, those who have demonstrated that quality of life improves early in the course of exercise training, and this improved level is maintained over the long term, even if the intensity of exercise decreases.[42,47]

Each of the studies in which the impact of exercise on quality of life was documented was either a randomized controlled trial or a random-

Table 6–3 Impact on Quality of Life of Exercise Training

Reference	Patients	Study Design	Intervention	Impact on Quality of Life	Quality of Life Measurement
Kostis et al[39]	• n = 20 • NYHAFC II, 95%; III, 5% • mean age 66 years • 70% male; 30% female	Randomized controlled trial (nonpharmacologic therapy vs digoxin vs placebo) with 3-month follow-up	Multimodal nonpharmacologic therapy • exercise training at cardiovascular rehabilitation center—steadily increasing intensity to 1 hour, 3–5 times per week at heart rate 40%–60% of functional capacity (walking, rowing, cycling, and stair climbing) • dietary control aimed at weight reduction for moderately obese patients and dietary sodium restriction • cognitive-behavioral group therapy—relaxation, stress reduction, and coping with adverse emotions	• Depression improved 52% in nonpharmacologic therapy group, compared with increase in depression by 15% in digoxin group and 25% in placebo group • Anxiety improved 39% in nonpharmacologic therapy group, compared with an increase in anxiety by 24% in the digoxin group and 45% increase in the placebo group	Factors that contribute to quality of life: • Beck Depression Inventory • Hamilton Anxiety and Depression Scales
Tyni-Lynné et al[41]	• n = 21 • NYHAFC II, 57%; III, 43% • mean age 60 years • 100% male	Randomized controlled trial (one-leg knee extensor training vs two-leg vs control) with 2-month follow-up	Local quadriceps femoris training (one-leg or two-leg) • 3 sessions per week for 8 weeks • continuous knee extensor at 60 repetitions per min on modified cycle ergometer for 15 min • 6 min of walking at self-selected speed for warm-up and 3 min for cool-down	• No change in Sense of Coherence Scale • Physical, psychosocial, home management, and sleep-rest subscales of Sickness Impact Profile improved with training in both one-leg and two-leg groups but deteriorated in control group	• Sickness Impact Profile (overall score, physical dimension, psychosocial dimension, remaining subscales) • Sense of Coherence Scale

continues

Table 6-3 continued

Reference	Patients	Study Design	Intervention	Impact on Quality of Life	Quality of Life Measurement
Kavanagh et al[42] and Shephard et al[43]	• n = 30 • NYHAFC III, 100% • mean age 62 ± 6 years • 83% male; 17% female	Randomized controlled trial (aerobic training vs usual care [usual care group, n = 9, followed only 12 weeks]) with 12 months' follow-up	Individualized aerobic training program in outpatient cardiac rehabilitation • walking at 50%–60% of peak VO_2 • for first 16 weeks, walked 5 times per week with rehabilitation therapist, covered ~ 10 km at a pace of ~ 13 min/km • after 16 weeks, once weekly visits to rehab center for walking for 20 weeks, then monthly for remainder of the 12 months • after 16 weeks, walk distance increased to ~ 21 km at 11.5 min/km • during reduced visit period, patients exercised to a total of 5 times per week	• Trend toward improvement in all subscales of Chronic Heart Failure Questionnaire in intervention group; no change in control group • 14% improvement in standard gamble compared with baseline; no change in control group	• Chronic Heart Failure Questionnaire (mastery, fatigue, dyspnea, emotional function) • Standard gamble
Tyni-Lynné et al[44]	• n = 16 • NYHAFC II, 56%; III, 44% • mean age 62 ± 10 years • 100% women	Randomized (training vs nontraining first) crossover (8 weeks training vs 8 weeks nontraining) trial with 16 weeks' follow-up	Hospital-based outpatient exercise supervised by physical therapist • 3 times per week • endurance training of leg muscles, 60 repeats/min for 15 min • walking with 6 min warmup, 3 min cool-down	• No change in Sense of Coherence Scale scores • Sickness Impact Profile scores improved after training	• Sense of Coherence Scale • Sickness Impact Profile

continues

Table 6–3 continued

Reference	Patients	Study Design	Intervention	Impact on Quality of Life	Quality of Life Measurement
Wielenga et al[45]	• n = 80 • NYHAFC not stated—classes II and III enrolled • mean age 64 years • 100% male	Randomized controlled trial (exercise vs usual care) with 3 months' follow-up	Standardized training program supervised by a physician • 3 10-min exercise series (bike, walk, ball game) with 5 min rest between each period • 3 times per week	• 26% improvement in feeling of being disabled subscale in Heart Failure Patients Psychological Questionnaire in intervention group vs 8% in control—no difference in other subscales • No difference in Sickness Impact Profile score (14% improvement in intervention vs 10% in control) • Self-Assessment of General Well-Being significantly better in intervention, compared with control group	• Heart Failure Patients Psychological Questionnaire with 4 subscales (well-being, feeling of being disabled, displeasure, social inhibition) • Sickness Impact Profile • Self-Assessment of General Well-Being
Willenheimer et al[46]	• n = 49 • NYHAFC I, 12%; II, 39%; III, 49% • mean age 64 years • 71% male; 29% female	Randomized, controlled trial (exercise training vs usual care) with 4 months' follow-up	Group exercise program supervised by a physiotherapist • interval training on a cycle ergometer • 90 seconds of exercise and 30 seconds of rest • exercise to 80% of VO_2 max during each interval for patients in sinus rhythm; patients in atrial fibrillation exercised to exhaustion grade 15 on the Borg scale	• Quality of life improved in intervention patients vs controls	• Global quality of life (one-item scale)

continues

Table 6-3 continued

Reference	Patients	Study Design	Intervention	Impact on Quality of Life	Quality of Life Measurement
Belardinelli et al[47]	• n = 99 • NYHAFC II, 47%; III, 34%; IV, 19% • mean age 59 ± 14 years • 89% male; 11% female	Randomized, controlled trial (exercise vs usual care) with 12 months' follow-up	Exercise supervised by a cardiologist • cycling at 60% of peak VO_2 • 3 times per week for 8 weeks • 2 times per week for remainder of 12 months • each session consisted of ~ 20 minutes of stretching warm-up, followed by ~ 40 minutes of cycling	• Improvement in quality of life in intervention group, compared with control (improvement sustained to 12 months)	• Minnesota Living with Heart Failure Questionnaire
Quittan et al[48]	• n = 27 • NYHAFC II, 60%; III, 40% • mean age 55 ± 9 years • 88% male; 12% female	Randomized controlled trial (exercise vs usual care) with 3 months' follow-up	Aerobic exercise supervised by physiotherapist • cycling 3 times per week for 1 hour each • each session consisted of 3–5 minutes warm-up, two 25-minute periods of aerobic exercise, 5 minutes cool-down	• Improvement in all domains of quality of life assessment greater in exercise vs control	• Medical Outcomes Study SF-36
Gottlieb et al[49]	• n = 33 • NYHAFC II, 36%; III, 64% • mean age 66 years • 87% male; 13% female	Randomized controlled trial (exercise vs usual care) with 6 months' follow-up	Supervised, graded aerobic exercise • cycling and treadmill 3 times per week intensity increased as tolerated	• No change in quality of life, depression, or functional status scores	• Minnesota Living with Heart Failure Questionnaire • CES-D (depression) • Medical Outcomes Study SF-36 • Functional Status Assessment

NYHAFC = New York Heart Association Functional Class.

ized crossover design, thus increasing our confidence in the validity of the findings and the magnitude of effect seen. The magnitude of improvement seen in this group of studies varies more widely than in the studies of heart failure disease management or biobehavioral therapy, ranging from a low of 14% to a high of approximately 50%. The wider range of magnitudes may reflect the varying intensities or types of exercise used, differences among the patients studied, or inability to compare directly quality of life findings across the number of different instruments used to measure quality of life.

In the one negative study in this group, Gottlieb and associates studied 33 elderly patients with moderate to severe heart failure.[49] Although patients randomized to the exercise program ($n = 17$, 11 of whom completed the program) demonstrated improved peak oxygen consumption and increased maximal and submaximal exercise capability, daily activities (measured by total-activity energy, using doubly labeled water technique and hip accelerometer) did not improve, nor did quality of life. This study was substantially smaller than most of the other studies in this group, and the quality of life measures were not assessed in randomized fashion, as were the primary exercise capacity end points. These factors may explain the lack of apparent impact on quality of life, but the quality of life measures showed no indication that quality of life changed with exercise. Thus, lack of adequate power may not be the only explanation for the negative finding.

Gottlieb and colleagues[49] speculate that elderly heart failure patients with more severe disease may not realize the same impact from exercise as do younger, relatively more "healthy" heart failure patients. This belief is supported by the number of patients who dropped from the exercise arm because they were "too sick" or felt that exercise made them feel worse. However, other investigators have enrolled elderly patients with moderate to severe heart failure and have demonstrated a positive impact on quality of life.[42,43,46] Nonetheless, it is likely that some subgroups of heart failure patients will not benefit from exercise training, and further investigations should attempt to identify those subgroups.

Potential Mechanisms of Action

Numerous investigators have demonstrated that exercise positively influences physical functioning, emotional well-being, and life satisfaction in individuals without disease, improving quality of life.[6] In this same way, exercise may improve quality of life in patients with heart failure. Patients with heart failure who participate in exercise training of a variety of types experience a marked improvement in exercise tolerance, functional status, and increased ability to perform activities without symptoms,[71,72] all of which enhance quality of life.[61] Although this is not the only mechanism whereby quality of life is improved, existing evidence indicates that it is a powerful mechanism. Even among patients who are trained using seated knee-extensor exercise versus whole body exercise and in whom, presumably, the mood-enhancing effect of exercise training might be less, quality of life improves.[41,44] For patients, improvement in functional capacity translates into increased ability to do the activities they desire, and this is associated with increased social competence and general health perception.[48]

Quality of life also may improve as a result of the impact of exercise on mood or due to the dynamics of the exercise environment. Although few investigators have examined the impact of exercise on mood, those who have measured it have demonstrated that, as in other populations, mood is substantially enhanced with exercise training.[39] Thus, quality of life also may improve as anxiety and depression decrease. Another possible mechanism related to the environment in which patients exercise is that the social support provided by health care providers who supervise the exercise or by fellow patients may result in improved quality of life. In each of the exercise studies in which quality of life was considered as an outcome, exercise training was supervised and conducted at rehabilitation centers or other health care environments with significant staff support; no studies reported to date involved home-based exercise. Thus, the role that social support might have played in the improved quality of life is unclear. Elucidation of increased social support as a possible mechanism awaits study of home-based exercise training.

AN INTEGRATED THEORY TO EXPLAIN MECHANISM

We have offered separate mechanisms whereby each nonpharmacologic therapy might improve quality of life. However, an integrated view that takes into account all of these explanations for how nonpharmacologic therapy may have a positive impact on quality of life comes from the work of several researchers,[84,85] who have suggested that quality of life outcomes are based on perceived discrepancies or "gaps" between the reality of one's present experience and what is expected. Discrepancy theory[85] offers an explanation for patient determinations of successful or unsuccessful coping and good or poor quality of life at the point of reappraisal. If actual experiences match expectations, evaluations of successful coping and good quality of life follow.

According to Cella,[86] there are four ways to close the gap (ie, reduce the discrepancy between reality and expectation) and improve quality of life: (1) treat the disease, (2) treat the symptoms, (3) enhance communication, and (4) reframe attitudes. In the context of discrepancy theory, nonpharmacologic therapy, such as heart failure disease management, biobehavioral therapy, or exercise training, can address all four, even though no "cure" of heart failure is possible. For example, in the case of exercise training, aerobic training can improve patients' physiologic state related to the disease by improving peripheral and pulmonary factors, as well as by improving peripheral muscle strength.[76] Second, the symptoms of fatigue and dyspnea, hallmarks of heart failure, decrease with physical conditioning.[77] Third, communication with health care providers often is enhanced during exercise training (at least in the case of supervised training) because patients have more frequent, prolonged contact with clinicians. Finally, patients may reframe their attitudes about the hopelessness of their health status as they experience increasing levels of physical function and activity.

CONCLUSION AND RECOMMENDATIONS FOR RESEARCH AND PRACTICE

The preponderance of evidence indicates that nonpharmacologic therapy positively influences quality of life in patients with heart failure. Participation in heart failure disease management, biobehavioral therapy, or exercise training, in combination with appropriate pharmacologic therapy, improves quality of life by approximately 30% (range 10%–50%). To date, no nonpharmacologic intervention has resulted in a decreased quality of life, a finding that is in contrast to pharmacologic or surgical interventions for heart failure.

Quality of life is a significant outcome to patients and health care providers for a number of reasons, including the following: (1) there is now a variety of therapeutic options with little difference in outcome except in terms of quality of life; (2) quality of life is a vital personal component to patients with chronic diseases with high morbidity and mortality; (3) patients need quality of life data to make decisions as they are asked to participate as partners in their own care[87]; and (4) quality of life affects morbidity and mortality.[10,11] As such, knowledge and use of those therapies that improve quality of life is essential in the management of heart failure.

Findings from the past decade of research provide clinicians with important data upon which to base a comprehensive approach to the management of patients with heart failure. Nonetheless, the research has been limited in significant ways, and these limitations should be addressed in future research. First, future researchers need to conduct their studies within the context of randomized controlled trials to delineate the impact and magnitude of effect. The true impact and magnitude are obscured in studies conducted without benefit of a control group, and, as a consequence, clinicians who must make decisions about implementation of new therapies are unable to determine the full cost/benefit ratio of doing so. Second, researchers should include methods of delineating the mechanisms whereby quality of life is affected by various interventions. Understanding mechanisms assists researchers and clinicians to calibrate nonpharmacologic therapies appropriately so that they are fully effective with the most efficient use of resources. Third, most longitudinal studies of the impact of nonpharmacologic therapy on quality of life include outcome measurement at only two time points—baseline and after the intervention—and the post-test is frequently short-term. Future research should include measurement of outcomes at some midpoints so that trends in change in quality of life across time are not missed. Such trends provide important information about the effect of changing intervention intensity or how soon effects can be expected. Post-testing should be conducted at various lengths of time (beyond 1 year) to determine whether the results are lasting or need periodic reinforcement. Fourth, certain populations may respond differently to various nonpharmacologic interventions. Research needs to be done to identify the subgroups that may not find such approaches beneficial.

A final suggestion for future research is the comparison of the impact of various nonpharmacologic treatment modalities. How does heart failure disease management compare to exercise training or biobehavioral therapy? Are these therapies synergistic? As resources available for health care shrink and competition for those resources increases, it is imperative that we discover the most optimal interventions for improving patients' quality of life.

In conclusion, many forces are converging to increase interest in the effect of nonpharmacologic approaches on the quality of life of patients with heart failure. As mortality rates from cardiovascular disease continue to decrease, quality of life as an outcome of treatment is increasingly recognized as important by clinicians and consumers, alike. Many pharmacologic treatments can have mixed or negative effects on patients' quality of life. The hope that nonpharmacologic treatment can influence quality of life positively is held by many patients and health care providers. Research on the interventions reviewed in this chapter—disease management programs, biobehavioral therapy, and exercise programs—suggest that such approaches may be beneficial and deserve further testing in systematic controlled clinical trials.

REFERENCES

1. Mills P. From shroud waving to quality of life. *Br Heart J.* 1993;69:371.
2. Williams RB, Chesney MA. Psychosocial factors and prognosis in established coronary artery disease. *JAMA.* 1993;270:1860–1861.
3. Dracup K, Walden JA, Stevenson LW, Brecht ML. Quality of life in patients with advanced heart failure. *J Heart Lung Transplant.* 1992;11:273–279.
4. Grady KL. Quality of life in patients with chronic heart failure. *Crit Care Nurs Clin North Am.* 1993;5:661–670.
5. Stewart AL, Greenfield S, Hays RD, et al. Functional status and well-being of patients with chronic conditions: Results from the Medical Outcomes Study. *JAMA.* 1989;262:907–913.
6. Walden JA, Stevenson LW, Dracup K, et al. Extended comparison of quality of life between stable heart failure patients and heart transplant recipients. *J Heart Lung Transplant.* 1994;13:1109–1118.
7. Hawthorne MH, Hixon ME. Functional status, mood disturbance and quality of life in patients with heart failure. *Prog Cardiovasc Nurs.* 1994;9(11):22–32.
8. Jaarsma T, Dracup K, Walden J, Stevenson LW. Sexual function in patients with advanced heart failure. *Heart Lung.* 1996;25:263–270.
9. Muirhead J, Meyerowitz BE, Leedham B, Eastburn TE, Merrill WH, Frist WH. Quality of life and coping in patients awaiting heart transplantation. *J Heart Lung Transplant.* 1992;11:265–272.
10. Bennett SJ, Pressler ML, Hays L, Firestine LA, Huster GA. Psychosocial variables and hospitalization in persons with chronic heart failure. *Prog Cardiovasc Nurs.* 1997;12(4):4–11.
11. Konstam V, Salem D, Pouler H, et al, for the SOLVD Investigators. Baseline quality of life as a predictor of mortality and hospitalization in 5,025 patients with congestive heart failure. *Am J Cardiol.* 1996;78:890–895.
12. Rich MW. Heart failure disease management: A critical review. *J Cardiac Failure.* 1999;5:64–75.
13. Rich MW, Vinson JM, Sperry JC, et al. Prevention of readmission in elderly patients with congestive heart failure: Results of a prospective, randomized pilot study. *J Gen Intern Med.* 1993;8:585–590.

14. Rich MW, Beckham V, Wittenberg C, Leven CL, Freedland KE, Carney RM. A multidisciplinary intervention to prevent readmission of elderly patients with congestive heart failure. *N Engl J Med.* 1995;333:1190–1195.

15. Stewart S, Pearson S, Horowitz JD. Effects of a home-based intervention among patients with congestive heart failure discharged from acute hospital care. *Arch Intern Med.* 1998;158:1067–1072.

16. Stewart S, Vandenbroek AJ, Pearson S, Horowitz JD. Prolonged beneficial effects of a home-based intervention on unplanned readmissions and mortality among patients with congestive heart failure. *Arch Intern Med.* 1999;159:257–261.

17. Stewart S, Marley JE, Horowitz JD. Effects of a multidisciplinary, home-based intervention on unplanned admissions and survival among patients with chronic congestive heart failure: A randomized controlled study. *Lancet.* 1999;354:1077–1083.

18. Paul S. Impact of a nurse-managed heart failure clinic: A pilot study. *Heart Lung.* 2000;9:140–146.

19. Dahl J, Penque S. The effects of an advanced practice nurse-directed heart failure program. *Nurse Pract.* 2000;25:61–77.

20. Tilney CK, Whiting SB, Horrar JL, Perkins BD, Vance RP, Reeves JD. Improved clinical and financial outcomes associated with a comprehensive congestive heart failure program. *Dis Manage.* 1998;1:175–183.

21. Fonarow GG, Stevenson LW, Walden JA, et al. Impact of a comprehensive heart failure management program on hospital readmission and functional status of patients with advanced heart failure. *J Am Coll Cardiol.* 1997;30:725–732.

22. West JA, Miller NH, Parker KM, et al. A comprehensive management system for heart failure improves clinical outcomes and reduces medical resources. *Am J Cardiol.* 1997;79:58–63.

23. Smith LE, Fabbri SA, Pai R, Ferry D, Heywood JT. Symptomatic improvement and reduced hospitalization for patients attending a cardiomyopathy clinic. *Clin Cardiol.* 1997;20:949–954.

24. Hanumanthu S, Butler J, Chomsky D, Davis S, Wilson JR. Effects of a heart failure program on hospitalization frequency and exercise tolerance. *Circulation.* 1997;96:2842–2848.

25. Moser DK, Macko MJ, Worster P. Community case management decreases rehospitalization rates and costs, and improves quality of life in heart failure patients with preserved and non-preserved left ventricular function: A randomized controlled trial. Under review.

26. Jaarsma T, Halfens R, Huijer A-SH, Dracup K, Diederiks J, Tan F. Self-care and quality of life in patients with advanced heart failure: The effect of a supportive educative intervention. *Heart Lung.* In press.

27. Cintron G, Bigas C, Linares E, Aranda JM, Hernandez E. Nurse practitioner role in a chronic congestive heart failure clinic: In-hospital time, costs, and patient satisfaction. *Heart Lung.*1983;12:237–240.

28. Karnowski R, Zeeli D, Averbuch M, et al. Intensive home-care surveillance prevents hospitalization and improves morbidity rates among elderly patients with severe congestive heart failure. *Am Heart J.* 1995;129:762–766.

29. Serxner S, Miyaji M, Jeffords J. Congestive heart failure disease management: A patient education intervention. *Congestive Heart Failure.* 1998;4:23–28.

30. Shah NB, Der E, Ruggerio C, Heidenreich PA, Massie BM. Prevention of hospitalizations for heart failure with an interactive home monitoring program. *Am Heart J.* 1998;135:373–378.

31. Weinberger M, Oddone EZ, Henderson WG, for the Veterans Affair Cooperative Study Group on Primary Care and Hospital Readmission. Does increased access to primary care reduce hospital readmissions? *N Engl J Med.* 1996;333:1190–1195.

32. Cline CMJ, Israelsson BYA, Willenheimer RB, Broms K, Erhardt LR. Cost effective management programme for heart failure reduces hospitalisation. *Heart.* 1998;80:442–446.

33. Moser DK, Worster PL. Effect of psychosocial factors on physiologic outcomes in patients with heart failure. *J Cardiovasc Nurs.* 2000;14:106–115.

34. Fergus I, Demopoulos LA, LeJemtel TH. Quality of life in older patients with congestive heart failure: Effects of ACE inhibitors. *Drugs Aging.* 1996;1:23–28.

35. Udelson JE, DeAbate CA, Berk M, et al. Effects of amlodipine on exercise tolerance, quality of life, and left ventricular function in patients with heart failure from left ventricular systolic dysfunction. *Am Heart J.* 2000;139:503–510.

36. Rogers WJ, Johnstone DE, Yusuf S, et al, for the SOLVD Investigators. Quality of life among 5,025 patients with left ventricular dysfunction randomized between placebo and enalapril: The Studies of Left Ventricular Dysfunction. *J Am Coll Cardiol.* 1994;23:393–400.

37. Townsend JN, Littler WA. Angiotensin converting enzyme inhibitors in heart failure: How good are they? *Br Heart J.* 1993;69:373–375.

38. Heidenreich PA, Ruggerio CM, Massie BM. Effect of a home monitoring system on hospitalization and resource use for patients with heart failure. *Am Heart J.* 1999;138:633–640.

39. Kostis JB, Rosen RC, Cosgrove NM, Shindler DM, Wilson AC. Nonpharmacologic therapy improves functional and emotional status in congestive heart failure. *Chest.* 1994;106:996–1001.

40. Moser DK, Kim KA, Baisden-O'Brien J. Impact of a nonpharmacologic cognitive intervention on clinical

and psychosocial outcomes in patients with advanced heart failure. *Circulation.* 1999;100:I-99.

41. Tyni-Lynné R, Gordon A, Sylven C. Improved quality of life in chronic heart failure patients following local endurance training with leg muscles. *J Cardiac Failure.* 1996;2:111–117.

42. Kavanagh T, Myers MG, Baigrie RS, Mertens DJ, Sawyer P, Shephard RJ. Quality of life and cardiorespiratory function in chronic heart failure: Effects of 12 months' aerobic training. *Heart.* 1996;76:42–49.

43. Shephard RJ, Kavanagh T, Mertens DJ. On the prediction of physiological and psychological responses to aerobic training in patients with stable congestive heart failure. *J Cardiopulm Rehabil.* 1998;18:45–51.

44. Tyni-Lynné R, Gordon A, Jansson E, Bermann G, Sylvé C. Skeletal muscle endurance training improves peripheral oxidative capacity, exercise tolerance, and health-related quality of life in women with chronic congestive heart failure secondary to either ischemic cardiomyopathy or idiopathic cardiomyopathy. *Am J Cardiol.* 1997;80:1025–1028.

45. Wielenga RP, Erdman RAM, Huisveld IA, et al. Effect of exercise training on quality of life in patients with chronic heart failure. *J Psychosom Res.* 1998;45:459–464.

46. Willenheimer R, Erhardt L, Cline C, Rydberg E, Israelsson B. Exercise training in heart failure improves quality of life and exercise capacity. *Eur Heart J.* 1998;19:774–781.

47. Belardinelli R, Georgiou D, Cianit G, Purcaro A. Randomized, controlled trial of long-term moderate exercise training in chronic heart failure. Effects on functional capacity, quality of life, and clinical outcomes. *Circulation.* 1999;99:1173–1182.

48. Quittan M, Sturm B, Wiesinger GF, Pacher R, Fialka-Moser V. Quality of life in patients with chronic heart failure: A randomized controlled trial of changes induced by a regular exercise program. *Scand J Rehabil Med.* 1999;31:223–228.

49. Gottlieb SS, Fisher ML, Freudenberger R, et al. Effects of exercise training on peak performance and quality of life in congestive heart failure patients. *J Cardiac Failure.* 1999;5:188–194.

50. Moser DK. Expert management of heart failure: Optimal health care delivery programs. *Annu Rev Nurs Res.* 2000;18:91–126.

51. Rector TS, Johnson G, Dunkman WB, et al. Evaluation by patients with heart failure of the effects of enalapril compared with hydralazine plus isosorbide dinitrate on quality of life. *Circulation.* 1993;87(suppl VI):VI-71–VI-77.

52. Rector TS, Cohn JN. Assessment of patient outcome with the Minnesota Living with Heart Failure Questionnaire: Reliability and validity during a randomized, double-blind, placebo-controlled trial of pimobendan. *Am Heart J.* 1992;124:1017–1025.

53. Rector TS, Kubo SH, Cohn JN. Patients' self-assessment of their congestive heart failure. *Heart Failure.* 1987;3198–3209.

54. Ware JE, Sherbourne CD. The MOS 36-item short-form health survey (SF-36). I. Conceptual framework and item selection. *Med Care.* 1992;30:473–483.

55. Ware JE, Snow KK, Kosinski M. *SF-36 Health Survey Manual and Interpretation Guide.* Boston: The Health Institute, New England Medical Center; 1993.

56. Gorkin L, Norvell NK, Rosen RC, et al. Assessment of quality of life as observed from the baseline data of the Studies of Left Ventricular Dysfunction (SOLVD): Trial quality-of-life substudy. *Am J Cardiol.* 1993;71:1069–1073.

57. Bennett SJ, Baker SL, Huster GA. Quality of life in women with heart failure. *Health Care Women Int.* 1998;19:217–229.

58. Martensson J, Karlsson J-E, Fridlund B. Male patients with congestive heart failure and their conception of their life situation. *J Adv Nurs.* 1997;25:579–586.

59. Grady KL, Jalowiec A, Grusk BB, White-Williams C, Robinson JA. Symptom distress in cardiac transplant candidates. *Heart Lung.* 1992;21:434–439.

60. Grady KL, Jalowiec A, White-Williams C, et al. Predictors of quality of life in patients with advanced heart failure awaiting transplantation. *J Heart Lung Transplant.* 1995;14:2–10.

61. Blackwood R, Mayou RA, Garnham JC, Armstron C, Bryant B. Exercise capacity and quality of life in the treatment of heart failure. *Clin Pharmacol Ther.* 1990;48:325–332.

62. Cleland JGF. Are symptoms the most important target for therapy in chronic heart failure? *Prog Cardiovasc Dis.* 1998;41:59–64.

63. Shapiro DH Jr, Schwartz CE, Astin JA. Controlling ourselves: Controlling our world. Psychology's role in understanding positive and negative consequences of seeking and gaining control. *Am Psychol.* 1996;51:1213–1230.

64. Moser DK, Dracup K. Psychosocial recovery from a cardiac event: The influence of perceived control. *Heart Lung.* 1995;24:273–280.

65. Moser DK. Social support in cardiac recovery. *J Cardiovasc Nurs.* 1994;9(1):741–785.

66. Friedman MM, King KB. The relationship of emotional and tangible support to psychological well-being among older women with heart failure. *Res Nurs Health.* 1994;17:433–440.

67. Baas LS, Fontana JA, Bhat G. Relationships between self-care resources and the quality of life of persons with heart failure: A comparison of treatment groups. *Prog Cardiovasc Nurs.* 1997;12(1):25–38.

68. Guzetta CE, Kessler CA, Dossey BM, Moser DK. Alternative/complementary therapies. In: Kinney MR, Dunbar SB, Brooks-Brun JA, Molter N, Vitello-Cicciu

JM, eds. *AACN Clinical Reference for Critical Care Nursing*. St. Louis, MO: Mosby; 1998.

69. Moser DK, Dracup K, Woo MA, Stevenson LW. Voluntary control of vascular tone using skin temperature biofeedback-relaxation in patients with advanced heart failure. *Altern Ther Health Med*. 1997;3(1):51.

70. Smith TW, Braunwald E, Kelly RA. The management of heart failure. In: Braunwald E, ed. *Heart Disease*. Philadelphia, WB Saunders Company; 1992:464–519.

71. Coats AJS. Exercise rehabilitation in chronic heart failure. *J Am Coll Cardiol*. 1993;22(suppl A):172A–177A.

72. McElvie RS, Teo KK, McCartney N, Humen D, Montague T, Yusuf S. Effects of exercise training in patients with congestive heart failure: A critical review. *J Am Coll Cardiol*. 1995;25:789–796.

73. Cohen-Solal A, Sellier P. Cardiac rehabilitation and chronic heart failure. *Heart Failure*. 1997;13:59–63,76.

74. Coats AJS, Adamopoulos S, Radaelli A, et al. Controlled trial of physical training in chronic heart failure: Exercise performance, hemodynamics, ventilation, and autonomic function. *Circulation*. 1992;85:2119–2131.

75. Dubach P, Myers J, Dziekan G, et al. Effect of high intensity exercise training on central hemodynamic responses to exercise in men with reduced left ventricular function. *J Am Coll Cardiol*. 1997;29:1591–1598.

76. Hambrecht R, Fiehn E, Yu Jet al. Effects of endurance training on mitochondrial ultrastructure and fiber type distribution in skeletal muscle of patients with stable chronic heart failure. *J Am Coll Cardiol*. 1997;29:1067–1073.

77. Meyer K, Schwaibold M, Westbrook S, et al. Effects of exercise training and activity restriction on 6-minute walking test performance in patients with chronic heart failure. *Am Heart J*. 1997;133:447–453.

78. Kiilavuori K, Sovijarvi A, Naveri H, Ikonen T, Leinonen H. Effect of physical training on exercise capacity and gas exchange in patients with chronic heart failure. *Chest*. 1996;110:985–991.

79. Keteyian SJ, Levine AB, Brawner CA, et al. Exercise training in patients with heart failure. A randomized, controlled trial. *Ann Intern Med*. 1996;124:1051–1057.

80. Kiilavuori K, Toivonen L, Naveri H, Leinonen H. Reversal of autonomic derangements by physical training in chronic heart failure assessed by heart rate variability. *Eur Heart J*. 1995;16:490–495.

81. Belardinelli R, Georgiou D, Scocco V, Barstow TJ, Purcaro A. Low intensity exercise training in patients with chronic heart failure. *J Am Coll Cardiol*. 1995;26:975–982.

82. Hambrecht R, Niebauer J, Fiehn E, et al. Physical training in patients with stable chronic heart failure: Effects on cardiorespiratory fitness and ultrastructural abnormalities of leg muscles. *J Am Coll Cardiol*. 1995;25:1239–1249.

83. Adamopoulos S, Coats AJ, Brunotte F, et al. Physical training improves skeletal muscle metabolism in patients with chronic heart failure. *J Am Coll Cardiol*. 1993;21:1101–1106.

84. Michalos AC. Job satisfaction, marital satisfaction, and the quality of life: A review and a preview. In: Andres FM, ed. *Research on the Quality of Life*. Ann Arbor, MI: Institute for Social Research, University of Michigan; 1986:57–83.

85. Linder-Pelz, S. Social psychological determinants of patient satisfaction: A test of five hypotheses. *Soc Sci Med*. 1982;16:583–589.

86. Cella DF. Functional status and quality of life: Current views on measurement and intervention. In: *Proceedings, Functional Status and Quality of Life in Persons with Cancer, Nov 30–Dec 2, 1989*. Atlanta, GA: American Cancer Society; 1–11.

87. Kinney MR, Burfitt SN, Stullenbarger E, Rees B, DeBolt MR. Quality of life in cardiac patient research: A meta-analysis. *Nurs Res*. 1996;45:173–180.

PART III

Improving Outcomes with Nonpharmacologic Management

CHAPTER 7

Nutritional Management of the Patient with Heart Failure

Susan J. Bennett, Laurie Hackward, and Sara A. Blackburn

The nutritional management of the patient with heart failure presents a special challenge for health care providers because of the complex problems that occur with heart failure, including sodium retention, malnutrition, and coexisting disorders such as diabetes mellitus. Nutritional management is focused on dietary sodium restrictions for all heart failure patients and treatment of malnutrition and cardiac cachexia in patients with advanced heart failure. Additional areas that may require nutritional intervention include hypovolemia and dehydration. A multidisciplinary team is necessary to optimize nutritional status because of the complexity of heart failure. Indeed, satisfactory nutritional management of patients with heart failure has the potential to minimize or prevent negative outcomes related to mortality, morbidity, and health-related quality of life.

In this chapter we discuss the major nutritional problems found in patients with heart failure. The nutrition assessment, including physical and clinical assessments to determine nutritional status, is described. Goals and interventions for the specific nutritional problems are presented. Compliance with the medical nutrition therapy is discussed in detail in Chapter 9.

NUTRITION ASSESSMENT

A complete evaluation and assessment by a dietitian are necessary on the initial diagnosis of heart failure for several compelling reasons. First, persons with heart failure are at high risk for sodium retention and malnutrition, both of which are associated with poor outcomes. As many as 60% of hospital admissions for heart failure are due to sodium retention.[1] Previous investigators reported that cachexia occurred in 16% of 171 patients with New York Heart Association (NYHA) Class I through IV heart failure,[2] whereas 50% of patients with severe heart failure were found to have malnutrition.[3] Cachexia is an independent predictor of mortality[2] and maybe a predictor of morbidity and poor quality of life, although this relationship has not been specifically documented through research. Second, the information obtained at initial diagnosis will provide a baseline on which to evaluate subsequent changes in nutritional status. Third, early detection of and intervention for the patient who has sodium retention or malnutrition developing might prevent or delay negative outcomes. Fourth, severe malnutrition is difficult to reverse once the process begins. Treatment of severe malnutrition is compounded by the accompanying severity of the heart failure among patients who have end-stage disease.

By use of the initial nutrition assessment of the patient with heart failure, the dietitian will develop a profile of the patient's current nutritional status, identify possible causes of existing nutritional disturbances, and recommend a medical nutrition plan. It is important to determine whether the patient is malnourished and, if so, the degree of malnourishment to develop a corrective medical nutrition therapy plan for him or her. Subsequent evaluations to monitor and/or correct the patient's nutritional status may be completed by another member of the multidisciplinary team who is knowledgeable about the assessment parameters.

Nutrition assessment is an indirect evaluation of body composition and cellular function.[4,5] An in-depth assessment includes evaluation of (1) anthropometric measurements (height, weight, and measurements of skeletal muscle mass); (2) selected biochemical serum markers; (3) clinical and physical examination; and (4) current dietary intake, medications, and symptoms. This assessment incorporates evaluation of the six body compartments: adipose tissue; skin and skeleton; extracellular; plasma protein; visceral protein mass; and skeletal muscle body cell mass. These compartments are assessed to determine the status of the protein and adipose tissues of the body. Depletion of plasma protein, visceral protein mass, and skeletal muscle body cell mass are of primary importance, because all proteins in the body are functional, and the loss of protein adversely affects body function.

For the patient with heart failure, changes in fluid and electrolyte balance complicate the assessment of nutritional status. Therefore, assessment of fluid and electrolyte balance is incorporated into the nutrition assessment of these patients.

Anthropometric Measurements

The health care professional should obtain an accurate baseline height and weight for each patient. Self-reported heights and weights are not reliable because women tend to underreport their weight and men to overreport their height.[6]

Height

Establishing an accurate baseline of height is important because evaluation of body mass index and body composition depends on height. Furthermore, it cannot be assumed that height is stable once adult height is achieved. Changes in height can occur with age and disease, and therefore height should be measured every 3 to 5 years in adults and annually in persons older than the age of 50.[7]

The arm span measurement is useful to estimate the height of wheelchair-bound or bedridden patients. Measure in inches from the patient's sternal notch to the longest finger on the dominant hand and double the measurement number. Convert this number to feet and inches to estimate the patient's height.[8]

Weight

Body weight is an indirect measure of total body energy stores and of protein mass.[5] Body weight should be monitored routinely because changes in body weight parallel changes in energy and protein balance and fluid volume.[5] Body weight may be influenced by the fluid and electrolyte status of the heart failure patient. A weight gain of greater than 0.5 kg/day is indicative of fluid volume increase rather than an increase in body mass. In the absence of caloric restriction, a weight loss of more than 0.5 kg/day indicates fluid volume decrease. In a person who is experiencing a gradual loss of lean body mass and fluid retention, body weight may be unchanged. The patient with heart failure may have episodes in which fluid shifts from the extracellular to the interstitial spaces, leading to the development of pulmonary edema without a change in body weight. Additional assessments, including a physical examination and a chest X-ray examination, are required to detect these changes.

In a clinic or hospital setting, the platform balance scale is the preferred method for obtaining an accurate weight. The scale must be on a firm and level surface, not a carpet, to ensure an accurate reading. Routinely calibrate the scale to maintain accuracy. In the hospital setting, it is important to have consistency in the types of scale available across multiple units to improve the comparison of the weights.

Patients with heart failure should weigh themselves daily at home. Clinicians should instruct patients to weigh themselves in the morning, after emptying the bladder, before eating or drinking, and while wearing light clothing without shoes.

For hospitalized patients, the intake and output records are useful to interpret significant weight changes. Fluctuations in fluid status, including edema or ascites, may mask loss in chemical or cellular body components. In addition, depleted protein stores caused by inadequate caloric and protein intake may cause the extracellular fluid volume to increase, which makes an assessment of the severity of lean tissue depletion more difficult.

On the initial visit to the clinic or office or on hospitalization, the patient should be asked his or her weight history. A comprehensive weight history can provide valuable information that gives a picture over time. A weight history might include weight over the past 6 months, preferred weight, highest and lowest adult weight, and patterns of weight fluctuations before the diagnosis of heart failure. Losses in lean muscle mass and adipose tissue may be missed if a weight history is not obtained.

Body Mass Index

Weight to height can be mathematically interpreted by the body mass index (BMI). The index, developed by Quetelet (weight in kilograms/[height in meters]^2)or ($704.5 \times$ [weight in pounds/height in inches^2]), is the most widely accepted method,[6] although it does not distinguish weight from lean muscle or adipose tissue. Other measures of body composition such as skinfold or muscle circumference may enhance the usefulness of BMI. A program to calculate BMI for varying heights and weights is available from the following Web site address: www.nhlbi.nih.gov/health/public/heart/obesity/lose_wt/index.htm.[9] A chart for determining BMI can be found in the *Clinical Guidelines on the Identification, Evaluation, and Treatment of Overweight and Obesity in Adults*.[10]

Biochemical Serum Markers

Selected biochemical serum markers are indicators of diminished nutrient intake and changes that occur in response to pathophysiological alterations.[11] Measurements of albumin, prealbumin, hemoglobin, and hematocrit can be used to evaluate the body protein. Cardiovascular disease risk status is assessed through examination of the lipid profile, including total serum cholesterol, low-density lipoprotein, high-density lipoprotein, and triglyceride levels.

Albumin and Prealbumin

Albumin has been used for many years as a measure of protein-calorie malnutrition.[12,13] In the clinical setting, it is generally thought that albumin is depressed in periods of stress and reduced dietary intake. Shifts in fluid status and alterations in albumin synthesis and degradation can affect albumin levels. Albumin may not be an accurate indicator for early protein depletion because of its 20-day half-life. Depression of serum albumin levels may reflect an acute metabolic response to fever and infection rather than depletion of body mass. Albumin values ranging from 3.5 to 5.0 g/dL are considered within normal limits for adults.[14]

Some clinicians are now using prealbumin levels rather than albumin as an assessment of changes in protein status. Prealbumin has a 2- to 3-day half-life and may more accurately reflect overall energy and nitrogen balance. Normal values are 0.2 to 0.4 g/dL.[15,16]

Serum Cholesterol and Triglycerides

Elevated total cholesterol, low-density lipoproteins, and triglycerides contribute to the development of coronary heart disease.[17,18] Hyperlipidemia may contribute to worsening heart failure in some patients, particularly those patients with underlying coronary heart disease. High-density lipoproteins are believed to have a protective effect against coronary heart disease.[18] The upper limits of cholesterol and triglycerides, as recommended by the National Cholesterol Education Panel[19] and the American Heart Association Task Force on Risk Reduction,[20] are presented in Table 7–1.

Although the lower limits for cholesterol and triglyceride levels have not been established, these levels may be depressed. Decreased cholesterol levels may indicate impaired cholesterol metabolism, malabsorption syndromes, acute or chronic inflammatory diseases, or a variety of anemias.[14] Decreased levels of triglycerides may be associated with protein malnutrition, hyper-

Table 7–1 Guidelines for Lipid Levels*

Lipid	Level
Total cholesterol	150–240 mg/dL, desirable level < 200 mg/dL to reduce cardio-vascular risk
Low-density lipoprotein (LDL)	60–160 mg/dL
For people without coronary heart disease and < 2 risk factors	< 160 mg/dL
For people without coronary heart disease and with 2 or more risk factors	< 130 mg/dL
For people with coronary heart disease	< 100 mg/dL
High-density lipoprotein (HDL)	> 35 mg/dL
Triglycerides	< 200 mg/dL

*National Cholesterol Education Panel.

thyroidism, or hyperparathyroidism.[14] In patients with decreased cholesterol or triglyceride levels, the management goal is to increase levels to within normal range for the patient's age and gender. Only one study was found that specifically assessed the impact of triglyceride levels among patients with heart failure. The authors found that triglycerides were significantly lower in patients who were malnourished.[3]

Hemoglobin and Hematocrit

Depressed levels of hemoglobin and hematocrit may represent inadequate diet, depressed protein synthesis, impaired absorption of nutrients (vitamin B_{12}, folic acid, pyridoxine, iron), or the anemia of chronic disease.[11,21] The anemia of chronic disease may occur in patients with heart failure, possibly as a metabolic response to stimulation of the cellular immune system involving macrophage activity and elevation of cytokines such as tumor necrosis factor-α and interleukin-1.[21] Hemoglobin and hematocrit levels are sensitive to alterations in fluid balance. With hypervolemia, hemoglobin and hematocrit may appear to be low because of a dilutional ef-

fect. With dehydration, these levels may appear to be elevated because of hemoconcentration. Normal values for hemoglobin are as follows: women, 12 to 15 g/dL; men, 13.5 to 17 g/dL.[14] The normal range for hematocrit values are 36%–46% for women and 40%–50% for men.[14]

Serum Glucose

Serum glucose is monitored to assess the patient for hyperglycemia, which is typically associated with diabetes mellitus, a known risk factor for coronary heart disease. Normal serum glucose (fasting blood sugar levels) ranges from 70 to 110 mg/dL.[14] Additional assessment of patients with suspected diabetes mellitus involves a detailed evaluation that is beyond the scope of this chapter.

Laboratory Tests for Fluid and Electrolyte Assessment

Measurements of serum electrolytes, blood urea nitrogen, creatinine, and osmolality are useful in assessing fluid and electrolyte balance. Urine values of electrolytes, particularly sodium and osmolality, are also used when assessing fluid and electrolyte balance. The main serum laboratory tests that are altered with hypervolemia and hypovolemia are presented in Table 7–2.

Serum Sodium

Sodium is a major cation in the body's extracellular fluid and is associated with regulation of water balance, regulation of acid-base balance, and neuromuscular conduction. The minimum daily requirement of sodium for healthy adults is 500 mg.[13] Elevated serum sodium, or hypernatremia, occurs when sodium intake is increased or when more water is lost than sodium, such as during dehydration. Diuretics may contribute to hypernatremia in heart failure patients. Hyponatremia, or low serum sodium, is associated with conditions in which sodium is lost (vomiting, diarrhea, gastric suction, burns, or tissue injuries) or restricted, such as reduced dietary intake. Heart failure patients may also experience decreased serum sodium levels as a re-

Table 7–2 Laboratory Values That May Be Altered with Hypervolemia and Hypovolemia

	Hypervolemia	*Hypovolemia*
Serum sodium	Within normal limits or decreased (hemodilution)	Within normal limits or increased (hemoconcentration)
Urine sodium	Decreased	Varies with condition
Serum osmolality	Decreased	Increased
Urine osmolality	Decreased	Increased
Blood urea nitrogen		Increased (hemoconcentration)
Creatinine		Within normal limits or increased
Hemoglobin and hematocrit	Decreased (hemodilution)	Increased (hemoconcentration)

sult of hypervolemia, which causes a dilutional hyponatremia. Normal serum sodium levels for adults are 135–145 mEq/L.[14]

Urine Sodium

Dietary sodium intake, aldosterone secretion, urine volume, and certain diseases influence urine sodium excretion. Elevated urine sodium may be noted in dehydration, hypertension, diabetes mellitus, or when sodium intake is high. Urine sodium is decreased when sodium is retained or sodium intake is reduced, which may occur in patients with heart failure and patients receiving diuretic therapy. Urine sodium levels are also decreased in hepatic and renal failure, chronic obstructive pulmonary disease, and Cushing's syndrome. Normal values of urine sodium in adults range from 40 to 220 mEq/L/24h.[14]

Serum Potassium

Potassium is a major intracellular cation. The daily potassium requirement is 40 mEq/day. Elevated serum potassium, or hyperkalemia, occurs when potassium is unable to be excreted from the kidneys (oliguria, renal failure), excess potassium is administered orally or parenterally, or when potassium is released from the cells (major tissue trauma, acidosis). Hypokalemia occurs when potassium is lost such as during vomiting, diarrhea, malnutrition, and physiologic stress. In patients with heart failure, hypokalemia may occur with diuretic therapy, and

careful assessment and replacement of potassium is essential. Serum potassium levels range from 3.5 to 5.3 mEq/L in the adult.[14]

Serum Osmolality

Serum osmolality indicates the concentration of the serum. Specifically, it is a measure of the number of dissolved particles within the serum. Normal serum osmolality ranges from 280–300 mOsm/kg. Elevated levels indicate hemoconcentration, often caused by dehydration. Decreased values indicate hemodilution and hypervolemia.[14]

Urine Osmolality

Urine osmolality provides assessment of the concentration of particles in the urine. Hemoconcentration results in elevated urine osmolality, whereas hemodilution and volume excess are associated with decreased urine osmolality. Diuretic therapy may be associated with decreased urine osmolality values when urine is dilute. Urine osmolality in the adult ranges from 50–1,200 mOsm/kg H_2O, with an average value of 200–800 mOsm/kg H_2O.[14]

Blood Urea Nitrogen and Serum Creatinine

Abnormalities of blood urea nitrogen (BUN) and creatinine further indicate the multiple metabolic factors that have an impact on patients with heart failure. Elevated BUN and creatinine may indicate impaired renal function and the need to modify the diet by reducing nitrogen intake to compensate for this dysfunction. Elevated BUN and creatinine may also be indicative of hypovolemia and dehydration that can occur with excessive diuresis. With hypervolemia, BUN may be decreased. The normal BUN is 5–25 mg/dL, and normal creatinine ranges from 0.5–1.5 mg/dL.[14]

Physical Examination

The physical examination is an important clinical method to detect nutritional status, particularly malnutrition, in the edematous patient when weight, biochemical measures, and other laboratory values may be skewed. Most of the areas assessed in the physical examination described in the following list are unlikely to be edematous. The characteristics of well-nourished, mild to moderately malnourished, and severely malnourished individuals are described in the following list.[22]

- Temples: Hollowing near the temple is a sign of muscle loss (see Figure 7–1).
- Clavicles: The clavicle is quite prominent in a malnourished patient. However, remember that women tend to have a more prominent clavicle even when well nourished.
- Shoulders: The shoulders of a well-nourished patient are rounded, whereas the shoulders are more square in someone with muscle loss.
- Scapulas and ribs: Like the clavicle, the scapula becomes more prominent as muscle loss occurs and the ribs are obvious (see Figure 7–2).
- Hands: The interosseous muscle is connected to the thumb and forefinger. When pressing the thumb and forefinger together, the muscle will bulge in a well-nourished person. If the person is malnourished, there will actually be a depression between the thumb and forefinger with no detection of the muscle present.
- Quadriceps and knees: Look at the inner thigh. Slight depressions indicate some degree of malnutrition. Grasp the thigh to feel the muscle and fat tissue. If malnourished,

the quadriceps will be reduced, and the knee and calf muscle will also show signs of decreased tissue.
- Eyes: Examine the fat pads of the eye. In well-nourished individuals, the fat pads underneath the eyes appear as a slight bulge. Fat loss around the eyes will make the eyes look hollow and/or dark (see Figure 7–3).
- Triceps/biceps: Pinch the skin where the triceps and biceps are located. If your fingers meet, there is subcutaneous fat loss in these areas (see Figure 7–4).

Other pertinent assessments that influence nutrition should also be noted at this time, such as poor dentition.

Signs of Sodium Retention and Hypervolemia

Peripheral signs of fluid retention include edema of the ankles and legs. The edema occurs in dependent areas such as the feet and ankles of patients who are mobile or sitting or the sacrum of patients who are recumbent. The face, eyelids, fingers, and hands may become edematous. In men, scrotal edema may occur. As fluid retention progresses, jugular venous distention, hepatomegaly, and ascites may develop. Other signs of fluid retention detected on physical examination include tachypnea, a dry hacking cough, crackles, increased pulse pressure, tachycardia, bounding pulse, and an S_3 gallop. In severe cases, pulmonary edema may develop, requiring immediate medical intervention.[23–25]

Signs of Hypovolemia and Dehydration

Decreased pulse volume and pulse pressure, hypotension, tachycardia, and decreased urine output are noted on physical examination in patients with hypovolemia and dehydration. The skin and mucous membranes are dry with poor skin turgor. The temperature may be elevated with severe dehydration. Patients may complain of thirst and mental status changes may be noted.[23–25]

Cardiovascular Risk Factors

During the physical examination, the presence of cardiovascular risk factors should be noted. For example, blood pressure and alter-

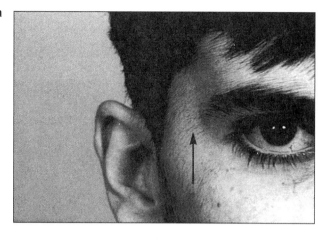

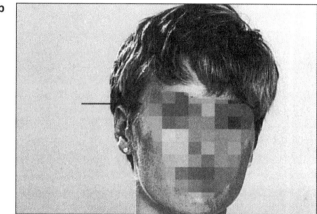

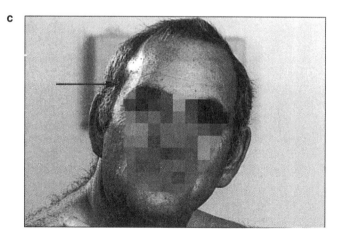

Figure 7–1 (a) Malnourished temple; (b) moderately malnourished temple; (c) well-nourished temple.

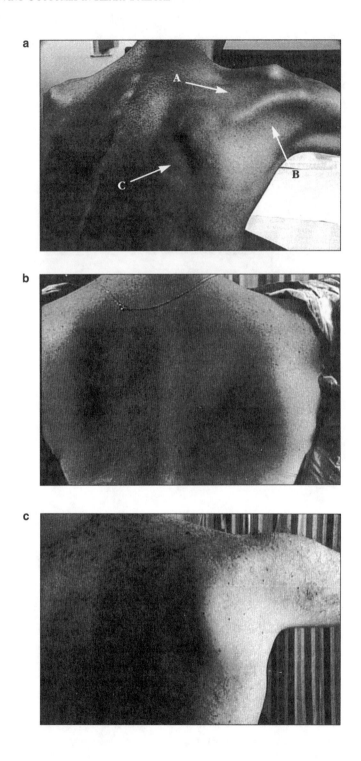

Figure 7–2 (a) Severely malnourished scapula; (b) moderately malnourished scapula; (c) well-nourished scapula. Arrows in figure (a) indicate evidence of tissue wasting.

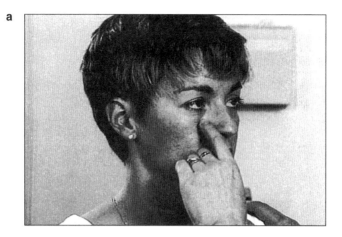

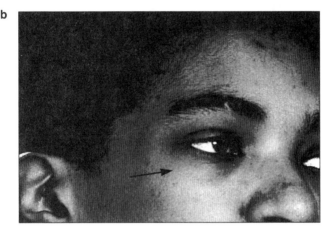

Figure 7–3 (a) Well-nourished eyes; (b) severely malnourished eyes.

ations resulting from hypertension or diabetes mellitus should be assessed.

Diet History

Current Dietary Intake Evaluation

A dietary evaluation is used initially to assess current dietary intake and routinely thereafter to assess compliance with the prescribed diet recommendations and monitor the nutritional status. The method used to assess dietary intake varies but may include obtaining a record of the foods and drinks consumed in the past 24 hours or the past 3 days or a food frequency question-naire. These methods can be used alone or in combination to evaluate dietary intake. Examples of two food frequency questionnaires are the Health Habits and History Questionnaire[26] and Willet's food frequency questionnaire.[27]

The Food Guide Pyramid[28] can be used as a tool for health care professionals in determining dietary intake. The Pyramid is a general population food guide, in which the recommended servings and appropriate portion sizes for different food items are shown. By comparing the patient's diet to the Guide, one can ascertain food group deficiencies and nutrients missing in the diet. A specific diet recommendation can be

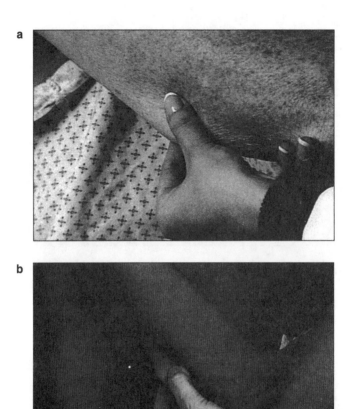

Figure 7–4 (a) Well-nourished triceps; (b) malnourished triceps; (c) nourished biceps; (d) malnourished biceps.

made if the patient is not eating enough nutritionally dense food sources.

Medical History

Coexisting medical conditions may have an independent effect on nutritional status and need to be evaluated as part of the patient's diet history. Comorbidities that commonly occur with heart failure and influence nutritional status include hypertension, hyperlipidemia, and diabetes mellitus. Recent surgery, food–drug interactions, and heart failure symptoms are other factors that suggest risk for malnutrition. Gastrointestinal symptoms lasting longer than 2 weeks are considered significant in a clinical nutrition examination. The more severe the coexisting medical condition the more food intake may be affected.

Symptoms of Heart Failure

The troublesome symptoms associated with heart failure can interfere with nutritional status and compliance with nutrition recommendations. When caring for the patient with heart failure, it is important to remember that symptoms are not always highly associated with the level of disease severity.[29]

c

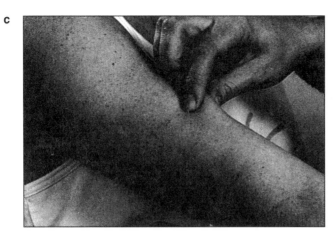

d

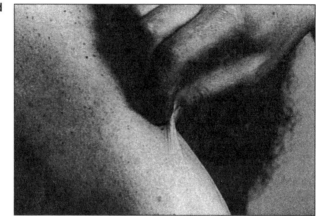

Figure 7–4 continued

Dyspnea and fatigue, the two most common symptoms of heart failure, can interfere with appetite, which limits the quantities of foods eaten and increases the risk of cachexia. This difficulty can establish a cycle in which less energy from food is available for the patient, which in turn reduces the body's energy stores even more. Dyspnea and fatigue may also interfere with nutritional status because patients may not have the physical energy required for shopping for food, carrying groceries, lifting arms over the head to place groceries in cabinets, and standing during meal preparation.[30] Likewise, cleaning, cutting, and cooking low-sodium foods (eg, fresh fruits and vegetables) may take more energy than

opening ready-to-eat foods and may not be possible for this patient.

Diminished cognitive function is another symptom of heart failure that may contribute to noncompliance with nutrition recommendations. Patients with heart failure report decreased concentration, attention, and memory as major problems.[30] Patients with diminished cognitive function may not be able to plan, shop for, or prepare nutritionally balanced meals. If patients cannot drive an automobile, their food supply may be limited. In addition, they may not understand the ways to prepare nutritious meals.

Patients with heart failure experience anorexia, nausea, and vomiting that reduce their appetite, decrease their food intake, and ultimately contribute to cachexia. Poor taste can contribute to patients not following dietary recommendations. Sodium-restricted diets do not taste good to many patients.[31] Patients identify altered taste, such as a metallic taste in the mouth, as a problem that influences their ability to eat.[30] The reason for the metallic taste is unclear. Many heart failure patients are elderly, and as patients age, taste buds are lost so food may taste bland and unappetizing.

Patients with heart failure report restricting activity as a primary way of dealing with dyspnea and fatigue.[30] Reduced activity may suppress appetite in some patients. Depression is commonly associated with heart failure[32] and may diminish a person's appetite, leading to inadequate food intake to meet daily energy needs and ultimately to loss of lean muscle and adipose tissue.

Finally, medication side effects may play a part in appetite. For example, a well-known side effect of digitalis toxicity is anorexia, nausea, and vomiting. Some patients who are required to take large doses of diuretics report difficulty shopping for foods because of urinary frequency or urgency.

Social and Cultural Factors

Eating is a social activity. The ability to participate fully in social and leisure activities is a major problem reported by patients with heart failure[33] that contributes to inadequate food intake. Decreases in social activity may contribute to inadequate food intake. Patients with heart failure are more likely to be elderly and live alone because the incidence of heart failure doubles each decade after age 40.[34]

The types of food eaten may be related to socioeconomic status. Foods required for a sodium-restricted diet (specially prepared canned items and fresh fruits and vegetables) may cost more than regular counterparts, thus making sodium-modified foods unavailable to patients with limited financial resources. Elderly patients with heart failure may be living on fixed incomes, be living in group facilities, or have multiple health problems, all of which restrict the types of food available to follow dietary sodium restrictions.

Finally, cultural and ethnic differences of patients require assessment to evaluate their influence on nutrition. Patients mention holidays as times when following a sodium-restricted diet is the most difficult. For example, ham is a food high in sodium that may be part of traditional meals at Christmas or Easter. People with particular religious or cultural backgrounds may not be willing to exclude some foods high in sodium from their diet.

The Subjective Global Assessment Tool

The Subjective Global Assessment (SGA)[35] is a brief clinical assessment questionnaire that can be used to assess nutritional status in busy practice settings. The SGA is a scoring method developed to quickly assess the nutritional status of surgical patients. It was shown by Lichtman[36] to be highly predictive of morbidity and mortality, and other investigators are now using this tool to assess malnutrition among patients with end-stage renal failure, cancer, and acquired immune deficiency syndrome.[37,38] The SGA is shown in Figure 7–5.

There are two parts to the SGA tool: the history and the physical examination. The history details the weight change, dietary intake, gastrointestinal symptoms, and nutritionally related functional capacity. The physical examination focuses on loss of adipose tissue and loss of lean muscle. The scores of the history and physical examination sections are reviewed and the patient is given an overall rating of A, B, or C to indicate the nutritional risk status of the patient.[35] For complete SGA scoring instructions, contact the authors of the SGA or Baxter Healthcare Corporation Renal Division.[22,35]

The well-nourished (A) rating is for those patients exhibiting no signs of malnutrition. Patients who have had some problems in the past but have improved may also receive an (A) rating. The (B) rating is the most ambiguous because it is for those patients who are not well-nourished or severely depleted. These patients may have (A), (B), or (C) ratings assigned be-

Subjective Global Assessment Scoring Sheet*

Patient Name: _____Patient ID: _____Date: _____

	SGA Score		
	A	B	C

Part 1: Medical History

1. Weight Change
   A. Overall change in past 6 months: _____ kgs.
   B. Percent change: _____ gain –<5% loss
                        _____ 5–10% loss
                        _____ >10% loss
   C. Change in past 2 weeks: _____increase
                                _____no change
                                _____decrease

2. Dietary Intake
   A. Overall change: _____no change
                        _____change
   B. Duration: _____weeks
   C. Type of change: _____suboptimal solid diet   _____full liquid diet
                        _____hypocaloric liquids   _____starvation

3. Gastrointestinal Symptoms (persisting for >2 weeks)
      _____none; _____nausea; _____vomiting; _____diarrhea; _____anorexia

4. Functional Impairment (nutritionally related)
   A. Overall impairment: _____none
                            _____moderate
                            _____severe
   B. Change in past 2 weeks: _____improved
                                _____no change
                                _____regressed

Part 2: Physical Examination

	SGA Score		
	Normal	Mild	Moderate	Severe

5. Evidence of: Loss of subcutaneous fat
                    Muscle wasting
                    Edema
                    Ascites

Part 3: SGA Rating (check one)
   A. ❏ Well Nourished B. ❏ Mildly Moderately Malnourished C. ❏ Severely Malnourished

*For complete SGA sheet scoring instructions, contact the authors of the SGA or Baxter Healthcare Corporation Renal Division.[22,35]

Figure 7–5 Subjective Global Assessment (SGA).

tween the different sections. Weight loss of 5% to 10% with a decrease in dietary intake may be seen. Some degree of muscle and fat wasting is usually observed. The patient may or may not experience gastrointestinal symptoms. The severely malnourished (C) rating is reserved for those patients showing obvious signs of malnutrition. These patients exhibit clear signs of significant muscle and fat loss, weight loss of greater than 10%, minimal dietary intake, and several gastrointestinal symptoms.

Summary

In conclusion, assessment of nutritional status of the heart failure patient requires a comprehensive approach to evaluate all factors that influence nutrition and fluid and electrolyte balance. The medical nutrition therapy is developed from this comprehensive assessment.

MANAGEMENT OF MALNUTRITION/ CACHEXIA

Malnutrition is a state that results from changes in diet intake, digestion, absorption, excretion, or metabolic requirements of nutrients.[39] Cachexia is defined as a state of protein-calorie malnutrition that:

> results from a calorie deficit that has extended over months or years. The patient experiences severe wasting of fat and muscle. Arm muscle circumference and skinfold thickness are diminished indicating a loss of muscle tissue and fat stores. The patient also has reduced immune function. Serum proteins may be moderately reduced or normal.[13(pp77,80)]

Cachexia has been termed "cytokine-induced malnutrition"[40(p645)] that is associated with wasting during periods of metabolic stress. Cachexia involves a loss of lean body mass that is metabolically active, and it results in a reduction in strength and immune competence. The weakness that occurs with loss of lean body mass in heart failure patients is a well-known syndrome called cardiac cachexia.[41]

National surveys of patients hospitalized with heart failure have demonstrated that 50% to 68% of these patients exhibit signs of malnutrition on the basis of body weight and on anthropometric and plasma protein measures.[42] Cachexia is known to affect outcomes of patients with heart failure.[2,43,44] In 171 patients with heart failure, Anker and colleagues[2] found cachexia to be an independent predictor of mortality and concluded that the influence of cachexia is so profound that it needs to be measured in all large clinical trials of heart failure patients. Cachexia was defined in the study as "a non-intentional documented weight loss of at least 7.5% of previous normal weight during at least 6 months."[2(p1050)]

The mechanisms that underlie heart failure, in combination with a gradual reduction in appetite and food intake, may lead to a decrease in body weight.[41] Continued weight loss may occur even when energy intake is adequate because of these mechanisms. The weight loss is accompanied by a proportional loss of lean body mass.[45] As lean muscle mass loss continues, functional status may decline. In the seriously ill patient, a significant correlation exists between the loss of body weight and changes in total body protein.[5] A loss of 10% of body weight in less than 6 months is clinically significant.

One mechanism that probably underlies the development of cachexia in patients with heart failure is the elevation of immune substances, particularly inflammatory cytokines. Cytokines elevated in patients with heart failure are tumor necrosis factor-α, interleukin-1, and interleukin-6.[46–48] Elevations in tumor necrosis factor-α were associated with increased physical symptoms, including dyspnea and fatigue, among 23 heart failure patients.[47] It is believed that tumor necrosis factor-α exacerbates a decline in nutritional status by decreasing appetite and food intake over an extended period of time. Tumor necrosis factor-α has been found to be associated with decreased free fatty acid synthesis, increased lipolysis, and accelerated protein catabolism in skeletal muscles. This accelerated protein catabolism may contribute to the fatigue experienced by patients with heart failure.[44,46]

Sympathetic activation leading to elevated catecholamines is another potential mechanism for cachexia in patients with heart failure. Anker and colleagues[49] found that heart failure patients who were cachectic had increased levels of norepinephrine, epinephrine, cortisol, tumor necrosis factor-α, and human growth hormone and decreased levels of plasma sodium. Patients who were not cachectic had levels of norepinephrine and epinephrine that were similar to patients in the control group.

During periods of cachexia, body fat is metabolized and ketoacids derived from fat are used by tissues as a fuel source.[50] With continued depletion of fat stores, there is increased muscle protein metabolism. The metabolic rate slows in proportion to the loss of body cell mass and adipose tissue. The body compensates for the reduced energy intake by decreasing energy expenditure until a new equilibrium is established between energy in and energy out. Previously, it was thought that these patients were hypermetabolic and had higher energy needs, and some evidence supports this view.[41] However, other investigators have recently demonstrated that patients with heart failure who were cachectic had significantly lower daily energy expenditure because of a decrease in physical activity and resting energy expenditure.[51,52]

Changes in the heart muscle itself may occur during periods of starvation. Silberman[53] reported reduced heart muscle volume and function in patients during starvation. In a classic study, Keys and colleagues[45] demonstrated that a 24% loss of body weight corresponded to a 17% reduction in heart volume during semistarvation (1500 kilocalorie diet).

Goals and Interventions

The long-term goals for the patient with heart failure who is well nourished and has an SGA (A) rating are to maintain lean body mass and prevent nutritional deficiency through intake of a well-balanced diet. Specifically, the goal is to strive for adequate protein and calories in the diet to maintain lean muscle mass. Educate the patient to eat a daily protein intake of 1.2 to 1.5 g/kg of body weight. This would be eating 6 to 8 ounces of lean meat, poultry, fish, low-fat dairy products, legumes, soy products, etc. per day. In patients with concomitant renal or hepatic disease, this recommendation would need to be altered. A sample menu for the patient with an (A) rating is presented in Exhibit 7–1.

Treatment of the patient with a (B) rating is critical to prevent him or her from progressing to a severely malnourished patient with a (C) rating. The goal for this patient is to restore nutritional status by improving protein and energy intake. To accomplish this goal, the patient needs to have a nutrition intake of 30 to 35 kcal/kg of body weight or 13.6 to 16 kcal/lb of body weight. Normal intake is 25 kcal/kg of body weight. This nutrition intake would include 1.5 to 1.8 g protein/kg of body weight or 0.68 to 0.82 g protein/lb of body weight. Normal protein intake is 0.8 g protein/kg of body weight or 0.36 g of protein/lb of body weight. A sample menu for the patient with a (B) rating is provided in Exhibit 7–1.

The primary goals for the heart failure patient with the compromised SGA (C) rating include preventing further loss of lean body mass and adipose tissue and gradually restoring the patient to adequate nutritional status. Correction of nutritional deficiencies is an additional goal. When planning interventions for this patient, match the patient's energy intake to his or her energy expenditure to avoid overfeeding. Overfeeding may result in gaining fat instead of muscle mass and development of fatty liver (see Exhibit 7–1).

A protein intake of 1.5 to 1.8 g protein/kg of body weight is recommended for this patient. The usual medical nutrition recommendation for this patient is 25 to 30 kcal/kg of body weight until weight is stabilized (adjusting for fluid status). After the weight is stabilized, slowly increase the patient to 30 to 35 kcal/kg of body weight to prevent overfeeding and cardiac stress.[40]

To help the patient meet energy and protein needs, encourage him or her to eat six to eight small meals daily. Consider meal replacements, either an oral supplement or tube feeding, if the

Exhibit 7–1 Sample Menus for Patients with Heart Failure

SGA Rating A:	SGA Rating B:	SGA Rating C:
Breakfast Cheerios—3/4 c 2% milk—1 c Bread, whole wheat—2 slices Banana—1 small Grape juice, unsweetened—1/3 c Margarine, tub, salted—2 tsp Jelly, regular—2 tsp	**Breakfast** Cheerios—3/4 c 2% milk—1 c Bread, whole wheat—2 slices Banana—1 small Margarine, tub, unsalted—1 TB	**Breakfast** Cheerios—1/2 c 2% milk—1 c
Lunch Turkey breast, unprocessed—4 oz Bread, whole wheat—2 slices Mayonnaise, regular—2 tsp Carrots, from frozen—1 c Pineapple, canned in juice—1 c 2% milk—1 c Animal crackers—8	**Snack** Grape juice, unsweetened—1/3 c Graham crackers—3 squares	**Snack** Bread, low sodium—1 slice Margarine, tub, unsalted—2 tsp Grape juice, unsweetened—1/3 c
	Lunch Turkey breast, unprocessed—4 oz Bread, whole wheat—2 slices Mayonnaise, regular—2 tsp Carrots, from frozen—1 c Pineapple, canned in juice—1 c 2% milk—1 c Animal crackers—8	**Lunch** 1/2 Turkey sandwich: Turkey breast, unprocessed—3 oz Bread, low sodium—1 slice Mayonnaise, regular—2 tsp Carrots, from frozen—1/2 c 2% milk—1 c
	Snack Frozen yogurt—1/2 c	**Snack** Frozen yogurt—1 c Pineapple, canned in juice—1/2 c

continues

Exhibit 7–1 continued

SGA Rating A:	SGA Rating B:	SGA Rating C:
Dinner	**Dinner**	**Dinner**
Cod—3 oz	Cod—4 oz	Cod—3 oz
Wild rice, regular—1 c	Wild rice, regular—1 c	Wild rice, regular—1/2 c
Asparagus, from fresh or frozen—1 c	Asparagus, from fresh or frozen—1 c	Asparagus, from fresh or frozen—1/2 c
Spinach salad—1 c	Spinach salad—1 c	2% milk—1 c
Oil-free Italian salad dressing—2 TB	Oil-free Italian salad dressing—2 TB	Margarine, tub, unsalted—2 tsp
Margarine, tub, unsalted—1 TB	Margarine, tub, unsalted—1 TB	
Dinner roll, whole wheat—1 medium	2% milk—1 c	**Snack**
2% milk—1 c		1/2 peanut butter sandwich:
	Snack	Peanut butter, regular—1 TB
	1/2 peanut butter sandwich:	Bread, low sodium—1 slice
	Peanut butter—2 TB	Spinach salad—1/2 c
	Bread, whole wheat—1 slice	Oil-free Italian salad dressing—1 TB
	2% milk—1/2 c	2% milk—1/2 c

continues

Exhibit 7–1 continued

SGA Rating A:	SGA Rating B:	SGA Rating C:
2056 kcal	2563 kcal	1661 kcal
2240 mg sodium	2627 mg sodium	1211 mg sodium
106 g or 19% protein	134 g or 20% protein	100 g or 24% protein
295 g or 56% carbohydrate	315 g or 49% carbohydrate	198 g or 48% carbohydrate
58 g or 25% fat	90 g or 31% fat	52 g or 28% fat
10% MFA	13% MFA	11% MFA
7% PFA	9% PFA	7% PFA
8% SFA	9% SFA	10% SFA
4053 mg potassium	4829 mg potassium	3494 mg potassium
1289 mg calcium	1585 mg calcium	1427 mg calcium
523 mg magnesium	635 mg magnesium	381 mg magnesium
191 mg cholesterol	248 mg cholesterol	205 mg cholesterol
29 g fiber	31 g fiber	13 g fiber
606 µg folate	644 µg folate	363 µg folate
108 mg vitamin C	109 mg vitamin C	65 mg vitamin C
1.9 mg thiamin	2.0 mg thiamin	1.4 mg thiamin
3.1 mg vitamin B_6	3.7 mg vitamin B_6	2.6 mg vitamin B_6
5.2 mg vitamin B_{12}	6.9 mg vitamin B_{12}	6.0 mg vitamin B_{12}
178 µg selenium	208 µg selenium	133 µg selenium

MFA, monounsaturated fatty acid; PFA, polyunsaturated fatty acid; SFA, saturated fatty acid.

patient is not able to meet his or her needs with oral food intake. Supplements that provide 1.5 to 2.0 kcal/mL will assist in accomplishing adequate nutrient intake. Another way to improve caloric intake is to advise the patient to take medications with a liquid nutrition supplement that provides 2.0 kcal/mL. A sample menu for the patient with a (C) rating is provided in Exhibit 7–1.

Cachexia and Sodium Restrictions

The patient with a (C) rating may require strict sodium restrictions if sodium retention is severe and cannot be controlled with medications. However, it is important not to restrict dietary sodium to less than 2 g/day if possible. With dietary restrictions of less than 2 g/day, it is very difficult to consume energy and protein in amounts or quantities required to prevent or treat loss of lean body mass.

Supplements

Supplemental nutrients may be prescribed to encourage a nutritionally balanced diet for some patients. A broad-based multivitamin supplement should be considered for patients with heart failure because of the potential benefits of supplementation with antioxidants, B vitamins, magnesium, potassium, calcium, and selenium. Additional supplements, including CoQ10, L-carnitine, taurine, and folic acid[54,55] have been found to be beneficial for some patients with cardiovascular disorders. However, at present the data are too limited to support their use in all patients with heart failure.

Further nutrition supplementation is recommended on an individual basis. However, given recent data that support cachexia as a predictor of mortality in patients with heart failure, research is urgently needed to identify specific nutritional supplementation that may prevent or delay the onset of malnutrition in these patients. For example, thiamine supplementation[56,57] has been shown to improve left ventricular ejection fraction in some heart failure patients who have a thiamine deficiency that is believed to be associated with furosemide.

MANAGEMENT OF SYMPTOMS

Goals and Interventions

The goal for patients with symptomatic heart failure is that symptoms will be managed at a level acceptable to the patient so that the patient is able to learn and follow the medical nutrition plan. Adequate symptom management by pharmacologic therapy is essential for the patient with heart failure before other nutrition interventions. Because patients with heart failure experience fatigue, dietary interventions can be implemented that assist in reducing the myocardial work load. Advise patients to eat small amounts frequently, such as minimeals of 350 to 500 kcal. This might also aid in food digestion. Educate patients to eat to promote an even distribution of calories and protein between meals and snacks. Soft, easy-to-chew foods should be eaten to decrease the energy expenditure of eating. The use of cardiac stimulants, such as caffeine, should be limited. Decaffeinated products should be substituted for caffeine products.

Gastrointestinal symptoms are problematic for patients with heart failure. Potential reasons for gastrointestinal symptoms include hypoxia, hepatic engorgement, or elevated immune substances, particularly tumor necrosis factor-α. Some patients feel better when foods are limited that cause gastric reflux, distention, and/or flatulence, such as beans, cabbage, onions, cauliflower, and Brussels sprouts. Soluble fiber (apples, applesauce, oatmeal, and oat fiber) can be used to reduce the constipation that may occur in patients who are required to follow fluid restriction. However, soluble fiber may not be effective with a reduced fluid intake, and a stool softener may be necessary.

Assessment of the patient's home environment, particularly the kitchen, may aid in educating the patient about ways to prepare meals efficiently to conserve personal energy. For example, patients can be taught to prepare foods while sitting rather than standing and store food items at a level that does not require reaching or bending. Heavy cans or appliances can be "scooted" across the counter rather than lifted.

Cordless telephones can be purchased so that patients do not have to leave the kitchen during meal preparation to answer the telephone. Assistance with meal preparation from organizations such as Meals on Wheels may be necessary for some patients. Inclusion of family members in meal preparation can help to ensure that the patient receives adequate nutrition.

Base education and behavior change interventions on an individualized assessment of the patient's symptoms, learning needs and abilities, and current dietary behaviors to match the education process and methods to each patient's needs and abilities. Include the patient and his or her family members in goal setting while developing the nutrition plan. Mutual goal setting is known to improve learning and behavior change. Incorporating the patient's goals has the potential to improve the person's satisfaction with nutrition recommendations.

MANAGEMENT OF SODIUM RETENTION AND HYPERVOLEMIA

Sodium retention and hypervolemia occur in patients with heart failure because of the pathophysiology of the disorder. The understanding of the pathophysiology, as well as management of heart failure, has changed over the past 50 years from viewing heart failure as a mechanical disorder associated primarily with edema and sodium retention to one of heart failure as a dynamic problem made up of ventricular remodeling and activation of the neurohormonal systems.[46,58] In addition to the hemodynamic derangements that occur with heart failure, it is now recognized that some neurohormonal substances activated during myocardial injury may have a direct negative effect on myocardial cell function.[58] For a detailed review of the pathophysiologic alterations that occur with heart failure, the reader is referred to Baig and colleagues.[46]

The sodium retention and hypervolemia that occur in these patients are believed to be due to elevations of aldosterone, angiotensin II, and atrial natriuretic factor.[46,59] Sodium retention influences mortality, morbidity, and health-related

quality of life in patients with heart failure by leading to hypervolemia and cardiac decompensation.[1,59,60] The Consensus Recommendations for the Management of Chronic Heart Failure[61] and the Agency for Health Care Policy and Research (AHCPR) Clinical Practice Guidelines for Heart Failure[60] recommend that assisting patients to (1) monitor signs of sodium retention, (2) comply with medication regimens, and (3) comply with dietary sodium restrictions should be part of routine care for persons with heart failure. The importance of these recommendations is supported by results from research studies. Inadequate prescription by health care providers of medications known to be effective in reducing sodium retention contributes to decompensation.[62,63] Sodium retention leading to volume overload and cardiac decompensation was the main reason for hospitalization in nearly two-thirds (59%) of 585 admissions for heart failure at two institutions.[1] Furthermore, lack of compliance with medication or diet therapy is associated with the sodium retention leading to decompensation.[64,65]

Currently, the AHCPR Guidelines[60] recommend that most patients with heart failure follow a 2-g sodium diet, and never more than a 3-g sodium diet. In addition, the Guidelines recommend that patients with heart failure avoid drinking excessive quantities of fluid and in selected cases fluid restrictions may become necessary. This recommendation is based on expert opinion because of lack of empirical research. Anecdotally, some patients do report noticeable differences such as increased dyspnea or swelling when they eat foods high in sodium.[30] However, no studies were found that specifically tested the effects of dietary sodium restrictions on patients with heart failure, thus optimal management of patients by a sodium-restricted diet is unclear. Until additional data become available, the recommendation of a 2- to 3-g sodium restriction is indicated.

An important factor in sodium retention may be the individual variation in sodium reabsorption that occurs within the kidneys. Age, comorbidity, and glomerular filtration rate likely influence reabsorption, as well as variable responses to medication therapy.[66] Health care providers need to be alert to the fact that patients may respond differently to the same medication regimens. Murray and colleagues[67] found great variability in renal absorption within and among 17 patients who received four different brands of oral furosemide for hypertension or heart failure. Newer products are being developed that have improved bioavailability and may be more consistently absorbed in patients.

Goals and Interventions

The main goals related to fluid and electrolyte balance for the patient with heart failure are to restore euvolemia, prevent further sodium retention and fluid retention, and maintain normal electrolyte balance. Interventions to achieve these goals are focused on educating the patient to adhere to pharmacologic therapies, follow dietary sodium restrictions, and self-monitor for signs and symptoms of fluid retention.

Patients are taught the importance of medications, particularly diuretics, in controlling sodium retention. Compliance with medication therapy should be monitored to assist in preventing sodium retention. Adjustments in therapies are indicated by changes in patients' conditions. In some settings, health care providers are now educating patients to adjust their own diuretic medications daily on the basis of weights, as indicated in the Consensus Recommendations.[61] This type of self-medication program promises improved outcomes but has not been prospectively tested. However, careful assessment of a patient's understanding of his or her condition and ability to self-medicate would be critical before implementing this type of intervention.

Patients need to be taught the importance of following their individualized, prescribed dietary sodium restrictions. Although guidelines are 2 to 3 g of sodium daily, it may be possible to liberalize sodium intake to 4 g daily. With a 2-g sodium restriction, it is difficult for patients to maintain adequate nutritional intake. Liberalization of the sodium restriction to up to 4 g daily may be beneficial by allowing the patient to focus on eating a well-balanced diet while still controlling sodium and fluid retention. Patients who are medically stable, have no signs of edema or fluid retention, are compliant with medications, and have difficulty following 2 or 3 g of sodium restriction may be considered for liberalization of the sodium restriction. Tips for controlling dietary sodium intake are presented in Exhibit 7–2.

If hypervolemia can be treated early, troubling symptoms and costly hospitalizations may be avoided. Teaching patients to self-monitor for signs of sodium retention, including a weight gain of greater than 0.5 kg/day and increasing edema, shortness of breath, and fatigue, has contributed to improved quality of life and reduced hospitalizations.[68,69] Strategies for assisting patients to learn self-monitoring skills are presented in Exhibit 7–3.

MANAGEMENT OF HYPOVOLEMIA AND DEHYDRATION

The patient with heart failure may be predisposed to hypovolemia as a result of diuretic therapy. If the hypovolemia becomes severe, the patient experiences dehydration. The combination of environmental conditions (ie, extremely high temperatures that cause increased perspiration) and loss of fluids because of fluid restrictions and large diuretic doses may increase the likelihood of dehydration in some patients. The problems of hypovolemia and dehydration are not commonly reported in the heart failure literature, perhaps because they are less commonly noted. In a study of 585 hospital admissions for heart failure, 9 (2%) were due to dehydration.[1]

Goals and Interventions

The main goals for the patient with hypovolemia and/or dehydration are to restore euvolemia, prevent further hypovolemia and dehydration, and maintain normal electrolyte balance. Review diuretic therapy requirements periodically and make adjustments on the basis of the patient's condition. Teach patients to self-monitor for signs and symptoms of hypovolemia

Exhibit 7–2 Tips for Controlling Dietary Sodium Intake

Avoid adding salt to foods during meal preparation.

Avoid adding salt to foods at the table.

Avoid processed foods (canned foods such as vegetables or meats; packaged foods such as potato chips, crackers; boxed foods such as macaroni and cheese).

Buy foods labeled "low sodium" when possible.

Give patients a list of low-sodium foods to keep on their refrigerator doors.

Educate patients to read the sodium content on food labels.

If patients cannot see the labels on foods, assist them with vision improvement (referral for eye examination, new glasses, or purchase magnifying glass).

When purchasing frozen meals, look for those meals with less than 600 mg of sodium for the total meal.

If purchasing a frozen entree, look for an entree with less than 300 mg of sodium.

Use a salt substitute that does not contain potassium (for example, *Mrs. Dash*).

Assist patients to alter the kitchen environment to conserve energy during food preparation. For example, keep a chair or stool in kitchen, keep items at levels where lifting or bending are unnecessary, use a cordless telephone to avoid having to go from the kitchen to other rooms to answer the telephone while cooking, etc.

Cook in large quantities and freeze in individual containers to be reheated later.

Check with local bakeries for low-sodium breads and health food stores for other low sodium products.

Check with local senior citizen center and meal delivery services, etc., to find out whether low-sodium foods are offered.

Educate patients about foods to eat at restaurants while following dietary recommendations.

Give patients a list of low-sodium foods available at nearby restaurants.

Invite patients to participate in cooking classes and demonstrations. These classes may be available at the institution or in the community (local grocery stores, etc.).

Exhibit 7–3 Ten Strategies for Teaching Patients with Heart Failure To Learn Self-Monitoring Skills for Weight and Edema Assessment

1. Evaluate the patient's ability to perform daily weight—visual problems, balance disturbances, cognitive function. Identify corrective actions as needed.
2. Provide the patient with a list of stores that carry bathroom scales and prices of the scales.
3. Obtain a bathroom scale for patients who cannot afford to purchase them (consider the need for a special scale if the patient weighs more than 300 pounds).
4. Maintain a list of community resources and volunteers for patients with special financial needs (eg, donation of bathroom scale by community retail merchant).
5. Assign each patient a weight range, based on BMI, to maintain.
6. Instruct the patient to notify his or her health care provider if he or she gains more than 5 pounds in 2 days.[60]
7. Instruct the patient to notify his or her health care provider if he or she notices increased edema, or swelling, after assessing legs and ankles. An easy sign that a patient can monitor for increasing edema is clothing or jewelry that becomes tight (shoes, belt on pants, rings on fingers).
8. Instruct the patient to record daily weights on a designated card or form. Provide the patient with a calendar or a card for the wallet on which to record his or her weight.
9. Instruct the patient to bring the weight record to visits with health care providers.
10. Include the family member(s) in self-monitoring.

and to notify their health care provider if these occur. During hospitalization, monitor patients' intake and output and electrolyte levels to prevent hypovolemia.

COMPLIANCE WITH MEDICAL NUTRITION RECOMMENDATIONS

The importance of education is widely recognized for people with heart failure who are required to follow prescribed nutrition recommendations. However, learning new behaviors and changing existing behaviors through patient education is often difficult to accomplish. A complete discussion of assisting patients with heart failure to make lifestyle changes, including dietary changes, is included in Chapters 11 and 12.

RECOMMENDATIONS FOR FUTURE RESEARCH

The nutrition problems associated with heart failure are associated with poor outcomes, including mortality. Thus, further research is needed to improve patient care in this area. Selected areas for future nutrition research are listed in the following.

1. Conduct a prevalence study to examine the extent and severity of cachexia among heart failure patients with varying degrees of disease severity.

2. Develop and test theoretically based interventions to improve compliance with medical nutrition recommendations in patients with heart failure.

3. Design and test nutritional education and behavior change interventions for heart failure patients with different levels of literacy skills.

4. Evaluate the reliability, validity, and clinical feasibility of the Subjective Global Assessment instrument and other assessment instruments in patients with heart failure.

5. Evaluate the Subjective Global Assessment instrument and other assessment instruments as predictors of outcomes in patients with heart failure.

6. Test the effects of specific medical nutrition recommendations (dietary sodium restrictions, improved dietary protein intake, supplements) on outcomes in patients with varying degrees of heart failure severity.

REFERENCES

1. Bennett SJ, Huster GA, Baker SL, et al. Characterization of the precipitants of hospitalization for heart failure decompensation. *Am J Crit Care.* 1998;7:168–174.

2. Anker SD, Ponikowski P, Varney S, et al. Wasting as independent risk factor for mortality in chronic heart failure. *Lancet.* 1997;349:1050–1053.

3. Carr JG, Stevenson LW, Walden JA, Heber D. Prevalence and hemodynamic correlates of malnutrition in severe congestive heart failure secondary to ischemic or idiopathic dilated cardiomyopathy. *Am J Cardiol.* 1989;63:709–713.

4. Blackburn GL, Bistrian BR, Maini BS, Schlamm HT, Smith MF. Nutritional and metabolic assessment of the hospitalized patient. *J Parenteral Enteral Nutr.* 1977;1:11–22.

5. Heymsfield SB., Baumgartner RN, Pan S. Nutritional assessment of malnutrition by anthropometric methods. In: Shils ME, Olson JA, Shike M, Ross AC, eds. *Modern Nutrition in Health and Disease.* 9th ed. Baltimore: Williams & Wilkins; 1999: 909.

6. Scott BJ, St. Jeor T, Feldman FB. Adult anthropometry. In: Simko MD, Cowell C, Gilbride JA, eds. *Nutrition Assessment: A Comprehensive Guide for Planning Intervention.* 2nd ed. Gaithersburg, MD: Aspen; 1995:117–134.

7. Grant JP, Custer PB, Thurlow J. Current techniques of nutritional assessment. Symposium on Surgical Nutrition. *Surg Clin North Am.* 1981;61:437–463.

8. American Dietetic Association. *Manual of Clinical Dietetics.* 5th ed. Chicago: The American Dietetic Association; 1996.

9. National Heart, Lung, and Blood Institute. National Heart, Lung, and Blood Institute. 1999. [On-line]. Available: www.nhlbi.nih.gov/health/public/heart/obesity/lose_wt/index.htm Accessed February 9, 2000.

10. National Heart, Lung, and Blood Institute. Clinical guidelines of the identification, evaluation, and treatment of overweight and obesity in adults: The evidence reports. June, 1998. [On-line]. Available: www.nhlbi.gov/health/public/heart/obesity/lose_wt/index.htm. Accessed February 9, 2000.

11. Russell MK, McAdams MP. Laboratory monitoring of nutritional status. In: Materese LE Gottschlich MM, eds. *Contemporary Nutrition Support Practice: A Clinical Guide.* Philadelphia: WB Saunders; 1998:47–63.

12. Pike R, Brown ML. *Nutrition: An Integrated Approach.* 3rd ed. New York: Macmillan; 1984.

13. Zeman FJ. Nutritional assessment. In: Zeman FJ, ed. *Clinical Nutrition and Dietetics.* 2nd ed. New York: Macmillan; 1991:64.

14. Kee JL. *Laboratory and Diagnostic Tests.* 4th ed. Norwalk, CT: Appleton & Lange; 1995.

15. Heymsfield SB, Tighe A, Wang Z. Nutritional assessment by anthropometric and biochemical methods. In: Shils ME, Olson JA, Shike M, eds. *Modern Nutrition in*

Health and Disease. 8th ed. Philadelphia: Lea & Febiger; 1994:839.

16. Alcock NW. Laboratory tests for assessing nutritional status. In: Shils ME, Olson JA, Shike M, Ross AC, eds. *Modern Nutrition in Health and Disease.* 9th ed. Baltimore: Williams & Wilkins; 1999:958.

17. Gulanick M, Cofer LA. Coronary risk factors: Influences on the lipid profile. *J Cardiovasc Nurs.* 2000;14:16–28.

18. Lamendola C. Hypertriglyceridemia and low high-density lipoprotein: risks for coronary artery disease? *J Cardiovasc Nurs.* 2000;14:79–90.

19. National Cholesterol Education Panel. Second report of the expert panel on detection, evaluation, and treatment of high blood cholesterol in adults (Adult Treatment Panel II). *Circulation.* 1994;89:1329–1445.

20. Grundy SM, Balady GJ, Criqui MH, et al. Guide to primary prevention of cardiovascular diseases. *Circulation.* 1997;95:2329–2331.

21. Lee GR. The anemia of chronic diseases. In: Lee GR, Bithel TC, Foerster J, Athens JW, Lukens JN, eds. *Wintrobe's Clinical Hematology.* 9th ed., Vol. 1. Philadelphia: Lea & Febiger; 1993:840–851.

22. Baxter Healthcare Corporation. *Assessing the Nutritional Status of Dialysis Patients Using Subjective Global Assessment.* Baxter Healthcare Corporation; 1993.

23. Bates B, Bickley LS, Hoekelman RA. *A Guide to Physical Examination and History Taking.* 6th ed. Philadelphia: JB Lippincott; 1995.

24. Braunwald E. *Heart Disease: A Textbook of Cardiovascular Medicine.* 4th ed. Philadelphia: WB Saunders; 1992.

25. Holloway NM. *Nursing the Critically Ill Adult.* 3rd ed. Menlo Park, CA: Addison-Wesley; 1988.

26. National Cancer Institute, Division of Cancer Prevention and Control. *Health Habits and History Questionnaire.* Bethesda, MD: National Institutes of Health; 1985.

27. Willet WC, Sampson L, Stampfer MJ, et al. Reproducibility and validity of a semiquantitative food frequency questionnaire. *Am J Epidemiol.* 1985;122:51–65.

28. United States Department of Agriculture. Food, Nutrition, and Consumer Services, Center for Nutrition Policy and Promotion. 1992. [On-line]. Available: www.usda.gov. Accessed February 16, 2000.

29. University of California, San Francisco School of Nursing Symptom Management Faculty Group. A model for symptom management. *Image.* 1995;26:272–276.

30. Bennett SJ, Cordes D, Westmoreland G, Castro R, Donnelly E. Self-care strategies for symptom management in patients with chronic heart failure. *Nurs Res.* 2000;49:139–145.

31. Bennett SJ, Milgrom LB, Champion V, Huster GA. Beliefs about medication and dietary compliance in people with heart failure: An instrument development study. *Heart Lung.* 1997;26:273–279.

32. Freedland KE, Carney RM, Rich MW, et al. Depression in elderly patients with congestive heart failure. *J Psychiatr Gerontol.* 1991;24:59–71.

33. Grady KL, Jalowiec A, Grusk B, White-Williams C, Robinson J. Symptom distress in cardiac transplant-candidates. *Heart Lung.* 1992;21:434–439.

34. Premen AJ. Research recommendations for cardiovascular aging research. *J Am Geriatr Soc.* 1996;44:1114–1117.

35. Detsky A, McLaughlin J, Baker J, et al. What is subjective global assessment of nutritional status? *J Parenteral Enteral Nutr.* 1986;11:8–13.

36. Lichtman T. What is the subjective global assessment, and has it been validated in renal population? *J Renal Nutr.* 1997;7:46–47.

37. Kalantar-Zadeh K, Kleiner M, Dunne E, et al. Total iron-binding capacity-estimated transferrin correlates with the nutritional subjective global assessment in hemodialysis patients. *Am J Kidney Dis.* 1998;31:263–272.

38. Bowers JM, Dols CL. Subjective global assessment in HIV-infected patients. *J Assoc Nurses AIDS Care.* 1996;7:83–89.

39. Newton JM, Halsted CH. Clinical and functional assessment of adults. In: Shils ME, Olson JA, Shike M, Ross AC, eds. *Modern Nutrition in Health and Disease.* 9th ed. Baltimore: Williams & Wilkins; 1999:895.

40. Hoffer LJ. Metabolic consequences of starvation. In: Shils ME, Olson JA, Shike M, Ross AC, eds. *Modern Nutrition in Health and Disease.* 9th ed. Baltimore: Williams & Wilkins; 1999:660–661.

41. Hughes C, Kostka P. Chronic congestive heart failure. In: Shils ME, Olson JA, Shike M, Ross AC. eds. *Modern Nutrition in Health and Disease.* 9th ed. Baltimore: Williams & Wilkins; 1999:1230–1231.

42. Freeman LM, Roubenoff R. The nutritional implications of cardiac cachexia. *Nutri Rev.* 1994;52:340–347.

43. Anker SD, Coats AJS. Cachexia in heart failure is bad for you. *Eur Heart J.* 1998;19:191–193.

44. Anker SD, Coats AJS. Cardiac cachexia: A syndrome with impaired survival and immune and neuroendocrine activation. *Chest.* 1999;115:836–847.

45. Keys A, Brozek J, Henschel A, Mickelsen O, Taylor HL. *The Biology of Human Starvation.* Minneapolis, MN: University of Minnesota Press; 1950.

46. Baig MK, Mahon N, McKenna WJ, et al. The pathophysiology of advanced heart failure. *Am Heart J.* 1998;I35:S216–S230.

47. Bennett SJ, Mohler ER, Sorensen LC, Huster G, Cropp AB, Pressler ML. Cytokines correlate with quality of life in severe chronic heart failure. *Circulation.* 1995;92(suppl.):1–116.

48. Levine B, Kalman J, Mayer L, Fillit HM, Packer M. Elevated circulating levels of tumor necrosis factor in severe chronic heart failure. *N Engl J Med.* 1990;323:236–241.

49. Anker SD, Chua TP, Ponikowski P, et al. Hormonal changes and catabolic/anabolic imbalance in chronic heart failure and their importance for cardiac cachexia. *Circulation.* 1997;96:526–534.

50. Smith MK, Lowry SF. The hypercatabolic state. In: Shils ME, Olson JA, Shike M, Ross AC eds. *Modern Nutrition in Health and Disease.* 9th ed. Baltimore: Williams & Wilkins; 1999:1560.

51. Toth MJ, Gottlieb SS, Goran MI, Fisher ML, Poehlman ET. Daily energy expenditure in free-living heart failure patients. *Am J Physiol.* 1997;272:E469–E475.

52. Toth MJ, Gottlieb SS, Fisher ML, Poehlman ET. Daily energy requirements in heart failure patients. *Metabolism.* 1997;46:1294–1298.

53. Silberman H. Parenteral and enteral nutrition. 2nd ed. Norwalk, CT: Appleton & Lange; 1989.

54. Kendler BS. Recent nutritional approaches to the prevention and therapy of cardiovascular disease. *Prog Cardiovasc Nurs.* 1997;12:3–23.

55. Futterman LG, Lemberg L. Homocysteine and coronary artery disease. *Am J Crit Care.* 1997;6:72–77.

56. Shimon I, Almog S, Vered Z, et al. Improved left ventricular function after thiamine supplementation in patients with congestive heart failure receiving long-term furosemide therapy. *Am J Med.* 1995;98:485–490.

57. Rieck J, Halkin H, Shlomo A, et al. Urinary loss of thiamine is increased by low doses of furosemide in healthy volunteers. *J Lab Clin Med.* 1999;134:238–243.

58. Packer M. How should physicians view heart failure? The philosophical and physiological evolution of three conceptual models of the disease. *Am J Cardiol.* 199371:3C–10C.

59. Cohn JN. Physiological variables as markers of symptoms, risk, and interventions in heart failure. *Circulation.* 1993;87(suppl VII):VII-110–VII-114.

60. Konstam M, Dracup K, Bake, D, et al. Heart failure: Evaluation and care of patients with left-ventricular systolic dysfunction. Clinical Practice Guideline No. 11. AHCPR Publication No. 94–0612. Rockville, MD: Agency for Health Care Policy and Research, Public Health Service, U.S. Department of Health and Human Services. June 1994.

61. Packer M, Cohn JN on behalf of the Steering Committee and Membership of the Advisory Council to Improve Outcomes Nationwide in Heart Failure: Consensus recommendations for the management of chronic heart failure. *Am J Cardiol.* 1999;83(suppl):1A–38.

62. Clinical Quality Improvement Network Investigators. Mortality risk and patterns of practice in 4606 acute care patients with congestive heart failure. *Arch Intern Med.* 1996;156:1669–1673.

63. Monane M, Bohn RL, Gurwitz JH, Glynn RJ, Avorn J. Noncompliance with congestive heart failure therapy in the elderly. *Arch Intern Med.* 1994;153:433–437.

64. Ghali JK, Kadakia S, Cooper R, Ferlinz J. Precipitating factors leading to decompensation of heart failure. *Arch Intern Med.* 1988;148:2013–2016.

65. Happ MB, Naylor MD, Roe-Prior P. Factors contributing to rehospitalization of elderly patients with heart failure. *J Cardiovasc Nurs.* 1997;11:75–84.

66. Hammarlund-Udenaes M, Benet LZ. Furosemide pharmacokinetics and pharmacodynamics in health and disease—an update. *J Pharmacokinet Biopharmaceut.* 1989;17:1–46.

67. Murray MD, Haag KM, Black PK, Hall SD, Brater DC. Variable furosemide absorption and poor predictability of response in elderly patients. *Pharmacotherapy.* 1989;17:98–106.

68. Rich MW, Beckham V, Wittenberg C, Leven CL, Freedland KE, Carney RM. A multidisciplinary intervention to prevent the readmission of elderly patients with congestive heart failure. *N Engl J Med.* 1995;333:1190–1195.

69. Rich MW, Vinson JM, Sperry JC, et al. Prevention of readmission in elderly patients with congestive heart failure. *J Gen Intern Med.* 1993;8:585–590.

CHAPTER 8

Exercise in Heart Failure

John R. Wilson, Don B. Chomsky, and Karen Dahle

Exercise intolerance is one of the most common problems experienced by patients with heart failure. Patients frequently are not able to perform certain normal daily activities or have to decrease the rate at which they carry out tasks. Even when patients report few symptoms during normal activities, their maximal exercise capacity is almost always reduced. Liang and colleagues, for example, measured peak exercise oxygen consumption in symptomatic and asymptomatic patients enrolled in the SOLVD treatment and prevention trials.[1] Patients who reported exertional symptoms had peak exercise $\dot{V}O_2$ levels that were only 40% of predicted normal levels (Figure 8–1). Patients who considered themselves asymptomatic actually had peak exercise $\dot{V}O_2$ levels 25% to 30% below normal levels.

Because exercise intolerance is such a major problem in heart failure, numerous research studies have been performed over the past three decades seeking to better understand why patients with heart failure are limited during exercise and to identify methods of treating this limitation. These studies have totally changed our views of why patients with heart failure have exercise intolerance. These efforts have also dramatically altered the way we evaluate and treat exertional symptoms in heart failure.

PATHOPHYSIOLOGY OF EXERCISE INTOLERANCE IN HEART FAILURE

Before 1985, exercise intolerance in heart failure was attributed exclusively to hemodynamic factors (Figure 8–2). Two symptoms were thought to limit most patients: exertional fatigue and dyspnea. Exertional fatigue was thought to be due to an inability of the heart to deliver adequate blood to the exercising skeletal muscle. Dyspnea was believed to be caused by an acute rise in intrapulmonary pressures during exercise and a consequent decrease in lung compliance.

The view that fatigue was due to inadequate skeletal muscle flow was based on studies showing reduced forearm blood flow during forearm exercise and reduced leg blood flow during bicycle exercise in patients with heart failure.[2-4] In these flow studies, it was also observed that blood lactate levels increased greater than in normal subjects. This finding was considered further evidence that skeletal muscle flow was impaired.[4,5] At the time, tissue lactate release was believed to be an unequivocal marker of tissue hypoxia.[5]

The concept that exertional dyspnea was due to acute increases in the pulmonary artery wedge pressure during exercise came primarily from hemodynamic studies performed on patients with mitral stenosis.[6-8] In these studies, pulmonary artery wedge pressure, minute ventilation, and lung compliance were monitored during exercise. During exercise, it was found that the pulmonary wedge pressure increased markedly accompanied by excessive ventilatory responses and decreased lung compliance. These abnormalities were partially corrected by mitral valvuloplasty, reinforcing the view that dyspnea in heart failure was due to elevated intrapulmonary pressures.

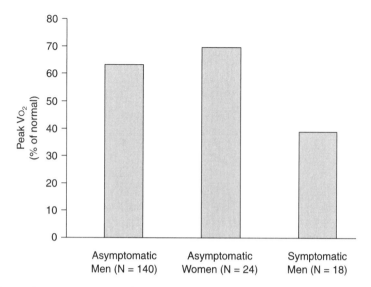

Figure 8-1 Peak exercise oxygen consumption in patients enrolled in the SOLVD trials.

Over the past two decades, it has become clear that these traditional explanations for exercise intolerance are overly simplistic. Although hemodynamic factors still are thought to limit exercise in some patients, recent observations suggest that the pathophysiology of exercise intolerance is far more complicated than originally thought.

The first hint that hemodynamic factors may not be as important as originally thought came from studies of inotropic and vasodilator agents.[9–11] In these studies, dobutamine, dopamine, and several different vasodilators were used to acutely increase the cardiac output and decrease the pulmonary artery wedge pressure during exercise in patients with heart failure. The investigators conducting these studies fully expected that such hemodynamic changes would improve the exertional symptoms and maximal exercise performance of patients. Surprisingly, the hemodynamic changes had no effect on exertional symptoms, maximal exercise performance, ventilatory responses to exercise, or blood lactate levels.

Further evidence that skeletal muscle fatigue in heart failure may not be due to skeletal muscle underperfusion came from studies using phosphorus-31 nuclear magnetic resonance.[12,13] This technology permits noninvasive assessment of inorganic phosphate, phosphocreatine, and hydrogen ion levels in working skeletal muscle.

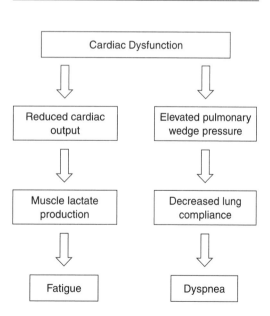

Figure 8–2 Traditional explanation for exercise intolerance in heart failure.

The ratio between inorganic phosphate and phosphocreatine provides an estimate of adenosine diphosphate concentrations and mitochondrial respiration.[14]

Using nuclear magnetic resonance, a number of groups compared forearm and calf metabolic responses to exercise in normal subjects and patients with heart failure.[12–14] These studies demonstrated markedly abnormal metabolic responses in the patients with heart failure. An example of such a response is shown in Figure 8–3. The top series of spectra are taken from the calf muscle of a normal subject during calf exercise. With progressive exercise, the inorganic phosphate concentration increased and the phosphocreatine concentration decreased, consistent with heightened oxidative phosphorylation. The bottom series of spectra is taken from a patient with heart failure. Much greater phosphocreatine depletion was noted in the patient than in the normal subject.

In several of these studies, limb blood flow and fatigability were also measured.[12,13] Despite the presence of markedly abnormal muscle me-

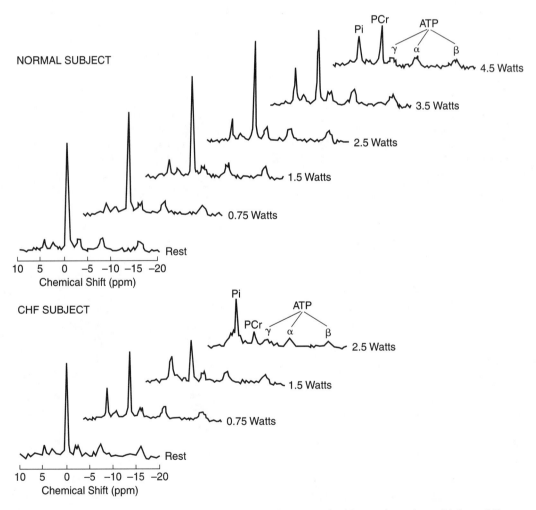

Figure 8–3 Changes in calf metabolism during exercise in a normal subject and a patient with heart failure as assessed with Phosphorus-31 nuclear magnetic resonance.

tabolism and increased fatigability, no reduction in limb blood flow was detected in the patients with heart failure. This finding strongly suggested that intrinsic skeletal muscle changes may play an important role in limiting the exercise capacity of patients with heart failure.

Since this original observation, numerous problems have been identified in the skeletal muscle of patients with heart failure (Exhibit 8–1). Minotti et al[16] have demonstrated that skeletal muscle endurance is decreased in heart failure. Skeletal muscle biopsy studies have demonstrated type II muscle fiber atrophy, decreased concentration of oxidative enzymes, and a reduction in mitochondrial volume. The study of mitochondrial volume by Drexler et al[19] is of particular interest. In this study, Drexler and his colleagues obtained muscle biopsy specimens from 57 patients with heart failure and 18 control subjects. These investigators noted a significant decrease in mitochondrial volume in patients with heart failure (Figure 8–4). These investigators also noted a relatively strong correlation between mitochondrial volume and peak exercise $\dot{V}O_2$.

Abnormalities of respiratory muscle have also been described in patients with heart failure. Mancini et al[20] compared maximal ventilatory capacity in 15 patients with heart failure and 8 normal subjects and observed close to a 50% reduction in ventilatory capacity in the patients. Others have reported significant decreases in inspiratory muscle strength in patients with heart failure.[21,22]

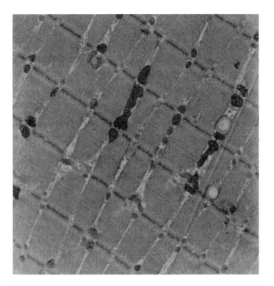

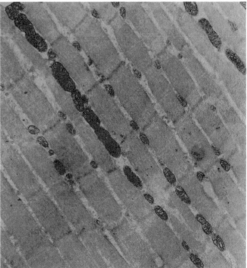

Figure 8–4 Electron micrographs of Cytochrome C Oxidase in a patient with severe heart failure (top) and in a normal subject (bottom). Enzyme activity within the mitochondria (black) is reduced in heart failure.

Exhibit 8–1 Skeletal Muscle Abnormalities in Heart Failure

- Abnormal skeletal muscle metabolism[12–14]
- Skeletal muscle atrophy[14,15]
- Decreased skeletal muscle endurance[16]
- Type II skeletal muscle atrophy and decreased oxidative enzyme concentration[17,18]
- Decreased mitochondrial volume[19]
- Reduced respiratory muscle endurance[20]
- Reduced respiratory muscle strength[21,22]

On the basis of such observations, it is now generally accepted that skeletal muscle abnormalities play an important role in limiting the exercise capacity of patients with heart failure. However, the extent to which these abnormalities limit exercise still is debated. Some patients with heart failure and severe exercise intolerance have normal skeletal muscle biopsy specimens, making it highly unlikely that exercise intolerance in heart failure can be explained totally by skeletal muscle abnormalities.

It is also not clear why patients with heart failure develop skeletal muscle changes. Several groups have shown that exercise training improves skeletal muscle metabolic responses to exercise in patients with heart failure.[23,24] Hambrecht et al[25] have demonstrated that 6 months of exercise training increases muscle mitochondrial volume. Such observations have led to a widespread assumption that the skeletal muscle abnormalities noted in heart failure are primarily due to inactivity and deconditioning.

Inactivity undoubtedly plays an important role in patients who have been extremely sedentary. However, it seems unlikely that activity is the only factor responsible for skeletal muscle changes in heart failure. Other factors that potentially could change skeletal muscle characteristics include malnutrition, chronic tissue underperfusion, and neurohormonal abnormalities, such as increased sympathetic activity, adrenocorticoids, and tissue necrosis factor.

What then is the cause of exercise intolerance in heart failure? On the basis of current information, it seems clear that multiple factors can limit the exercise ability of patients with heart failure (Figure 8–5). However, individual patients are probably limited by different combinations of these factors. For example, some patients may be limited primarily by hemodynamic factors, whereas others may be limited by muscle deconditioning.

Hopefully, techniques will be developed in the future that will allow the clinician to determine why an individual patient is limited during exertion. Unfortunately, there are at present no noninvasive methods to determine the cause of exercise intolerance in any given patient. Hemodynamic monitoring during exercise often provides useful information but is not available in most medical centers.[26-30]

EXERCISE TRAINING AND HEART FAILURE

How can you improve exertional symptoms in heart failure? Over the past three decades, nu-

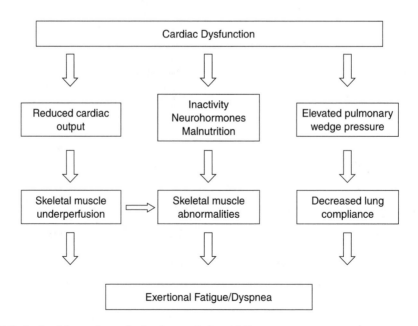

Figure 8–5 Pathophysiology of exercise intolerance in heart failure.

merous pharmacologic interventions have been used to treat these exertional symptoms, including angiotensin-converting enzyme inhibitors, inotropic agents, ß-blocking agents, and calcium antagonists. Unfortunately, very few of these pharmaceutical interventions significantly improve exercise performance. Moreover, even when exercise performance does improve, the effect is typically slight.

For example, in the early 1980s the Captopril Multicenter Research Group conducted a pivotal randomized trial of captopril.[31] In this study, patients with symptomatic heart failure were randomly assigned to either captopril therapy (50 patients) or placebo therapy (42 patients). Exercise testing using a modified Naughton protocol was performed at baseline and again at 2, 4, 8, and 12 weeks of therapy. Placebo therapy had no significant impact on maximal exercise duration. In contrast, patients placed on captopril exhibited a highly significant 24% increase in exercise time, from 494 to 614 seconds.

On first glance, this change in exercise time appears to represent a major improvement in exercise performance. However, a change of 120 seconds on the Naughton protocol actually represents a very small absolute change in exercise capacity. Moreover, even after receiving captopril therapy, patients continued to have markedly reduced maximal exercise capacity.

Such findings have led clinicians to seek alternative methods of treating exercise intolerance in heart failure. One method that has attracted particular attention is the use of exercise training programs.

Widespread interest in the use of exercise training programs to treat patients with heart failure was first stimulated by two events: the demonstration that local forearm training can reverse forearm muscle metabolic abnormalities in heart failure[23] and a comprehensive study of exercise training conducted at Duke University by Sullivan and colleagues.[32,33] In the Duke study, 12 patients with chronic heart failure and peak exercise $\dot{V}O_2$ levels of 16.8 ± 3.8 mL/min/kg underwent 16 to 24 weeks of exercise training. Patients exercised in a supervised cardiac rehabilitation program 3 to 5 h/week at 75% of peak exercise $\dot{V}O_2$.

Cardiopulmonary exercise testing and hemodynamic monitoring during exercise were performed at baseline and at the end of training. As shown in Figure 8–6, training significantly increased peak exercise $\dot{V}O_2$ to 20.6 ± 4.7 mL/min/kg, reduced the heart rate response to exercise, decreased lactate levels during exercise, and increased oxygen extraction at the end of exercise.[32] The cardiac output and pulmonary wedge pressure during exercise was unchanged when compared at matched workloads.[32] This study provided the first convincing evidence that training can improve the exercise performance of patients with heart failure.

Several years later, Coats et al[34] extended these observations by conducting a controlled crossover trial of 8 weeks of training in 17 men with heart failure. Exercise was performed at home using a training bicycle provided by the research group. Patients were encouraged to exercise at least 5 days each week. During the exercise part of the study, patients increased their peak oxygen uptake from 13.2 ± 0.9 to 15.6 ± 1.0 mL/min/kg. Minute ventilation and norepinephrine spillover also decreased with training.

This study served to further emphasize the potential benefits of exercise training. However, in addition, this study demonstrated that the response to training was highly variable. Almost half of the patients exhibited little or no change in maximal bicycle exercise duration during the training period (Figure 8–7).

Since these two initial studies, multiple additional studies have been published. These more recent studies have in general confirmed the findings of the two initial studies and have also shown that exercise training improves endothelial function in heart failure, as measured by vascular responses to the infusion of acetylcholine.[35,36] However, all of the studies have included relatively small numbers of patients and variable exercise protocols, making interpretation of the findings somewhat difficult.

Recently, two larger studies have been completed, one in Canada and one in Italy. The Canadian study (EXERT) has thus far only been published in abstract form.[37] In this study, 181 patients were randomly assigned to usual care or

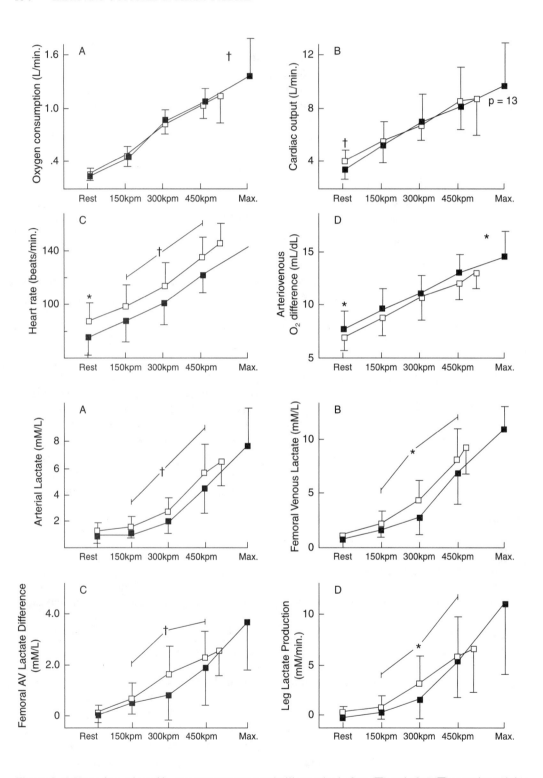

Figure 8–6 Hemodynamic and lactate responses to treadmill exercise before (□) and after (■) exercise training.

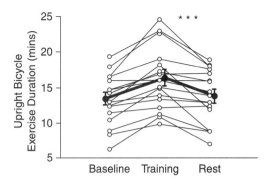

Figure 8–7 Individual and mean patient upright exercise durations for baseline, training, and detraining periods. ***$P < 0.001$ for comparison between training and detraining periods, $n = 17$.

to a supervised exercise training program that lasted for 3 months. No significant changes were observed in the control group. The training groups exhibited a 10% increase in peak exercise $\dot{V}O_2$ and a 15% increase in muscle strength. However, no significant change in quality of life was observed.

The Italian study randomized 99 patients to a training program versus usual care.[38] Patients in the training program exercised three times a week for 8 weeks and then twice a week for 1 year. In this study, patients randomly assigned to the training group exhibited a significant increase in peak exercise $\dot{V}O_2$ from 15.7 ± 2 to 18.6 ± 1 mL/min/kg, whereas patients in the control group had no significant change in peak $\dot{V}O_2$. The training group also had improved quality of life, a lower mortality rate, and a lower hospital readmission rate for heart failure (Figure 8–8).

These studies indicate that exercise training substantially improves the exercise tolerance of at least some patients with heart failure. In addition, training may have several additional major benefits, including a beneficial effect on mortality and hospitalization frequency.

EXERCISE PRESCRIPTIONS IN CLINICAL PRACTICE

Given these findings, should all patients with heart failure and exercise intolerance be enrolled in a cardiac rehabilitation program? A number of expert groups have provided recommendations regarding exercise and heart failure. In 1994, the Agency for Health Care Policy and Research released clinical practice guidelines for the management of heart failure.[39] These guidelines recommended: "Regular exercise such as walking or cycling should be encouraged for all patients with stable NYHA Class I–III heart failure. There is insufficient evidence at this time to recommend the routine use of supervised rehabilitation programs for patients with heart failure, although such programs may be of benefit to patients who are anxious; are dyspneic at a low work level; or have angina, a recent MI, or a recent CABG."

In 1995, a combined American Heart Association and American College of Cardiology task force published *Guidelines for the Evaluation and Management of Heart Failure*.[40] Little specific attention was given to exercise, except for the following brief statement: "Dynamic exercise as tolerated should be encouraged."

The most recent recommendations for the management of heart failure were published in 1999.[41] These recommendations were based on the consensus opinion of a large number of heart failure experts. The following recommendations were made regarding exercise: "Although most patients should not participate in heavy labor or exhaustive sports, aerobic activity should be encouraged (except during periods of acute decompensation), since the restriction of activity promotes physical deconditioning. Indeed, in patients with mild-to-moderate symptoms, aerobic training alone (carried out in the context of a supervised program) may improve symptoms and exercise capacity and may decrease the risk of disease progression."

Similar statements have been made by exercise specialists. For example, a consensus American Heart Association statement on Exercise Standards published in 1995 recommended the following: "Medically stable subjects with compensated heart failure may participate in exercise training programs. Benefits that accrue from conditioning of the musculoskeletal system include increased skeletal muscle vascular

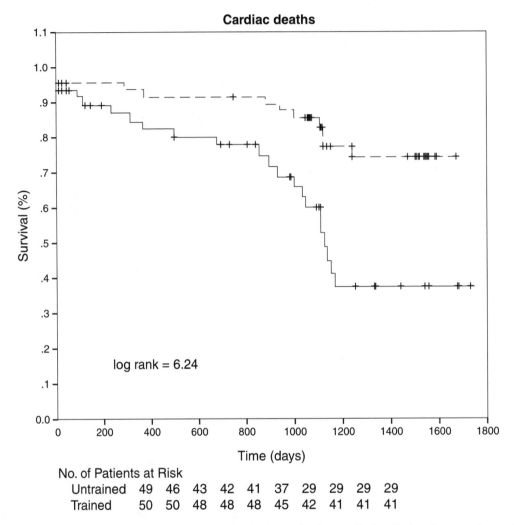

Figure 8–8 Kaplan-Meier survival curves of cardiac death in trained group (broken line) and untrained control group (solid line) during follow-up. The cross marking (+) indicates censored cases.

conductance and oxygen extraction and decreased skeletal muscle lactate production."[42]

Taken together, these consensus documents do not specifically indicate whether patients with heart failure should be enrolled in cardiac rehabilitation programs or not. These documents also provide no specific recommendations regarding home exercise programs, such as the types, duration, and intensity of exercise. Therefore, most cli-

nicians use exercise prescription strategies that have been developed for cardiac patients and published by the American College of Sports Medicine and American Heart Association.[42-44] These recommendations can be obtained from a variety of publications.[42-44]

Cardiac rehabilitation programs usually involve three exercise sessions a week on nonconsecutive days. Programs typically last 12 weeks.

The primary emphasis is on large muscle group exercise, such as walking, cycling, rowing, and stair climbing.

Before enrollment in the rehabilitation program, patients should undergo a maximal exercise test. The intensity of exercise is then set on the basis of the peak exercise heart rate. The intensity of exercise is set lower at the beginning of the rehabilitation program and then gradually adjusted upward. For example, during the first 2 weeks of a rehabilitation program, patients usually exercise at 40% to 50% of peak exercise heart rate. Exercise intensity is advanced to 60% to 75% of peak heart rate by 4 to 6 weeks into the program. Maximal exercise testing sometimes is repeated during the program to reassess peak exercise heart rate.

Each exercise session usually lasts 60 minutes. However, at the beginning of a cardiac rehabilitation program, shorter exercise periods may be used. Patients who are severely deconditioned may also benefit from frequent, shorter exercise sessions.

At the end of 3 months, maximal exercise testing is usually repeated to document improvement in the patient's functional capacity. Patients are then encouraged to undertake a home exercise program. Ideally, this program should involve 30 minutes of moderate-intensity exercise on most if not all days of the week.

Patients should be taught to take their own pulse or be encouraged to purchase a cardiotachometer. Exercise should be set at 60% to 75% of peak treadmill heart rate or at a perceived exertion level of 12 to 13, using a scale of 6 to 20. Exercise should consist of walking, treadmill exercise, or cycling.

Patients who do not participate in a formal cardiac rehabilitation program can be encouraged to undertake a home exercise program. Before embarking on such a program, all patients should undergo a maximal cardiopulmonary exercise test. This test should be used to develop an exercise prescription. Patients with angina, significant ischemic electrocardiogram changes, hypotension, or arrhythmias during exercise should be fully evaluated before undertaking any type of exercise program. If it is believed that the patient can safely participate in an exercise program, such patients should be enrolled in some type of monitored cardiac rehabilitation program before embarking on a home exercise program.

Patients should be encouraged to keep a log of their exercise sessions and to show the log to their physicians. Patients should start with 10- to 15-minute exercise sessions three to five times each week. The exercise intensity should be set at 40% to 60% of peak heart rate. Exercise duration should be increased gradually until the patient is exercising 30 to 60 minutes most days of the week at 50% to 70% of their maximal heart rate.

Which patients with heart failure should be enrolled in formal cardiac rehabilitation programs? Such programs appear to pose little risk to patients. Therefore, it could be argued that all patients with heart failure should be enrolled in some type of supervised exercise program. However, the cost of such programs is relatively large. In addition, no large randomized trials of cardiac rehabilitation have been conducted in patients with heart failure, although several trials are in process.

At present, it would seem prudent to reserve cardiac rehabilitation for patients most likely to benefit from this intervention. This group would include patients who have been deconditioned by prolonged bed rest or repeated hospitalizations and patients who are inactive because of a fear of exertion. Other patients with heart failure should probably be encouraged to participate in a home exercise program.

CONCLUSION

In summary, exercise intolerance is a major problem in heart failure. This exercise intolerance can be caused by multiple factors. Pharmaceutical agents have only a modest impact on exertional symptoms. Exercise training potentially is a useful adjunct to pharmaceutical agents. Patients who have been deconditioned by prolonged bed rest or repeated hospitalizations and patients who are inactive because of a fear of exertion should be enrolled in a formal cardiac rehabilitation program. Other patients with heart failure should be encouraged to participate in a home exercise program.

REFERENCES

1. Liang C, Stewart DK, LeJemtel TH, et al. Characteristics of peak aerobic capacity in symptomatic and asymptomatic subjects with left ventricular dysfunction. *Am J Cardiol.* 1992;69:1207–1211.

2. Wade OL, Bishop JM. *Cardiac Output and Regional Blood Flow.* Oxford, England: Blackwell Publishers; 1962.

3. Zelis R, Longhurst J, Capone RJ, Mason DT. A comparison of regional blood flow and oxygen utilization during dynamic forearm exercise in normal subjects and patients with congestive heart failure. *Circulation.* 1974;50:137–143.

4. Wilson JR, Martin JL, Schwartz D, Ferraro N. Exercise intolerance in patients with chronic heart failure: role of impaired nutritive flow to skeletal muscle. *Circulation.* 1984;69:1079–1087.

5. Huckabee WE, Judson WE. The role of anaerobic metabolism in the performance of mild muscular work. I. Relationship to oxygen consumption and cardiac output, and the effect of congestive heart failure. *J Clin Invest.* 1959;37:1577–1592.

6. Christie RV, Meakins JC. The intrapleural pressure in congestive heart failure and its clinical significance. *J Clin Invest.* 1934;13:323–346.

7. Marshall R, McIlroy MB, Christie RV. The work of breathing in mitral stenosis. *Clin Sci.* 1954;13:137–146.

8. Reed JW, Ablett M, Cotes JE. Ventilatory responses to exercise and to carbon dioxide in mitral stenosis before and after valvulotomy: causes of tachypnoea. *Clin Sci Mol Med.* 1978;54:9–16.

9. Maskin CS, Kugler J, Sonnenblick EH, LeJemtel TH. Acute inotropic stimulation with dopamine in severe congestive heart failure: Beneficial hemodynamic effect at rest but not during maximal exercise. *Am J Cardiol.* 1983;52:1028–1032.

10. Wilson JR, Martin JL, Ferraro N. Impaired skeletal muscle nutritive flow during exercise in patients with congestive heart failure: Role of cardiac pump dysfunction as determined by the effect of dobutamine. *Am J Cardiol.* 1984;53:1308–1315.

11. Fink LI, Wilson JR, Ferraro N. Exercise ventilation and pulmonary artery wedge pressure in chronic stable congestive heart failure. *Am J Cardiol.* 1986;57:249–253.

12. Wilson JR, Fink L, Maris J, Ferraro N, Power-Vanwqart J, Eleff S, Chance B. Evaluation of skeletal muscle energy metabolism in patients with heart failure using gated phosphorus-31 nuclear magnetic resonance. *Circulation.* 1985;71:57–62.

13. Massie B, Conway M, Yonge R, et al. Skeletal muscle metabolism in patients with congestive heart failure: Relation to clinical severity and blood flow. *Circulation.* 1987;76:1009–1019.

14. Mancini DM, Walter G, Reichek N, et al. Contribution of skeletal muscle atrophy to exercise intolerance and altered muscle metabolism in heart failure. *Circulation.* 1992;85:1364–1373.

15. Minotti JR, Pillay P, Oka R, Wells L, Christoph I, Massie BM. Skeletal muscle size: relationship to muscle function in heart failure. *J Appl Physiol.* 1993;75:373–381.

16. Minotti JR, Christoph I, Oka R, Weiner MW, Wells L, Massie BM. Impaired skeletal muscle function in patients with congestive heart failure. Relationship to systemic exercise performance. *J Clin Invest.* 1991;88:2077–2082.

17. Mancini DM, Coyle E, Coggan A, et al. Contribution of intrinsic skeletal muscle changes to 31P NMR skeletal muscle metabolic abnormalities in patients with chronic heart failure. *Circulation.* 1989;80:1338–1346.

18. Sullivan MJ, Green HJ, Cobb FR. Skeletal muscle biochemistry and histology in ambulatory patients with long-term heart failure. *Circulation.* 1990;81:518–527.

19. Drexler H, Riede U, Munzel T, Konig H, Funke E, Just J. Alterations of skeletal muscle in chronic heart failure. *Circulation.* 1992;85:1751–1759.

20. Mancini DM, Henson D, LaManca J, Levine S. Evidence of reduced respiratory muscle endurance in patients with heart failure. *J Am Coll Cardiol.* 1994;24:972–981.

21. Hammond MD, Bauer KA, Sharp JT, Rocha RD. Respiratory muscle strength in congestive heart failure. *Chest.* 1990;98:1091–1094.

22. McParland C, Resch EF, Krishnan B, Wang Y, Cujec B, Gallagher CG. Inspiratory muscle weakness in chronic heart failure: role of nutrition and electrolyte status and systemic myopathy. *Am J Respir Crit Care Med.* 1995;151:1101–1107.

23. Minotti JR, Johnson EC, Hudson TL, et al. Skeletal muscle response to exercise training in congestive heart failure. *J Clin Invest.* 1990;86:751–758.

24. Adamopoulos S, Coats AJS, Brusnotte F, et al. Physical training improves skeletal muscle metabolism in patients with chronic heart failure. *J Am Coll Cardiol.* 1993;21:1101–1106.

25. Hambrecht R, Neibauer J, Fiehn E, et al. Physical training in patients with stable chronic heart failure: effects on cardiorespiratory fitness and ultrastructural abnormalities of leg muscles. *J Am Coll Cardiol.* 1995;25:1239–1249.

26. Wilson JR, Rayos G, Yeoh TK, Gothard P, Bak K. Dissociation between exertional symptoms and circulatory function in patients with heart failure. *Circulation.* 1995;92:47–53.

27. Wilson JR, Rayos G, Yeoh TK, Gothard P. Dissociation between peak exercise oxygen consumption and hemodynamic dysfunction in potential heart transplantation candidates. *J Am Coll Cardiol.* 1995;26:429–435.

28. Wilson JR, Groves J, Rayos G. Circulatory status and response to cardiac rehabilitation in patients with heart failure. *Circulation.* 1996;94:1567–1572.

29. Chomsky DB, Lang CC, Rayos GH, et al. Hemodynamic exercise testing: A valuable tool in the selection of cardiac transplantation candidates. *Circulation.* 1996;94:3176–3183.

30. Chomsky DB, Lang CC, Rayos G, Wilson JR. Treatment of subclinical fluid retention in patients with symptomatic heart failure: Effect on exercise performance. *J Heart Lung Transplant.* 1997;16:846–853.

31. Captopril Multicenter Research Group. A placebo-controlled trial of captopril in refractory chronic congestive heart failure. *J Am Coll Cardiol.* 1983;2:755–763.

32. Sullivan MJ, Higginbotham MB, Cobb FR. Exercise training in patients with severe left ventricular dysfunction. Hemodynamic and metabolic effects. *Circulation.* 1988;78:506–515.

33. Sullivan MJ, Higginbotham MB, Cobb FR. Exercise training in patients with chronic heart failure delays ventilatory anaerobic threshold and improves submaximal exercise performance. *Circulation.* 1989;79:324–329.

34. Coats AJS, Adamopoulos S, Radaelli A, et al. Controlled trial of physical training in chronic heart failure. *Circulation.* 1992;85:2119–2131.

35. Hambrecht R, Fiehn E, Weigl C, et al. Regular physical exercise corrects endothelial dysfunction and improves exercise capacity in patients with chronic heart failure. *Circulation.* 1998;98:2709–2715.

36. Katz SD, Yuen J, Bijou R, LeJentel TH. Training improves endothelium-dependent vasodilation in resistance vessels of patients with heart failure. *J Appl Physiol.* 1997;82:1488–1492.

37. McKelvie RS, Teo KK, McCartney N, et al. Randomized controlled trial of exercise training in patients with congestive heart failure (EXERT) [abstract]. *J Am Coll Cardiol.* 1998;31(Suppl A):508A.

38. Belardinelli R, Georgiou D, Cianci G, Purcaro A. Randomized, controlled trial of long-term moderate exercise training in chronic heart failure. *Circulation.* 1999;99:1173–1182.

39. Heart failure: evaluation and care of patients with left-ventricular systolic dysfunction. Agency for Health Care Policy and Research. Rockville, Maryland. Publication No. 94–0612, 1994.

40. ACC/AHA Task Force Report. Guidelines for the evaluation and management of heart failure. *Circulation.* 1995;92:2764–2784.

41. Consensus recommendations for the management of chronic heart failure. *Am J Cardiol.* 1999;83:1A–38A.

42. ACC/AHA Task Force Report. Exercise standards. *Circulation.* 1995;91:580–615.

43. American College of Sports Medicine. *ACSD's Guidelines for Exercise Testing and Prescription.* Baltimore: Williams & Wilkins; 1995.

44. American College of Sports Medicine. *Resource Manual for Guidelines for Exercise Testing and Prescription.* 3rd ed. Philadelphia: Lea & Febiger; 1998.

CHAPTER 9

Risk Factor Modification in Heart Failure

Lynn V. Doering, Susan J. Bennett, Laurie Hackward,
Sara A. Blackburn, and Karol E. Watson

INTRODUCTION

Recent increases in the incidence of heart failure can be traced primarily to the increased incidence of its most common etiologies, coronary heart disease (CHD) and hypertension. From large epidemiologic studies,[1–4] clinicians and scientists have identified "cardiac risk factors," which are commonly evaluated in heart failure patients, as well as other cardiac populations. Coronary heart disease and hypertension are the most common contributing factors to the development of heart failure, and individuals who survive a myocardial infarction or develop hypertension remain at increased risk for heart failure as they age. Therefore, attention to management of cardiac risk factors is vital for these special patient populations.

There is increasing awareness in the general population of the importance of the reduction of cardiac risk factors in preventing cardiovascular diseases. Unfortunately, appreciation and attention to cardiac risk factors is often lacking once an individual develops heart failure because it is such a chronic, life-altering disease. However, attention to cardiac risk factors can be vital in preventing deaths both by preventing initial left ventricular dysfunction and by reducing the likelihood of additional myocardial injury. The purpose of this chapter is to summarize findings and treatment recommendations regarding reduction of key cardiac risk factors in the heart failure population. The chapter will focus on control of hypertension, hyperlipidemia, diabetes mellitus,

obesity, smoking and alcohol consumption, and lack of exercise. For each of these risk factors, the evidence regarding its influence on heart failure progression or exacerbation will be reviewed. Recommendations for clinical management, based on evidence-based guidelines and clinical studies, will be presented. Also, where available, evidence regarding the efficacy of strategies to improve compliance with risk factor modification recommendations will be evaluated. This chapter will focus on tertiary prevention (intervention to prevent disease progression through identification, treatment, and rehabilitation), as opposed to primary prevention (intervention in asymptomatic individuals to prevent disease) or secondary prevention (intervention to improve outcomes in patients with existing but preclinical disease).[5]

BEHAVIORAL HEALTH ASSESSMENT IN HEART FAILURE

Risk factor evaluation in heart failure patients requires a systematic behavioral health assessment. Gordon's Functional Health Patterns has been suggested as a logical framework for health assessment in other cardiac populations.[6] Gordon identifies 11 health patterns that incorporate health behaviors and related perceptions, beliefs, and attitudes.[7] The functional health patterns, related general examples, and specific assessment data associated with cardiac risk factors are presented in Table 9–1.

Table 9–1 Functional Health Patterns and Specific Assessment in Heart Failure

Functional Health Pattern	General Assessment	Specific Assessment
Health perception—health management	General health care pattern Perceived health pattern Health risk	History of heart failure progression Satisfaction with care Quality of life Specific behavioral assessment (smoking, alcohol, activity)
Nutrition—metabolic	Patterns of food/fluid intake Food preferences	Daily weight assessment Food diary Fingerstick glucose log (for diabetics)
Elimination	Bowel and bladder function	Urine output (daily weights indirectly indicate) Problems with elimination
Activity—exercise	Activities of daily living Patterns of activity	NYHA classification Number, type, and intensity of activities
Sleep—rest	Sleep, rest, relaxation patterns Use of sleep aids	Number, timing, duration of naps Type and frequency of sleep disturbances
Cognitive—perceptual	Sensory acuity Pain Memory and language Decision making	Vision acuity, adequacy of correction with glasses or contacts, hearing acuity, adequacy of correction Frequency/duration of angina or dyspnea Cognitive function Reading ability Knowledge of behavioral recommendations re: smoking, alcohol, fat/calorie intake, blood pressure, weight control, activity
Self-perception—self-concept	General emotional pattern Body image Attitude about self	Presence of mood disorders Self-efficacy
Role—relationship	Major roles and responsibilities Social relationships	Individual's perception of roles Identification of social support network
Sexuality—reproductive	Reproductive stage Satisfaction with sexuality	Presence/absence of sexual dysfunction Type/frequency of activity. Use of low energy-expenditure activities
Coping—stress tolerance	Capacity to handle stress Modes of handling stress	Identification of coping style Identification of activities/situations associated with angina or dyspnea
Value—belief	Values, goals, beliefs Quality-of-life decisions	Importance of specific health outcomes Attitudes/concerns re: transplantation End-of-life decisions

NYHA, New York Heart Association.

Because so many cardiac risk factors, such as hypertension, diabetes, hypercholesterolemia, and alcohol consumption, are influenced by the patient's dietary intake and habits, a comprehensive nutritional assessment provides an additional framework for risk factor modification in heart failure patients. Nutrition assessment is an indirect evaluation of body composition and cellular function.[8] An in-depth assessment includes evaluation of (1) anthropometric measurements; (2) selected biochemical serum markers; (3) clinical and physical examination; and (4) current dietary intake, medications, and symptoms. This assessment incorporates evaluation of the six body compartments: adipose tissue; skin and skeleton; extracellular; plasma protein; visceral protein mass; and skeletal muscle body cell mass. These compartments are assessed to determine the status of the protein and adipose tissues of the body. Depletion of plasma protein, visceral protein mass, and skeletal muscle body cell mass are of primary importance, because all proteins in the body are functional, and the loss of protein adversely affects body function. A summary of key components of the nutritional assessment is included in Table 9–2.

HYPERTENSION

Systemic hypertension is a frequent cause of heart failure in the United States. Left ventricular dysfunction occurs six times more frequently in hypertensive versus normotensive patients,[9] and data from the Studies of Left Ventricular Dysfunction (SOLVD) registry underscore the importance of hypertension in the development of heart failure, particularly in the African-American community. In the SOLVD registry, information was collected on patients with left ventricular dysfunction over a 14-month period. In this registry, hypertension was responsible for 32% of heart failure cases in African Americans and 4% of heart failure cases in Caucasians.[10] Furthermore, systemic hypertension may contribute to exacerbation of the syndrome in patients with established heart failure or precipitation of heart failure in cases of clinically latent left ventricular dysfunction.

Hypertension is important in exacerbation of heart failure in several ways. Elevated arterial pressure increases myocardial oxygen demand, thereby adversely affecting the myocardial oxygen supply/demand ratio. This occurs by increasing both left ventricular end-systolic wall stress (afterload) and left ventricular diastolic pressure.

Management of Hypertension

The goals of antihypertensive therapy in heart failure are to prevent further myocardial injury, prevent other cardiovascular morbidity, and optimize cardiac performance. To affect these goals, the Joint National Committee on Prevention, Detection, Evaluation, and Treatment of High Blood Pressure recommends maintaining blood pressure below 130/80 mm Hg in the presence of heart failure, diabetes, or renal failure.[11] In many instances, myocardial performance is optimal at even lower pressures. In fact, current vasodilator therapy is often tailored to achieve hemodynamic goals that focus on lowering of systemic vascular resistance (< 1,200 dyne/sec) and pulmonary capillary wedge pressure (< 15 mm Hg).[12] If these goals are achieved, systolic blood pressure < 130 mm Hg is acceptable, as long as the patient remains asymptomatic.

In low-risk hypertensives with no major risk factors, target organ disease, or clinical cardiovascular disease, a 3- to 6-month period of individualized life-style modification is usually recommended prior to the initiation of antihypertensive drug therapy.[11] However, because heart failure patients with hypertension are at high risk, life-style modification and drug therapy should be started together.[11,13] Individualized life-style modification is important because it has been shown to complement drug therapy, reduce the dosage and number of medications needed to control blood pressure, and contribute to reductions in all-cause mortality.[11] Because many life-style modifications are directed at lowering cardiac risk factors, they will be addressed in more detail throughout the chapter. Specific recommendations for life-style modification as an adjunct therapy for hyperten-

Table 9–2 Key Components of Nutritional Assessment

Assessment Category	Component	Measurements
Anthropometric	Height Weight Skeletal muscle mass	Body mass index Triceps skinfold thickness
Biochemical markers	Protein markers Lipids Glucose metabolism Fluid/electrolyte balance	Albumin/prealbumin Hgb/hct Total cholesterol, LDL, HDL, triglycerides Glucose Serum and urine sodium, potassium, BUN, creatinine, serum and urine osmolality
Physical examination	Overall assessment Cardiac assessment Pulmonary assessment Assessment for peripheral edema	Subjective Global Assessment Elevated JVD, S4 Crackles Pretibial edema, periorbital edema
Diet history	Food frequency assessment	Willet's Food Frequency Questionnaire Health Habits and History Questionnaire Food Guide Pyramid
Medical history	Diabetes Hypertension Hyperlipidemia Recent surgery Food–drug interactions GI symptoms > 2 weeks	Subjective Global Assessment
Heart failure symptoms	Dyspnea, fatigue, anorexia, nausea, vomiting Altered cognitive function	Patient report Minimental status exam
Social/cultural factors	Eating environment Food preferences Religious/cultural needs	

sion, together with the rationale for each modification, are presented in Table 9–3.

Drug therapy for hypertension control in heart failure centers focuses on the use of diuretics and angiotensin-converting enzyme (ACE) inhibitors. These types of drugs, along with β blockers, are often indicated even when patients are not hypertensive. There are few studies of optimal diuretic therapy for heart failure, but patients with mild heart failure can usually be managed with thiazide diuretics.[14] For patients with severe volume overload, severe renal insufficiency, or persistent edema, loop diuretics are preferable.[15] ACE inhibitors are considered critical for management of hypertension because resultant vasodilation is associated with interruption of the neurohormonal activation that exacerbates heart failure progression. Their use results in increased survival.[16] Many researchers suspect that ACE inhibitors may be underused

Table 9–3 Lifestyle Modifications for Hypertension Management

Modification	Rationale Related to Hypertension Management
Lose weight if overweight	1. Weight reduction of as little as 10 lbs reduces BP in a large proportion of overweight persons with hypertension.[95] 2. Weight reduction enhances BP-lowering effect of concurrent antihypertensive agents.[96]
Limit alcohol intake to < 1 oz ethanol per day or 0.5 oz in women and lighter individuals	1. Excessive alcohol intake can cause resistance to antihypertensive therapies.[97]
Increase physical activity to 30–45 minutes most days of the week	1. Regular physical activity can enhance weight loss and functional health status, and reduce the risk for all-cause mortality.[98]
Reduce sodium intake to < 100 mmol/day	1. Sodium intake is positively correlated with BP.[99] 2. A reduction to 75–100 mmol/day in sodium intake lowers BP over periods of weeks to a few years.[100]
Maintain adequate intake of dietary potassium (approximately 90 mmol/day)	1. High dietary potassium intake may improve BP control in patients with hypertension.[101]
Stop smoking	1. A significant rise in BP accompanies the smoking of each cigarette.[102]

because of clinicians' concerns regarding excessive blood pressure reduction.[15] However, maximum benefit from ACE inhibitors is realized when the largest-tolerated dose is used. Doses of ACE inhibitors should be titrated upward over a 2- to 3-week period, with the goal of reaching the doses used in large-scale clinical trials: captopril 50 mg TID or enalapril 10 mg BID.[15] Doses of diuretics should be titrated to achieve euvolemia while maintaining maximal ACE inhibitor dosages.

A third category of drugs, β blockers, may be useful for control of hypertension in heart failure. Although β blockers are potentially harmful to some patients because of their negative inotropic effect, they are helpful for stable patients. They have been shown to increase ejection fraction, reduce risk of hospitalization, and reduce all-cause mortality.[17]

Management of sodium retention and fluid overload, although critical for symptom management for all heart failure patients, is also an important element of hypertension management. The Consensus Recommendations for the Management of Chronic Heart Failure[18] and the Agency for Health Care Policy and Research (AHCPR) Clinical Practice Guidelines for Heart Failure[15] recommend that assisting patients to (1) monitor signs of sodium retention, (2) comply with medication regimens, and (3) comply with dietary sodium restrictions should be part of routine care for persons with heart failure. The importance of these recommendations is supported by results from research studies. Inadequate prescription by health care providers of medications known to be effective in reducing sodium retention contributes to decompensation.[19] Sodium retention leading to volume overload and cardiac decompensation was the main reason for hospitalization in nearly two-thirds (59%) of heart failure admissions.[20] Lack of compliance with medication or diet therapy was associated with the sodium retention that led to decompensation.[21]

Currently, the AHCPR Guidelines recommend that most heart failure patients follow a 2- to 3-g sodium diet.[15] Additionally, the Guidelines recommend that patients avoid drinking excessive quantities of fluid and, in selected cases, fluid restrictions may become necessary. No studies have specifically tested the effects of dietary sodium restrictions on fluid balance in heart failure; therefore, optimal management of patients by a sodium-restricted diet is unclear. Until additional data become available, the recommendation of a 2- to 3-g sodium restriction is indicated.

The main goals related to fluid and electrolyte balance for the patient with heart failure are to restore euvolemia, prevent further sodium retention and fluid retention, and maintain normal electrolyte balance. Interventions to achieve these goals are focused on educating the patient to adhere to pharmacologic therapies, follow dietary sodium restrictions, and self-monitor for signs and symptoms of fluid retention.

Patients should be taught the importance of medications, particularly diuretics, in controlling sodium retention. Compliance with medication therapy should be monitored to assist in preventing sodium retention. Adjustments in therapies are indicated by changes in patients' conditions. In some settings, health care providers are now educating patients to adjust their own diuretic medications daily, based on weights, as indicated in the Consensus Recommendations.[18] This type of self-medication program promises improved outcomes but has not been prospectively tested. However, careful assessment of a patient's understanding of his or her condition and ability to self-medicate would be critical prior to implementing this type of intervention. Patients need to be taught the importance of following their individualized, prescribed dietary sodium restrictions. With a 2-g sodium restriction, it is difficult for patients to maintain adequate nutritional intake. Cautious liberalization of the sodium restriction may be beneficial by allowing the patient to focus on eating a well-balanced diet while still control-

ling sodium and fluid retention. Patients who are medically stable, have no signs of edema or fluid retention, are compliant with medications, and have difficulty following 2 or 3 g of sodium restriction may be considered for liberalization of the sodium restriction. Tips that patients can use to control dietary sodium are presented in Exhibit 9–1.

Outcomes of Hypertension Management

Appropriate management of hypertension can have significant benefits in heart failure. In the Systolic Hypertension in the Elderly Program (SHEP)[22] 4,735 patients older than 50 years of age with isolated systolic hypertension were randomized to placebo or antihypertensive therapy for an average of 4.5 years. In this study in pa-

Exhibit 9–1 Tips for Controlling Dietary Sodium Intake

- Avoid adding salt to foods during meal preparation or at the table.
- Avoid processed foods (canned foods, such as vegetables or meats; packaged foods, such as potato chips, crackers; boxed foods, such as macaroni and cheese).
- Buy foods labeled *low-sodium* when possible.
- Post a list of low-sodium foods to keep on the refrigerator door.
- Read the sodium content on food labels.
- Purchase frozen meals with < 600 mg sodium for the total meal.
- Use a salt substitute that does not contain potassium (for example, *Mrs. Dash*).
- Cook in large quantities and freeze in individual containers to be reheated later.
- Check with local bakeries for low-sodium breads and with health food stores for other low-sodium products.
- Check with local senior citizen center and Meals on Wheels, etc., to find out if low-sodium foods are offered.
- For dining out, carry a list of low-sodium foods available at nearby restaurants.

tients with a history of prior myocardial infarction, antihypertensive therapy decreased the risk of developing heart failure by 81%.[22] Also, in the Veterans Affairs Cooperative Study on Antihypertensive Agents,[23] 380 patients with diastolic hypertension were randomized to placebo or antihypertensive therapy. In this study, antihypertensive therapy also decreased the risk of developing heart failure.[23] Therefore, appropriate treatment of systemic hypertension would be expected to have enormous benefit, not only in preventing new cases of heart failure, but also in limiting progression of existing heart failure.

HYPERLIPIDEMIA

Coronary heart disease is the etiology of heart failure in approximately two-thirds of cases, and hyperlipidemia is one of the major contributors to CHD.[24] Therefore, appropriate management of hyperlipidemia is essential. Lipid disorders are quite common in the general population and perhaps even more common in heart failure populations. Numerous recent studies have documented the benefits of reducing serum low-density lipoprotein (LDL) cholesterol levels in patients both with and without known CHD.[25–28] The benefits that have been documented in cholesterol-lowering trials are primarily in the form of reduced coronary heart disease mortality and, in some studies, reduced total mortality. In at least one study, the risk of developing heart failure was also found to be decreased with lipid-lowering medication. In the Scandinavian Simvastatin Survival Study (4S), 4,444 patients with hypercholesterolemia and known CHD were randomized to placebo or the lipid-lowering agent simvastatin for approximately 5 years. In this study, treatment with simvastatin decreased coronary mortality by 42%, all-cause mortality by 30%, and the risk of developing heart failure by 20%.[24,29] The observed benefits in heart failure reduction were likely secondary to a decrease in cardiac events and, therefore, myocardial injury.

Lipid and Triglyceride Management

In patients with known CHD, the National Cholesterol Education Panel Adult Treatment Panel II recommends an LDL target of less than 100 mg/dL. Specific recommendations for lipid targets in patients with CHD are presented in Table 9–4.[30] In many patients, achieving these goals will require the use of lipid-lowering medications. The most prevalent lipid-lowering medications in current use are the HMG-CoA reductase inhibitors, also known as the *statins*. Therapy with statins has been found to be highly efficacious in lowering serum LDL and is extremely safe and well tolerated; thus, their use should be considered in all patients with heart failure and hyperlipidemia. This should result in fewer recurrent cardiac events in patients with known CHD and fewer primary cardiac events in patients with other etiologies of heart failure.

Current dietary recommendations are to encourage well-nourished heart failure patients to follow a low-fat diet, which means 30% of the total calories should be from fat. However, no studies have investigated the relationship of low-fat diets to the development or progression

Table 9–4 Lipid Targets for Patients with and without Coronary Heart Disease

Target	Patients with CHD	Patients without CHD
Total cholesterol	160	200
LDL	100	130
HDL	> 45	> 3
Triglycerides	< 200	< 200

LDL, low-density lipoprotein; HDL, high-density lipoprotein.

of cachexia in heart failure. Basic information for following a low-fat diet includes educating patients to consume lean meats and low-fat dairy products. Avoiding fried foods is beneficial. Patients should be counseled to limit adding fat, such as margarine, butter, oils, and salad dressings with a high fat content. In addition to following a low-fat diet, using fats such as omega-3-rich foods (flax seed, salmon, cod) and monounsaturated fats (olive oil, canola oil) may help to decrease serum cholesterol and triglycerides.[31]

To assist with maintaining normal triglyceride levels, patients should avoid using table sugar, using a sugar substitute if desired. Desserts high in sugar contribute to elevated triglycerides, and these foods should be avoided. Some patients who are very sensitive to refined carbohydrates and alcohol would need closer monitoring than would other patients.

DIABETES MELLITUS AND INSULIN RESISTANCE

Both Type I and Type II diabetes mellitus are powerful and independent risk factors for development of CHD.[32] CHD is the leading cause of death among patients with Type II diabetes, regardless of duration of diabetes. There is no obvious association between the extent or severity of cardiovascular complications and the duration of diabetes or the degree of hyperglycemia. In fact, even impaired glucose tolerance and insulin resistance carry an increased cardiovascular risk, despite minimal hyperglycemia,[33,34] and in individuals who are prone to develop Type II diabetes, insulin resistance is the earliest detectable defect and can occur up to 25 years prior to the onset of overt hyperglycemia.[35] Several atherogenic metabolic changes occur in Type II diabetes, including elevated serum triglycerides, reduced high-density lipoprotein (HDL) cholesterol levels, often with normal LDL cholesterol levels but with abnormal LDL particle composition, resulting in an abundance of smaller, denser (more atherogenic) LDL particles. In addition, diabetes has been seen as a prothrombotic state with a variety of alterations in the coagulation and fibrinolytic systems that include increased platelet adhesiveness,[36] elevated levels of coagulation factors,[37] and elevated fibrinogen levels.[38]

Risks for heart failure and idiopathic cardiomyopathy are greatly increased in diabetic patients.[39] In the Framingham Heart Study, diabetes conferred more than twice the risk of developing heart failure in men and more than five times the risk for developing the syndrome in women. In addition to increased risk of developing heart failure, diabetes mellitus is also one of the parameters associated with a worse prognosis in patients who have heart failure.

Because of the dismal prognoses in regard to development of heart failure and development of heart failure in patients with diabetes, in particular, aggressive risk factor modification is clearly warranted in this group of patients. Screening for asymptomatic hyperglycemia is warranted in all patients with heart failure, and, once identified, aggressive management of not only hyperglycemia but also hyperlipidemia, hypertension, obesity, and other cardiac risk factors is essential. Furthermore, diabetics with end-organ damage are almost always excluded as candidates for cardiac transplantation. Thus, strict management of hyperglycemia and attention to end-organ complications, such as diabetic nephropathy and retinopathy, is essential in the event that cardiac transplantation is considered.

OBESITY

Obesity is defined[40] as a Body Mass Index (BMI) 30 kg/m^2. Obesity is an independent risk factor for the development of CHD. Furthermore, there is a strong correlation between obesity and other cardiovascular risk factors, such as hypertension, diabetes, and hyperlipidemia.[40] Excess adipose tissue demands an increase in oxygen, and the usual adaptive response is an increase in the cardiac output, achieved by increases in stroke volume without significant change in heart rate. To achieve these needs, the heart in response to obesity both dilates and thickens, and total blood volume increases. Left ventricular hypertrophy can be seen in approximately 50% of patients who are more than 50% overweight.[41,42] Weight reduction results in several beneficial effects in heart failure. With weight reduction, mean arterial pressure decreases, left ventricular mass decreases, and total blood volume decreases.[43] In addition, weight loss is accompanied by a decrease in plasma norepinephrine levels, plasma rennin activity, and aldosterone levels.[44]

Management of Obesity

Current recommendations are to aim for a weight loss of 5%–10% in obese and overweight patients, because this achievable level of weight loss has been shown to improve outcomes.[45] For BMI > 25 kg/m^2 (overweight), placing the patient in a weight loss program to achieve a 5%–10% weight loss may help to relieve heart failure symptoms while maintaining lean body mass. Prior to beginning a weight loss regimen, patients should have a thorough nutritional assessment to ensure that a positive nitrogen balance is achieved because obese patients may be malnourished. Diet, exercise, behavior modification, and drug therapy are options for the management of obesity in heart failure. Attempts to treat obesity through dietary restriction alone have been disappointing, with an enormously high recidivism rate.[44] Long-term results of behavioral treatment are also discouraging, with less than 5% of subjects remaining lean for more than 4 years.[46] When diet and exercise are combined, the most encouraging results in the treatment of obesity are obtained.[47] There is increasing interest in the use of fat replacers that are not absorbed as a strategy to reduce obesity. Longer-term safety studies are needed before these can be recommended. The final consideration is the use of medication to treat obesity. However, these drugs have not been extensively studied in patients with heart failure; thus, their use must be considered only following a careful weighing of risk, benefits, and other available treatment options.

SMOKING

Smoking is a major risk indicator for the development of CHD.[48] Population studies have linked smoking with heart failure.[49,50] Among patients with CHD, smoking significantly increases the risk of developing the syndrome, and cessation is associated with improved prognosis.[51,52] Using data from the Coronary Artery Surgery Study (CASS) to identify predictors of heart failure, researchers used a case-control design in which all patients who developed heart failure were identified as cases, and patients who did not develop the syndrome were identified as controls. Patients who were current smokers had a 50% increased risk of developing heart failure, compared with nonsmokers, even after adjustment for the extent of CHD and myocardial infarction.[52]

Investigators have established the mechanism of action of smoking in the development of CHD, in general, and heart failure, in particular. Smoking increases heart rate and blood pressure, both important determinants of myocardial oxygen consumption.[53] In patients with angina, stroke index has been shown to decrease after smoking. This decrease is believed to result from increased levels of carboxyhemoglobin, which have a negative inotropic effect and increase left ventricular end diastolic pressure.[54] In patients with moderate (New York Heart Association [NYHA] functional Class III) heart failure, smoking is associated with hemodynamic changes, including increases in heart rate, systemic blood pressure, pulmonary artery pressure, ventricular filling pressures, and systemic and pulmonary vascular resistance.[55] Together, these changes contribute to decreased stroke volume and increased afterload in heart failure patients.[55] Therefore, smoking increases oxygen demand via increased heart rate and increased afterload but decreases oxygen supply via reduced diastolic filling time and higher carboxyhemoglobin levels.[56] In heart failure patients, the effects of smoking on oxygen supply and demand may be critical.

Although these hemodynamic data suggest that smoking may be associated with heart failure exacerbations, studies of precipitating factors of relapse in heart failure have not specifically investigated the role of tobacco use. Heart failure exacerbations have been associated with lack of adherence to the medical regimen, dietary noncompliance, arrhythmias, angina, emotional and environmental issues, iatrogenic factors, infections, and other causes.[56,57] Because smoking may serve as a catalyst for heart failure decompensation, further study is needed to evaluate the role of smoking in heart failure exacerbations.

Both epidemiologic and hemodynamic evidence, therefore, underscore the importance of smoking cessation in heart failure patients. Patients should be advised strongly to stop smoking and should be informed that continued smoking is associated with poorer outcomes. Although this may seem obvious, it does not appear to be a regular part of routine management for heart failure. Two studies have reported that the heart failure patients who smoke receive documented advice to quit in only 9%–11% of cases.[58,59]

The efficacy of specific smoking cessation methods has been studied widely in healthy individuals. Several studies have focused on cardiac patients, in general, but none have focused on heart failure patients, specifically.[60–64] Approaches to smoking cessation that have been tested in cardiac patients include nicotine replacement (patch), behavioral counseling, and simple advice and encouragement from a health care provider. At least three studies have shown that the use of the nicotine patch is safe in cardiac patients, and two of these also have shown that, with use of the nicotine patch, short-term smoking abstinence (6 months) increases, compared with controls.[63–65] However, the long-term efficacy of nicotine replacement treatment remains unknown in cardiac patients. Behavioral counseling in cardiac patients has shown equivocal results. In two studies, nurse-delivered therapies were effective in reducing some unhealthy behaviors, such as reducing dietary fat intake and increasing exercise, but showed little effect on smoking cessation.[60,61] A third study showed that a nurse-delivered smoking cessation intervention that included three months of telephone follow-up increased self-reported smoking cessation by 15%, compared with controls.[62]

More rigorous studies, including biochemical validation of smoking abstinence, are needed in cardiac patients. Additional interventions also warrant rigorous study. Specifically, the use of antidepressants in smoking cessation has shown promise in healthy smokers.[66–68] Antidepressants

have been associated with longer abstinence rates, when combined with cognitive behavioral therapy,[66] particularly in patients with mild depression. Time-sustained antidepressants have been shown to be superior to nicotine patch or placebo[67] and to be associated with reduced weight gain.[68] Because depression is common among both smokers and heart failure patients, the use of antidepressants alone or in combination with nicotine replacement therapies may hold particular promise.

An acute event or new diagnosis, especially in light smokers, represents a key opportunity for health care providers to initiate smoking cessation measures because patients may be more receptive to making a decision to stop smoking. In a study of CHD patients who were smokers and who were admitted to a coronary care unit, 6-month and 12-month cessation rates of more than 30% and 25%, respectively, have been reported.[69] In these patients, smoking cessation was more likely if patients had no prior history of CHD, smoked less than one pack of cigarettes daily, and had heart failure during hospitalization. A past history of heart failure was not related to successful smoking cessation, nor was a discharge diagnosis of acute myocardial infarction.[69]

Clinicians should be particularly aware of how instrumental their advice to stop smoking can be in inducing patients to change their behavior. Following personal advice and encouragement to stop smoking given by physicians during a single routine consultation, an estimated 2% of all smokers stopped smoking and did not relapse for up to 1 year, as a direct consequence of the advice.[70] Furthermore, advice and encouragement are even more effective for smokers at special risk, including those with ischemic heart disease.[70] Physician advice and encouragement is as effective as behavior modifications techniques in achieving smoking cessation.[70] Therefore, all clinicians should take time to advise their cardiac patients—especially heart failure patients—who smoke to quit. The patient's plans for quitting should be discussed, and additional support, including nicotine replacement, should be considered. Overall low success rates for long-term (1-year) smoking cessation of 2%–8% make it important that clinicians reevaluate smoking habits periodically in these high-risk patients.[70]

ALCOHOL

Alcohol has a definitive, acute negative inotropic effect, and chronic overuse leads to decreased contractile function of the heart related to myocyte hypertrophy, interstitial fibrosis, and myocytolysis.[71,72] Abstention may be effective in limiting the progression of dysfunction only up to a certain stage of the disease.[72] There is evidence that mild heart failure may be reversible if patients abstain from alcohol. However, there is no consensus that disease progression can be halted once structural myocardial dilation has evolved.[73]

In patients with confirmed alcoholic cardiomyopathy, abstention from alcohol is essential.[74] Echocardiographic studies show that major clinical improvement and normalization of left ventricular function can be achieved after abstention from alcohol in these patients.[75] Resumed alcohol intake may precipitate heart failure relapse in patients with alcoholic cardiomyopathy.[56]

Most clinicians have adopted a conservative approach and recommend complete alcohol abstention in patients with severe heart failure of all etiologies. The practice of recommending alcohol abstinence to all heart failure patients stems from the belief that it may exacerbate already existing cardiac depression. However, there is no clear evidence regarding the efficacy of alcohol abstention in heart failure patients with nonalcoholic etiologies.[71,74,76] However, initial studies show that alcohol consumption may contribute to heart failure progression in patients with other heart failure etiologies.[77] Moreover, anecdotal evidence indicates that some patients with nonalcoholic-induced heart failure may have significant improvement after complete alcohol abstention. Therefore, an evaluation of alcohol abstention in severe heart failure patients of all etiologies is prudent.[56]

Noncompliance to recommendations for complete alcohol abstinence appears to be common. Although there has been little study in this area,

there have been recent reports of up to 40% noncompliance to alcohol abstention in heart failure patients.[77,78] Furthermore, alcohol consumption frequently is coupled with cigarette smoking, and smoking cessation is not always associated with alcohol abstention.[79,80] Therefore, continued alcohol consumption places heart failure patients at especially high risk.

Continued alcohol consumption, along with continued smoking, has been implicated in the need for multiple hospital admissions in heart failure patients.[79] The fact that alcohol use is far higher among patients with multiple readmissions has important implications. Continued alcohol use after a heart failure diagnosis may be critical to the progression or exacerbation of the disease process. Therefore, it seems more likely that continued alcohol use may be a general marker for health care usage, either because heart failure patients experience more health problems and seek help or because they engage in other high-risk behaviors. In fact, other investigators have reported a relationship between alcohol use and health care usage. In a report of 2,546 heart failure and myocardial infarction patients from the Medical Outcomes Study, a longitudinal observational study of patients with chronic medical problems, alcohol consumption was shown to increase outpatient doctor visits.[81]

Reducing alcohol consumption in heart failure patients may be difficult because medically ill alcoholics often do not respond to conventional alcoholism treatment or decline physician referrals.[82] However, a recent study showed that standard medical care alone was surprisingly effective in inducing abstinence in medically ill alcoholic veterans.[82] Together with this report, the finding that alcohol use is prevalent in heart failure patients with multiple hospital admissions[79] underscores how important it is for clinicians to emphasize a simple recommendation to abstain from alcohol use as part of routine medical care for heart failure patients.

INACTIVITY

The role of inactivity in the progression of heart failure has been the focus of considerable recent study. Inactivity as a risk factor for progression of the syndrome has gained recognition with the study of exercise as a treatment intervention to improve functional ability in heart failure patients. To date, several randomized trials have shown that both in-hospital and home exercise training programs are associated with positive clinical outcomes, including increased exercise capacity, decreased resting catecholamines, and improved heart rate variability and quality of life.[83–85] Additional studies have shown various exercise regimens, including walking or bicycle ergometry, to be safe in patients with compensated heart failure and in elderly heart failure patients.[86,87] In a small feasibility study, the addition of strength training has been shown to be safe and to increase muscle endurance and total muscle work.[88] Improvements have been noted as early as 2 months after training, with sustained, but not improved, benefit for up to 14 months.[85]

Whether heart failure patients are instructed to exercise and to remain physically active is unclear. Many specialists now recommend regular, progressive exercise for compensated heart failure patients. Cardiac rehabilitation for patients after an acute event is included in national guidelines.[89] However, no more than 40% of all cardiac patients are referred for training.[90] Although the percentage of heart failure patients referred for cardiac rehabilitation has not been reported, it is fair to assume that it is even lower because recommendations for exercise training for heart failure patients is relatively recent. Whereas over 80% of heart failure patients at academic medical centers are counseled to be as physically active as possible, only 61% of elderly heart failure patients received similar instructions.[71,72]

Compliance to activity instructions among heart failure patients is not well documented. Up to one-third of heart failure patients, most of whom were NYHA Class II–III, report no regular physical exercise.[78] When compared by functional status, more NYHA Class I–II patients reported regular exercise than did NYHA Class III–IV patients.[78] Predictors of exercise compliance have been reported in a broader sample of cardiac rehabilitation patients. Perceived self-efficacy, perceived benefits of exercise, interpersonal support for exercise, and perceived barriers to exercise were significant predictors of compliance.[91] Together, these findings suggest that heart failure patients may need more careful and detailed instruction regarding activity as an essential part of risk management and treatment. Based on experience from cardiac rehabilitation patients, heart failure patients may benefit from specific discussions regarding how they perceive exercise and physical activity fitting into their lives.

Enrollment in exercise programs as a means of developing and maintaining regular physical activity habits has not been reported in heart failure patients. However, heart failure patients enrolled in clinical trials have demonstrated respectable mean compliance rates of approximately 85%.[84,85] In broader samples of cardiac patients, evidence indicates that, even after exercise training, many cardiac patients do not develop long-term physical activity patterns. Three months after cardiac rehabilitation training following an acute cardiac event, only 50% of women continued to remain physically active.[92] These findings are discouraging and stress the importance of considering interventions to enhance long-term compliance in high-risk populations.

Several investigators have evaluated behavior modification programs to enhance physical activity compliance in cardiac patients. In general, life-style modification interventions have shown improvement in physical activity. Intensive interventions have resulted in improved physical activity behaviors at 1 year[61] and at 5 years.[93] However, these programs are expensive and involve significant commitment from the patient. More modest counseling interventions, including brief nurse-administered behavioral counseling based on the Stage of Change model, were effective in improving self-reported exercise compliance at 4 months and at 1 year.[60] In heart failure patients, there have been no reports regarding the effects of counseling interventions on exercise compliance. However, a single study of pharmacist-directed counseling related to medications showed improved medication compliance in elderly patients who received the intervention.[94] This study suggests that heart failure patients may benefit from brief, specific counseling about the importance of exercise, along with clear instructions for exercise duration and intensity.

CONCLUSION

Hypertension and CHD are the most common causes of heart failure in the United States. Because risk factors for CHD have been well established, continued attention to controlling them in heart failure patients is an essential strategy for reducing morbidity and mortality. Control of hypertension, especially following myocardial infarction, is particularly important. Therapeutic goals of blood pressure less than 130/80 mm Hg are recommended. However, goals for blood pressure should be individualized to ensure that optimal myocardial performance is attained. Likewise, hyperlipidemia is more common in heart failure patients than in the general population. Cholesterol-lowering agents should be prescribed in all patients with heart failure and hyperlipidemia, with an LDL target of less than 100 mg/dL. The dismal prognosis of heart failure patients who develop diabetes warrants aggressive risk factor modification. Screening for asymptomatic patients and aggressive blood sugar control for affected patients is imperative.

Treatment of obesity is difficult, with high recidivism rates for both dietary management and behavior modification. Modification of diet combined with exercise has yielded the most promising results.

Compliance of heart failure patients to recommended behaviors associated with cardiac risk is discouraging. Many heart failure patients continue to smoke and drink, and less than half report engaging in regular exercise. Studies indicate that clinicians should be more vigilant in counseling patients regarding smoking, alcohol, and exercise, because there is evidence that most patients do not receive adequate instruction. Intensive life-style modification programs have been effective in broader samples of cardiac patients but require considerable patient commitment and are resource-intensive. Brief counseling sessions, including telephone follow-up, have shown equivocal results. The most effective intervention in promoting compliance to risk factor modification in high-risk patients, including heart failure patients, may be the firm recommendation of the patient's care provider that they abstain from tobacco and alcohol and stay physically active with regular exercise. Such a recommendation, followed by a brief discussion to help the patient make individual plans to comply, holds promise as a powerful clinical tool to control behavioral risk factors in heart failure patients.

REFERENCES

1. Dawber TR, Meadors GF, Moore FEJ. Epidemiological approaches to heart disease: The Framingham Study. *Am J Public Health*. 1951;41:279–286.

2. Kannel WB, Feinleib M, McNamara PM, et al. An investigation of coronary heart disease in families: The Framingham Offspring Study. *Am J Epidemiol*. 1979;110:281–290.

3. Dawber TR, Moore FEJ, Mann GV. Coronary heart disease in the Framingham Study. *Am J Public Health*. 1957;47(2):4–24.

4. Kannel WB, Dawber TR, Kagan A, et al. Factors of risk in the development of coronary heart disease—six-year follow-up experience: The Framingham Study. *Ann Intern Med*. 1961;55:33–50.

5. United States Preventive Services Task Force. The periodic health examination of older adults: The recommendations of the U.S. Preventive Services Task Force. *J Am Geriatr Sci*. 1990;38:817–823.

6. Doran K, Sampson B, Staus R, Ahern C, Schiro D. Clinical pathway across tertiary and community care after an interventional cardiology procedure. *J Cardiovasc Nurse*. 1997;11:1–14.

7. Gordon M. *Nursing Diagnosis: Process and Application*. New York: McGraw-Hill, 1987.

8. Heymsfield, SB, Baumgartner RN, Pan S. Nutritional assessment of malnutrition by anthropometric methods. In: M.E. Shils, JA Olson, M Shike, A Ross. eds. *Modern Nutrition in Health and Disease*. 9th ed. Baltimore: Williams & Wilkins, 1999:909.

9. Thom T, Kannel W. Congestive heart failure: Epidemiology and cost of illness. *Dis Manage Health Outcomes*. 1997;1:75–83.

10. Centers of Disease Control. Changes in mortality from heart failure—United States, 1980–1985. *MMWR*. 1998;30:633–637.

11. National High Blood Pressure Education Program. *The Sixth Report of the Joint National Committee on Prevention, Detection, Evaluation, and Treatment of High Blood Pressure*. National Heart, Lung, and Blood Institute. Bethesda, MD: U.S. Department of Health and Human Services (DHHS), 1997.

12. Stevenson L, Massie B, Francis G. Optimizing therapy for complex or refractory heart failure: A management algorithm. *Am Heart J*. 1998;135(Suppl):S292–S309.

13. National High Blood Pressure Education Program Working Group. *Report on Hypertension in Diabetes*. National Heart, Lung and Blood Institute. Bethesda, MD: DHHS, 1995.

14. Kupper AJ, Fintelman H, Huige MC, et al. Cross-over comparison of the fixed combination of hydrochlorothiazide and triamterene and the free combination of furosemide and triamterene in the maintenance of congestive heart failure. *Eur J Clin Pharmacol*. 1986;30: 341–343.

15. Konstam MA, Dracup K, Baker DW, et al. Heart failure: Evaluation and care of patients with left-ventricular systolic dysfunction. *Agency for Health Care Policy and Research*. Rockville, MD: DHHS, 1994.

16. Garg R, Yusuf S, for the Collaborative Group on ACE Inhibitor Trials. Overview of randomized trials of angiotensin-converting enzyme inhibitors on mortality and morbidity in patients with heart failure. *JAMA*. 1995;273:1450–1456.

17. Packer M, Bristow MR, Cohn JN, et al., for the U.S. Carvedilol Heart Failure Study Group. The effect of carvedilol on morbidity and mortality in patients with chronic heart failure. *N Engl J Med*. 1996;334:1349–1355.

18. Packer M, Cohn JN, on behalf of the Steering Committee and Membership of the Advisory Council to Improve Outcomes Nationwide in Heart Failure: Consensus recommendations for the management of chronic heart failure. *Am J Cardiol*. 1999;83(Suppl):1A–38.

19. Clinical Quality Improvement Network Investigators. Mortality risk and patterns of practice in 4606 acute care patients with congestive heart failure. *Arch Intern Med*. 1996;156:1669–1673.

20. Bennett SJ, Huster GA, Baker SL, et al. Characterization of the precipitants of hospitalization for heart failure decompensation. *Am J Crit Care*. 1998;7:168–174.

21. Happ MB, Naylor MD, Roe-Prior P. Factors contributing to rehospitalization of elderly patients with heart failure. *J Cardiovasc Nurs*. 1997;11:75–84.

22. SHEP Cooperative Research Group. Prevention of stroke by antihypertensive drug treatment in older persons with isolated systolic hypertension: Final results of the Systolic Hypertension in the Elderly Program (SHEP). *JAMA*. 1991;265:3255–3264.

23. Veterans Administration Cooperative Study Group on Antihypertensive Agents. Effects of treatment on morbidity in hypertension. II. Results in patients with diastolic blood pressure averaging 90 through 114 mm Hg. *JAMA*. 1970;213:1143–1152.

24. Kannel WB, Castelli WP, Gordon T. Cholesterol in the prediction of atherosclerotic disease: New perspectives based on the Framingham study. *Ann Intern Med*. 1979;90:85–91.

25. Scandinavian Simvastatin Survival Study Group. Randomized trial of cholesterol lowering in 4444 patients with coronary heart disease. The Scandinavian Simvastatin Survival Study (4S) *Lancet*. 1994;44:1383–1389.

26. Sacks FM, Pfeffer MA, Moye L, et al. The effect of pravastatin on coronary events after myocardial infarction in patients with average cholesterol levels. *N Engl J Med*. 1996;335:1001–1009.

27. Tonkin AM. Management of the long-term intervention with pravastatin in ischaemic disease (LIPID) study after the Scandinavian Simvastatin Survival Study (4S). *Am J Cardiol*. 1995;76:107C–112C.

28. Shepard J, Cobbe SM, Ford I, et al. Prevention of coronary heart disease with pravastatin in men with hypercholesterolemia. *N Engl J Med*. 1995;333:1301–1307.

29. Kjekshus J, Pederson TR, Olsson AG, Faergeman O, Pyorala K. The effects of simvastatin on the incidence of heart failure in patients with coronary heart disease. *J Cardiac Failure*. 1997;3:249–254.

30. National Institutes of Health National Cholesterol Education Program (NCEP) ATP-II Guidelines: Summary of the Second Report of the NCEDP Expert Panel on Detection, Evaluation, and Treatment of High Blood Cholesterol in Adults (Adult Treatment Panel II). *JAMA*. 1993;269:3015–3023.

31. Ney DM. The cardiovascular system. In: FJ Zeman, ed. *Clinical Nutrition and Dietetics*. 2nd ed. New York: Macmillan Publishing USA; 1991, 373.

32. Schwartz CJ, Valente AJ, Sprague EA, et al. Pathogenesis of the atherosclerotic lesion: Implications for diabetes mellitus. *Diabetes Care*. 1992;15:1156–1167.

33. Yamasaki Y, Kawamore R, Matsuhima H, et al. Asymptomatic hyperglycemia is associated with increased intimal plus medial thickness of the carotid artery. *Diabetologia*. 1995;38:585–591.

34. Crub JD, Rodriguez BL, Burchfiel CM, et al. Sudden death, impaired glucose tolerance, and diabetes in Japanese American men. *Circulation*. 1995;91:2591–2595.

35. Kahn CR. Insulin action, diabetogenes, and the cause of type II diabetes. *Diabetes*. 1994;43:1066–1084.

36. Winocour PD. Platelet abnormalities in diabetes mellitus. *Diabetes.* 1992;41(Suppl 2):26–31.

37. Ceriello A, Giugliano D, Quatraro A, et al. Blood glucose may condition factor VII levels in diabetic and normal subjects. *Diabetologia.* 1988;31:889–891.

38. Ganda OP, Arkin CF. Hyperfibrinogenemia: An important risk factor for vascular complication in diabetes. *Diabetes Care.* 1992;15:1245–1250.

39. Couglin SS, Pearle DL, Baughman KL, et al. Diabetes mellitus and risk of idiopathic dilated cardiomyopathy: The Washington Diabetes Care Dilated Cardiomyopathy Study. *Ann Epidemiol.* 1994;4:67–74.

40. National Institutes of Health Consensus Development Panel. Health implications of obesity. *Ann Intern Med.* 1985;103:147–151.

41. Messerli FH, Sundgaard-Riise, Eeisin ED, et al. Dimorphic cardiac adaptation to obesity and arterial hypertension. *Ann Intern Med.* 1983;99:757–761.

42. Reisin E, Frohlich ED, Messerli FH, et al. Cardiovascular changes after weight reduction in obesity hypertension. *Ann Intern Med.* 1983;98:315–319.

43. MacMahon SW, Wilcken DEL, MacDonald GJ. The effect of weight reduction on left ventricular mass. *N Engl J Med.* 1986;314:334–338.

44. Grodstein F, Levine R, Troy L, et al. Three-year follow-up of participants in a commercial weight loss program: Can you keep it off? *Arch Intern Med.* 1996;156:1302–1306.

45. National Heart, Lung, and Blood Institute. *Clinical Guidelines of the Identification, Evaluation, and Treatment of Overweight and Obesity in Adults: The Evidence Reports.* Bethesda, MD: DHHS, 1998.

46. Kramer FM, Jeffrey RW, Forster HI, Sell MK. Long-term follow-up of behavioral treatment for obesity: Patterns of weight regain among men and women. *Int J Obes.* 1989;13:123–136.

47. Tremblay A, Despres JP, Maheux J, et al. Normalization of the metabolic profile in obese women by exercise and a low fat diet. *Med Sci Sports Exerc.* 1991;23:1326–1331.

48. Doll R, Peto R. Mortality in relation to smoking: Twenty years observations on male British doctors. *Br Med J.* 1979;2:1525–1536.

49. Kannel WB, Sorlie P, McNamara PM. Prognosis after initial myocardial infarction: The Framingham study. *Am J Cardiol.* 1979;44:53–59.

50. Eriksson H, Svardsudd K, Larsson B, et al. Risk factors for heart failure in the general population: The study of men born in 1913. *Eur Heart J.* 1989;10:647–656.

51. Salonen JT. Stopping smoking and long-term mortality after acute myocardial infarction. *Br Heart J.* 1980;43:463–469.

52. Herlitz J, Bengtson A, Hjalmarson A, Karlson BW. Smoking habits in consecutive patients with acute myo-

cardial infarction: Prognosis in relation to other risk indicators and to whether or not they quit smoking. *Cardiology.* 1995;86:496–502.

53. Rabinowitz BD, Thorp K, Huber GL, et al. Acute hemodynamic effects of cigarette smoking in man assessed by systolic time intervals and echocardiography. *Circulation.* 1979;60:752–670.

54. Aronow WS, Cassidy J, Vangrow JS, et al. Effect of cigarette smoking and breathing carbon monoxide on cardiovascular hemodynamics in anginal patients. *Circulation.* 1974;50:340–347.

55. Nicolozakes AW, Binkley PF, Leier CV. Hemodynamic effects of smoking in congestive heart failure. *Am J Med Sci.* 1988;296:377–380.

56. Feenstra J, Grobbee DE, Jonkman FAM, Hoes AW, Stricker BHC. Prevention of relapse in patients with congestive heart failure: The role of precipitating factors. *Heart.* 1998;80:432–436.

57. Ghali JK, Kadakia S, Cooper R, Ferlinz J. Precipitating factors leading to decompensation of heart failure: Traits among urban blacks. *Arch Intern Med.* 1988;148:2013–2016.

58. Nohria A, Chen YT, Morton DJ, Walsh R, Vlasses PH, Krumholz HM. Quality of care for patients hospitalized with heart failure at academic medical centers. *Am Heart J.* 1999;137:1028–1034.

59. Krumholz HM, Wang Y, Paent EM, Mockalis J, Petrillo M, Radford MJ. Quality of care for elderly patients hospitalized with heart failure. *Arch Intern Med.* 1997;157:2242–2247.

60. Steptoe A, Doherty S, Rink E, Kerry S, Kendrick T, Hilton S. Behavioral counseling in general practice for the promotion of healthy behavior among adults at increased risk of coronary heart disease: Randomised trial. *Br Heart J.* 1999;319:943–947.

61. Toobert DJ, Glasgow RE, Nettekoven LA, Brown JE. Behavioral and psychosocial effects of intensive lifestyle management for women with coronary heart disease. *Patient Educ Counsel.* 1998;35:177–188.

62. Johnson JL, Budgz B, Mackay M, Miller C. Evaluation of a nurse-delivered smoking cessation intervention for hospitalized patients with cardiac disease. *Heart Lung.* 1999;28:55–64.

63. Tzivoni D, Keren A, Meyler S, Khoury Z, Lerer T, Brunel P. Cardiovascular safety of transdermal nicotine patches in patients with coronary artery disease who try to quit smoking. *Cardiovasc Drug Ther.* 1998;12:239–244.

64. Joseph AM, Morman SM, Ferry LH, et al. The safety of transdermal nicotine as an aid to smoking cessation in patients with cardiac disease. *N Engl J Med.* 1996;335:1792–1798.

65. Zevin S, Jacob P III, Benowitz NL. Dose-related cardiovascular and endocrine effects of transdermal nicotine. *Clin Pharmacol Ther.* 1998;64:87–95.

66. Hitsman B, Pingitore R, Spring B, et al. Antidepressant pharmacotherapy helps some cigarette smokers more than others. *J Consult Clin Psychol.* 1999;67:547–554.

67. Jarenby DE, Leschow SJ, Nides MA, et al. A controlled trial of sustained-release bupropion, a nicotine patch or both for smoking cessation. *N Engl J Med.* 1999;340:685–691.

68. Hurt RD, Sachs DP, Glover ED, et al. A comparison of sustained-release bupropion and placebo for smoking cessation. *N Engl J Med.* 1997;337:1195–1202.

69. Rigotti NA, Singer DE, Mulley AG, Thibault GE. Smoking cessation following admission to a coronary care unit. *J Gen Intern Med.* 1991;6:305–311.

70. Law M, Tang JL. An analysis of the effectiveness of interventions intended to help people stop smoking. *Arch Intern Med.* 1995;155:1933–1941.

71. Waldenstrom A. Alcohol and congestive heart failure. *Alcohol Clin Exp Res.* 1998;22:315S–317S.

72. Morris N, Kim CS, Doye AA, Hajjar RJ, Laste N, Gwathmey JK. A pilot study of a new chicken model of alcohol-induced cardiomyopathy. *Alcohol Clin Exp Res.* 1999;23:1668–1772.

73. Prazak P, Pfisterer M, Osswald S, Buser P, Burkart F. Differences of disease progression in congestive heart failure due to alcoholic as compared to idiopathic dilated cardiomyopathy. *Eur Heart J.* 1996;17:251–257.

74. Dracup K, Baker DW, Dunbar SB, et al. Management of heart failure. II. Counseling, education, and lifestyle modifications. *JAMA.* 1994;272:1442–1446.

75. Molgaard H, Kristensen BO, Baadrup U. Importance of abstention from alcohol in alcoholic heart disease. *Int J Cardiol.* 1990;26:373–375.

76. Dargie HJ, McMurray JJ. Diagnosis and management of heart failure. *Br Med J.* 1994;308:312–328.

77. Olubodun JO, Lawal SO. Alcohol consumption and heart failure in hypertensives. *Int J Cardiol.* 1996;53:81–85.

78. Ni H, Nauman D, Burgess D, Wise K, Crispell K, Hershberger RE. Factors influencing knowledge of and adherence to self-care among patients with heart failure. *Arch Intern Med.* 1999;159:1613–1619.

79. Evangelista L, Doering L, Dracup K. Noncompliance in heart failure patients with multiple hospital admissions. *Am Heart J.* 1999, in press.

80. Nothwehr F, Lando HA, Bobo JK. Alcohol and tobacco use in the Minnesota Heart Health Program. *Addict Behav.* 1995;20:463–470.

81. Jackson CA, Manning WG Jr, Wells KB Impact of prior and current alcohol use on use of services by patients with depression and chronic medical illnesses. *Health Serv Res.* 1995;30:687–705.

82. Willenbring ML, Olson DH. A randomized trial of integrated outpatient treatment for medically ill alcoholic men. *Arch Intern Med.* 1999;159:1946–1952.

83. Sullivan MJ, Higginbotham MB, Cobb FR. Exercise training in patients with severe left ventricular dysfunction: Hemodynamic and metabolic effects. *Circulation.* 1988;78:506–515.

84. European Heart Failure Training Group. Experience from controlled trials of physical training in chronic heart failure: Protocol and patient factors in effectiveness in the improvement in exercise tolerance. *Eur Heart J.* 1998;19:466–475.

85. Belardinelli R, Georgiou D, Cianci G, Purcaro A. Randomized, controlled trial of long-term moderate exercise training in chronic heart failure: Effects on functional capacity, quality of life, and clinical outcome. *Circulation.* 1999;99:1173–1182.

86. Gottlieb SS, Fisher ML, Freudenberger R, et al. Effects of exercise training on peak performance and quality of life in congestive heart failure patients. *J Cardiac Failure.* 1999;5:188–194.

87. Keteyian Sj, Levine AB, Brawner CA, et al. Exercise training in patients with heart failure: A randomized, controlled trial. *Ann Intern Med.* 1996;124:1051–1057.

88. Delagardelle C, Feiereisen P, Krecke R, Essamri B, Beissel J. Objective effects of a 6 months endurance and strength training program in outpatients with congestive heart failure. *Med Sci Sports Exerc.* 1999;31:1102–1107.

89. Wenger NK, Froelicher ES, Smith LK, et al. Cardiac rehabilitation as secondary prevention. Agency for Health Care Policy and Research and National Heart, Lung, and Blood Institute. *Clin Pract Guideline. Quick Reference Guide for Clinicians.* 1995;17:1–23.

90. Mark D, Naylor CD, Hlatky MA, et al. Use of medical resources and quality of life after acute myocardial infarction in Canada and the United States. *N Engl J Med.* 1994;331:1130–1135.

91. Helman EA. Use of the stages of change in exercise adherence model among older adults with a cardiac diagnosis. *J Cardiopulm Rehabil.* 1997;17:145–155.

92. Moore SM, Ruland CM, Pashkow FJ, Blackburn GG. Women's patterns of exercise following cardiac rehabilitation. *Nurs Res.* 1998;47:318–324.

93. Ornish D, Scerwitz LW, Billings JH, et al. Intensive lifestyle changes for reversal of coronary heart disease. *JAMA.* 199;280:2001–2007.

94. Goodyer LI, Miskelly F, Milligan P. Does encouraging good compliance improve patients' clinical condition in heart failure? *Br J Clin Pract.* 1995;49:173–176.

CHAPTER 10

Biobehavioral Therapy in the Management of Patients with Heart Failure

Debra K. Moser and Lynne W. Stevenson

In the past decade, heart failure has emerged as a significant public health threat.[1–6] As our population ages, the incidence and prevalence of heart failure are expected to increase in the United States and worldwide, and its impact is expected to worsen dramatically.[5,7] As a consequence, it is crucial that we determine optimal pharmacologic and nonpharmacologic methods of managing heart failure patients. The role of nonpharmacologic intervention in the management of patients with heart failure has received considerably less attention than that of pharmacologic therapy.

An optimally effective treatment option should have a beneficial impact on both the pathophysiologic and psychologic manifestations of the target condition. This goal is especially important for a condition such as chronic heart failure, which has a profoundly negative impact on physical and psychologic function. Hallmark pathophysiology in heart failure includes intense neuroendocrine activation with marked vasoconstriction.[8,9] Characteristic psychologic manifestations of chronic heart failure include feelings of helplessness or loss of control with subsequent dysphoria, poor psychoso-

cial adjustment, and poor overall quality of life.[10–16] Biobehavioral therapies such as biofeedback and relaxation may be effective adjuncts to pharmacologic therapy in the management of patients with heart failure because they have a beneficial impact on neuroendocrine activation and vasoconstriction, and on perceived helplessness, dysphoria, and poor quality of life.[17–20] In this chapter the research on these therapies in patients with related cardiovascular disorders will be discussed. One promising nonpharmacologic approach is biofeedback-relaxation therapy, a type of biobehavioral intervention, and this is discussed in some detail. Although the research on the possible role of such therapies specifically in the management of heart failure is limited, it suggests the potential of these therapies, and that research also will be discussed.

One may argue that pharmacologic therapy is effective enough that resources need not be expended on research and development of nonpharmacologic therapies. However, two points argue against this stance. First, despite substantial advances made in heart failure treatment with drug therapy, morbidity and mortality remain unacceptably high.[5,21–23] Second, although drug therapy frequently provides significant improvement in symptoms and functional ability, quality of life may not improve (see Chapter 5).[24] Quality of life is an important outcome for patients with heart failure, and recent evidence that poorer quality of life independently is predictive of morbidity and mortality adds to its importance.[25,26] Thus, ad-

Acknowledgments: Some of the research reported in this chapter supported by grants or aid to D.K. Moser from an AACN-Sigma Theta Tau Research Grant; an American Heart Association Grant-in-Aid, The Ohio State University Seed Grant Program; The Ohio State University, General Clinical Research Center, M01RR00034.

ditional treatment options to combat this serious condition should be explored.

BIOBEHAVIORAL THERAPY: BIOFEEDBACK AND RELAXATION IN PATIENTS WITH CARDIOVASCULAR DISEASE

Biofeedback and relaxation are two distinct biobehavioral techniques that often are used together to achieve voluntary control of some aspects of the autonomic nervous system such that sympathetic nervous system activation is decreased. Biofeedback is the use of feedback of output such as skin temperature, respiratory rate and pattern, or blood pressure that is detected by an external sensor and displayed to an individual so that the individual can exert a measure of voluntary control over that output.[27–29] When individuals can see or hear a signal representing the output of the organ system, such as a digital display of their skin temperature or an auditory tone indicating their heart rate, the ability to attain voluntary control of that output is increased. Relaxation is the active elicitation of a calming response that involves visceral and somatic responses and that is characterized by relative sympathetic nervous system withdrawal and parasympathetic nervous system tone predominance.[29]

Physiologic effects of biofeedback or relaxation (or their combination) in patients with hypertension, arterial occlusive disease, diabetic vascular insufficiency, Raynaud's, and coronary artery disease include vasodilation, increased peripheral blood flow, reduced systemic vascular resistance, reduced sympathetic nervous system activity, and increased parasympathetic nervous system tone.[30–36] Psychologic effects that have been demonstrated include increased perceived control, decreased dysphoria, and increased quality of life.[37–42]

Physiologic Outcomes

In a series of well-designed and executed studies, Freedman[31,43] and associates[44–48] demonstrated the use of biofeedback for the treatment of Raynaud's disease, a vasospastic disorder of complex origin in which finger blood flow is decreased compared with individuals without Raynaud's.[49] The vasospastic attacks of Raynaud's can be painful and debilitating, and in extreme cases can produce ischemic damage. Freedman and associates trained patients to increase their skin temperature voluntarily through the use of skin-temperature biofeedback alone, which led to reduction in the number of vasospastic attacks by up to 92%.[44] In addition, they used injected radioisotope sodium iodine-131 and venous occlusion plethysmography to demonstrate increases in finger capillary blood flow and total finger blood flow.[48,49] The effects seen were sustained when retested up to 2 years after initial biofeedback training.

Several investigators have demonstrated clinically significant reductions in blood pressure after biofeedback-relaxation training in hypertensive patients, which may be related to direct or indirect effects on central autonomic tone and peripheral vascular tone.[30,50–54] In well-controlled studies, treatment of essential hypertension with biofeedback-relaxation techniques resulted in mean decreases in (1) systolic blood pressure of 7 to 30 mm Hg, (2) diastolic blood pressure of 4 to 17 mm Hg, and (3) mean arterial pressure of 5 to 15 mm Hg.[30,42,50–57] Moreover, use of biofeedback-relaxation techniques can reduce the requirements for antihypertensive drugs and has been associated with decreased morbidity as reflected in decreased number of cardiovascular events,[56] decreased left ventricular mass,[42,57] improved capacity for work,[30] and fewer sick days taken from work.[42]

Further evidence that alteration of the autonomic nervous system and vascular tone is possible with biobehavioral therapies comes from studies in patients with peripheral vascular disease, diabetes, and migraine headaches. After biofeedback-relaxation therapy, patients with claudication and chronic arterial occlusive disease exhibited enhanced peripheral blood flow as evidenced by increased symptom-free walking time and improved exercise ankle blood pressure.[35] After foot skin temperature biofeedback-relaxation training, diabetic patients both with and without peripheral vascular disease demonstrated enhanced blood flow to the extremities.[36,58] Patients with migraine headaches who received biofeedback-relaxation training reported a reduction in headache intensity, duration, and frequency; used less medication; and had positive changes in cerebral blood flow as measured by transcranial Doppler ultrasonography.[59,60]

Changes in biochemical indicators of neuroendocrine status provide further evidence for the impact of biobehavioral therapies, and evidence of decreased sympathetic nervous system activation as a result of biofeedback-relaxation has been demonstrated in several studies. In controlled studies, investigators have shown significant reductions in plasma norepinephrine and epinephrine,[38,57] plasma dopamine-β-hydroxylase, renin activity,[34] plasma aldosterone, and urinary cortisol[52,61,62] after biofeedback-relaxation training.

Autonomic tone has been assessed using heart rate variability, which is decreased in heart failure and reflects increased risk for both sudden death and death from progressive heart failure. Improved prognosis has been seen with therapies that increase heart rate variability such as angiotensin-converting enzyme (ACE) inhibitor therapy or exercise training. Increased heart rate variability was associated with use of relaxation therapy in healthy volunteers[63] and with the use of biofeedback in hypertensive patients with and without organ damage.[55] Using feedback of heart rate in phase with tidal volume and respiratory rate to increase respiratory sinus arrhythmia, Cowan and associates demonstrated that survivors of cardiac arrest could increase their heart rate variability.[64]

Psychologic Outcomes

Psychologic benefits also may result from biofeedback-relaxation techniques because an individual exerts voluntary control over what are traditionally thought of as involuntary processes. This process engenders feelings of increased personal control that can decrease feelings of helplessness or loss of control[37,65] that can occur in advanced heart failure. As a consequence, dysphoria may be decreased and psychosocial adjustment increased. Biofeedback-relaxation training has been associated with decreased anxiety[38,39,41,61] and depression.[39] In addition, improved psychologic adaptation and quality of life have been documented as an effect of biofeedback-relaxation training.[30] Relaxation training plus exercise was substantially more effective than exercise training alone in decreasing anxiety and increasing well-being after myocardial infarction.[66]

Specific benefits for patients with cardiac disease were demonstrated in a randomized crossover trial of 10 weeks of relaxation training with stress management instruction for patients after acute myocardial infarction or coronary artery bypass grafting.[67] Compared with their own baseline and the control group, patients in the intervention group demonstrated significant improvements that were sustained at 6 months' follow-up in anxiety, depression, psychologic well-being, activities of daily living, number of days restricted by illness, quality of interactions, sexual relationships, and satisfaction with health. In addition, more patients in the intervention group were angina free on follow-up.

Maintenance of Effects

The question of long-term effectiveness is particularly important to address with biobehavioral therapies, for which there is concern that patients will not continue after the initial intensive training period. However, there is good evidence from biofeedback-relaxation studies in hypertension that the early effects can be sustained at 1- and 2-year follow-up.[50,68] Evidence from 24-hour ambulatory blood pressure monitoring has demonstrated that reduced blood pressure is sustained even while patients are in a natural environment with usual daily stresses operating.[69]

Evidence of the long-term effectiveness of biofeedback-relaxation is further strengthened by demonstrated reductions in clinical events. Patel and associates[56] studied 204 subjects 4 years after initial biofeedback-relaxation training. These investigators found that subjects in the intervention group maintained significantly lower blood pressures and had fewer cardiovascular events (angina, ischemic heart disease, fatal myocardial infarctions, electrocardiographic evidence of ischemia, and treatment of hypertension and its complications) than controls.

Cost-Effectiveness

Limited evidence indicates that biofeedback-relaxation therapy is also a cost-effective method of treatment. Ginsberg and associates[70] estimated a nationwide $80.8 million savings over 10 years based on reduced drug costs alone from a nonpharmacologic hypertension control program in Israel that included biofeedback-relaxation techniques. In this nationalized system, this savings represents over twice the cost of such a program.

BIOBEHAVIORAL THERAPY: BIOFEEDBACK AND RELAXATION IN PATIENTS WITH HEART FAILURE

On the basis of the evidence from other cardiovascular conditions, there is reason to believe that biobehavioral therapy might supplement usual management strategies in heart failure by helping patients achieve conscious self-regulation of certain physiologic systems, particularly the autonomic nervous system. Biofeedback and relaxation can decrease the negative manifestations of sympathetic nervous system arousal caused by both cardiac pathophysiology and psychologic stress. These effects may be especially beneficial in heart failure, where overactivation of the sympathetic nervous system is a major underlying pathophysiologic mechanism and where psychologic stress can contribute to overactivation of the sympathetic nervous system.

Thus far, only two groups of investigators have reported their experiences using biobehavioral therapies in patients with heart failure.[17–20] The first group, Kostis and associates,[17] randomly assigned 20 New York Heart Association Class II and III patients with left ventricular ejection fraction less than 40% to one of three groups: (1) a 12-week nonpharmaco-

logic group-based intervention; (2) digoxin therapy; or (3) double-blind placebo. The nonpharmacologic therapy group received instruction in salt restriction, weight reduction if overweight, graduated exercise training, and structured cognitive-behavioral strategies that included relaxation training, positive imagery, stress management, and coping with negative emotions. All patients were maintained on ACE inhibitors as background therapy along with their other drug therapy, which for most patients included diuretics and nitrates.

At 12 weeks, patients in the digoxin group had a significant improvement in ejection fraction (mean increase $4.4\% \pm 6.5\%$) compared with the placebo and nonpharmacologic therapy groups. Patients in the nonpharmacologic therapy group had significantly improved exercise tolerance as evidenced by a 37% increase in exercise stress test time compared with a 3% increase in the digoxin group and a 22% increase in the placebo group. Patients in the nonpharmacologic therapy group demonstrated greater weight loss than those in the other two groups. In addition, anxiety decreased 39% and depression decreased 52% in nonpharmacologic therapy patients, whereas anxiety increased by 24% and depression by 15% for patients on digoxin, and anxiety increased by 45% and depression by 25% for patients on placebo. This study was small, however, and not designed to isolate the components of the nonpharmacologic intervention responsible for the beneficial effects.

The second group of investigators to examine the impact of biobehavioral therapy in heart failure, Moser and associates,[18] studied the effect of biofeedback-relaxation in 40 patients with advanced chronic heart failure (NYHA Class III and IV; mean left ventricular ejection fraction 21%) on hemodynamics, catecholamines, and oxygen consumption. Patients undergoing elective evaluation for cardiac transplantation and optimization of medical therapy guided by pulmonary artery catheterization pressures were randomly assigned to receive no intervention or a single in-hospital biofeedback-relaxation training session. Biofeedback-relaxation was associated with the following significant changes in the intervention group: (1) increase in finger skin temperature of 3.1 ± 2.8°F and foot skin temperature of 1.5 ± 5.2°F; (2) increase in cardiac output of 0.30 ± 0.33 L/min; (3) decrease in systemic vascular resistance of 152 ± 225 dyne-sec-cm^{-5}; and (4) decrease in respiratory rate of 4.5 ± 3.2 breaths/minute (Table 10–1). These changes were transient as would be expected from a short-term intervention, and values returned to baseline within 30 minutes of the end of the intervention. There were no changes across time in the control group. Neither oxygen consumption nor catecholamine changes were evident in either group. The major limitation of this study is the use of a one-time only intervention.

This study demonstrated that despite the pathophysiology driving them to a state of intense vasoconstriction, patients with advanced heart failure could successfully use biofeedback-relaxation to voluntarily increase skin temperature, decrease vascular tone, and increase cardiac output. In addi-

tion, respiratory rate was significantly decreased. Even though biofeedback was confined to finger temperature, the early response to biofeedback-relaxation in this group was generalized as evidenced by the effect on systemic vascular resistance and foot temperature.

Plasma catecholamines did not change as a result of the intervention. Other investigators have demonstrated that biofeedback can produce vasodilation without withdrawal of sympathetic tone, but this effect occurs in patients without prior sympathetic nervous system activation.[70] The lack of acute changes in catecholamine levels does not rule out withdrawal of sympathetic tone. Although plasma norepinephrine is frequently used to measure acute response to intervention, heterogeneity of tissue response may obscure changes when blood is sampled at only one site. As most studies in which decreased plasma catecholamines were reported as a result of similar interventions included inter-

Table 10–1 Comparison of Outcomes between Groups across Time

	Preintervention		Postintervention		
	Time 1	Time 2	Time 3	Time 4	Time 5
Finger skin (°F) temperature					
Biofeedback-relaxation	91.5 ± 4.7	91.4 ± 4.7*	94.6 ± 3.1*†	93.1 ± 3.5*‡	91.3 ± 4.4*
Control	91.1 ± 4.9	90.6 ± 5.9	90.4 ± 5.5†	90.4 ± 5.4‡	90.8 ± 5.5
Systemic vascular resistance (dyne•sec•cm^{-5})					
Biofeedback-relaxation	1672 ± 389	1678 ± 385*	1510 ± 309*	1679 ± 282*	1676 ± 305
Control	1647 ± 414	1627 ± 450	1721 ± 539	1768 ± 597	1690 ± 432
Cardiac output (L/min)					
Biofeedback-relaxation	3.8 ± 1.0	3.7 ± 1.1*	4.1 ± 1.0*	3.8 ± 1.0*	3.9 ± 1.0
Control	3.9 ± 1.1	3.9 ± 1.2	3.8 ± 1.1	3.8 ± 1.2	3.8 ± 1.1
Respiratory rate (breaths/min)					
Biofeedback-relaxation	22 ± 5	22 ± 4*	17 ± 5*†	21 ± 4*‡	22 ± 5
Control	23 ± 4	23 ± 4	25 ± 3†	24 ± 4‡	24 ± 4

Values are means ± standard deviations. Time 1 and Time 2 are the times at which data were collected before intervention. Time 1 is 30 minutes between the intervention, and Time 2 is immediately before the intervention. Times, 3, 4, and 5 are the times at which data were collected after the intervention. Time 3 is immediately after the intervention. Time 4 and Time 5 are 15 and 30 minutes, respectively, after the intervention. No between-groups or within-groups differences were found unless indicated as follows:

*$P < 0.005$ for within-group differences across time periods.
†$P < 0.001$ for between-group differences at this time period.
‡$P < 0.05$ for between group differences at this time period.

ventions of at least a week[33] or more,[34,38,57] the relaxation component of the intervention in this study may have been of inadequate length to produce changes in catecholamines. Further studies are needed that include more direct measures of sympathetic nerve activity to clearly determine the cause of vasodilation with biofeedback. It has been suggested that some of the profound effects of exercise programs on clinical function and outcomes may reflect sustained benefits of brief alterations in hemodynamics and autonomic tone.

The vasodilation produced by the one-time biofeedback-relaxation intervention was transient as would be expected for a short-term intervention. However, many patients did exhibit clinically significant changes in cardiac output and systemic vascular resistance, and it is likely that even relatively minor degrees of sustained improvement could be advantageous in heart failure.

To examine the effects of a longer intervention, a second study by this group tested the hypothesis that patients who received biofeedback-relaxation training would have significantly greater perceived control, less dysphoria, better quality of life, fewer rehospitalizations, better

functional status, lower catecholamine levels, and higher heart rate variability on follow-up than patients in a usual care control group (Figure 10–1).[19,20] In this randomized controlled trial, 90 patients with advanced heart failure were assigned to one of two groups: (1) usual care plus biofeedback-relaxation training; or (2) usual care only. All patients were followed for 6 months. Patients in the biofeedback-relaxation training group received 6 weeks of training consisting of weekly sessions of skin temperature biofeedback augmented by progressive muscle relaxation. They were asked to practice twice daily at home for 15 to 20 minutes each time during the training period and then to continue performing the biofeedback-relaxation exercises at least once daily during the follow-up period.

Compared with patients in the control group, patients in the biofeedback-relaxation training group experienced significantly fewer rehospitalizations (Figure 10–2), greater perceived control (Figure 10–3), decreased anxiety and depression (Figure 10–4), and improved quality of life (Figure 10–5). In the control group across time, anxiety and depression increased and quality of life decreased. There were no differences in functional status assessed by the

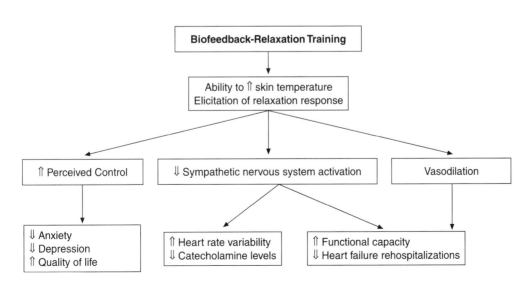

Figure 10–1 Hypothesized effects of biofeedback-relaxation training in patients with heart failure.

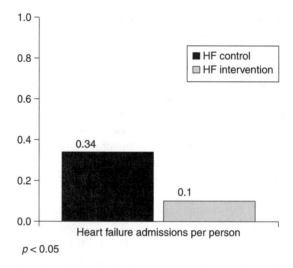

Figure 10–2 Comparison of number of hospitalizations per person between heart failure intervention and heart failure control patients.

6-minute walk test between the two groups. Among patients in the intervention group, norepinephrine levels were unchanged across time, whereas they increased significantly in the control group. Finally, intervention patients demonstrated less sympathetic nervous system responsiveness as assessed by spectral analysis of heart rate variability response to a standardized physical stressor. These findings indicate that clinical, physiologic, and psychologic outcomes can be improved with biofeedback-relaxation therapy in patients with advanced heart failure.

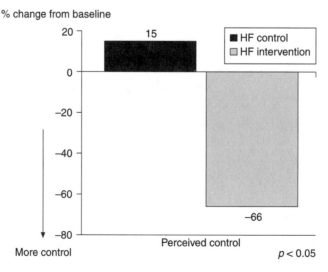

Figure 10–3 Comparison of person change in perceived control between heart failure (HF) intervention and HF control patients.

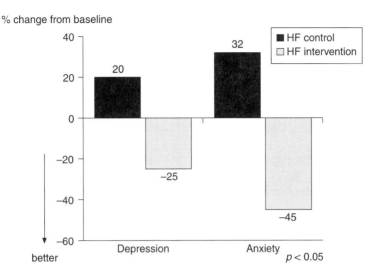

Figure 10–4 Comparison of percent change in anxiety and depression between heart failure (HF) intervention and HF control patients.

CONCLUSION

Biobehavioral therapy, such as biofeedback-relaxation, holds promise as an adjunct strategy to pharmacologic treatment in patients with heart failure. On the basis of the evidence available at this time, these therapies may be safe and effective to help reduce the morbidity, dysphoria, and poor quality of life common in these patients. However, more research needs to be done to define their optimal clinical application.

Further research is required to answer unresolved questions about which patients are the best candidates for biobehavioral therapy.

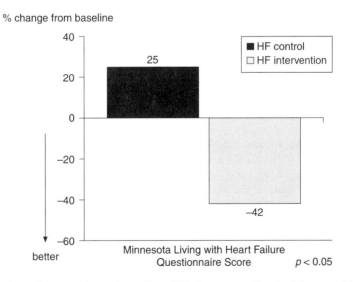

Figure 10–5 Comparison of percent change in quality of life (as measured by the Minnesota Living with Heart Failure Questionnaire) between heart failure (HF) intervention and HF control patients.

Therapy that decreases sympathetic tone has been effective in heart failure but is sometimes difficult to institute and individualize because some patients rely on increased sympathetic tone for maintenance of hemodynamic stability. For these patients, biobehavioral therapy with a substantial relaxation component may not be indicated. Clinicians do not yet have the ability to predict accurately either those patients who will be able to perform biofeedback-relaxation procedures or those who will experience a significant clinical response.[71]

Another unresolved issue is how to ensure long-term adherence to a therapy that requires patient commitment to practice the technique. Many patients are initially drawn to try biofeedback-relaxation therapies because they are intrigued by the possibility of exerting some personal control in a situation that frequently seems completely out of their control and may not appreciate the commitment involved. Although adherence to a practice schedule has been reported to be high (at least by self-report diary and continuation in the project) within the context of a research study,[19–20] there are concerns that adherence might decrease outside of an intensive research environment that has multiple incentives to continue with the protocol. Clearly, adherence to heart failure management strategies is a problem, and the request to add another treatment modality may tax and overburden some patients.

Other potential limitations to use of biobehavioral interventions in clinical practice include lack of clinician or patient acceptance of such therapy and the need for clinician training and equipment to implement some of the modalities (ie, biofeedback). Furthermore, still unresolved is the issue of which components are necessary to produce an effect. For example, is a combination of biofeedback and relaxation necessary or will biofeedback or relaxation alone be effective? The answers to these questions have important implications for the potential clinical application of biobehavioral therapies. The evidence that biofeedback-relaxation therapy has a positive impact on clinical and psychosocial outcomes in patients with heart failure warrants further investigation to determine whether it has use as a widespread clinical management strategy for patients with heart failure.

REFERENCES

1. Hoes AW, Mosterd A, Grobbee DE. An epidemic of heart failure? Recent evidence from Europe. *Eur Soc Cardiol.* 1998;19(suppl L):L2–L8.

2. Massie BM, Shah NB. The heart failure epidemic. *Curr Opin Cardiol.* 1996;11:221–226.

3. McMurray JJ, Petrie MC, Murdoch DR, Davie AP. Clinical epidemiology of heart failure: Public and private health burden. *Eur Heart J.* 1998;19(suppl):9–16.

4. O'Connell JB, Bristow MR. Economic impact of heart failure in the United States: time for a different approach. *J Heart Lung Transplant.* 1994;13:S107–S112.

5. O'Connell JB. The economic burden of heart failure. *Clin Cardiol.* 2000;23:III-6–III-10.

6. Garg R, Packer M, Pitt B, Yusuf S. Heart failure in the 1990's: Evolution of a major public health problem in cardiovascular medicine. *J Am Coll Cardiol.* 1993;22 (suppl A): 3A–5A.

7. Lenfant C. Report of the task force on research in heart failure. *Circulation.* 1994;90:1118–1123.

8. Packer M. The neurohormonal hypothesis: A theory to explain the mechanism of disease progression in heart failure. *J Am Coll Cardiol.* 1992;20:248–254.

9. Francis GS, McDonald K, Chu C, Cohn J. Pathophysiologic aspects of end-stage heart failure. *Am J Cardiol.* 1995;75:11A–16A.

10. Dracup K, Walden JA, Stevenson LW, Brecht ML. Quality of life in patients with advanced heart failure. *J Heart Lung Transplant.* 1992;11:273–279.

11. Grady KL. Quality of life in patients with chronic heart failure. *Crit Care Nurs Clin N Am.* 1993;5:661–670.

12. Stewart AL, Greenfield S, Hays RD, et al. Functional status and well-being of patients with chronic conditions: Results from the Medical Outcomes Study. *JAMA.* 1989;262:907–913.

13. Walden JA, Stevenson LW, Dracup K, et al. Extended comparison of quality of life between stable heart failure patients and heart transplant recipients. *J Heart Lung Transplant.* 1994;13:1109–1118.

14. Hawthorne MH, Hixon ME. Functional status, mood disturbance and quality of life in patients with heart failure. *Prog Cardiovasc Nurs.* 1994;9(11):22–32.

15. Jaarsma T, Dracup K, Walden J, Stevenson LW. Sexual function in patients with advanced heart failure. *Heart Lung.* 1996;25:263–270.

16. Muirhead J, Meyerowitz BE, Leedham B, Eastburn TE, Merrill WH, Frist WH. Quality of life and coping in patients awaiting heart transplantation. *J Heart Lung Transplant.* 1992;11:265–272.

17. Kostis JB, Rosen RC, Cosgrove NM, et al. Nonpharmacologic therapy improves functional and emotional status in congestive heart failure. *Chest.* 1994;106(4):996.

18. Moser DK, Dracup K, Woo MA, Stevenson LW. Voluntary control of vascular tone using skin temperature biofeedback-relaxation in patients with advanced heart failure. *Altern Ther Health Med.* 1997;3(1):51.

19. Moser DK, Kim KA, Baisden-O'Brien J. Impact of a nonpharmacologic cognitive intervention on clinical and psychosocial outcomes in patients with advanced heart failure. *Circulation.* 1999;100:I–99.

20. Moser DK, Nelson SD. Impact of biofeedback-relaxation training on hemodynamics, neuroendocrine function and rehospitalizations in advanced heart failure. *Am J Crit Care.* 1999;8:202.

21. Ho KKL, Pinsky JL, Kannel WB. The epidemiology of heart failure: The Framingham study. *J Am Coll Cardiol.* 1993;22(4 suppl A):6A–13A.

22. Goldberg RJ, Konstam MA. Assessing the population burden from heart failure. Need for sentinel population-based surveillance systems. *Arch Intern Med.* 1999;159:15–17.

23. Cohn JB, Bristow MR, Chien KR, et al. Report of the National Heart, Lung, and Blood Institute Special Emphasis Panel on Heart Failure Research. *Circulation.* 1997;95:766–770.

24. Townsend JN, Littler WA. Angiotensin converting enzyme inhibitors in heart failure: How good are they? *Br Heart J.* 1993;69:373–375.

25. Konstam V, Salem D, Pouler H, et al, for the SOLVD Investigators. Baseline quality of life as a predictor of mortality and hospitalization in 5,025 patients with congestive heart failure. *Am J Cardiol.* 1996;78:890–895.

26. Bennett SJ, Pressler ML, Hays L, Firestine LA, Huster GA. Psychosocial variables and hospitalization in persons with chronic heart failure. *Prog Cardiovasc Nurs.* 1997;12(4):4–11.

27. Schwartz GE. A systems analysis of psychobiology and behavior therapy: implications for behavioral medicine. *Psychother Psychosom.* 1981;36:159–184.

28. Basmajian JV. *Biofeedback: Principles and Practices for Clinicians.* 3rd ed. Baltimore: Williams & Wilkins; 1989.

29. Guzetta CE, Kessler CA, Dossey BM, Moser DK. Alternative/complementary therapies. In: Kinney MR, Dunbar SB, Brooks-Brun JA, Molter N, Vitello-Cicciu JM, eds. *AACN Clinical Reference for Critical Care Nursing.* St. Louis, MO: Mosby; 1998.

30. Aivazyan TA, Zaitsev VP, Salenko BB, Yurenev AP, Patrusheva IF. Efficacy of relaxation techniques in hypertensive patients. *Health Psychol.* 1988;7(Suppl): 193–200.

31. Freedman RR. Quantitative measurements of finger blood flow during behavioral treatments for Raynaud's disease. *Psychophysiology.* 1989;26:437–441.

32. Messerli FH, Decarvalho JGR, Christie B, Frohlich ED. Systemic haemodynamic effects of biofeedback in borderline hypertension. *Clin Sci.* 1979;57:437s–439s.

33. Davidson DM, Winchester MA, Taylor CB, Alderman EA, Ingels NB. Effects of relaxation therapy on cardiac performance and sympathetic activity in patients with organic heart disease. *Psychosom Med.* 1979;41:303–309.

34. Stone RA, DeLeo J. Psychotherapeutic control of hypertension. *N Engl J Med.* 1976;294:80–84.

35. Greenspan K, Lawrence PF, Esposito DB, Voorhees AB. The role of biofeedback and relaxation therapy in arterial occlusive disease. *J Surg Res.* 1980;29:387–394.

36. Rice BI, Schindler JV. Effect of thermal biofeedback-assisted relaxation training on blood circulation in the lower extremities of a population with diabetes. *Diabetes Care.* 1992;15:853–858.

37. Chen WW. Enhancement of health locus of control through biofeedback training. *Percept Mot Skills.* 1995;80:395–398.

38. Mathew R, Ho B, Kralik P, et al. Catechol-O-methyltransferase and catecholamines in anxiety and relaxation. *Psychiatry.* 1980;3:418–426.

39. Bohachick P. Progressive relaxation training in cardiac rehabilitation: effect on psychologic variables. *Nurs Res.* 1984;33:283–287.

40. Rice KM, Blanchard EB, Purcell M. Biofeedback treatment of generalized anxiety disorder: preliminary results. *Biofeed Self Regul.* 1993;18:93–105.

41. Gift AG, Moore T, Soeken K. Relaxation to reduce dyspnea and anxiety in COPD patients. *Nurs Res.* 1992;41:242–246.

42. Aivazyan TA, Zaitsev VP, Yurenev AP. Autogenic training in the treatment and secondary prevention of essential hypertension: Five-year follow-up. *Health Psychol.* 1988;7(Suppl):201–208.

43. Freedman RR. Long-term effectiveness of behavioral treatments for Raynaud's treatment. *Behav Ther.* 1987;18:387–399.

44. Freedman RR, Lynn S, Ianni P, Hale P. Biofeedback treatment of Raynaud's disease and phenomenon. *Biofeed Self Regul.* 1981;6:355–365.

45. Freedman RR, Ianni P. Self-control of digital temperature: Psychophysiological factors and transfer effects. *Psychophysiology.* 1983;20;682–689.

46. Freedman RR, Ianni P, Wenig P. Behavioral treatment of Raynaud's phenomenon in scleroderma. *J Behav Med.* 1984;7;343–353.

47. Freedman RR, Ianni P, Wenig P. Behavioral treatment of Raynaud's disease: long-term follow-up. *J Consult Clin Psychol.* 1985;53:136.

48. Freedman RR, Sabharwal SC, Ianni P, Desai N, Wenig P, Mayes M. Nonneural beta-adrenergic vasodilating mechanism in temperature biofeedback. *Psychosom Med.* 1988;50:394–401.

49. Freedman RR, Ianni P, Wenig P. Behavioral treatment of Raynaud's disease. *J Consult Clin Psychol.* 1983;51;539–549.

50. Agras WS, Taylor CB, Kraemer HC, Allen RA, Schneider JA. Twenty-four hour blood pressure reductions. *Arch Gen Psychiat.* 1980;37:859–863.

51. Cooper MI. Effect of relaxation on blood pressure and serum cholesterol. *Act Nerv Super.* 1982;3(Suppl.):428–436.

52. McGrady A, Woerner M, Bernal GAA, Higgins JT. Effect of biofeedback-assisted relaxation on blood pressure and cortisol levels in normotensives and hypertensives. *J Behav Med.* 1987;10:301–310.

53. Hatch JP, Klatt KD, Supik JD, et al. Combined behavioral and pharmacological treatment of essential hypertension. *Biofeed Self-Regul.* 1985;10:119–138.

54. Nazzaro P, Mudoni A, Manzari M, et al. Efficacy of biofeedback treatment compared with drug therapy in hypertensive patients. *Functional Neurol.* 1991;6:49–57.

55. Nakao M, Nomura S, Shimosawa T, Fujita T, Koboki T. Blood pressure biofeedback treatment, organ damage and sympathetic activity in mild hypertension. *Psychother Psychosom.* 1999;68:341–347.

56. Patel C, Marmot MG, Terry DJ, et al. Trial of relaxation in reducing coronary risk: Four year follow-up. *Br Med J.* 1985;290:1103–1106.

57. McCoy GC, Fein S, Blanchard EB, Wittrock DA, McCaffrey RJ, Pangburn L. End organ changes associated with the self-regulatory treatment of mild essential hypertension. *Biofeed Self Regul.* 1988;13:39–46.

58. Saunders JT, Cox JD, Teates CD, Pohl SL. Thermal biofeedback in the treatment of intermittent claudication in diabetes: a case study. *Biofeed Self Regul.* 1994;19:337–345.

59. Wauquier A, McGrady A, Aloe L, Klauser T, Collins B. Changes in cerebral blood flow velocity associated with biofeedback-assisted relaxation treatment of migraine headaches are specific for the middle cerebral artery. *Headache.* 1995;35:358–362.

60. McGrady A, Wauquier A, McNeil A, Gerard G. Effect of biofeedback-assisted relaxation on migraine headache and changes in cerebral blood flow velocity in the middle cerebral artery. *Headache.* 1995;34:424–428.

61. Holden-Lund C. Effects of relaxation with guided imagery on surgical stress and wound healing. *Res Nurs Health.* 1988;11:235–244.

62. McGrady A. Effects of group relaxation training and thermal biofeedback on blood pressure and related physiological and psychological variables in essential hypertension. *Biofeedback Self Regul.* 1994;19:51–66.

63. Sakakibara M, Takeuchi S, Hayano J. Effect of relaxation training on cardiac parasympathetic tone. *Psychophysiology.* 1994;31:223–228.

64. Cowan MJ, Kogan H, Burr R, Hendershot S, Buchanan L. Power spectral analysis of heart rate variability after biofeedback. *J Electrocardiol.* 1990;23:85–94.

65. Nelson DV, Baer PE, Cleveland SE, Revel KF, Montero AC. Six-month follow-up of stress management versus cardiac education during hospitalization for acute myocardial infarction. *J Cardiopulmonary Rehabil.* 1994;14:384–390.

66. Van Dixhoorn J, Duivenvoorden HJ, Pool J, Verhage F. Psychic effects of physical training and relaxation therapy after myocardial infarction. *J Psychosom Res.* 1990;34: 327–337.

67. Trzcieniecka-Green A, Steptoe A. The effects of stress management on the quality of life of patients following acute myocardial infarction or coronary bypass surgery. *Eur Heart J.* 1996;17:1663–1670.

68. Fahrion S, Norris P, Green A, Green E, Snarr C. Biobehavioral treatment of essential hypertension: a group outcome study. *Biofeed Self-Regul.* 1986;11:257–277.

69. Southam TA, Agras WS, Taylor CB, Kraemer HC. Blood pressure lowering during the working day. *Arch Gen Psychiat.* 1982;39:715–717.

70. Ginsberg GM, Viskoper RJ, Oren S, Bregman L, Mishal Y, Sherf S. Resource savings from non-pharmacological control of hypertension. *J Hypertension.* 1990;4:375–378.

71. Weaver MT, McGrady A. A provisional model to predict blood pressure response to biofeedback-assisted relaxation. *Biofeed Self Regul.* 1995;20:229–240.

PART IV

Improving Outcomes by Enhancing Treatment Compliance

CHAPTER 11

Extent of the Problem of Noncompliance in Patients with Heart Failure

Martha N. Hill

THE COMPLIANCE CHALLENGE

Dramatic advances in medical treatments over the past four to five decades have led to impressive improvements in outcomes for chronic illness. In addition to demonstrating the effectiveness of new interventions, clinical trials have established the importance of the extent to which patients participate in their care, providers follow intervention protocols, and systems of care maximize anticipated outcomes. In practice and in research, compliance or adherence increasingly is seen as a major contributor to improved outcomes. Moreover, the traditional definition of compliance—the extent to which patients follow doctors' recommendations[1]—has been recognized as limited. In a recent scientific statement, the American Heart Association suggested a broader definition that recognizes improved outcomes require a commitment from providers and health care organizations, as well as patients to follow recommendations or advice.[2] Noncompliance is defined as not following recommendations based on efficacious or best evidence-based practices. The American Heart Association scientific statement reviews numerous factors that contribute to the problem of noncompliance and the evidence-based strategies that reduce noncompliance and consequently improve patient outcomes (Table 11–1).[2] Although the authors of the statement did not specifically focus on the heart failure literature, their framework is a useful one for organizing this chapter.

Compliance is important because it is a mediator of improved clinical outcomes. As such, it determines the extent to which successful prevention and treatment programs are effective in individuals. Furthermore, noncompliance is important because it is a major contributor to the morbidity and mortality associated with heart disease, including heart failure. In the research literature on heart failure, as in most conditions, the majority of studies focus on a health outcome and presume compliance is mediating in nature. Nonetheless, the problem of noncompliance is recognized in both clinical practice and research as a major contributor to the increasing prevalence of heart failure and its associated morbidity and mortality. This chapter will review the impact of noncompliance and how patient, family, provider, and health care organization factors contribute to noncompliance.

IMPACT OF NONCOMPLIANCE

Concerns about the quality and cost of health care, especially in the past decade, have stimulated an imperative to demonstrate improved outcomes for patients, providers, health care organizations, and payers. Large, well-controlled trials have demonstrated the benefit of primary and secondary prevention of coronary heart disease through the modification of risk factors and use of effective lifestyle, pharmacologic, and surgical interventions. But, because these effective interventions have not been implemented fully in practice, similar outcomes have not been

Table 11–1 Actions to Increase Compliance with Prevention and Treatment Recommendations

Actions by Patients	*Specific Strategies*
Patients must engage in essential prevention and treatment behaviors • Decide to control risk factors. • Negotiate goals with provider. • Develop skills for adopting and maintaining recommended behaviors. • Monitor progress toward goals. • Resolve problems that block achievement of goals.	• Understand rationale, importance of commitment. • Develop communication skills. • Use reminder systems. • Use self-monitoring skills. • Develop problem-solving skills, use social support networks.
Patients must communicate with providers about prevention and treatment services. —	• Define own needs on basis of experience. • Validate rationale for continuing to follow recommendations.

Actions by Providers	*Specific Strategies*
Providers must foster effective communication with patients. • Provide clear, direct messages about importance of a behavior or therapy. • Include patients in decisions about prevention and treatment goals and related strategies. • Incorporate behavioral strategies into counseling.	• Provide verbal and written instruction, including rationale for treatments. • Develop skills in communication/counseling. • Use tailoring and contracting strategies. • Negotiate goals and a plan. • Anticipate barriers to compliance and discuss solutions. • Use active listening. • Develop multicomponent strategies (ie, cognitive and behavioral).
Providers must document and respond to patients' progress toward goals. • Create an evidence-based practice. • Assess patient's compliance at each visit. • Develop reminder systems to ensure identification and follow-up of patient status.	• Determine methods of evaluating outcomes. • Use self-report or electronic data. • Use telephone follow-up.

Actions by Health Care Organizations	*Specific Strategies*
Health care organizations must • Develop an environment that supports prevention and treatment interventions.	• Develop training in behavioral science, office set-up for all personnel. • Use preappointment reminders. • Use telephone follow-up. • Schedule evening/weekend office hours. • Provide group/individual counseling for patients and families.

continues

Table 11–1 continued

Actions by Health Care Organizations	Specific Strategies
• Provide tracking and reporting systems.	• Develop computer-based systems (electronic medical records).
• Provide education and training for providers.	• Require continuing education courses in communication, behavioral counseling.
• Provide adequate reimbursement for allocation of time for all health care professionals.	• Develop incentives tied to desired patient and provider outcomes.
Health care organizations must adopt systems to rapidly and efficiently incorporate innovations into medical practice.	
—	• Incorporate nursing case management.
	• Implement pharmacy patient profile and recall review systems.
	• Use electronic transmission storage of patient's self-monitored data.
	• Obtain patient data on lifestyle behavior before visit.
	• Provide continuous quality improvement training.

References provide evidence from studies and key articles to support the recommendations of the panel.

achieved in practice.[3] More than half of all Americans with chronic diseases do not follow their doctors' recommendations for lifestyle changes and medication. More than half of Americans report sedentary lifestyles, 25% continue to smoke, and 40% of men and 25% of women are obese.[4] Approximately 50% of prescriptions are taken improperly and nearly a third are never filled. The result is that tens of thousands of people die each year and many more become or remain ill. One major reason for the gap between what is effective in clinical trials and what happens in practice and in patients' daily lives is that the scope of the compliance problem and the complexity of the compliance challenge have not been widely recognized. Typically, the compliance problem is seen only as "Patients failing to follow doctors' orders." Another major reason for the gap is that the multidisciplinary team approach to improved care and management demonstrated in clinical trials is not sufficiently incorporated into practice.[5]

A variety of important issues have been identified in evaluation of the extent to which behavioral noncompliance, the discrepancy between what is recommended and what is done, is a problem. These include the numerous recommended behaviors; the degree of compliance required to get the desired treatment effect; the types of noncompliance; and the need to assess noncompliance at the patient, provider, and system levels.[2,6] Another important issue in evaluation of the extent to which noncompliance is a problem is how compliance, and thus noncompliance, is measured. Patient recall, for example, although commonly used in practice, is a less than reliable method. The validity of self-report is uncertain, because both patients and providers overestimate the extent to which patients take their medications as prescribed.[7] In a recent meta-analysis, Roter and colleagues[8] summarized 153 studies published between 1977 and 1994 that evaluated the effectiveness of interventions to improve patient compliance with medical regimens. The authors concluded that compliance interventions had a weak to moderate effect but were generally efficacious and practical, although no single intervention strategy appeared consistently stronger than any other. The effects of the interventions varied widely according to the patient's condition. These investigators also concluded that studies have been much too narrow and limited. No mention was made in the review of interventions specifically designed to increase compliance of patients with heart failure.

The potential for preventing heart failure and improving the outcomes for heart failure patients is associated in large part with the control of high blood pressure. The dramatic reduction in heart failure incidence caused by control of blood pressure was first demonstrated in the Veterans Administration Cooperative Trials.[9,10] More recently, further evidence of the benefit of hypertension control in people age 60 and older with isolated systolic hypertension was provided. The Systolic Hypertension in the Elderly Program (SHEP)[11] demonstrated that a regimen of diuretic medication, compared with the same regimen of placebos, lowered the risk of stroke by 36% and other major cardiovascular complications by 32% in a sample of 4736 men and women.[12] In a secondary analysis of the data, diuretic treatment of systolic hypertension in older people was shown to reduce the risk of heart failure. Participants in the SHEP study who took active medications were half as likely to have heart failure develop after an average of 4.5 years of follow-up compared with those who took placebos. In addition, it was shown that the risk reduction was 80% among the people who had previous heart attacks.[12] The literature on strategies to improve compliance with hypertension care is relatively extensive and is summarized in review articles and chapters.[13–16]

It is difficult to document the extent to which noncompliance is a problem in heart failure. This is because most studies designed to improve outcomes in heart failure were designed to test the efficacy of interventions, such as new pharmacologic agents or regimens or systems of heart failure management, on primary and secondary heart failure outcomes. These outcomes have included mortality from various causes, morbidity, ejection fraction and other biologic variables, medical resource use and costs, and health-related quality of life. Improving compliance, in the process of improving care, rarely has been identified as a main study aim. Few studies in heart failure patients explicitly mention measuring compliance with lifestyle recommendations and medications, and few of those that do measure compliance describe how compliance is measured. Thus, explicit reports of the method for operationalizing and measuring compliance (or its inverse, noncompliance) and the contribution of compliance to heart failure care outcomes are scant. One study in heart failure patients, the DIG Study, compared two methods of estimating patient adherence with medication: actual pill count or calibrated graduated cylinders along with a conversion chart. Of the 302 participating sites, 47 used both methods simultaneously. The comparison of the two methods was highly correlated (Pearson's $r = 97$, $n = 168$). The mean difference in pill count was 6.2, standard deviation (SD) ± 17.2, and the range of differences was from 117 to 52. A subsequent comparison of on-site pill counts with coordinating center counts on corresponding bottles was not as highly correlated. Possible explanations for the findings include dispensing of the bottles for more than one patient visit, misreading the cylinder, and data entry errors.[17]

PATIENT AND FAMILY FACTORS CONTRIBUTING TO NONCOMPLIANCE

Most compliance research focuses on patient compliance. Many factors have been identified that significantly influence compliance and explain why individuals do not comply with medical recommendations. The characteristics of patient noncompliance are well described in a review of the research on compliance with cardiovascular disease prevention strategies.[6] To examine the compliance challenge, it is important to recognize that patients must learn and apply multiple skills to adopt, or cease, and then maintain recommended behaviors. The general skills include decision making, goal setting, self-monitoring, creating and responding to prompts and reminders, and problem solving.

Patient noncompliance can take many forms. In regard to participating in care, noncompliance includes not making appointments, not attending or rescheduling appointments, and not seeking recommended screening tests. In regard to lifestyle, noncompliance can include not following physical activity and dietary recommendations, continuing to smoke cigarettes, and drinking alcohol excessively. In regard to medication taking, noncompliance includes not having a prescription filled, taking incorrect dosage (over- or underdosing), taking medication at the wrong time or in the wrong way, missing doses, and stopping the medication too soon. Noncompliance with other self-care measures includes not keeping logs, not weighing or measuring blood pressure, and not managing insurance and other paperwork. Moreover, noncompliance patterns vary by recommended behaviors, the complexity of the regimen, and ease of incorporating recommendations into daily routines. It is difficult to predict which patients will comply. Noncompliance may occur at any age. It crosses all age, racial, gender, and socioeconomic groups. Noncompliance varies across behaviors and time and increases over time. Much noncompliance occurs early after recommendations are made, and early rates predict long-term rates. Successful strategies to improve compliance include cognitive aids, appointment reminders, persuasive communication, convenient care settings, and nurse-managed interventions.

Early studies in heart failure identified a number of issues thought to contribute to patient noncompliance. Most of these studies focused on the elderly in whom heart failure is increasingly prevalent and identified common problems including the prescription of multiple medications, high rates of readmission, and short length of life. Luther and colleagues[18] questioned 156 elderly patients with heart failure about adherence to medications. They reported the following factors contributed to problems with nonadherence: difficulty remembering to take medication(s) (20%), medication too expensive (16%), too many medications (10%), dislike taking medication (10%), and uncertain how to take medication (9%). Other factors were medication side effects (8%), regimen too much trouble (7%), bottle too difficult to open (7%), medication not explained (6%), medication difficult to swallow (6%), and too sick to take (4%).

Factors that contribute to noncompliance with angiotensin-converting enzyme (ACE) inhibitors and dosing were examined in a sample of 869 patients with heart failure, most of whom were employed outside of the home.[19] This study indicated that patients had ACE inhibitors available 71% of the time they were prescribed. Participants who had their medication available more often were more likely to be men, have lower chronic disease scores, have a greater number of outpatient visits, and be ongoing users of ACE inhibitors. At 180 days after the index prescription, 88% of patients continued to take their ACE inhibitor. By 300 days after the index prescription, the continuation of therapy rate had dropped to 78%. Variability in daily dosing and dispensing also was documented. The authors recommended that new users of medication, women, and the elderly be targeted for enhanced compliance interventions.

Noncompliance with congestive heart failure therapy in the elderly has been estimated to be approximately 50%.[20] To better understand this phenomenon, Monane and colleagues[20] evaluated a population-based cohort of elderly patients beginning use of digoxin and followed them longitudinally. The investigators carried out retrospective follow-up visits in the complete New Jersey Medicaid prescription claims file data between 1981 and 1991. The measure of compliance was number of days during the 12-month period after the initial digoxin prescription in which no congestive heart failure medication was available to the patient. Patients who started digoxin were without it or a common alternative congestive heart failure drug 111 of 365 days. Only 10% of the sample filled enough prescriptions to have their prescribed daily congestive heart failure medication available every day. Compliance rates were higher in patients older than 85 years of age, women, those taking multiple medications, and those in a hospital or nursing home before therapy was started. Additional studies, conducted by Rich and colleagues,[21–23] were undertaken to prospectively assess medication compliance rates, identify factors associated with reduced compliance in elderly patients with heart failure, and intervene to improve outcomes. These studies are described under provider factors because they tested the impact of multidisciplinary interventions.

Patient and family factors that influence compliance are implicit in consensus guidelines for evaluation and management of heart failure.[24] Guidelines are developed for physicians and other health professionals to help them with what they are supposed to do. Typically, practice guidelines do not provide explicit recommendations on how health care professionals can help patients and families incorporate behaviors recommended for them into their lives. Studies that examine explicit patient and family behaviors, such as increasing physical activity by exercising three times a week and weighing daily, provide important information.[25,26] Careful reading of research articles may provide practical information of the facilitators and barriers to patient and family compliance. However, page restrictions on length of manuscripts may cause authors to abbreviate methods sections and it may be necessary to contact the investigators to learn the strategies that succeeded in implementing the behavioral intervention.

The increasing pressure to contain costs by decreasing emergency department visits and hospital admissions has stimulated assessment of factors that influence resource use. The long-term goal of reducing utilization and costs will depend on targeted interventions for patients at high risk for readmission. In most of the limited research in this area, compliance was not specifically evaluated. For example, in a study of factors that precipitated hospitalization in patients with decompensated heart failure, the most common reason for decompensation by far was fluid overload with sodium retention.[27] Although the authors speculated on the basis of their review of patient medical records that noncompliance contributed to many or most of these cases, they acknowledge that, "Compliance with

cardiac medications and dietary sodium restrictions was evaluated from history obtained by dietitians, nurses, and medical personnel. However, because of inconsistencies in the records, compliance was difficult to determine through retrospective review."

The study by Chin and colleagues,[28] who undertook a study to identify correlates of early hospital readmission or death within 60 days of discharge in patients with congestive heart failure, is an exception to the limited research specifically examining compliance. They prospectively enrolled 257 patients in 1993 and 1994 and assessed access to care, compliance, social support, primary insurance, and demographic data at baseline. At 60 days after discharge from the hospital, the patient or proxy completed a mailed questionnaire that inquired about hospital readmission during the time since discharge and compliance. These investigators used a compliance scale that was composed of seven items that asked a patient to rate his or her adherence to the treatment regimen over the preceding 4 weeks on a 5-point scale ranging from "all of the time" to "none of the time."[29] Within 60 days of discharge, 5% of patients died ($n = 13$), and 31% were readmitted ($n = 80$). Patient compliance, as well as ejection fraction and sickness at discharge, were not correlated with readmission or death. The authors comment that the compliance scale was not sufficiently sensitive or discriminating in their study population.

Michalsen and colleagues[30] in Berlin, Germany, conducted a second study that specifically examined patient compliance with heart failure treatment recommendations. They interviewed a consecutive sample of 179 patients admitted to the hospital with acute decompensation of heart failure to determine factors associated with admission. Lack of adherence to the medical regimen was the most commonly identified factor (41% of cases). Noncompliance with drugs was acknowledged by 23.5% of patients. Other common factors included coronary ischemia (13.4%), cardiac arrhythmias (6.1%), uncontrolled hypertension (5.6%), and inadequate preadmission treatment (12.3%). Admission was regarded as preventable in 54.2% of patients.

PROVIDER FACTORS CONTRIBUTING TO NONCOMPLIANCE

At the provider level, noncompliance refers to not following recommendations or guidelines for practice behavior. This could include not asking patients whether they smoke, and if they do, not working with the patient to stop, or not providing patient education that addresses behavioral expectations and knowledge. The extent to which providers follow evidence-based consensus recommendations regarding the diagnosis, evaluation, and treatment of heart failure is being assessed with increasing frequency. Evidence exists that there is a significant discrepancy between state-of-the-art practice shown to be efficacious in improving patient outcomes in clinical trials and actual care being given to patients.

In an editorial entitled "Addressing the Heart Failure Management Gap," Cohn (1999) wrote "By most objective evidence and personal experience it appears that the management of heart failure in the community is inadequate."[31] In part the gap between what is known to be efficacious in heart failure clinical trials and in practice is due to a pattern of physicians not prescribing effective medications in adequate doses. Cohn continues "Drugs that should be used—including angiotensin-converting enzyme (ACE) inhibitors and now β-blockers—are not prescribed in all eligible patients, and drugs that probably should not be used—most calcium antagonists and antiarrhythmics as well as nonsteroidal inflammatory drugs—are often prescribed. Diuretic therapy, when indicated, often is not titrated to the optimal dose. Nonpharmacologic management, including appropriate coronary reperfusion and patient education, often is inadequate." Cohn also comments that it is difficult to quantify the magnitude of the gap between what should be done, based on well-controlled trial data, and what is being done in the community. This is in part because data from surveys of prescription patterns for ACE inhibitors provide conflicting information. As is seen in other diagnoses, such as hypertension,[32] about half of the

patients with heart failure are receiving such drugs and often at doses less than those shown to optimally improve outcomes.

Numerous studies provide evidence that physicians should be prescribing β-blockers to treat well-established heart failure and improve mortality and morbidity. A recent study, the CIBIS II Trial, provided evidence of the benefit of β-blockers in stable patients (those whose condition is not worsening) with mild to moderate heart failure.[33] In this trial, investigators recruited 2647 participants who had stable symptomatic heart failure (New York Heart Association Class II–IV). All individuals had left ventricular systolic dysfunction with an ejection fraction less than 35% and were treated with standard therapy for heart failure that included diuretics and ACE inhibitors. Half of the participants were randomly assigned to bisoprolol at a dose starting at 1.25 mg/day and increased to a maximum dose of 10 mg/day during the 6 months of follow-up. The other half of the participants received a placebo (instead of the bisoprolol). The trial was stopped prematurely because of a benefit in favor of the group receiving the bisoprolol. During an average follow-up period of 1.3 years, 11.8% of the patients on bisoprolol died compared with 17.3% of those who received the placebo. The patients who received the bisoprolol lived longer and were admitted to the hospital less often. As Krumholtz stated in the editorial that accompanied the article, "The drugs are inexpensive and the benefits are substantial."[34] It is important to note that many patients feel worse for a while when started on β-blockers. Repeated adjustment of doses, teaching, and time—things physicians may not have or be skilled at doing—are needed to minimize or eliminate troublesome adverse effects that may contribute to noncompliance with medication regimens.

Unfortunately, little evidence exists to determine why appropriate pharmacologic therapy has not been prescribed for most patients with heart failure. One supposition about why physicians are not prescribing appropriate drugs at optimal doses is that they are unaware of the evidence supporting such practices. Familiarity with the original clinical trial studies, consensus recommendations for the management of heart failure, or physician's beliefs in the appropriateness of the consensus recommendations may be limited. However, in the absence of research findings, these suppositions are purely speculative.

The evidence that providers can improve outcomes for patients with heart failure by enhancing their own and/or patients' compliance is largely implied. However, a few studies were identified that address the issue directly. Goodyear and colleagues[35] designed a study to determine whether improved compliance by intensive medication counseling, given by a pharmacist, to elderly patients with chronic, stable heart failure could influence both objective and subjective measures of heart failure. Patients were randomized to 3 months' follow-up with or without counseling. To assess changes in functional status, as well as compliance, measurements included submaximal 6-minute walk test, the Nottingham Health Profile, clinical signs of heart failure, tablet count, and medication knowledge. The changes in the special intervention and usual care groups were significantly different with the exception of medication knowledge. The distance walked during the 6-minute walk test increased as did the distance before breathlessness occurred in the intervention group, while they decreased in the control group. Edema scores increased in the intervention group but did not change in the control group. Breathlessness measured by visual analog score decreased in the intervention group but did not change in the control group. Finally, compliance increased 32% in the intervention group, but there was no change in the control group.

Rich and colleagues[19,21–23,36] have undertaken a series of studies to assess prospectively medication compliance rates, identify factors associated with reduced compliance, and evaluate the effects of a multidisciplinary treatment approach. The interventions are described in detail in Chapter 20. In 1993, Rich reported on a study to determine the feasibility and potential impact of a study of a nonpharmacologic multidisciplinary intervention for reducing hospital read-

missions in elderly patients with congestive heart failure. In this prospective pilot study of the intervention, 96 patients, whose average age was 70 years, were randomized in a 2:1 ratio to either special intervention or usual care. The special intervention consisted of intensive teaching by a nurse specialist in geriatrics and cardiology, detailed review of medications by a cardiologist with specialization in geriatrics, recommendations to increase compliance and decrease side effects, early consultation with social services, dietary teaching, and close follow-up after discharge by a home nurse and the study team. Overall, in the total study sample lower rates in 90-day readmission were seen between the intervention versus usual care group (33% to 46%, respectively). Although compliance was presumed to be improved and to contribute to the lower rehospitalization rate seen in the intervention group, it was not explicitly tested.

In 1996, Rich and colleagues did test explicitly the impact of their multidisciplinary intervention on medication compliance in 156 patients whose mean age was 70 years and of whom 67% were women and 65% nonwhite. Before discharge, they were randomly assigned to conventional care or the intervention. Compliance was assessed by pill count at 30 days after discharge. The compliance rates, 88% for the special intervention group and 81% for the conventional care group, were significantly different on follow-up. Three predictors of compliance identified by multivariate analysis were special intervention treatment group, Caucasian race, and not living alone.

SYSTEM FACTORS CONTRIBUTING TO NONCOMPLIANCE

At the level of the system, or health care organization, noncompliance can be defined as not following recommendations based on efficacious or best practices. Clinical trials have demonstrated the importance of individualized appointment schedules at times convenient to the patient, short waiting times, preappointment reminders, scheduling a return appointment before the patient leaves the office, telephone follow-up, tickler systems, use of electronic record keeping and communication, rapid response to data collected by home monitoring, and nurse case management.[6,16,37,38] Because of the urgency surrounding efforts to reduce costs associated with the management of heart failure, numerous studies have been undertaken to increase understanding of the factors that influence utilization of medical services so that interventions can be developed to reduce emergency department visits and hospital admissions.

One of the earlier studies in this area examined factors related to hospitalization for decompensation of heart failure among urban African-Americans to identify factors that directly precipitated admission.[39] Patients were included in the study if they had been hospitalized three times in the past year. The 101 participants, average age 59 and 97% African-American, were interviewed, a physical examination was performed, and their medical records were reviewed. The participants were divided into 10 subgroups according to potential heart failure–precipitating factors. Noncompliance, defined as patient discontinuation of medications or taking medications intermittently, was one category. Other categories included inadequately prescribed drug therapy, iatrogenic causes, uncontrolled hypertension, acute myocardial infarction, arrhythmias, environmental factors, emotional distress, endocrine disorder, and miscellaneous. The three most common factors in decreasing order of frequency were lack of adherence to the medical regimen (65%; diet, 22%; medication, 6%; and both diet and medication, 37%); uncontrolled hypertension (44%); and cardiac arrhythmias (29%). This was the first study, to the best of this author's knowledge that reported data that specifically addressed the importance of compliance in heart failure care at the multiple levels—patient, provider, and organization.

The most promising organization or systems-level strategies to improve compliance in trials of heart failure management and in trials of primary and secondary prevention of coronary heart disease[11,40–43] and other chronic diseases[8] demonstrate that combinations of, rather than single, interventions are most promising. These include patient education and skill building,

contracting, self-monitoring, social support, telephone follow-up, and tailoring. Implementing these strategies calls for commitment to follow guidelines and provide state-of-the-art services at the system and provider levels.

Large multisite, randomized trials in heart failure such as SOLVD, support a multilevel approach in which multidisciplinary teams operating within systems of health care delivery have been successful in modifying risk factors.[44] However, because the primary aim of these studies was to demonstrate the benefit of various pharmacologic therapies, publications have not described the team approach and the associated organizational and systems supports in any detail. Thus, the importance of the health care organization incorporating the positions of clinical specialist, nurse practitioner, or on-site nurse case manager has not appeared in the literature. The development and testing of disease management strategies, including nurse case management such as the MULTIFIT System,[45] has been a major focus of heart failure clinical research. The considerable data describing the improvement on patient outcomes is described elsewhere in this book in Chapters 17–20.

RESEARCH RECOMMENDATIONS TO ENHANCE COMPLIANCE

Research to enhance compliance is urgently needed at the levels of the patient, the provider, and the health care organization. There is a great need for studies designed with compliance improvement as the primary outcome. Studies are needed that develop accurate methods for measuring compliance and providing feedback on progress toward goals and outcomes. Studies also are needed to assess the economic impact of compliance enhancing interventions including cost utility, cost-effectiveness, and cost benefit. In addition to developing their own studies, clinician researchers can take advantage of the opportunities that exist within other studies by incorporating ancillary studies and substudies within clinical trials testing new interventions to improve the outcomes for heart failure patients.[46] Researchers working with investigators who are testing new interventions for heart failure patients have the opportunity to suggest additional questions or variables at the time of protocol development.[13]

Patient Level

Self-monitoring, symptom recognition, and interpretation and symptom management, and their relationships with compliance are promising areas for research. Heart failure is a condition that fluctuates. Patients' perceptions and behavior also may vary as their functional and cognitive capacities fluctuate with changes in physiologic status. This is an obvious area for integrating biologic and behavioral research. It will be important to better understand how heart failure patients and their caregivers understand the cause-and-effect relationships between prevention and treatment of symptoms. Multiple drug regimens, with changes in the number and type of drugs (that are easily confounded by substitution of generic preparations), and the correct dose and times of administration are complex. It is important that patients and their caregivers understand the principles of combined therapy and gradual incremental dosing.

We also need to understand better cultural differences affecting barriers to compliance, skill-building interventions, patient satisfaction, and patient and family understanding of the need for long-term change for future health benefit. Studies are needed to identify and test new methods to improve long-term compliance and relapse prevention with life-style modification and medication. Valid and reliable methods of assessing compliance in the home and clinical practice settings are needed. Research is needed, especially in the elderly, about behaviors important for effective management of heart failure. Self-care behaviors include appointment making and keeping, obtaining and taking medications, exercising, eating, smoking cessation, and weight monitoring.[26,27] Critical patient behaviors also include making the decision to reach treatment goals, following treatment recommendations, monitoring progress toward treatment goals, and resolving problems that interfere with achieving treatment goals.[16]

Provider Level

Physicians recognize the problem of noncompliance, yet they have little time to implement the necessary strategies to facilitate compliance. They report that they lack the skills needed to enhance compliance. Skill training to enhance their success is needed. Effective communication between patients and physicians is critical, but limited time requires that physicians must be cued, and peer support is necessary. In addition, physicians benefit by practicing in collaboration with other health professionals whose competencies supplement and complement their own.[5] Research is needed to understand better how to give providers the necessary skills to assess the feasibility of patients and their caregivers being able to implement the recommended regimen. Studies also are needed to help providers efficiently and effectively assess the following: (1) cost of medications and patients' ability to pay for them; (2) patients' ability to read labels, open caps, and follow dosing schedules; (3) need for cognitive aids, such as pill boxes and reminder phone calls; and (4) need for home assistance. Studies are needed urgently to learn how to help providers identify those individuals at highest risk for difficulty with compliance behaviors and to intervene appropriately.

The importance of provider–patient communication and collaboration in improving outcomes is receiving increasing recognition. Active sensitive listening and open communication have been shown to improve patient compliance and clinical outcomes, increase satisfaction with care, save clinicians' time, and lower the risk of malpractice suits.[47] Actively involving patients in the management of their chronic illness with shared decision making and responsibility has been shown to improve compliance. Effective provider strategies include offering options, recommending simple therapeutic regimens, decreasing patients' reluctance to take medication, helping a patient control the pace of change, and planning a strategy for self-care.[8,48] In the meta-analysis of the compliance literature by Roter and colleagues, the significant predictors of patient compliance were length of visit, amount of information given, degree of partnership building, amount of positive talk, and fewer questions asked, but more questions asked about compliance. Further studies are needed of how these strategies can be implemented in a cost-effective manner to improve the quality and the length of life for heart failure patients.

Systems Level

Systems for disease prevention and improvement of outcomes have enhanced compliance rates; however, factors to enhance their adoption and sustained use need to be understood better. If organizations are to improve compliance with recommendations for best practices, they need to respond to documented need and evaluate progress toward improved patient outcomes. Randomized trials are needed to demonstrate the effectiveness, feasibility, and cost-effectiveness of organizing systems for secondary prevention in heart failure patients. Follow-up studies to determine factors that maximize delivery of health services and maintenance of beneficial primary and secondary prevention systems also are needed. For example, the practicality and sustainability of telephone contact and home visits to enhance patient self-sufficiency, self-care, and social support need to be evaluated. In addition, the clinical and economic consequences of noncompliance with life-style modification, medication, and continuation in care need to be determined in parallel with evaluation of the process of care and achieved outcomes.

Another important question that needs to be examined is whether case management systems in managed care are superior to nondirective, physician-based management of patients with heart failure. Finally, the pharmaceutical industry could collaborate in studies of product labeling to enhance the effectiveness of medication taking.

CONCLUSION

Noncompliance at the patient, provider, and system levels is a major contributor to poor outcomes in patients with heart failure. Numerous beneficial therapies, such as exercise, ACE inhibitors, and β-blockers, are inexpensive, and the benefits are substantial. Their use needs to increase. All clinicians can help with the issue of noncompliance. Providers need to look for opportunities to use these therapies and follow evidence-based consensus guidelines. Patients and their families need to be educated to inquire about therapies from which they might benefit and helped to develop the skills to appropriately integrate these therapies into their daily lives. Health care organizations and policy makers need to commit to implementing beneficial therapies in a convenient, considerate, and affordable manner. Outcomes for heart failure patients will improve if therapies now known to be effective are implemented. Patient outcomes will improve as research indicates which new therapies are beneficial and how to maximize compliance to recommendations at the level of the patient, provider and system.

REFERENCES

1. Haynes RB, Taylor DW, Sackett DL, eds. *Compliance in Health Care.* Baltimore: Johns Hopkins University Press; 1979.
2. Miller N, Hill MN, Kottke T, Ockene IS. The multilevel compliance challenge: Recommendations for a call to action. *Circulation.* 1997;95:1085–1090.
3. Hill MN. Behavior and biology: The basic sciences for AHA action. *Circulation.* 1998;97:807–810.
4. National Institutes of Health, NHBLI Obesity Education Initiative Expert Panel. *Clinical Guidelines on the Iden-*

tification, Evaluation, and Treatment of Overweight and Obesity in Adults: The Evidence Report. June 1998.
5. Hill MN, Miller NH. Compliance enhancement: A call for multidisciplinary team approaches. *Circulation.* 1998;93:4–6.
6. Burke LE, Dunbar-Jacob JM, Hill MN. Compliance with cardiovascular disease prevention strategies: A review of the research. *Ann Behav Med.* 1997;19:239–263.
7. Burnier M, Schneider MP, Chiolro A, et al. Objective monitoring of drug compliance: An important step in the

management of hypertension resistant to drug therapy. *Am J Hypertens.* 1999;12:129A.

8. Roter DL, Hall JA, Merisca R, Nordstrom B, et al. Effectiveness of interventions to improve patient compliance: A meta-analysis. *Medical Care.* 1998;36:1138–1159.

9. Veterans Administration Cooperative Study Group on Antihypertensive Agents. Effects of treatment on morbidity in hypertension. Results in patients with diastolic blood pressures averaging 115 through 129 mm Hg. *JAMA.* 1967;202:1028–1034.

10. Veterans Administration Cooperative Study Group on Antihypertensive Agents. Effects of treatment on morbidity in hypertension. Results in patients with diastolic blood pressures averaging 90 through 114 mm Hg. *JAMA.* 1970;213:1143–1152.

11. SHEP Cooperative Research Group. Prevention of stroke by antihypertensive drug treatment in older persons with isolated systolic hypertension: final results of the Systolic Hypertension in the Elderly Program (SHEP). *JAMA.* 1991;265:3255–3264.

12. Kostis JB, Davis BR, Cutler J, et al. Prevention of heart failure by antihypertensive drug treatment in older persons with isolated systolic hypertension. SHEP Cooperative Research Group. *JAMA.* 1997;278:212–216.

13. Cowley SM, Somelofski C, Hill MN, et al. Nursing and cardiovascular clinical trial research: Collaborating for successful outcomes. *Cardiovasc Nurs.* 1988;24:25–30.

14. Hill MN. Adherence to antihypertensive therapy. In: Izzo J Jr, Black, H, eds. *Hypertension Primer.* 2nd ed. Baltimore: Williams & Wilkins; 1998.

15. Hill MN, Bone LR, Levine DM. (2000). Community outreach. In: Oparil S, Weber M, eds. *Hypertension.* Philadelphia: WB Saunders Company; 2000.

16. Working Group to Define Critical Patient Behaviors in High Blood Pressure Control, National High Blood Pressure Education Program, National Heart, Lung, and Blood Institute. Patient behavior for blood pressure control. *JAMA.* 1979;241:2534–2537.

17. Fye CL, Raisch DW, Gagne WH, et al. Comparison of tablet measure by calibrated cylinder versus tablet count in the DIG Study. Abstract presented at the Sixteenth Annual Meeting Society for Clinical Trials, Seattle, Washington; 1995.

18. Luther P, Baldus D, Beckham V, et al. Adherence to prescribed medications in elderly patients with congestive heart failure. *Cardiovascular Reviews and Reports.* 1995;33–40.

19. Roe CM, Motheral BR, Teitelbaum F, et al. Angiotensin-converting enzyme inhibitor compliance and dosing among patients with heart failure. *Am Heart J.* 1999;138:818–825.

20. Monane M, Bohn RL, Gurwitz JH, et al. Noncompliance with congestive heart failure therapy in the elderly. *Arch Intern Med.* 1994;154:433–437.

21. Rich MW, Vinson JM, Sperry JC, et al. Prevention of readmission in elderly patients with congestive heart failure: Results of a prospective, randomized pilot study. *J Gen Intern Med.* 1993;8:585–590.

22. Rich MW, Baldus DG, Beckham V, et al. Effect of a multidisciplinary intervention on medication compliance in elderly patients with congestive heart failure. *Am J Med.* 1996;101:270–276.

23. Vinson JM, Rich MW, Sperry JC, et al. Early readmission of elderly patients with congestive heart failure. *J Am Geriatr Soc.* 1990;38:1290–1295.

24. Guidelines for the Evaluation and Management of Heart Failure: A Report of the American College of Cardiology/American Heart Association Task Force on Practice Guidelines Committee on Evaluation and Management of Heart Failure. *Circulation.* 1995;92:2764–2784.

25. Belardinelli GD, Georgiou D, Cianci G, Purcaro A. Randomized, controlled trial of long-term moderate exercise training in chronic heart failure: Effects on functional capacity, quality of life, and clinical outcome. *Circulation.* 1999;19:1173–1182.

26. Sulzbach-Hoke LM, Kagan SH, Craig K. Weighing behavior and symptom distress of clinic patients with CHF. *MEDSURG Nurs.* 1997;6:288–293.

27. Bennett SJ, Huster GA, Baker SL, et al. Characterization of the precipitants of hospitalization for heart failure decompensation. *Am J Crit Care.* 1998;7:168–174.

28. Chin MH, Goldman L. Correlates of early hospital readmission or death in patients with congestive heart failure. *Am J Cardiol.* 1997;79:1640–1644.

29. DiMatteo MR, Hays RD. Adherence to cancer regimens: Implications for treating the older patient. *Oncology.* 1992;6:50–57.

30. Michalsen A, König G, Thimme W. Preventable causative factors leading to hospital admission with decompensated heart failure. *Heart.* 1998;80:437–441.

31. Cohn JN. Addressing the heart failure management gap [editorial]. *J Card Fail.* 1999;5:1–2.

32. Burt VL, Cutler JA, Higgins M, et al. Trends in the prevalence, awareness, treatment and control of hypertension in the adult US population. Data from the Health Examination Surveys, 1960–1991. *Hypertension.* 1995;26:60–69.

33. CIBIS-II Investigators and Committees. The Cardiac Insufficiency Bisoprolol Study II (CIBIS-II): a randomised trial. *Lancet.* 1999;353:9–13.

34. Krumholz HM. Beta-blockers for mild to moderate heart failure. *Lancet.* 1999;353:2–3.

35. Goodyear LI, Miskelly F, Milligan P. Does encouraging good compliance improve patients' clinical condition in heart failure? *Br J Clin Psychol.* 1995;49:173–176.

36. Rich MW, Beckham V, Wittenberg C, et al. A multidisciplinary intervention to prevent the readmis-

sion of elderly patients with congestive heart failure. *N Engl J Med.* 1995;333:1190–1195.

37. Finnerty FA Jr, Mattie EC, Finnerty FA 3rd. Hypertension in the inner city. Part I. Analysis of clinic dropouts. *Circulation.* 1973;47:73–75.

38. Finnerty FA Jr, Shaw LW, Himmelsbach CK. Hypertension in the inner city. Part II. Detection and follow-up. *Circulation.* 1973;47:1973.

39. Ghali JK, Kadakia S, Cooper R, Ferlinz J. Precipitating factors leading to decompensation of heart failure: Traits among urban blacks. *Arch Intern Med.* 1998;148:2013–2016.

40. Hypertension Detection and Follow-up Program Cooperative Group (HDFP). Five-year findings of the hypertension detection and follow-up program, I: reduction in mortality of persons with high blood pressure, including mild hypertension. *JAMA.* 1979;242:2562–2571.

41. Multiple Risk Factor Intervention Trial Research Group (MRFIT). Multiple risk factor intervention trial: risk factor changes and mortality results. *JAMA.* 1982;248:1465–1477.

42. Treatment of Mild Hypertension Study Research Group (TOHP I). Treatment of mild hypertension study: final results. *JAMA.* 1993;270:713–724.

43. Whelton PK, Buring J, Borhani NO, et al. The effect of potassium supplementation in persons with a high-normal blood pressure. Results from phase I of the Trials of Hypertension Prevention (TOHP). Trials of Hypertension Prevention Collaborative Research Group (TOHP II). *Ann Epidemiol.* 1995;5:85–95.

44. The SOLVD Investigators. Effect of enalapril on survival in patients with reduced left ventricular ejection fractions and congestive heart failure. *N Engl J Med.* 1991;325:293–302.

45. DeBusk RF, Miller NH, Superko R, et al. A case-management system for coronary risk factor modification after acute myocardial infarction. *Ann Intern Med.* 1994;120:721–729.

46. Hill MN, Schron EB. Opportunities for nurse researchers in clinical trials. *Nurs Res.* 1992;41:114–116.

47. Levinson W, Roter DL, Mullooly J, et al. Physician–patient communication: the relationship with malpractice claims among primary care physicians and surgeons. *JAMA.* 1997;277:553–559.

48. Kushner PR, Smith SY. Collaboration and compliance: Improving outcomes in older women. *Women's Health in Primary Care.* 1999;2:288–300.

CHAPTER 12

Heart Failure Patient and Family Education

Deborah Knox, Lisa Mischke, and Randall E. Williams

The diagnosis of heart failure can be disconcerting and perplexing to patients and their loved ones. They often feel fear, a loss of freedom, and powerless as control shifts from the patient to the health care provider. Education can restore a sense of control by helping the patient and family to understand the nature of the diagnosis and the lifestyle changes that can help them live successfully, despite having heart failure.

Educating patients and their families or other caregivers can help to achieve several objectives. At the most basic level, knowledge is increased. With knowledge comes empowerment and an increased sense of personal control and confidence. Confidence or self-efficacy has been shown to influence persistence and subsequent success when new behaviors are attempted.[1] Providers who integrate patients and families into the "treatment team" increase patient satisfaction and create excitement and motivation about learning how to manage heart failure. Motivation to comply with treatment recommendations and learning effective strategies are the goals of patient and family education.

Noncompliance has been referred to as "America's other drug problem."[2] Noncompliance is particularly problematic and damaging in patients with heart failure. Repeated exacerbations of symptoms result in a 17% national readmission rate for heart failure within 30 days after discharge.[3] Noncompliance with the prescribed regimen is thought to contribute to an alarming number of these heart failure readmissions. By some estimates, as many as 50% of hospital admissions

for heart failure may be preventable; failure to adhere to the following recommendations contributes to most preventable readmissions[3–5]:

- Sodium-restricted diet
- Prescribed medications
- Exercise and activity guidelines
- Daily weight monitoring
- Notification of health care personnel regarding symptom changes
- Timely follow-up within 2–4 weeks after discharge

There are many reasons for patient noncompliance, but failure of providers to educate and counsel patients and their families or caregivers adequately is paramount among them.[2] Simply imparting knowledge, however, without providing patients and families with the requisite skills, strategies, and support to initiate change and adopt lifestyle changes results in failure of the educational process. Appropriate patient education and counseling that addresses knowledge attainment, successful behavioral strategies, patient problem solving—as well as the social and emotional factors that promote behavior change—may significantly improve compliance with treatment recommendations and lifestyle changes and, thus, reduce readmissions for heart failure.[3] In this chapter, traditional methods of providing heart failure patient education are critiqued. Strategies for teaching heart failure patients and their family members are explored, and essential components of heart failure education are detailed.

TRADITIONAL HEART FAILURE EDUCATION

Patients frequently are diagnosed with heart failure after they develop severe symptoms and require hospitalization.[3] Once discharged, symptoms may worsen, but patients often feel reluctant to alert their provider or, more commonly, fail to recognize the need for notification. Often, the earliest sign of a heart failure exacerbation is increased body weight. However, due to lack of appropriate or adequate education, patients frequently do not weigh themselves daily or identify weight gain as an early warning sign.[6] Subsequently, heart failure symptoms such as extreme lower extremity swelling and paroxysmal nocturnal dyspnea develop and become severe enough to trigger a call to the provider. If the primary physician's office cannot effectively treat an acute heart failure exacerbation, the patient may be sent to the emergency department. When patients with heart failure are seen in the emergency department for worsening symptoms, most are admitted to the hospital, thus beginning a cycle of dependence (Figure 12–1).[7] This cycle contributes to high readmission rates and cost of care, lowers patients' perception of control and self-efficacy, and lowers motivation for self-management.

The cycle of dependence illustrates the need for appropriate and adequate education, reinforcement of treatment objectives, and timely follow-up. Unfortunately, deficiencies in the current health care system affects patient and family education, which contributes substantially to poor patient adherence and frequent hospitalizations.[8] These problems include premature discharge of patients from the hospital, teaching in a stressful environment, ineffective communication patterns, and failure to include

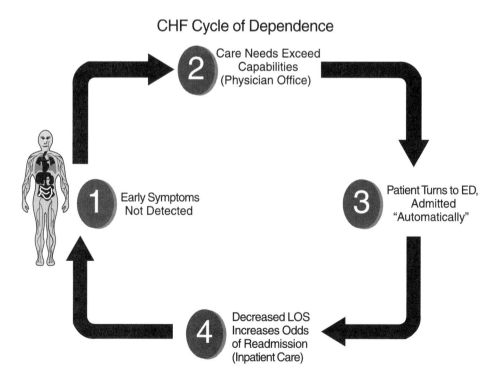

Figure 12–1 Congestive Heart Failure (CHF) Cycle of Dependence.

family, caregivers, or other supporters in patient teaching efforts.

Premature Discharge from the Hospital

Traditionally, education of patients with heart failure has occurred solely in the hospital at the time of the initial diagnosis or after a disease exacerbation. Thus, health care systems largely have been reactive instead of proactive in responding to the educational needs of patients with heart failure. During a typical hospitalization, providers attempt to accomplish all educational objectives but must do so in shorter periods of time as lengths of stay decrease nationally.[3] An initial heart failure hospitalization may not provide sufficient time to optimize the treatment regimen and teach the patient and family about their condition and new treatment. Several new medications may be initiated in a short period of time, and these, along with exercise and diet recommendations, may need to be adjusted in the following weeks. Decreases in length of stay may limit the opportunity to cover all the necessary material, evaluate adequacy of the education provided, assess information retention, and negotiate needed life-style changes. Therefore, patients frequently are sent home without a full comprehension of their illness and the necessary life-style changes needed to avoid an exacerbation.

Several investigators have evaluated the link between inpatient education, premature hospital discharge, and readmission. In one such study, patients who felt they were discharged too soon were more likely to be readmitted than were patients who felt they were ready for discharge.[9] Both caregivers and patients have cited premature hospital discharge as a common contributory factor (58%) in unplanned readmission within 28 days of discharge.[10] Recognizing that inpatient education and counseling have been ineffective, other investigators have demonstrated the importance of individualizing a discharge plan of care prior to discharge that includes home care follow-up by advanced practice nurses for assessment, problem solving, and provision of long-term education and coun-

seling.[11] Such interventions result in improved patient outcomes that include fewer rehospitalizations and lower health care costs.[11]

Teaching in a Stressful Environment

The hospital setting is stressful for most patients, especially during an exacerbation of heart failure. It is difficult to learn and integrate information under such conditions. A positive learning experience is not likely to be possible during the initial hospitalization, when the patient and family are faced with the stress of an unfamiliar environment, as well as a new diagnosis or worsening chronic heart failure.[12]

For these and other reasons, management of the patient with heart failure who is experiencing symptoms in the acute care setting is a multifaceted and daunting challenge for even the experienced provider. A primary objective in the inpatient setting is to lay the groundwork for subsequent educational efforts. Small quantities of information should be conveyed upon admission and daily thereafter, depending on the patient's readiness to learn. However, experts agree that the majority of education should be completed and evaluated in the less stressful outpatient setting.[13] Numerous investigators have examined different health care delivery models in which patient and family education and counseling are given in a variety of outpatient settings, once the acute exacerbation has cleared and the patient is stabilized. The models and their beneficial outcomes are described in Chapters 16–20.

Ineffective Communication Patterns

Coordination and communication between constituents of the health care team often are lacking. Lack of coordination becomes especially pronounced as patients make the transition from one site of care to another. Communication between the specialist and primary care physician often is lacking. For example, a primary care physician may alter medications or dosages without being aware of medication changes made by the heart failure specialist, with the result that the patient is confused about the ultimate regimen. Compounding this problem, patient education in the physician's office often is abbreviated or omitted, due to lack of resources and time.

Communication in the hospital setting is similarly problematic. Patients with heart failure require education on many topics, such as medications, dietary sodium restriction, activity levels, and psychologic responses.[14] Advance directives should be discussed with heart failure patients, as well. Communication among providers in the hospital often is poor, due to excessive demands on their time. Providers are challenged to complete all of the educational objectives, despite nursing shortages, lower staffing ratios, and decreased lengths of hospital stay. The result is that educational efforts are inadequately coordinated. As a consequence, providers frequently view the educational process as overwhelming and time-consuming, and, therefore, impossible to carry out effectively.

One function of critical pathways is to assist clinicians to complete appropriate education. Pathways can provide guidance to maximize patient education by detailing criteria and specific educational goals (see Figure 12–2). Although helpful for hospital care, clinical pathways are usually limited to the inpatient setting, with minimal transition to the outpatient environment. As a result, seamless communication between inpatient and outpatient settings is lacking. An educational tool is needed for providers to utilize in patient education across the health care continuum.

Failure To Include Supporters

Many patients with advanced heart failure are dependent on their spouses, children, or significant others for meal preparation, administration of medications, and daily activities such as bathing, dressing, and ambulating. According to Agency for Health Care Policy and Research (AHCPR) guidelines, patients should be discharged only when they and their caregivers have been educated about medications, diet, activity, exercise recommendations, symptoms of worsening heart failure, and when adequate follow-up care has been arranged.[15] Inadequate social support contributes significantly to many heart failure readmissions.[3,11] It is imperative, therefore, that caregivers be identified, taught, and supported.[16] Family members who participate in heart failure education can reinforce the information with the patient. However, family members may not be available or invited when the patient receives education in the hospital. Further, the inpatient setting often is not conducive to family, caregivers, or members of a patient's support system involvement.

New Models of Heart Failure Education

Few investigators have examined directly issues related to patient and family or caregiver education; however, education is often the intervention assumed to mediate the outcome achieved by an intervention, such as telephonic case management. Those who have studied patient teaching have demonstrated that, although patients with heart failure perceive education to be important, most either do not receive adequate education or do not retain what they are taught. Three groups of investigators have studied the perceived learning needs of patients with heart failure by having them rank the importance of specific learning categories.[17–19] Their findings demonstrate that patients with heart failure perceive education as important. Education related to signs, symptoms, and medications is perceived as most important by these patients.

Although patients may believe that education is important, Dunbar and associates demonstrated limited knowledge about heart failure among 67 patients with heart failure.[14] The majority reported limiting sodium and fluids, but none weighed themselves daily, and most patients could not recite the signs of worsening heart failure. These findings suggest that patients with heart failure do not have adequate knowledge and comprehension of self-management strategies important in heart failure. Bushnell studied 41 patients and found that almost none could define heart failure, less than half could identify their medications, and two-

EMERGENCY DEPARTMENT STAFF COMPLETE 1–6

Point of entry (1):   ☐ 1 = ER ☐ 2 = Direct

Pathway initiated in ER (2): ☐ No ☐ Yes

ENH EVANSTON
NORTHWESTERN
HEALTHCARE

EVANSTON HOSPITAL & GLENBROOK HOSPITAL

		Symptomology If any are checked, start patient on CHF pathway				
	No	**Yes**		**No**	**Yes**	
Fluid overload requiring IV diuretics (3)	☐	☐	Increased ankle edema (5)	☐	☐	
CXR with Volume overload (4)	☐	☐	Jugular vein distension (6)	☐	☐	

Admit Date (7): ____/____/____   Expected LOS: 5 days, Date pathway started (8): ____/____/____

Discharge Date (9): ____/____/____

D/C'd from pathway (10): ☐ No or ☐ Yes (Variance Code (11)_____)

Discharge delay (12): ☐ No or ☐ Yes (Variance Code(s) (13)_____(14)_____)

Discharge destination (15): ☐ 1 = Home, self-care   ☐ 4 = Extended care, skilled (TCC)   ☐ 7 = Acute care specialty

☐ 2 = Home with home health care (ENH) ☐ 5 = Extended care, skilled (other) ☐ 8 = Assisted living

☐ 3 = Home with home health care (other) ☐ 6 = Nursing home   ☐ 9 = Rehab

Patient's Needs	Outcomes: Indicate dates outcomes achieved **and/or** variance codes for those not achieved using variance legend on back of this sheet. Outcomes to be met by patient's discharge unless otherwise indicated. Key daily outcomes are **bold** and denoted with a ➜. Achievement or variances of these items must be documented.		Date Achieved/ Initials (a)	Variance Codes/ Initials (b)
Clinical	• Decreased shortness of breath since admission	16		
	• Increased activity tolerance since admission	17		
	➜ Off IV inotropes (by day 4)	18		
	➜ Off IV diuretics (by day 4)	19		
	• Stable renal function (creatinine not increasing at discharge)	20		
	• Off oxygen	21		
	• Baseline weight established	22		
	• LV function measured and documented (within last 12 months)	23		
Educational	➜ Patient views CHF video (by day 3)	24		
	• Patient identifies own risk factors and develops plan to control them	25		
	• Patient explains the diagnosis of CHF including signs and symptoms	26		
	• Patient describes 2000 mg Na diet and label reading	27		
	• Patient demonstrates understanding of concepts related to activities of daily living, limitations, activity pacing, energy conservation and stress reduction	28		
	• Patient agrees to weigh him- or herself daily upon discharge			
	• Patient states weight gain parameters	30		
	• Patient has scale at home	31		
	• Patient discusses medications and food/drug interactions	33		
	• Patient states indications to call MD	34		
	• Patient agrees to follow-up with primary MD in 1 week	35		
Medications	• Medications: Patient received information and discharged home on the following			
	• ASA (36)		No Yes	
	• Digoxin (37)		No Yes	
	• Diuretics (38)		No Yes	
	• ACE Inhibitor (39)		No Yes	
	• Angiotensin receptor blockers (40)		No Yes	
	• Carvedilol (41)		No Yes	
	• Hydralazine (42)		No Yes	
	• Coumadin (43)		No Yes	
	• Statin (44)		No Yes	
Health Care Team Signatures				

Figure 12–2 Critical Pathway Guideline for Congestive Heart Failure.

thirds did not weigh themselves regularly.[20] Friedman demonstrated that older adults with heart failure experienced symptoms such as dyspnea, edema, and a cough for 7 days on average before seeking care, and this delay frequently resulted in hospitalization.[21]

The findings from these studies highlight two issues in care—the lack of timely follow-up, compounded by a deficit of knowledge. The AHCPR guidelines suggest that education become a standard part of management plans and that both content and counseling be included (Exhibit 12–1).[17] Counseling involves an active, two-way process that involves an exchange of information between the provider and the patient, not simply the delivery of facts and rules. Due to the complexity of heart failure management, patients require a comprehensive, tailored, and systematic approach to education.[3,8,22]

The current literature on compliance focuses on prevention and treatment of the patient, as well as provider and system factors that contribute to noncompliance.[2] The American Heart Association multilevel approach for increasing compliance provides suggested actions for patient, provider, and health care organization to improve compliance (see Chapter 11).[2] Patients should be helped to become motivated to learn and have potential barriers to learning removed. Multiple strategies are needed to address noncompliance.[23] Heart failure disease management programs generally have demonstrated improved patient outcomes and health care resource use that likely are the result of improved patient education and increased patient adherence to the treatment regimen.[24–31] Although sparse, the available literature is optimistic for using and implementing successful educational strategies to enhance compliance and improve outcomes.

Provider and Patient Factors that Contribute to Noncompliance

Health care education is fraught with breakdowns in the lines of communication between patients and clinicians.[2] For example, many patients are instructed to weigh themselves, notify the clinician of weight gains, and adjust their medications accordingly. However, clinicians often fail to ask whether patients own or can afford to purchase a scale. A patient may be considered noncompliant with the recommendations when resources such as lack of access to a scale, a telephone, or medications are the culprits. Commonly, noncompliance results from a lack of true comprehension or an understanding of the importance of a particular recommendation. Dunbar and associates described desired outcomes with possible reasons for noncompliance (Table 12–1).[14] This information is useful for counseling patients because it suggests potential reasons for noncompliance that are crucial for tailoring education. For example, if a patient is noncompliant because of financial difficulties, efforts to obtain medication samples or a scale would be helpful. Other patients may need to be referred to an indigent program.[32–34]

Exhibit 12–1 Suggested Patient and Family Caregiver Heart Failure Education and Counseling

---

Patient, family, and caregiver counseling and education are critical to treatment and care.

Patients hospitalized for heart failure should be discharged only when symptoms have been adequately controlled and reversible causes of morbidity have been treated.

Patients and caregivers have been educated about medications, diet, activity, and exercise recommendations, symptoms of worsening heart failure; adequate outpatient support and follow-up care have been provided.

Specific guidelines for the following:
- Restrict sodium intake
- Consult dietitian
- Limit use of alcohol
- Instigate individualized exercise program
- Measure daily weights, reporting weight gain of 3–5 pounds

Education programs and support programs for patients and families

Table 12–1 Noncompliance Issues and Desired Treatment Outcomes

Desired Outcome	Possible Reasons for Noncompliance
Verbalizes signs and symptoms Verbalizes contact and phone number	Denial, anxiety, pain, fatigue, communication barriers
Weighs and records or phones daily	Does not own scale. Vision difficulties reading scale, financial difficulties, no phone.
Verbalizes 2,000-mg diet restriction Understands label reading	Cultural influences Inability to shop or perform culinary tasks Family member unaware of sodium restriction Eating fast foods, frequent dining out
Verbalizes medications and side effects Carries medication list	Financial limitations Literacy problems
Verbalizes how alcohol affects the heart	Alcohol addiction, social environment
Verbalizes the benefits of exercise, target heart rate Warning signals of when to stop activity	Physical disability, reconditioning, fatigue, anxiety

Improving Health Care Systems

Providing education across the full continuum of care is essential in the management of patients with heart failure. Currently, many health care systems neither incorporate adequate education into daily care nor provide outpatient resources for delivering education. A different approach to care for patients with chronic illness that addresses these problems is termed *disease management*. Disease management is described as the process of overseeing the patient with chronic disease across the continuum of care.[35] The spectrum of disease management encompasses health promotion and disease prevention through diagnosis, treatment, and rehabilitation to long-term care.[35] Programs designed to administer disease management interventions to a specific patient population have a higher number of patients achieving the expected outcomes, such as decreased admissions.[5,36–38] The disease management approach appears to prevent or limit heart failure exacerbation, improve quality of life, and optimize resource utilization. Al-

though considered the panacea of heart failure care ills, disease management programs remain to be proven effective in diverse, unselected, large patient populations.[39] Chapters 16 through 20 deal specifically with various disease management modalities.

Promoting Behavior Change

The provision of information is essential but not sufficient to encourage a patient to change behavior. Making a life-style change involves learning about the need for a change, becoming motivated to make a change, identifying resources needed to support the change, making the change, then maintaining the change.[40] Change is recognized as a process, and individuals perform these tasks in stages that have been labeled:[40]

- Precontemplation
- Contemplation
- Preparation
- Action
- Maintenance

These stages do not always proceed in an orderly, linear fashion. When a provider first sees a patient, the patient may be in any one of these stages and may later progress forward or revert to an earlier stage. Individualized interventions designed according to the patient's stage of change have been demonstrated to promote behavioral change with smoking, exercise, and a variety of other behaviors.[40] Although not yet tested in patients with heart failure, adaptation of the stage of change model may be an effective approach to heart failure patient education (Table 12–2).[40]

Another approach to behavioral change focuses on the cognitive processes that persons with heart failure must engage in if they are to be successful in managing their illness. Riegel and colleagues[41] described the heart failure self-management process as one requiring that patients be able to recognize that a change in their signs and/or symptoms has occurred. Once recognized, patients need to be able to judge the importance of the change. There are actions that patients can take to treat those signs and symptoms (eg, an extra diuretic for shortness of breath or weight gain). The person adept at self-management is adventuresome in intervening early, before the change has reached a critical or severe level. For example, patients with heart failure should be taught to monitor their weight daily and to modify their diet, fluid intake, or diuretic dose if a 3-pound weight gain has occurred in a

Table 12–2 Stages of Behavior Change

Behavior Change	Nurse	Patient
Precontemplation	Teach patient that some aspect of present behavior has possible negative consequences.	Patient may dine out and exceed 2,000-mg sodium diet, leading to weight gain and swelling the next day.
Contemplation	Assist patient to identify the pros of limiting sodium, offering dining out tips and recipes. Identify cultural, financial, social, and other barriers to high sodium intake.	Patient is weighing the benefit of change with pros and cons. Patient needs to make own decision that limiting sodium is a good choice.
Preparation	Offer encouragement and reinforcement of positive effects of changed behavior. Set goals for weight range, setting realistic expectations for dining out.	Begin to weigh and report daily. Initiate 2,000-mg diet.
Action	Continue encouragement. Initiate monitoring behavior, such as weight and symptoms.	Continue to weigh and report daily. Continue 2,000-mg diet. Take prescribed medications.
Maintenance	Offer reminders through telephone or clinic visits. Monitor progress of patient by tracking weight and symptoms. Show patient graph of successful weights	Stay out of hospital. Continue weighing, reporting, diet, and medications.

short period of time. The final phase of the self-management process is evaluation of the action taken. True self-management occurs when a patient is able to recognize a problem, understand its importance, take action to treat it early in the process, and note the effectiveness of that action for later use. Patient education that teaches this decision-making process will be more useful to patients than will a lecture on the function of the heart or the coronary anatomy.

Strategies for Patient Education

Sound principles of patient education should be incorporated into all education plans. These principles include repetition and use of multiple methods (eg, printed information, oral communication, visual presentations, audio and videotapes, television, and Internet resources).[42] Information should be provided in small quantities and repeated to avoid overwhelming the patient. Education should be scheduled at times that are convenient for the patient and family.

Principles of adult learning include recognition that adults must feel a need for the information if learning is to occur. Thus, educators working with heart failure patients should concentrate on linking the material to be learned with symptoms experienced. Individualizing and tailoring education to incorporate the patient's past learning experiences is essential to successful educational efforts aimed at adults, for example, to assist a patient in learning how to adopt a sodium-restricted diet, review food labels and make sure that the patient knows the relationship between sodium and salt.

Heart failure patients are typically elderly. Recognition that the normal changes of aging may interfere with learning will facilitate educational efforts. For example, patients need to be able to see food labels if they are to learn how to read them. Patients may need to be referred for a vision evaluation if it becomes evident that they are unable to see the labels adequately. Use of a magnifying glass may be helpful.

Educational materials that are tailored to individual beliefs and characteristics are most effective. For example, methods of adapting food preferences, including cultural or ethnic practices, into the medical nutrition plan will help patients to comply because the pleasure of eating can be maintained. Identification of individual patient barriers to compliance and open discussion of ways to minimize or remove those barriers are essential. Strengthening and reinforcing the benefits of following a regimen can enhance or maintain compliance. For example, working with a patient to find a diuretic dosing schedule that does not interfere with normal activities may enhance compliance and teach the patient important lessons about self-management.

A tool available to assist educators to address cultural, socioeconomic, and social support barriers to improve education effectiveness is the Monitoring and Educating using Disease Management to Improve Compliance Instrument (MEDICI) (see Appendix 12–A). Elements of the educational process that are incorporated into MEDICI include:

- understanding heart failure
- signs and symptoms
- who to notify in an emergency
- medications
- restricted sodium diet
- exercise guidelines
- alcohol restrictions

At Evanston Northwestern Healthcare, MEDICI is initiated upon consultation, and heart failure team members document completed sections as educational goals are met. Using MEDICI, heart failure team members are able to continue education to patients across the continuum of care, to reinforce educational goals, and to document goal achievements.

Environmental barriers decrease the effectiveness of education provided in the hospital. Unless adequate resources already exist or there is money available to purchase materials, providers will require time to design and produce patient educational materials. It may be necessary to allot additional time so that providers can effectively teach and evaluate patients to assess the effectiveness of that teaching. Physical space for education should be available for use at times convenient for families and patients. Dedicated physical space that is conducive to learning and counseling will enhance outcomes. That space should be private, comfortable, quiet, and free from interruptions.

If staff members lack knowledge about specific treatment requirements or skills in patient education strategies, trained personnel (eg, dietitians, pharmacists, advanced practice nurses) should be recruited to educate staff, assemble materials, intervene with complex patients, and evaluate programs. The social worker may be enlisted to develop a list of community resources for patients. Resources are available in most communities for patients who need to obtain scales and/or medications; such assistance can decrease the overwhelming financial burden that many patients with heart failure face.

Telemanagement

It is clear that simply imparting information is not sufficient to promote behavioral change, self-management, or treatment compliance. Patients and their families or caregivers need continuing assistance as they struggle to implement what they have learned. In our heart failure program, telemanagement is used as a means of daily reinforcement of education for patients at high risk for rehospitalization (Exhibit 12–2). A core component of our follow-up is constant communication among patients and providers.

Managing patients by phone may be as advanced as using video technology or as simple as having patients phone in their weight and symptoms. Telephonic weight monitoring and daily reporting of symptoms have been shown to have a compliance rate of 90%, to decrease heart failure rehospitalization rates, and to reduce health care costs.[43] Empowering the patient to initiate the daily call may promote behavioral change and assist in self-management because it returns control to the patient. In the Evanston Northwestern Healthcare telemanagement program, patients call daily into an automated voice system that records their weight and symptoms (Exhibit 12–3). Nurses receive variance reports on patients who fluctuate from their set weight range or have positive symptoms. If a patient

Exhibit 12–2 Characteristics of Patients at High Risk for Hospitalization

Myriad comorbidities
  Coronary artery disease
  Diabetes
  Hypertension
  Chronic renal insufficiency
Medications
  Medication noncompliance
  Adverse drug reactions
Dietary noncompliance
Psychosocial concerns
  Social isolation
  Depression
Financial constraints
  Lack of scale, medications
Cognitive dysfunction
  Neglecting to notify health care providers

dines out and the next day experiences a weight gain of 3 pounds, he or she will receive a call from a provider that reinforces the need to request low-sodium choices and the wisdom of taking an extra diuretic. As a consequence, patients begin to correlate their actions with health consequences, and true learning occurs. Providers react to important symptom changes and take quick action to prevent further physiologic deterioration that can lead to a hospitalization. Daily

Exhibit 12–3 Telemanagement Daily Symptom and Weight Survey Questions

1. Have you felt more short of breath in the last day?
2. Have you noticed more swelling in the last day?
3. Did you wake up from sleep short of breath last night?
4. Did you sleep in a chair or prop up with pillows more than usual last night?
5. Have you had any light-headedness or dizziness in the last day?
6. Have you had to rest more in the last day?

patient tracking can identify noncompliance problems, thereby allowing targeting of education.

One simple technologic advance will markedly improve telemanagement in the future—interactive voice response or computer telephony. This telephone-based computer technology has allowed the nearly instantaneous feedback of important patient status information to the providers. It has also allowed for educational content and reinforcement of treatment goals from the providers to the patient. This two-way interaction promises to be even more robust and effective as newer technologies are applied. Advances such as voice response, where patient input can be done by voice, rather than touchpad, have begun to be tested in clinical applications for chronic diseases. In addition, several companies are now evaluating the Internet as a low-cost platform for multimedia communications between providers and patients with chronic illness. Some may believe that these technologies are useful only with younger heart failure patients, but senior citizens who completed a training session on searching the Internet to discuss issues with their physicians remained satisfied with and interested in using the Internet.[44] This approach to disease management, sometimes called *e-Health*, promises to change forever the way patients and providers communicate and exchange information.

Telemanagement provides patients with opportunities for self-directed behavior, active participation, and reinforcement of education. Telemanagement can be applied in any practice setting—a primary physician's office, heart failure clinic, or nurse-managed heart failure program—as a means of reinforcing education and promoting compliance. In the Stanford Multi-Fit program, as few as three telephone calls between scheduled office visits improved compliance and reduced the utilization of medical services in a sample of 500 patients.[45] For severely ill patients, telephone contact may reduce mortality.[46] Heart failure patients who were aggressively telemanaged in one clinical trial experienced substantially reduced heart failure admissions, decreased costs, and improved quality of life.[47] Although apparently beneficial, telemedicine requires assessment for effectiveness, efficiency,

and safety before its use becomes widespread.[48] Chapter 19 provides an in-depth description of telephonic case management.

Outpatient Education Seminars

Another option for effective education is the outpatient education seminar. Outpatient education seminars allow patients to interact actively with peers, and the seminars also reinforce the information that has been taught.[49] The seminar should incorporate various activities and learning sessions. Patients often share coping strategies and offer support and encouragement, increasing motivation for complying with the treatment plan. In one such group, topics from a "Heart Failure Handbook" (see Exhibit 12–4) provide the necessary educational components for heart failure patients and families. The group setting provides opportunities for discussion and questions to clarify misconceptions and ensure understanding. Opting to participate in an outpatient seminar acknowledges that the patient and family are motivated and ready to learn. Rotating the time of seminars may allow various family members the opportunity to attend. Learning from peers such information as the names of local restaurants with low-sodium menu selections, the brands of low-sodium foods, various books and web sites, and tips for tolerating medication side effects may be helpful and will provide camaraderie.

Although helpful for many patients, outpatient seminars or support groups cannot be the sole method of delivering heart failure education. Many patients lack transportation, are home bound, prefer not to attend education provided in a group, or do not learn well in the group setting. Other organizations have developed cable television programs for inaccessible patients. However, these education strategies are fatal unless coupled with a plan for follow-up care by a health care provider.

Other Sources of Educational Materials

An important objective for providers is to educate and inform patients using the variety of resources available. Patients can read books or

Exhibit 12–4 Evanston Northwestern Healthcare Heart Failure Handbook

This handbook is designed to help you and your family better understand, manage, and track your congestive heart failure. The following topics are covered in this handbook:

Your heart and how it works
- Puzzle

Causes of heart failure
- Successfully managing your heart failure

Tracking your heart failure
- Daily weight record
- Vital signs/laboratory record

CHF telemanagement program
- Instructions using telemanagement

Medications
- Ace inhibitors
- Nitrates
- Diuretics
- Digoxin
- β blockers
- Coumadin
- Amiodarone
- Calcium channel blockers

Activity and Exercise
- Becoming active
- Exercise guidelines
- Stretching exercises
- Taking your pulse
- Target heart rate

Diet
- Tips for limiting sodium
- Tips for limiting cholesterol and fats
- Cooking healthy meals
- Reading labels
- Recipes for low-sodium, low-fat, and low-cholesterol meals
- Dining out

Diagnostic testing
- Electrocardiogram
- Chest X-ray
- Echocardiogram
- MUGA
- Cardiac catheterization
- Laboratory work
- 24-hour Holter
- Stress test
  Thallium stress
  Cardiopulmonary stress
  Cardiopulmonary stress, sestamibi

search the Internet in their own environments and without distractions if they are provided with books and web sites. Discovering resources and learning about heart failure can empower patients, helping to transform them into informed consumers who successfully use available resources to improve their health. Appendix 12–B provides a list of recommended books and web sites for heart failure patients.

CONCLUSION

Over the last decade, research has led to an improved understanding of the pathophysiology of heart failure and to innovative treatments that dramatically improve outcomes. These therapeutic advances, however, are fruitless if patients lack the education and motivation necessary to achieve optimum success. Patient empowerment through increased knowledge and promotion of self-care is now the core objective in managing this troublesome syndrome. Further research and outcomes tracking will facilitate understanding of the education needed to enhance compliance and self-management. Education is the cornerstone of every successful heart failure program in existence.

REFERENCES

1. Bandura A. Self-efficacy mechanism in human agency. *Am Psychol.* 1982;37(2): 122–147.

2. Miller NH, Hill M, Kottke T, Ockene IS. The multilevel compliance challenge: Recommendations for a call to action. A statement for health care professionals. *Circulation* 1995;1085–1090.

3. Cardiology Pre Eminence Roundtable. *Beyond Four Walls: Cost Effective Management of Chronic Congestive Heart Failure.* Washington, DC: The Advisory Board Company; 1994.

4. Ghali JK, Kadakia S, Cooper R, Ferlinz J. Precipitating factors leading to decompensation of heart failure: Traits among urban blacks. *Arch Intern Med.* 1998;148:2013–2016.

5. Rich MW, Beckham V, Wittenberg C, Leven CL, Freedland KE, Carney RM. A multidisciplinary intervention to prevent the readmission of elderly patients with congestive heart failure. *N Engl J Med.* 1995;333: 1190–1195.

6. Bertel O. Effects of patient information, compliance and medical control on prognosis in chronic heart failure. *Herz.* 1991;1:294–977.

7. ACC/AHA Task Force Report. Guidelines for the evaluation and management of heart failure. *J Am Coll Cardiol.* 1995;26:1376–1398.

8. Pearson TA, McBride PE, Miller NH, Smith SC. 27th Bethesda Conference: Matching the intensity of risk factor management with the hazard for coronary disease events: Task Force 8: Organization of preventive cardiology service. *J Am Coll Cardiol.* 1996;27:1039–1047.

9. Williams EL, Fitton F. Factors affecting early unplanned readmission of elderly patients to hospital. *Br Med J.* 1988;297:784–787.

10. Andrews K, Relevance of readmission of elderly patients discharged from a geriatric unit. *J Am Geriatr Soc.* 1986;34:15–21.

11. Naylor MD, Brooten D, Campbell R, et al. Comprehensive discharge planning and home follow-up of hospitalized elders. *JAMA.* 1999;281:613–620.

12. Harrison MB, Toman C, Logan J. Hospital to home: Evidence-based education for heart failure. *Can Nurs.* 1998;94:36–42.

13. Falvo D. *Effective Patient Education.* Rockville, MD: Aspen Publishers; 1985: 34.

14. Dunbar SB; Jacobson LH; Deaton C. Heart failure: Strategies to enhance patient self-management. *AACN Clin Issues.* 1998;9:244–256.

15. Konstam M, Dracup K, Baker D, et al. *Heart Failure: Evaluation and Care of Patients with Left-Ventricular Systolic Dysfunction.* Rockville, MD: Agency for Health Care Policy and Research; Public Health Service, US Dept. of Health and Human Services, 1994. Clinical practice guideline #11. AHCPR Publication No. 94–0612.

16. Stewart S, Pearson S, Horowitz JD. Effects of a home-based intervention among patients with congestive heart failure discharged from acute hospital care. *Arch Intern Med.* 1998;158:1067–1072.

17. Hagenhoff BD, Feutz C, Conn VS, Sagehorn KK, Moranville-Hunziker M. Patient education needs as reported by congestive heart failure patients and their nurses. *J Adv Nurs.* 1994;19:685–690.

18. Wehby D, Brenner, PS. Perceived learning needs of patients with heart failure. *Heart Lung.* 1999;28:31–40.

19. Frattini E, Lindsay P, Kerr E, Park YJ. Learning needs of congestive heart failure patients. *Prog Cardiovasc Nurs.* 1998;13(2):77–82.

20. Bushnell FK. Self care teaching for congestive heart failure patients. *J Gerontol Nurs.* 1992;18:27–32.

21. Friedman MM. Older adults' symptoms and their duration before hospitalization for heart failure. *Heart Lung.* 1997;26:169–176.

22. Stanley M. Current trends in the clinical management of an old enemy: Congestive heart failure in the elderly. *AACN Clin Issues.* 1997;8:616–626

23. Lasseleben M, Cullen MJ, Wilson AJ. Compliance by collaboration: Effectively addressing problems of treatment adherence. *Aust Fam Physician.* 1999;28:850–853.

24. Kornowski R, Zeeli D, Averbuch M, et al. Intensive home care surveillance prevents hospitalization and improves morbidity and mortality rates among elderly patients with severe congestive heart failure. *Am Heart J.* 1995;129:762–766.

25. Knox D, Mischke L. Implementing a congestive heart failure disease management program to decrease length of stay and cost. *J Cardiovasc Nurs.* 1999;14:55–74.

26. Cintron G, Bigas C, Linares E, Aranda JM, Hernandez E. Nurse practitioner role in a chronic congestive heart failure clinic: In-hospital time, costs, and patient satisfaction. *Heart Lung.* 1983;12:237–240.

27. Laster M. The effect of a nurse-managed heart failure clinic on patient readmission and length of stay. *Home Healthcare Nurse.* 1996;14:351–356.

28. West JA, Miller NH, Parker KM, et al. A comprehensive management system for heart failure improves clinical outcomes and reduces medical resource utilization. *Am J Cardiol.* 1997;79:58–63

29. Fonarow GC, Stevenson LW, Walden JA, et al. Impact of a comprehensive heart failure management program on hospital readmission and functional status of patients with advanced heart failure. *J Am Coll Cardiol.* 1997;30:725–732.

30. Smith LE, Fabbri SA, Pai R, Ferry D, Heywood JT: Symptomatic improvement and reduced hospitalization for patients attending a cardiomyopathy clinic. *Clin Cardiol.* 1997;20:949–954.

31. Rich MW. Effect of a multidisciplinary intervention on medication compliance in elderly patients with congestive heart failure. *Am J Med.* 1996;101:270–276.

32. Vinson JM, Rich MW, Sperry JC, et al. Early readmission of elderly patients with congestive heart failure. *J Am Geriatr Soc.* 1990;38:1290–1295.

33. Kegel LM. APNs can refine the management of heart failure. *Clin Nurs Specialist.* 1995;9:76–81.

34. Goodyer L, Milligan P. Does encouraging good compliance improve patients' clinical condition in heart failure. *Br J Consult Psychol.* 1995;49(36):173–176.

35. Roark MK. Critical Pathways. *Health Care Resource Manage.* 1997;12–15.

36. Shah N, Der E, Ruggerio C, Heidenreich PA, Massie BM. Prevention of hospitalizations for heart failure with an interactive home monitoring program. *Am Heart J.* 1998;3:373–378.

37. Jaarsma T, Halfens R, Huijer Abu-Saad H, et al. Effects of education and support on self care and resource utilization in patients with heart failure. *Eur Heart J.* 1999;20:673–782.

38. Schneider JK, Hornberger S, Booker J, Davis A, Kralicek R. A medication discharge planning program: Measuring the effect on readmissions. *Clin Nurs Res.* 1993;2:41–53.

39. Rich MW. Heart failure disease management. *Cardiac Failure.* 1999;5:64–75.

40. Prochaska JO, Velicer WF, Rossi JS, et al. Stages of change and decision balance for 12 problem behaviors. *Health Psychol.* 1994;13:39–46.

41. Riegel, B, Carlson, B, Glaser, D. Development of an instrument to measure self-management of heart failure. *Heart Lung.* 2000;29(1): 4–12.

42. Bond WS, Hussar DA. Detection methods and strategies for improving medication compliance. *Am J Hosp Pharm.* 1991;48:1978–1988.

43. Williams RE, Keller L, Sprang M, Mehan C. Telemanagement of congestive heart failure: Results of daily weight and symptom tracking. *J Am Coll Cardiol.* 1997;2(Suppl A):247A.

44. Leaffer T, Gonda B. The Internet: An underutilized tool in patient education. *Comput Nurs.* 2000;18(1):47–52.

45. DeBusk RF, Miller NH, Superko HR, et al. A case management system for coronary risk factor modification after acute myocardial infarction. *Ann Intern Med.* 1994;120:721–729.

46. Wasson J, Gaudette C, Whaley F, Sauvigne A, Barbeau P, Welch G. Telephone care as a substitute for routine clinic follow-up. *JAMA.* 1992;267:1788–1793.

47. Schiller AE Jr., Bondmass M, Avitall B. Technology-based home care for disease management. *Health Serv Adm J.* 1997;5:10–12.

48. Currell R, Urquhart C, Wainwright P, Lewis R. Telemedicine versus face-to-face consultations: Effect on professional practice and health care outcomes. *The Cochrane Database of Systematic Reviews.* 2000.

49. English M, Mastream MB. Congestive heart failure: Public and private burden. *Crit Care Nurs* 1995;18(1):1–6.

Monitoring and Educating Using Disease Management To Improve Compliance Instrument (MEDICI)

Demographics

Name_____ Date_____

Address _____

Home Phone _____ Work Phone _____

Date of Birth _____ SS# _____

Sex : ☐ Male ☐ Female

Can patient follow and understand directions? ☐ Yes ☐ No

Is patient/family motivated to learn? ☐ Yes ☐ No

Race ☐ Caucasian ☐ African American ☐ Hispanic ☐ Asian
      ☐ Other _____

Primary language ☐ English ☐ Spanish ☐ French ☐ Polish
      ☐ German ☐ Other _____
      Specific cultural issues _____

Religion ☐ Christian ☐ Jewish ☐ Muslim ☐ Buddhist
      ☐ Other _____
      Specific Religious issues: _____

Educational Level ☐ Elementary ☐ High School ☐ College
      ☐ Graduate or above

Living Situation ☐ Alone ☐ Spouse/family ☐ Caretaker ☐ Extended care facility

Support System Name _____
      Relation _____
      Phone number _____

Socioeconomic Status   ☐ Employed   ☐ Disabled   ☐ Retired   ☐ Unemployed

Physical Limitations   ☐ HOH   ☐ Blind   ☐ Dementia

Social History

Smoking   ☐ Current   ppd_____

☐ Previous   ppd_____   Years smoked_____

Quit (Date)_____

☐ None

Alcohol   ☐ Current   ☐ Beer   ☐ Wine   ☐ Liquor

☐ Daily   ☐ Weekly   ☐ Socially

☐ Previous   ☐ Beer   ☐ Wine   ☐ Liquor

☐ Daily   ☐ Weekly   ☐ Socially

Quit (Date)_____

☐ None

MEDICI—Diet

Problem	Recommendations	Date/Initials
Lack of knowledge	Obtain food diary	_____
	Consult dietitian	_____
	Explain 2 gram sodium diet (ie, reading labels)	_____
	Distribute written material—CHF Handbook	_____
	Low sodium choices	_____
	Dining out tips	_____
	Low sodium and cholesterol recipes	_____
	Instruct importance of daily weight	_____
	View CHF video	_____
	Encourage to attend support group	_____
	Enroll in telemanagement training	_____
	Follow-up by home care agency (cabinet inspection)	_____
Cultural issues	Become familiar with various diets	_____
	Provide CHF Handbook in native language (at ENH, Spanish material available)	_____
	Assess patient and family's willingness to change (if unwilling, increase medications?)	_____
	Follow by home care agency—cupboard assessment and counseling	_____

Dining out	Assess frequency	
	Provide names of accommodating local restaurants	
	Encourage to attend support group (tips for dining out)	
	Suggestions for requesting low sodium meals	
Inadequate social support/resources	Assess living situation (ie, cook, Meals on Wheels, transportation to grocery store)	
	Educate person responsible for culinary tasks	
	Follow-up with home care agency (pill counts, safety concerns)	
	Assess affordability of low sodium foods	

MEDICI—Medications

Problem	Recommendations	Date/Initials
Lack of knowledge	Assess baseline knowledge	
	Teach purpose of medications	
	Carries list of medications/schedule	
	Aware of side effects	
	Create medication schedule to alleviate nocturia and hypotension	
	Consult with pharmacist at clinic visit	
	Encourage to attend support group	
	Distribute written material on all medications	
	Distribute written material—CHF Handbook	
	Follow with home care agency (fill pillboxes, verify dose/schedules)	
Lower socio-economic status	Assess insurance coverage (if inadequate—indigent programs, drug samples, drug company programs)	
Inadequate social support/resources	Assess living situation (ie, alone, incapacitated, demented)	
	Assess vision/hearing loss	
	Identify status/availability of support system (if necessary, supervision provided)	
	Educate resources on medication regimen	
	Follow with home care agency (pill counts, safety concerns, IV diuretics/inotropes, if necessary)	

MEDICI—Neglecting To Notify Health Care Provider

Problem	Recommendations	Date/Initials
Lack of knowledge	Obtain baseline knowledge of CHF	_____
	Instruct patient to verbalize signs and symptoms to notify health care providers:	_____
	Sudden weight gain	_____
	Breathing more difficult	_____
	Waking up at night out of breath	_____
	Chest pain	_____
	Increased fatigue	_____
	Increased swelling	_____
	Reduced appetite	_____
	Lightheadedness/Dizziness	_____
	Weigh daily and record	_____
	Provide education CHF handbook by topic	_____
	Review CHF handbook and have patient verbalize understanding	_____
	Enroll patient in telemanagement	_____
	Home care to reiterate education	_____
	Provide emergency phone number, contacts	_____
	Provide follow-up appointment	_____
Culture	Provide education materials in native language	_____
	Provide translator if possible	_____
Lack of support system	Assess knowledgebase of CHF	_____
	Include family in all education	_____
	Invite family to clinic, support group	_____
	If patient is alone, assess need for 24-hour caretaker, nursing home for safety	_____

MEDICI—Exercise

Problem	Recommendations	Date/Initials
Lack of knowledge	Assess baseline knowledge of exercise	_____
	Teach signs and symptoms to STOP	_____
	Instruct on palpating heart rate	_____

	Provide target heart rate	_____
	Instruct warm up and cool down exercises	_____
	Consult with exercise physiologist	_____
	Encourage to attend support group	_____
	Distribute written material on exercise—CHF Handbook	_____
Lower socio-economic status	Assess insurance coverage for rehabilitation	_____
	If lacking, enroll in Phase 3 or home exercises	_____
Inadequate social support/resources	Assess living situation (ie, alone, incapacitated, demented)	_____
	Educate support system about exercise	_____
	Encourage participation in exercise	_____
	Identify status/availability of support system (if necessary, supervision provided)	_____

Consumer Information

The following is a compiled list of recommended books and web sites for heart failure patients.

BOOKS

A Resource Directory for Older People, published by the National Institute on Aging. Phone (301) 496–1752.

American Heart Association Low-Salt Cookbook: A Complete Guide To Reducing Sodium and Fat in the Diet by Rodman Starke.

Get the Salt Out: 501 Simple Ways To Cut the Salt Out of any Diet by Ann Gittleman.

How To Live between Office Visits by Bernie S. Siegel, MD.

Love, Medicine, and Miracles by Bernie S. Siegel, MD.

Success with Heart Failure by Marc Silver, MD

WEB SITES

American Heart Association: www.amhrt.org

Heart Failure Society of America: www.hfsa.org

Jon's Place: www.jonsplace.org/heartforum.htm

PART V

The Role of Family in Heart Management

CHAPTER 13

Supportive Resources for the Patient with Heart Failure

Linda S. Baas, Robin Trupp, and William T. Abraham

Heart failure is a major public health problem in the United States that afflicts more than 5 million persons at an estimated national economic cost of nearly 40 billion dollars.[1,2] However, the full burden of this disorder is personal and not quantifiable. Heart failure reduces functional status and the quality of life of those who bear the diagnosis. In addition, it has a profound effect on family, friends, and other members of patients' immediate social circle.[3–5] Social support is the most commonly thought of form of supportive resource, but many other external and internal factors may serve the same capacity in terms of assisting the person with heart failure.

This chapter will review the myriad supportive resources that people with heart failure may need to promote self-care, maintain an acceptable functional status, promote quality of life, and achieve personal goals.[3–9] The supportive resources will be discussed from the perspective of a theoretical approach to understanding the varied types of resources that are available. The Modeling and Role Modeling (MRM) theory has been applied as a framework for research and a useful guide for practice.[7–13] A general review of research related to external and internal resources will be presented, followed by specific research conducted with persons with heart failure. Finally, practice implications for the multidisciplinary heart failure treatment team will be discussed.

OVERVIEW OF SUPPORTIVE RESOURCES

The contemporary view of support is that it is an individual perception or experience. Thus, all discussions of supportive resources should recognize that support is a subjective rather than an objective determination. In discussing support in this chapter, the reference is to perceived support, unless indicated otherwise. Within this framework, perceived support often is differentiated into two categories, based on the source of the resource.[7,10–12,14] External resources are those social factors that are separate from the individual and are derived from social interactions with others or from their environment. Examples of external resources include social support, social network, financial assistance, support of health care providers, and tangible support, such as help with driving or shopping.[7–10,14] Internal resources are derived from those inner psychologic, cognitive, and physiologic factors that make people unique. Hope, control, self-efficacy, a future orientation, and knowledge of the illness and treatment are examples of internal resources that may be useful for the person with a chronic health problem.[7–10,14]

Some identified resources may be difficult to categorize as derived from either external or internal sources. In reality, the supportive resource may have a mixed source. One example of that is spirituality, which is recognized as an important resource for the person adjusting to a chronic illness such as heart failure.[10,15,16] In a thorough review of measures of spirituality, distinctions have been made between the more internal aspect that is the spiritual belief system and the more external aspect that includes participation in religious practices and services.[16] In a sample of 31 persons with heart failure treated medically and 41 who underwent heart transplantation, subjects reported their participation in religious activities, as well as more internal beliefs about spirituality.[17] There were no differences between the two treatment groups. Both variables were positively related to a global measure of quality of life, but the stronger relationship was found with the measure of internal spirituality (r = .77).

Modeling and Role Modeling is one theoretical framework that incorporates both internal and external resources as factors that can promote positive outcomes in persons with health problems and other stressors. A brief description of MRM theory is provided as a guide for understanding the relationship of the two forms of supportive resources. Research based on this framework is presented.

A THEORETICAL APPROACH TO FACILITATING SUPPORTIVE RESOURCES

Erickson, Tomlin, and Swain derived the MRM theory from their extensive years in practice and an integration of extant theories of development, basic and growth needs, attachment and loss, stress, and coping.[10] Subsequent research by these theorists and others has provided support for many of the theoretical relationships described in the paradigm.[7–13,15] The title of the theory is derived from the approach to assessment and intervention. Modeling is the process of building an understanding or "model" of the person's world through an individualized assessment of self-care knowledge, needs, and resources. It is important to stress that this model is derived from the personal perception of the client, not the perceptions of the health care pro-

vider. Role modeling refers to the individualized interventions that are designed to regain health or provide restorative care.[10,11] Within the framework of MRM, there are four major constructs: affiliated-individuation, self-care, developmental residual, and the adaptive potential assessment model. These constructs have been recognized as being the core of different middle-range theories, and each will be briefly described and applied to the care of the patient with heart failure.[18]

Affiliated–Individuation

Affiliated–individuation describes how one has simultaneous needs to be both connected and affiliated with others while also being autonomous or individuated from others.[10] Affiliation represents the need to be connected for the purposes of obtaining support and maintaining social connections. Thus, affiliation is the need for the external supportive resources previously discussed. Attachment to others is essential to our sense of being. When attachments are lost, we grieve. If grief is prolonged, depression may ensue. When new attachments are formed, grief is resolved.

Individuation represents the need to be able to rely on internal resources to maintain autonomy and control. The ability to be individuated requires adequate internal resources. Those with a greater degree of individuation may be able to manage better when attachments are lost. They have more of the internal strength needed to form new attachments.

The dynamic nature of change in the environment requires the person to be open and responsive to evolving, situational-based needs for both affiliation and individuation; thus, these concepts can be viewed along two parallel continuums. One continuum is for affiliation needs, and the other continuum for individuation. Both continuums would have a range from low to high levels of needs. There are times when a person has greater needs for affiliation and other times when the need for individuation is greater. The person moves along these continuums, based on the current stressors or needs that he or she faces. For example, within a single day, one may have numerous examples of behaviors that demonstrate affiliation, such as inviting a friend to visit or calling a friend to talk about family problems. Similarly, the same person may feel the need to sit alone after hearing the results of his or her echocardiogram. Taking control over the situation in this way, the patient is able to reflect on the meaning of the information, review the situation, and regain control over the health plan.

In a study of caregivers of persons with Alzheimer's disease, the measures of affiliation and individuation had a mediating effect on stress.[19] Research conducted in persons with heart failure demonstrated positive outcomes when external (affiliation) needs were met for both the patient with heart disease and their caregivers.[20] Both internal and external resources were significant predictors of global quality of life in persons with heart failure treated medically or with transplant. Neither treatment group nor gender differences were found.[8] Similar results were found in a larger convenience sample ($n = 317$) of persons with various cardiovascular diagnoses.[13] Whereas most studies examine affiliation, individuation was the focus of one study of 73 persons with heart failure.[21] Perceived enactment of autonomy was examined as a measure of individuation. A moderately strong ($r = .41$) and significant relationship with global quality of life was found.[21] This study was interesting and provided support for examining the degree of individuation in persons with heart failure. An interesting future study might include both measures of affiliation and individuation in predicting quality of life.

Self-Care Model

Another middle-range theory within MRM is the Self-Care Model. In this paradigm, self-care is the ability to mobilize sufficient resources to cope with the stress of a health-related problem. These resources can be derived from either external or internal sources, such as social support, support from health care providers, self-esteem, control, resilience, and spirituality. The actual model of self-care depicts self-care resources and self-care knowledge as the requisites of self-care action.

Self-care resources include all of the various internal and external resources that the person perceives to be available. These resources can be relied upon to be available so that they can be used to cope with the stress of the health care problem. It is important, as with all other components of this theory, that the perception of resources must come from the perspective of the patient. Thus, building a model of the client's world includes an assessment of the perception of resources available.

Self-care knowledge is what the person believes has caused the illness or has lessened ability to cope with the situation. Furthermore, it includes what the person believes is needed to regain or maintain health, functional status, and quality of life. Again, it is important to recognize that this is the person's perception of the event, state of health, and desired outcomes—not a reflection of his or her understanding of the disease process. For instance, if one asks a patient with heart failure why their weight is up, the patient may indicate that he or she has been stressed by the upcoming marriage of a child. This is that patient's understanding of the event. As health care providers, we recognize that this stressful period led to an increase in fluid intake or decrease in fluid removal for various reasons that can be explored. Teaching about the role of sodium, amount of fluid intake, or need to take scheduled medications is not the appropriate intervention. The way to deal with this situation is through recognition of the stress of this event and advising on ways to deal with the fluid excess within the context of the person's life. Recognizing and targeting the stress response may have a beneficial effect by blunting the sympathetic stimulation that worsens heart function.

Self-care actions are those behaviors or activities that are done to promote, maintain, or regain health. When internal and external resources are adequate, one can mobilize the resources to perform the self-care actions needed to meet health-related goals. However, this must be viewed within the context of what the person feels is necessary. Thus, both self-care resources and self-care knowledge contribute to the self-care actions.

The Self-Care Resource Inventory was developed to measure the array of internal and external resources identified in the theory. Over a series of studies, the reliability and validity of the instrument was determined to be acceptable for use in larger studies.[13] This tool has 35 items, rated from 0 (none) to 4 (a lot) on two dimensions. Respondents first rate each item in terms of how much is needed. Based on the definition of self-care knowledge in this theory, the needs score provides a measure of this concept. Next, the item is rated in terms of the amount that is perceived to be available, representing self-care resources. In a study of 81 persons who were between 3 and 6 months after myocardial infarction, self-care resources predicted 22% of the variance of life satisfaction. Activity level predicted an additional 8% of the variance, and resources needed added another 4% to the model. The measure of self-care knowledge was not significantly related to life satisfaction, which was determined to be the outcome of self-care action. However, self-care knowledge (needs) acted as a suppressor variable in the analysis and was important to include because of the relationship with resources available. It is of interest that, when the need scores were subtracted from the resources available, a self-care deficit score was derived. When the deficit score was entered into a regression model, it predicted only 17% of the variance in life satisfaction. This can actually be viewed as a test of two theories. The original and better predictive model used both self-care knowledge and resources and tested the MRM theory of self-care. Using the deficit score could be considered to be a test of Orem's model of Self-Care Deficits.[13] Similar results were found in a sample of 317 persons with various cardiac disorders and 153 persons with heart failure treated medically or with transplant.[7,13]

Developmental Residual

A third middle-range theory within MRM is that of developmental residual. Many of these internal resources can be viewed as the positive residual strengths that are developed as a result of repeated successful achievement of developmental challenges. Nearly half a century ago, Maslow identified eight stages of development with bipolar outcomes of successful versus unsuccessful outcomes.[22] The stages are: trust–distrust, autonomy–shame, initiative–guilt, industry–inferiority, identity–role confusion, intimacy–isolation, generativity–self absorption, and integrity–despair.[22] Erikson also defined strengths and virtues that arise from successful resolution of a developmental challenge.[23] These include hope, drive, purpose, self-control, fidelity, and wisdom. For each stage that is completed successfully, the person accumulates strengths that can be internal supportive resources in times of need. Although we often think of these stages as sequential, in fact, Erikson proposed that these stages may be an overwhelming challenge that coincides with certain age groups, but that the same challenges recur throughout life. If one has positive residual from facing the challenge in the past, there is more residual strength to make the current challenge less stressful and easier to resolve.

In one study of 138 adults with heart failure, qualitative analysis of goal statements supported the hypothesis that these patients faced a variety of developmental challenges representing the eight stages identified by Erikson.[9] Subjects also completed the Index of Well-Being to assess quality of life and the Profile of Mood States to assess levels of anger and depression. Of interest, the subjects under age 45 years had the highest levels of depression and anger. This may have been related to a realization of premature death. The older subjects reported the highest well-being, perhaps indicating more positive residual related to later adulthood developmental challenges, as well as goal achievement over their lifetimes. The quantitative data related to negative or positive moods were supported when triangulated with qualitative data obtained from the same individuals.

Adaptive Potential Assessment Model

The fourth middle-range theory, the Adaptive Potential Assessment Model, is based on Selye's physiologic and Engel's psychosocial response to stress.[23,24] Stressors may be real or perceived, but either can result in a state of arousal. When coping resources are mobilized, the person adapts and returns to a state of equilibrium. If unable to muster the resources needed to manage the stress, impoverishment results. Long-term impoverishment also leads to depression and morbid grief.

The stage of equilibrium is identified by a high degree of hope but a lack of tension, fatigue, sadness, and anxiety. The arousal state is characterized by increased motor activity, tension, anxiety, and sensory awareness while demonstrating a low level of fatigue or sadness. The impoverished state is one in which there is a high degree of anxiety, sadness, fatigue, and hopelessness. These states and the associated characteristics have been validated in studies of adolescents and adults.[25] Whereas the state of impoverishment is undesirable, the state of arousal also can be detrimental to the person with heart failure. The additional neurohormonal stimulation can worsen cardiac function and perhaps lessen the effectiveness of medications prescribed to modulate the sympathetic nervous system and the associated chemical activation. Thus, interventions to reduce arousal are beneficial and should be a major thrust of care provided by the multidisciplinary team.

Many of the studies conducted using other theoretical frameworks focused on the role of supportive resources in reducing stress, improving coping, and facilitating adaptation or self-management of the disease. A summary of these studies will be presented in the review of external and internal supportive resources.

Interrelationships of the Component Theories of Modeling and Role Modeling

Affiliated–individuation, self-care resources, developmental residual, and adaptive potential are all examples of what can enable the person with a stressor or health problem to have more positive outcomes. The process of mobilizing resources is a self-care action. Thus, all of these components of MRM theory can be linked through propositions and relational statements (Figure 13–1). The four middle-range theories of affiliated–individuation, self-care, developmental residual, and adaptive potential are all applied from the perspective of the individual. These key concepts within the framework of the overall theory provide dimensions that can be used to assess each person's "model of the world." Complete assessment guides based on MRM theory have been published and could easily be adapted for special populations such as those with heart failure.[10,11,26]

The MRM theory provides a framework for future research and perhaps more specific theory development for persons with heart failure. However, much research has been conducted in the areas of social support; social networks; supportive benefits of information, groups, and health care providers; and various internal resources. To understand the current knowledge about the broad perspective of supportive resources, it is important to review key research findings about supportive resources in other populations, and to discuss research specifically conducted with persons with heart failure.

SUPPORTIVE EXTERNAL RESOURCES

This section begins with a discussion of social support because it is the most frequently dis-

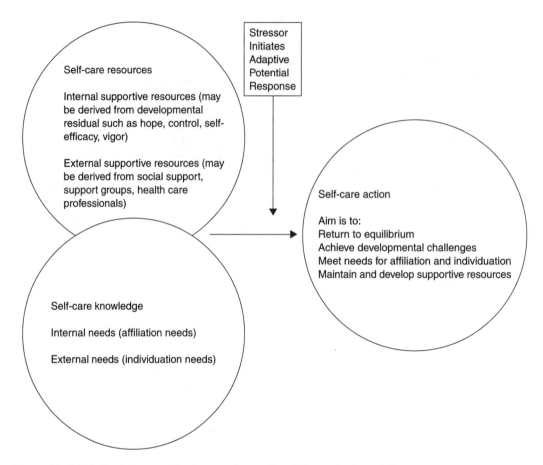

Figure 13–1 Relationship among the four constructs of modeling and role modeling.

cussed external supportive resource. Historical perspective on the development of social support research and the relationship of social support and health will be presented.[27–31] This will provide a foundation for understanding the current work in social support for persons with heart failure. The progression of social support definitions, research, and theory development will be traced by describing general literature reviews, seminal studies, and, finally, research specific to heart failure. Discussions of the quantity and quality of the social network and reciprocity will be presented. The recent studies that demonstrate the supportive role of health care professionals for persons with heart failure also will be discussed.

Overview of Social Support Research and Theory Development

Early social support investigations focused on the role of a spouse or significant other who could help the individual in many ways. It was assumed that the spouse provided the emotional and tangible support to assist the person with a health problem, to speed recovery, or to achieve better outcomes. Objective measures of social support were used instead of describing support from the perceptions of the individual with the health problem. Despite the fact that these investigations were not of perceived support, the unmarried or the socially isolated person with a health problem had higher mortality and morbidity.[3,27–31] This was found in persons with noncardiovascular problems, as well as those with coronary artery disease and myocardial infarction.[32,33] In the Tecumseh Community Health Study, the 9- to 12-year survival was increased in persons who had higher levels of social integration. The rates of death were 2.3 (men)–2.8 (women) times higher in the groups with less social integration.[34]

Although the results of these studies were impressive, neither the quantity nor the quality of the support obtained from the marital relationship was evaluated. Furthermore, the degree of social integration or isolation was not assessed. Thus, a person with a spouse but in a stressful, unwanted, or even abusive relationship would be seen as having social support. Likewise, an unmarried person with a large social network and a confidante to turn to might be seen as having no social support. Despite these problems with the measurement of social support, marriage, cohabitation, and social integration have been strongly associated with survival in samples of people with a variety of acute and chronic illnesses.

The next focus of social support research was on the size of the social network, as investigators assumed that a larger number of people in the network meant more social support.[27–30] Many instruments were developed to assess the social network.[28–30] Although some surveys included only the number of persons in the work, community, and family circles, others included evaluative information on the quality of these networks. Of interest, studies of the social network revealed conflicting results. Early researchers found positive outcomes associated with a larger social network; however, further investigation found that the ill person might feel indebted to the person providing support. This was described as the "dark side of social support."[35,36] The ability to provide some form of repayment to the supporter was important. Reciprocity could take many forms, such as doing some sort of task or favor for the supporter. The size of the repayment was not as important as the meaning behind it. This concept has been widely studied in persons with various chronic diseases.

The quality of social networks and support also has been examined. Measurement tools were developed to assess this dimension of social support.[28,30] As one might expect, the quality of the support added another layer of complexity to the understanding of social support but refined the construct further and added precision to measurement. By incorporating a personal appraisal of the quality of social support, researchers could begin to study support from the perspective of the individual. Oxman and Berkman proposed a model that expanded the understanding of the nature of the social network.[33–37] They advocated for evaluating both quality and quantity of the social network and described how these factors influenced the function of the type and amount of social support received. In this model, the social network was defined as patterns of ties that would link people together. Furthermore, this social network was characterized by its range, density, reachability, and homogeneity. The strength of the relationship, frequency of contact, multiple roles provided, duration of relationship, reciprocity of support, and degree of closeness could further describe each individual member of the network.

Social support is now conceptualized as a multifaceted construct. Stewart[27] provided a thorough review of the definitions of social support and found many commonalities, including measures of emotional support to share feelings and thoughts; tangible support to perform activities of daily living and tasks such as shopping, cleaning, or transportation; and information to understand the experience. Another common component of the definitions is the subjective appraisal of support. It is the individual's perspective of what is and what is not support that is important. Most of the definitions included a description of the social interaction that is foundational for social support. Of interest, one definition described how social support enhanced internal resources such as self-esteem and confidence.[35] Most definitions include an implicit or explicit relationship between social support and the ability to cope with the health problem.

In a review of 81 studies of social support and health outcomes, significant positive relationships were found in clinical descriptive or experimental studies, as well as laboratory simulations.[3] Across the studies, positive changes occurred in cardiovascular, neurologic, and immunologic markers. This review provided evidence for a strong link between social support and health outcomes. The strength of this meta-analysis is the consistency of findings across many different health problems, thus providing health care professions some support for generalizing results to the heart failure population.[3]

Several theoretical explanations are offered to describe the relationship between social support and health. Lazarus and Folkman see social support as one of a number of factors from the social environment that can facilitate coping and, thus, relieve stress.[38] However, preferred coping strategies employed by an individual will influence the amount and type of support sought and perceived as received. Heller et al. emphasized that social activity and social support enhanced self-esteem.[35] He described social support as providing stress-reducing personal aid. Festinger[39] proposed the social comparison theory that describes how people make constant comparisons of their positions to the positions of others who they perceive to have better or worse situations. These comparisons include perceived amount of social support, health status, illness severity, and coping stage.[39]

Three relationships between social support and health have been described. The first relationship explains that social support has a direct, main effect on health. An increase in social support will have a direct and proportional increase in health-related outcomes. A second approach is that social support buffers the individual from the harmful outcomes of the stressful event and, thus, promotes healthier outcomes. In this view, social support is protective. The final relationship described is the mediating model, in which social support acts as an intervening variable to reduce the effects of stress. Results from numerous investigators support each of these relationships. Whether one model is superior to the others is not known; however, the positive results found with the use of each model provide a foundation for viewing this relationship as situation-based.[27]

Social Support Research in Persons with Cardiovascular Disease and Heart Failure

Several authors published integrative reviews of social support in persons with cardiovascular disease that appeared approximately five to six years ago. Moser[40] reviewed the literature examining the complexity of social support, mechanisms of support and recovery, and suggested implications for practice. Meagher-Stewart[41] reviewed the literature by study design. This review included qualitative studies and quantitative studies that were descriptive, correlational, and experimental.[41] McCauley[42] reviewed the literature and applied the combined Oxman/Berkman and Jacobsen model of social support to the care of patients with cardiovascular disease. Yates, Skaggs, and Parker[43] discussed the status of theory and research related to optimal matching of support, appropriate timing, nature of the relationship, personality characteristics, coping assistance, and costs and conflicts of support. The final groups of authors included the role of the health care professional in their discussion of support.

In all of these reviews, most of the nursing research on social support pertained to persons with coronary artery disease undergoing medical management, percutaneous transluminal coronary angioplasty, or surgical revascularization. The analysis of overall results mirrored findings from general studies of social support in noncardiac populations. However, at the time of these reviews, little research had been conducted in persons with heart failure. As the decade progressed, so did the interest in studying persons with heart failure; thus, we find most of the studies of social support in heart failure published within the past 6 years.

In one of the early nursing studies, 50 persons with cardiomyopathy were recruited for a study of psychosocial adjustment, based on the Lazarus and Folkman model.[44] The mean age was 54 years, and the average duration of time since diagnosis was 2 months. Subjects were categorized into the better or poorer adjustment groups. Those with poorer adjustment had a higher number of other health problems, more symptoms, lower functional status, and greater changes in interpersonal relationships. These relationships were more strained and perceived to be suffering from the demands imposed by the diagnosis. Furthermore, there were significant differences in the frequency that assistance was required. This study provided insights into the strains on social relations and support systems that were associated with heart failure. Also, it confirmed the general opinion that heart failure places great demands on social structures and supported generalizing findings from other studies to patients with heart failure.

A group of investigators have reported the quality of life of persons with heart failure as they waited for and eventually recovered from a heart transplant. A sample of 359 subjects was recruited for this multicenter study.[45] Prior to transplant, subjects described that they were most satisfied with their health care, emotional support from others, their children, their family's health, relationship with spouse/partner, and faith in God. Subjects also reported the amount of emotional and tangible support needed. In this sample, neither form of support was among the 11 of 20 variables that entered the regression model to predict quality of life. The sheer volume of variables in the model and the possibility of strong correlations among the variables may be responsible for the failure of support to be a predictor of quality of life. However, many external and internal sources of support were included in the list of areas of life with which subjects were most satisfied.

In a sample of 64 men and 1 woman with heart failure, the effect of social support on hospitalization was examined.[46] At the end of 6 months, 23 subjects had been rehospitalized. There was no significant difference ($P = 0.69$) in scores on the MOS Social Support Survey between those who were hospitalized and those who were not hospitalized (mean scores 59.3 vs 57.2). However, two significant group differences were found. First, those who had been hospitalized

had a higher impact of emotional symptoms on quality of life. Second, those who had been hospitalized reported more cognitive symptoms, such as problems concentrating and remembering. Other areas in which the hospitalized group did not significantly differ from the nonhospitalized group were impact of physical symptoms, left ventricular ejection fraction, coping, and health perceptions.

Two groups of investigators specifically focused on social support in the elderly with heart failure.[47,48] In a recent retrospective, epidemiologic study of 292 patients with heart failure, persons who reported low levels of social support had higher rates of recurrent cardiac events and mortality 1 year after hospitalization for an exacerbation of heart failure symptoms.[47] Of interest, no significant relationship was found between social support and depression. An adjustment for clinical severity, comorbidity, functional status, social ties, and instrumental support was made in the sample. The absence of emotional support significantly increased the overall mortality (odds ratio = 3.2; 95% CI 1.4–7.8). When gender differences were examined, lack of emotional support was a stronger predictor of mortality for women (odds ratio = 8.2). The mean age of this sample was 80 years, and functional impairment was reported in 80% of the subjects.[47] This sample required a high degree of instrumental support or tangible assistance to enable them to live independently; however, it was the emotional support that was the significant predictor of mortality. Perhaps there are ways to provide emotional support through peer groups or pairing with another person if other friends and family are no longer present.

Elderly people with heart failure have a unique set of problems related to obtaining adequate supportive resources. One study described that one-third of the caregivers of elderly with heart failure had cardiovascular illnesses also.[48] Their own physical limitations imposed barriers to their ability to provide supportive care to the elderly person with heart failure.

Two additional studies focused on social support in elderly women. In a qualitative study of

57 women, interviews were done after hospital discharge and again 18 months later.[49] Emotional and tangible support sources were stable over that time period. Those who reported a loss of tangible support had a less positive affect during the interview. In another study, 80 older women were surveyed after hospitalization for an episode of heart failure.[50] Subjects who reported a higher level of emotional support had higher positive affect and satisfaction with life. However, it was a high degree of tangible support that was associated with less negative affect. Neither emotional nor tangible support was found to buffer the severity of symptom impact. Despite advanced age and severe chronic heart failure, these elderly women maintained quality of life with stable emotional and tangible support systems.

Support Groups

Support groups provide another example of an external resource. An individual may derive a number of benefits from meeting with others who have the same health problem. Group dynamics may provide opportunities for imparting information, sharing common experiences, providing a sense of belonging, learning from others, and perhaps teaching peers.[51] The group may fulfill an individual's need to feel attached and socially integrated. Support groups may exist as national organizations, such as Mended Hearts for cardiac surgical patients; community-based support groups that might be found with a cardiac rehabilitation program; or as computer chat rooms. Although support groups are generally assumed to have a positive effect, the literature in this area is scant.

A total of 134 Swedish elderly persons with coronary heart disease participated in 10 self-help heart groups located throughout the country.[52] Ten subjects volunteered to be interviewed as part of a qualitative study, describing the lived experience of participating in the group. Participants described social support as a genuine understanding of their troubles. The group provided a shared solidarity and fellowship that encouraged them to keep going. In summary, the group provided "a sharing of experience among confident equals, thanks to mutual feelings of caring and belonging, which in turn strengthens confidence."[52(p227)] This information is valuable to consider as more heart failure support groups are formed. Support groups can be organized to ensure adequate time for sharing and developing fellowship. Also, when studying the outcome of support groups, it is worthwhile to include both qualitative and quantitative data collection methods.

Information As a Supportive Resource

Information or knowledge about disease processes and self-care management strategies has been identified as a component of social support. The MOS Social Support Survey was specifically designed to include a scale that measured information, based on the investigators' review of the literature.[53] Using factor analysis of the instrument, the investigators found that the information and emotional items formed a single scale, but all items were retained. The other scales in the instrument are tangible support, affectionate support, and positive social interactions.

In a previously described study of 50 persons with cardiomyopathy, Lazarus and Folkman's theory was used as a framework.[44] Resources, defined as information about the disease process, were added to the interpersonal factors and found to be a significant predictor of psychosocial adjustment. Information provided by health care providers is essential for self-care management in the face of a chronic disorder such as heart failure.

To determine the information needs of patients with heart failure, 50 subjects and 47 cardiac nurses were surveyed.[54] The instrument listed 43 learning needs that were categorized into seven scales. The patients ranked the following scales in order of highest to lowest need: medications, risk factors, anatomy and physiology, psychologic factors, other topics, activity, and diet. In all categories, nurses ranked the relative importance slightly lower than did the patients. Nurses also ranked medications as the most important topic, and the remaining topics were ranked in the following order: diet, risk factors, activity, anatomy and physiology, other topics, and psychologic factors. It is striking that nurses saw psychologic factors as being of the lowest importance, whereas patients ranked that in the middle. This speaks to the need to ensure that the topic of psychosocial factors is covered in patient education.

A study of 179 persons with severe heart failure examined the effect of education and support provided by a nurse on self-care and resource.[55] Subjects who were hospitalized for treatment of an exacerbation of heart failure symptoms were randomized to the usual care or intervention group. The intervention consisted of an intense, systematic education program that started in the hospital and continued after discharge with home nursing visits. Although both groups had increased their self-care behaviors at 1 month after discharge from the hospital, the effect was significantly greater in the education group. Both groups experienced a decrease in self-care behaviors over the next 8 months, but this was significantly less in the intervention group. No difference in resource use was found.

Support Provided by Health Care Professionals

A final form of support is that provided by health care professionals. Conceptually, this form of support has been included in the development of many social support instruments. Any clinical health care program that broadly examines ways to improve patient care is probably examining new ways to provide and evaluate the supportive services of the professional health care team. For instance, the growing number of patients with heart failure and the associated demand for health care services led to the development of specialized centers for heart failure treatment, community-based heart failure clinics, and innovative programs for home care delivery of services to persons with heart failure.

In one of the early studies, 142 elderly patients with heart failure were randomized to either usual care or a comprehensive multidisciplinary inpatient teaching and postdischarge telephone follow-up intervention.[56] The nurse case managers provided the intervention that reduced the readmissions for heart failure by 56%. In another study, 42 elderly persons with heart failure undergoing an intensive home surveillance program significantly reduced hospitalizations and hospital days.[57] In a much larger sample ($n = 301$), similar results were found.[58] Likewise, results from a study with a 1-year follow-up were also strong.[59]

Outcomes of such programs have consistently reduced hospital readmission rates and cost of services while at the same time improving the functional status and other outcomes for those with heart failure.[5-8,55-59] Although the initial intent of these programs was to provide comprehensive and coordinated health care that reflected current standards of practice, the focus on case management and on patient-oriented nonpharmacologic interventions shaped these programs so that they became supportive resources for the person with heart failure.

One study of support provided by the health care team reported equivocal results in a sample of persons after myocardial infarction.[60] A total of 1,376 subjects were randomized to usual care or a program of supportive and educational home nursing intervention. At the end of a year, there was no difference in survival. The group differences in depression and anxiety were small and not significant. Subjects in this study had a mean age of 59 years and a left ventricular ejection fraction of .49. Mortality in the intervention group was 5.5% but only 3.9% in the control group. The lack of significant difference may have been related to the nearly normal cardiac function. Although many patients who have a myocardial infarction do develop heart failure, the subjects in this study may not have experienced the need for prolonged support that patients with more impaired cardiac function require. The studies that were conducted in persons with heart failure included subjects with greater cardiac dysfunction, and they may have had greater needs.

A growing body of evidence supports the development of specialized heart failure centers.[5,6] One strong advantage of these programs is improved pharmacologic management of the disease. In addition, these programs have improved patient outcomes while reducing costs of care. Furthermore, patient satisfaction and functional status are increased. Heart failure treatment programs usually include advanced practice nurses providing case management in concert with heart failure physicians. Social workers, pharmacists, dietitians, exercise physiologists, and financial counselors are usually included in the multidisciplinary team. Continued management by the same care providers enables the patient to know and trust the health care team. Disease management is coordinated. More importantly, the patient becomes empowered to be more involved in the plan of care as skills are acquired and supportive resources developed.

Currently, most of the care of persons with mild heart failure continues to take place under the management of primary care physicians, with referral to community-based cardiologists as needed. Those with more severe heart failure can benefit from referral to a specialized heart failure center for consultation and/or continued management. A recent innovation in care delivery is the nurse practitioner-managed community heart failure program that is operated as a satellite of the specialized heart failure center. This type of program may provide more patients who have heart failure with the supportive resources of the multidisciplinary health care providers who have the most expertise in individualizing their care to achieve mutual goals.

Summary of External Supportive Resources

Until recently, most knowledge of social support and other forms of external supportive resources were derived from studies of persons with other health problems. Although some investigators explored social support in persons after myocardial infarction or percutaneous coronary angioplasty, only a few actually examined social support in persons with heart failure. A growing body of knowledge related to the broader spectrum of external supportive resources has recently begun to emerge. The almost unanimous positive outcomes of the stud-

ies warrant continued research in this model of examining resources. Health care providers can and should continue to work with individuals to facilitate external supportive resources. Furthermore, systems and health care programs should be designed to encourage health care professionals to accept and develop the role of support provider for patients with heart failure.

SUPPORTIVE INTERNAL RESOURCES

An array of internal resources may help the person with heart failure to cope and adapt to the chronic illness. Hope, control, and self-efficacy are but a few of the factors that provide strength to all people. When faced with a diagnosis of heart failure, these positive affective traits can enhance resilience, well-being, and quality of life. Each will be discussed in more detail.

Hope

Hope is a positive expectation about the future. Hopeful thoughts can include desirable events related to relationships, daily occurrences, occupational goals, sporting events, and, more importantly, one's health status. Hope focuses on events or abstract goals deemed important by the person. Research over several decades has demonstrated that a loss of hope and depression is strongly associated with mortality in chronic illness.[61–64] Two forms of hope have been described. Generalized hope is more of a global outlook, whereas particularized hope is related to a very specific event in one's life. In a study of community-based elderly people, generalized hope was related to spirituality, frequency of family visits, number of support systems, and trust. Particularized hope was related to control.[65]

In 23 subjects with heart failure, hope was significantly related to morale ($r = .57$) and social function ($r = .50$) but not to physical function ($r = .15$).[66] This sample had a mean age of 66 years and was primarily comprised of men (66%). Most were married (61%) and lived with family (74%). The authors proposed that, although physical functioning was not associated with hope, there was an adaptive mechanism that allowed more hopeful subjects to adjust better to the physical limitations imposed by heart failure.

Depression is often described as a state of hopelessness. A sample of 542 consecutive patients over the age of 60 years admitted to an inpatient service was interviewed for depression.[67] Of these, 107 had a diagnosis of heart failure. Major depression was diagnosed in 36.5% of the heart failure patients, and 21.5% had minor depression. Those with either major or minor depression had more comorbid psychiatric disorders, more medical diagnoses, and more severe functional impairment. Most (60%) of those with depression and heart failure improved their mood state over the year following the intensive care admission, even though few received treatment with either antidepressants or psychotherapy. Perhaps the individuals with more developmental residual and stronger attachments were able to reduce depression through their own self-care management strategies that did not require traditional psychiatric intervention with either drugs or therapy.

Control

Control is also viewed as an internal resource. Several qualitative studies of recovery identified regaining control as an important process that was required to recoup physical and emotional health.[68,69] Control can be real or perceived. For instance, patients may not have real control over their pharmacologic health care regimens because the general guideline for medications and treatments essential to maintain cardiac function have been determined through rigorous investigation. Many patients accept the imposed pharmacologic regimen to achieve overall health goals. However, they may have perceived control over some aspects of when specific treatments or tests are done. Significant differences in recovery after acute myocardial infarction were found between those with high and low levels of perceived control. Those with high levels of perceived control had less anxiety, depression, and hostility 6 months after the event.[70] As previously described, autonomy was found to be

significantly correlated with global quality of life in persons with heart failure.[21] Examples of common nursing interventions designed to give clients more control in the management of their health are contracting, mutual goal setting, and provision of information.

Self-regulatory theory proposed by Johnson and Morse[69] explains how one gains control over a situation by developing a cognitive scheme that guides incoming information. The premise is that teaching patients factual information regarding health problems or treatment that also includes the sensory experience surrounding the event will increase the accuracy of the cognitive scheme. With cognitive and sensory information, the person has a wider scope of information that provides more control over the situation. Two decades of research supports this theoretical approach to patient education for a variety of health problems, including coronary artery disease and cardiac surgery.[70–74] Most of Johnson and Morse's work was in the area of gaining control in acute situations. However, there may be some applicability in a disorder such as heart failure that is characterized by exacerbations of symptoms that can lead to perceptions of loss of control for the patient.

Self-Efficacy

Another internal resource is self-efficacy, which is the belief that one has the knowledge and skill to perform some behavior.[75] In the context of persons with chronic illness such as heart failure, self-efficacy is related to specific activities needed to manage their lives in the face of an often-complex treatment regimen. As one develops self-efficacy, positive reinforcement further enhances perceived control and self-esteem. Self-efficacy has been studied and applied in the clinical management of persons with many forms of chronic illness, including cardiac disease.[20,76,77]

Forty-three persons with heart failure were recruited into a descriptive study to examine predictors of activity level in heart failure.[78] Subjects were primarily male (78%) with a mean age of 56 years. The number of people who were married or cohabitating ($n = 22$, 56%) was slightly higher than that of those who were unmarried and living alone ($n = 17$, 44%). Mean peak oxygen consumption was 17.7 mL/kg body weight/minute. Scores on walking and stair climbing self-efficacy measures were significantly related to peak oxygen consumption (.58 and .51, respectively). The authors suggested that self-efficacy scores could be used to assess fitness in persons with low activity levels, such as are found in heart failure.

Vigor

Vigor is an internal resource that has been associated with quality of life in persons with heart failure. In a pilot study of elderly patients with severe heart failure, vigor was identified as being related to quality of life and not related to severity of illness.[79] Despite severe cardiac dysfunction, those individuals with high levels of vigor had high perceived general health. In a subsequent study, 54 persons with severe heart failure completed surveys, and a subset was interviewed. Predictors of vigor included: general health perceptions, mental health, and energy expenditure in planned exercise.[80] Triangulation of the data supported the relationships found in the pilot study. Developing a sense of vigor may serve to be a valuable resource that facilitates adaptation to the physical limitations of heart failure.

Summary of Internal Resources

The range of potential internal resources that may facilitate recovery may not be fully recognized because this is a more recent area of study. Despite the lack of clear definition, the variables of hope, control, self-efficacy, and vigor have demonstrated a statistically and clinically significant role as facilitating supportive resources associated with recovery in persons with heart failure. These resources may be the result of positive developmental residual, as described in the MRM theory.

THE ROLE OF HEALTH CARE PROVIDERS IN ENHANCING SUPPORTIVE RESOURCES

The MRM theory can provide a framework for care of those with heart failure. This particular disorder has multiple etiologies and multiple human responses to the pathology. It would seem that an appropriate approach to the patient is to individualize care to truly meet patient needs.

Pharmacologic interventions in heart failure are aimed at blunting the neurohormonal responses that arise from the attempts to compensate for an inadequate cardiac output. Angiotensin-converting enzyme inhibitors and β-adrenergic blocking agents are the mainstay of current treatment of heart failure. Investigational drugs are targeting other neurologic or hormonal foci.[2,4] Interventions based on MRM provide a nonpharmacologic approach to achieve the same effect. Thus, the blend of pharmacologic and nonpharmacologic interventions may be particularly synergistic in promoting functional status, symptom management, and quality of life.

A client-focused approach to holistic care that is based on MRM begins with the assessment, or building a model of the client's world. This initial assessment should include more than the usual information obtained in the history and physical exam. The personal and social history should focus on the supportive resources needed and available. The resources assessed should include social support from family and friends, the scope of social network, importance and use of support groups, and support needed and obtained from health care providers. Next, focus on the internal resources that the person possesses. Ask the persons to share what they think are their particular strengths and how they typically manage stress. In addition, determine how they have participated in self-monitoring or self-management of health care. A person who actively seeks opportunities for self-monitoring or self-management is likely to have high levels of control, self-regulation, and self-efficacy. Valid and reliable tools used to measure these concepts in persons with heart failure may be useful for the clinician coordinating care of the patient with heart failure.[13,30,53,70,77,78,81]

Throughout the interview, focus on comments that relate to a future orientation, generalized hope, or particularized hope.[64,66] On the other hand, a person may express low levels of self-esteem, hopelessness, and powerlessness. Negative affectivity or a persistent level of depression is indicative of a lack of internal resources. As presented earlier, depression is underrecognized and undertreated in persons with heart failure.[67] These red flags should help the clinician to recognize that the person may not have the internal resources to mobilize adequately any external resources that are available, due to morbid grief or an attitude of "giving in and giving up."[62] Many patients may also benefit from antidepressants until they are able to return to their usual mood state.

Assessment of affiliation and individuation can be obtained by determining the external and internal resources available.[11,13] A review of the external resources that one perceives to be available reflects the ability to meet affiliation needs.[7,13] Individuation needs are derived from the internal resources, such as control and hope.[13,21] In addition to knowing what internal and external resources are available, it is important to see whether the needs for individuation and affiliation are somewhat balanced overall. However, during exacerbations of symptoms and worsening of the heart failure syndrome, it is anticipated that affiliation needs prevail. After the acute situation is resolved, individuation needs may be greater.

AIMS OF INTERVENTION

The theory of MRM prescribes five general aims of intervention.[10] These aims provide a framework for interventions that will enhance supportive resources, promote self-care, aid in facilitating affiliated-individuation, and promote adaptation to stress. The aims are not specific prescriptions of therapeutic interventions; instead, they provide broad categories that must be individualized to the specific needs of the individual.

The first aim of intervention is to build trust. Trust is derived from the first stage of development. Building trust is essential for the development of a good relationship between the patient and the health care provider. Maintaining open and honest communication between the patient and all health care providers is a cornerstone for developing trust. Other actions that can promote a trusting relationship are: maintaining confidentiality, providing consistent messages, and giving realistic information regarding condition. Trust also entails following through on all promises made by the health care team.

The second aim of intervention is to provide control. Encourage self-monitoring and self-management as the person expresses interest and demonstrates the ability to participate in self-care. When teaching, provide factual information with sensory preparatory information so that the client better understands what to expect. This empowers the person while reducing fears and concerns related to uncertainty.

The next aim of intervention is to promote a positive orientation. In the face of a chronic disorder such as heart failure, it can be difficult to see something positive in the situation. One way to maintain a positive orientation for the patient is to use the method reframing. This technique is built on seeing the positive side of a situation. For instance, the glass can be viewed as half full instead of half empty. Or the need for periods of rest may be necessary to conserve energy to do some other desired activity. A positive orientation promotes hope for the best possible future.

The fourth aim of intervention is to promote strengths. Applaud correct decisions regarding self-monitoring or self-management. This will increase self-esteem and self-efficacy. The entire multidisciplinary team can find ways to promote client strengths along the many dimensions of self-care.

The final aim of intervention is to set mutual goals. The most important aspect of this aim is to ensure that the goals are really mutual. If the client is asked to share long- and short-term goals, the health care team can see how treatment goals can be congruent with personal goals. This aim is based on a very individualized approach to treatment goals. In heart failure, there are many lifestyle changes that must be made. Setting goals that are realistic will help to facilitate goal achievement and to promote feelings of self-efficacy.

CONCLUSION

Heart failure management provides an ideal practice area to apply a theoretical and research-based approach to the care of patients. The commitment of the team to understanding and individualizing support for patients with heart failure is key to the success of any practice. The health care team can become a supportive resource for the patient who can depend on them for the provision of individualized care. In addition, the health care team helps the patient to recognize and mobilize other external and internal resources.

In summary, the multidisciplinary team approach to heart failure care improves outcomes in persons afflicted with the disease. Although the improved outcomes undoubtedly derive in part from improved pharmacologic treatment, enhanced process of care and nonpharmacologic management, which promote achievement of growth needs and developmental challenges by facilitating supportive internal and external resources, must also play a vital role. This latter observation underscores the need for team commitment to understanding and individualizing support for heart failure patients. It is important to recognize that the specific requirements for supportive resources vary from person to person. Thus, the inclusion of a broad range of specialties into the multidisciplinary team is essential to meet the supportive needs of clients.

REFERENCES

1. *2000 Heart and Stroke Statistical Update.* Dallas, TX: American Heart Association; 1999.

2. Packer M, Cohn JN. Consensus recommendations for the management of chronic heart failure. *Am J Cardiol.* 1999;83(2A):1A–38A.

3. Uchino BN, Cacioppo JT, Kiecolt-Glaser, JK. The relationship between social support and physiological processes: A review with emphasis on underlying mechanisms and implications for health. *Psychol Bull.* 1996;119:488–531.

4. Havranek EP, Mcgovern KM, Weinberger J, Brocato A, Lowes BD, Abraham WT. Patient preferences for heart failure treatment: Utilities are valid measures of health-related quality of life in heart failure. *J Cardiac Failure.* 1999;5(2):85–91.

5. Riegel B, Thomason T, Carlson B, et al. Implementation of a multidisciplinary disease management program for heart failure patients. *Congestive Heart Failure.* 1999;5:164–170.

6. Fonarow GC, Stevenson LW, Walden JA, et al. Impact of a comprehensive heart failure management program on hospital readmission and functional status of patients with advanced heart failure. *J Am Coll Cardiol.* 1997;30:725–732.

7. Baas LS, Fontana JA, Bhat G. Relationships between self care resources and the quality of life of persons with heart failure: A comparison of treatment groups. *Prog Cardiovasc Nurs.* 1997;12(1):25–38.

8. Baas LS, Fontana JA, Hess DA, Bhat G. The impact of physical and emotional symptoms on type of activity performed in heart failure. *J Cardiopulm Rehabil.* 1996;16:300.

9. Baas LS, Beery TA, Fontana JA, Wagoner LE. An exploratory study of development growth in adults with heart failure. *J Holistic Nurs.* 1999;17:117–138.

10. Erickson HC, Tomlin E, Swain MA. *Modeling and Role-Modeling: A Theory and Paradigm for Nursing.* Lexington, SC: Pine Press of Lexington; 1988.

11. Erickson HC. Self-care knowledge: An exploratory study. In: Erickson HC, Kinney C eds. *Modeling and Role-Modeling: Theory, Practice and Research.* Austin, TX: The Society for the Advancement of Modeling and Role-Modeling; 1990, 178–202.

12. Erickson HC, Swain MAP. Mobilizing self-care resources: A nursing intervention for hypertension. *Issues Ment Health Nurs,* 1990;11:217–235.

13. Baas LS, Curl ED, Hertz JE, Robinson KR. Innovative approaches to theory-based measurement: Modeling and role-modeling research. *ANS: Advances in Methods*

of Inquiry for Nursing. Gaithersburg, MD: Aspen Publishers; 1994:147–159.

14. Rowe MA. The impact of internal and external resources on functional outcomes in chronic illness. *Res Nurs Health*, 1996;19:485–497.

15. Landis BJ. Uncertainty, spiritual well-being, and psychosocial adjustment to chronic illness. *Issues Ment Health Nurs.* 1996;17(3):217–232.

16. Ellerhorst-RJ. Instruments to measure aspects of spirituality. In: Frank-Stromberg M, Olsen SJ, eds. *Instruments for Clinical Health-Care Research.* 2nd ed. Boston: Jones and Bartlett Publishers; 1997, 202–212.

17. Fowler, C. Religious and existential well-being in patients with heart failure who have and have not undergone cardiac transplantation. Master's Research Project, University of Cincinnati College of Nursing, 1999.

18. Liehr P, Smith MJ. Middle range theory: Spinning research to practice to create knowledge for the new millennium. *Adv Nurs Sci.* 1999;21(4):81–91.

19. Acton GJ, Miller EW. Affiliated-individuation in caregivers of adults with dementia. *Issues Ment Health Nurs.* 1996;17:245–260.

20. Hickey ML, Owen SV, Froman RD. Instrument development: Cardiac diet and exercise self-efficacy. *Nurs Res.* 1992;41:347–351.

21. Hoffman, R. *Relationship of global quality of life and health related quality of life and the perceived enactment of autonomy in persons with severe heart failure.* Thesis, University of Cincinnati College of Nursing and Health, 1997.

22. Maslow AH. *Toward a Psychology of Being.* New York: Van Nostrand Reinhold; 1968.

23. Erikson, E. *Identity, Youth and Crisis.* New York: WW Norton; 1968.

24. Selye H. *Stress without Distress.* Philadelphia: JB Lippincott Co.; 1974.

25. Barnfather JS, Ronis DL. Test of a model of psychosocial resources, stress, and health among undereducated adults. *Research in Nursing and Health.* 2000;23(1):55–66.

26. Frisch NC, Kelley J. *Healing Life's Crises: A Guide for Nurses.* Albany, NY: Delmar Publishers; 1996.

27. Stewart MJ. *Integrating Social Support in Nursing.* Newbury Park, CA: Sage Publications; 1993.

28. Norbeck, JS. Social support. *Annu Rev Nurs Res.* 1998;6:85–105.

29. Stewart MJ. Social support intervention studies: A review and prospectus of nursing contributions. *Int J Nurs Stud.* 1989;26(2):93–114.

30. Lindsey AM. Social support: Conceptualization and measurement instruments. In: Frank-Stromberg M, Olsen SJ, eds. *Instruments for Clinical Health Care Research.* 2nd ed. Boston: Jones and Bartlett Publishers; 1997, 149–176.

31. Bruhn JG, Phillips BU. Measuring social support: A synthesis of current approaches. *J Behav Med.* 1994;7(2):151.

32. Blazer DG. Social support and mortality in an elderly community population. *Am J Epidemiol.* 1982;115:684–689.

33. Berkman LF, Syme SL. Social networks, host resistance and mortality: A year follow-up study of Alameda County residents. *Am J Epidemiol.* 1979;109(2):186–204.

34. House JS, Robbins C, Metsner HL. The association of social relationships and activities with mortality: Prospective evidence from the Tecumseh Community Health Study. *Am J Epidemiol.* 1982;116:123–140.

35. Heller K, Swindle R, Dusenbury L. Component social processes: Comments and integration. *J Consulting Clin Psychol.* 1986;54:466–470.

36. Tilden VP, Galen RD. Costs and conflict: The darker side of social support. *West J Nurs Res.* 1987;9(1):9–18.

37. Oxman T, Berkman L. Assessment of social relationships in elderly patients. *Int J Psychiatry Med.* 1990;20:65–84.

38. Lazarus RS, Folkman S. *Stress, Appraisal, and Coping.* New York: Springer-Verlag Publishing Company, 1984.

39. Festinger L. A theory of social comparison. *Hum Relations.* 1954;1:117–140.

40. Moser D. Social support and cardiac recovery. *J Cardiovasc Nurs.* 1994;9(1):27–36.

41. Meagher-Stewart D. The role of social support in recovery from cardiovascular illness. *Can J Cardiovasc Nurs.* 1994;5(2):19–29.

42. McCauley KM. Assessing social support in patients with cardiac disease. *J Cardiovasc Nurs.* 1995;10(1):73–81.

43. Yates BC, Skaggs BG, Parker JD. Theoretical perspectives on the nature of social support in cardiovascular illness. *J Cardiovasc Nurs.* 1994;9:1–15.

44. Frost MH, Kelly AN, Mangan DB, Zarling KK. An analysis of factors influencing psychosocial adjustment to cardiomyopathy. *Cardiovasc Nurs.* 1994;30(1):1–7.

45. Grady KL, Jalowiec A, White-Williams C, et al. Predictors of quality of life in patients with advanced heart failure awaiting transplantation. *J Heart Lung Transplant.* 1995;14:2–10.

46. Bennett SJ, Pressler ML, Hays L, Firestine LS, Huster GA. Psychosocial variables and hospitalization in persons with chronic heart failure. *Prog Cardiovasc Nurs.* 1997;12(4):4–11.

47. Krumholz HM, Butler J, Miller J, et al. Prognostic importance of emotional support for elderly patients hospitalized with heart failure. *Circulation.* 1998;97:958–964.

48. Karmilovich SE. Burden and stress associated with spousal caregiving for individuals with heart failure. *Prog Cardiovasc Nurs.* 1994;9(1):33–38.

49. Friedman MM. Social support sources among older women with heart failure: Continuity versus loss over time. *Res Nurs Health*. 1997;20:319–327.

50. Friedman MM, King KB. The relationship of emotional and tangible support to psychological well-being among older women with heart failure. *Res Nurs Health*. 1994;17:433–440.

51. Kinney CK, Mannetter R, Carpenter MA. Support groups. In: Bulechek GM, McCloskey JC, eds. *Nursing Interventions: Essential Nursing Treatments*. 2nd ed. Philadelphia: WB Saunders Company; 1992, 326–339.

52. Hildingh C, Fridlund B, Segesten, K. Social support in self-help groups, as experienced by persons having coronary heart disease and their next of kin. *Int J Nurs Stud*. 1995;32:224–232.

53. Sherbourne CD, Stewart AL. The MOS social support survey. *Soc Sci Med*. 1991;32:705–714.

54. Frattini E, Linddsay P, Kerr E, Park YJ. Learning needs of congestive heart failure patients. *Prog Cardiovasc Nurs*. 1998;13(2):11–16,33.

55. Jaarsma T, Halfeens R, Abu-Saad JJ, et al. Effects of education and support on self-care and resource utilization in patients with heart failure. *Eur Heart J*. 1999;20:673–682.

56. Rich MW, Becham V, Wittenberg C, Leven CL, Freedland KE, Carney RM. A multidisciplinary intervention to prevent the readmission of elderly patients with congestive heart failure. *N Engl J Med*. 1995;333:1190–1195.

57. Kornowski R, Zeel D, Auerbach M, Kinkelstein A, Schwartz D, Moshkovitz M, Weinreb B, Hershkovitz R, Eyal D, MIller M, Levo Y, Pines A. Intensive home-care surveillance prevents hospitalization and improves mordibity among elderly patients with severe congestive heart failure. *Am Heart J*. 1995;129:762–766.

58. Roglieri J, Futterman R, McDonough K. Disease management intervention to improve outcomes in congestive heart failure. *Am J Managed Care*. 1997;3:1831–1839.

59. Hanmanthu S, Butler J, Chomsky D, Davis S, Wilson JR. Effect of a heart failure program on hospitalization frequency and exercise tolerance. *Circulation*. 1997;96:2842–2848.

60. Frasure-Smith N, Lesperance F, Prince RH, et al. Randomised trial of home-based psychosocial nursing intervention for patients recovering from myocardial infarction. *Lancet*. 1997;350:473–457.

61. Farran CJ, Herth KA, Popovich MJ. *Hope and Hopelessness: Critical Clinical Constructs*. Newbury Park, CA: Sage Publications; 1995.

62. Engel GL. A life setting conducive to illness: The giving-up given-in complex. *Ann Intern Med*. 1968;69:293–300.

63. Ruberman W, Weinblatt E, Goldberg J, Chardhary B. Psychosocial influences on mortality after myocardial infarction. *N Engl J Med*. 1984;311:552–559.

64. Curl ED. Hope in the elderly: Exploring the relationship between psychosocial developmental residual and hope. *Dissertation Abstracts Int*. 1992;53(4):1782.

65. O'Malley P, Menke E. Relationship of hope and stress after MI. *Heart Lung*. 1988;17:184–190.

66. Rideout E, Montemuro M. Hope, morale and adaptation in patients with chronic heart failure. *J Adv Nurs*. 1986;11:429–433.

67. Koening HG. Depression in hospitalized older patients with congestive heart failure. *Gen Hosp Psychiatry*. 1998;20:29–43.

68. Baker, C. A. Recovery: A phenomenon extending beyond discharge. *Schol Inq Nurs Pract Int J*. 1989;3:181–197.

69. Johnson JL, Morse JM. Regaining control: The process of adjustment after myocardial infarction. *Heart Lung*. 1990;19:126–135.

70. Moser DK, Dracup K. Psychosocial recovery from a cardiac event: The influence of perceived control. *Heart Lung*. 1995;24:273–280.

71. Johnson JE, Fuller SS, Endress MP, Rice VH. Altering patients' responses to surgery: An extension and replication. *Res Nurs Health*. 1978;1:111–121.

72. Suls J, Wan CK. Effects of sensory and procedural information on coping with stressful medical procedures and pain: A meta-analysis. *J Counseling Clin Psychol*. 1989;57:372–379.

73. Keeling AW. Health promotion in coronary care and step-down units: Focus on the family-linking research to practice. *Heart Lung*. 1988;17:28–34.

74. Moore SM. CABG discharge information: Addressing women's recovery. *Clin Nurs Res*. 1996;5:97–104.

75. Bandura A. Self-efficacy mechanism in human agency. *Am Psychol*. 1982;37:122–147.

76. Sotile WM. *Psychosocial interventions for cardiopulmonary patients*. Champaign IL: Human Kinetics. 1996.

77. Gortner S, Jenkins L. Self-efficacy and activity levels following cardiac surgery. *J Adv Nurs*. 1990;15:1132–1138.

78. Oka RK, DeMarco T, Haskell WL. Perceptions of physical fitness in patients with heart failure. *Prog Cardiovasc Nurs*. 1999;14(3):97–102.

79. Fontana JA. A consideration of vigor as an outcome measure of exercise therapy in chronic illness. *Rehabil Nurs Res*. 1995;4(3):75–81.

80. Fontana JA. The emergence of the person-environment interaction in a descriptive study of vigor in heart failure. *Adv Nurs Sci*. 1996;18(4):75–82.

81. Reigel B, Glaser D, Thomas V, Gocka I, Gillespie TA. Development of an instrument to measure cardiac illness dependency. *Heart Lung*. 1997;26:448–457.

CHAPTER 14

Transitioning Heart Failure Care to the Family

Peggy M. O'Connor

INTRODUCTION

The care of heart failure patients takes place in many settings (eg, the outpatient clinic, the physician's office, the acute care hospital) with the contributions of many health professionals (eg, nurses, social workers, physicians, dietitians, exercise physiologists). Emphasis has been placed on the optimum management of these patients by this interdisciplinary team in these settings. However, the actual "management" of these patients takes place on a daily basis within the four walls of their homes by themselves and their families. It is in the home setting that heart failure must be successfully managed. To accomplish this, our care, knowledge, and skill must be transitioned to patients and their families.

This chapter will examine the role of family in heart failure management. It will explore both the impact of the family on management of the illness and the impact of the illness on the family, specifically the caregiver. The needs of the caregiver will be discussed with interventions for health professionals to support and empower the caregiver. The home care needs of heart failure patients will be addressed along with opportunities to intervene in the home setting.

FAMILY THEORY

Most clinicians would agree that families play a role in the health and illness of individuals. However, the importance of this role, especially in the management of chronic illness, has not been taken seriously enough. Family theory and research can shed some light on the basis of this importance.

Early on, sociologists studied the role of the family in society. Later, theorists in family sociology and psychology became interested in the interaction of family and illness. Initial focus of this research looked at the impact of illness on the family and encouraged health professionals to broaden their care from individuals to families. More recently, as attention has been drawn to improving outcomes of chronic illness, there has been much interest in the impact of the family on illness.

Research on the family and illness has been described as "atheoretical."[1] It has shown the presence of a relationship between the family and illness but has not explained the covariation between variables well or tied the assumptions or findings to a theory. However, examination of one model and some related research may be helpful in understanding some basic concepts about families and illness.

The cognitive-behavioral transactional model of family functioning[2-4] pulls together constructs of many family theories and places them within a cognitive-behavioral framework. It draws on the family adjustment/adaptation model,[5] the family paradigm model,[6] and modern models of stress and coping. The model provides a "framework for examining the role of the family in influencing the ongoing adaptation and adjustment of the chronically-ill individual."[3(p120)] It views the family and its members "as active processors of information" who seek out information or sources of stress, evaluate resources available, act on the environment, and evaluate the effectiveness of the response.[2] The appraisal-coping process is an important aspect of this model. The family members appraise the stress (ie, illness) and also appraise their resources (ie, coping ability) to respond to the stress. The family's appraisal of their own resources will have an impact on their confidence in their ability to respond, which will influence the successfulness of the response in managing the stress. How the family then evaluates the success of the response determines whether the response will be reinforced or discontinued. The transactional nature of this model suggests that the family response to the perceived stress (ie, illness) and the evaluation of the level of success of the response will form the experience of the stress. For example, if the family perceives they have coped effectively with a stress, the stress will be less threatening in the future, and they will feel more confident and deal more successfully with the stress.

Kerns applies this model to families experiencing chronic illness by looking at four domains of chronic illness.[2] His approach is interesting because it provides a framework for how family has an impact on chronic illness. He suggests that the family can actually determine the course of the chronic illness in regard to (1) the disease process itself, (2) symptomology, (3) the amount of disability, and (4) the affective response or distress of the affected individual (see Figure 14–1). Research on this model has been limited primarily to patients with chronic pain, but some research on other chronically ill populations supports the model.[7–10]

The main way a family influences the disease process itself is by its ability to help the patient adhere to the prescribed medical regimen. The importance of patient compliance is widely recognized by clinicians, but surprisingly, the family has not been a central component in compliance models or compliance research,[11] although some investigators have described the role of the family in compliance. A small study of 23 chronic hemodialysis patients found a significant relationship between healthy family func-

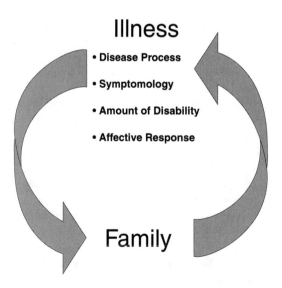

Figure 14–1 Graphic depiction of Kerns'[2] model of families experiencing chronic illness.

tioning behaviors and overall compliance with care.[7] An exploratory study of 95 non-insulin-dependent diabetic patients found that one factor that contributed to successful adherence to medical regimens was the capacity to use family support.[8] A few experimental studies have included family in interventions aimed at improving patient compliance with prescribed medical regimens. In a longitudinal study of 400 hypertensive patients, adult family members in the home were instructed in hypertension management and ways to help the patient follow the treatment plan. This specific intervention (one of many) resulted in increased patient compliance with medication and was effective in increasing the percentage of patients who maintained blood pressure control.[9] A follow-up study at 5 years found that the family intervention demonstrated a positive impact on appointment-keeping behavior and medication compliance.[10] Blood pressure control was found to be the result of a combination of interventions, with involvement of the family members in the patient's care having a greater effect on the outcomes than the other interventions. Although these results are encouraging, research is not consistent on the value of family involvement in programs of treatment compliance. Some studies have found no differences in compliance outcomes between groups with and without family involvement, and more research is needed to clarify this hypothesis.[11] The potential benefit, however, is clear enough to warrant incorporation of family in interventions of illness management.

Also of great interest is the assumption that the family's response to the symptoms of a disease may determine the frequency, severity, and impact of the symptoms and the resulting level of disability. Kerns[2] suggests that individuals may be more likely to take on the "sick role" when the response they get from those around them (family) is solicitous or overprotective. Family patterns that overprotect the ill person and reduce his or her roles in the family and the outside world could lead to progressive declines in activity.

There is evidence of this phenomenon with patients with chronic pain.[12–14] This chronic pain research has demonstrated a positive relationship between spouse behaviors and pain symptoms. One study used direct observation to examine the relationship between patient pain behaviors and spouse responses[14] and found significant relationships between spouse solicitous behavior and patient pain behavior. This suggests that solicitous behavior may be a reinforcer of chronic pain behavior. Another study of 106 married chronic pain patients found similar results.[13] A significant proportion of variance in pain severity was accounted for by pain-contingent attention from the spouse. This was particularly significant in the context of satisfying marital relationships. It is not known, however, whether these results can be applied to other illnesses. Many believe that overprotectiveness may lead to increased disability in cardiac patients, but a study on postmyocardial infarction (MI) patients found the opposite.[15] Patients who considered themselves "overprotected" (defined by a patient's perception of receiving more social support from family and friends than desired) were less likely to be emotionally reliant on others 4 months after MI than those with inadequate support. This study also suggested that the timing of support may be important. The ability to return to work after acute MI was facilitated by overprotectiveness within the first month of illness, but by decreasing levels of support afterward.[15] It may be that symptoms and disability are impacted positively by high levels of support in initial illness, but in chronic illness overly supportive family behaviors may be detrimental.

The family context also affects a person's affective state or the level of depression or anxiety they experience related to their illness. Lower levels of depression are found in chronic pain patients when their spouses were viewed as supportive.[13,16] This was also true for the post-MI sample[15] referred to earlier. Overprotected patients experienced less anxiety, depression, anger, and confusion and higher self-esteem 1 month after acute MI. Because one's affective state can have such an impact on illness management and quality of life, the role of the family in this regard demands attention.

In summary, the cognitive-behavioral transactional model of family functioning suggests that families are not only impacted by the illness of a family member, but they also play a role in determining the course of illness, symptoms, disability, and distress of the affected member. Therefore, health care professionals working to promote healthy adaptation and optimum management of heart failure patients need to include the family in their care and consider the role families play in the manifestation and course of the illness. At the same time, it is important to address the needs of the families and caregivers.

CARING FOR THE CAREGIVER

Heart failure is a debilitating illness. The symptoms of weakness, fatigue, and shortness of breath result in an inability to perform normal activities. As the course of illness progresses, many persons with heart failure are no longer able to live independently and must rely on others for assistance.[17,18] This assistance may include help with activities of daily living (ADLs) such as dressing, bathing, mobility, and meal preparation; with instrumental activities such as shopping, transportation, finances, and housework; and with disease management activities such as medication management, weighing, and monitoring and reporting of symptoms. For many heart failure patients, this assistance is provided by family members.[19] Frail elders who need caregiving assistance usually rely first on a spouse, then on children and other family members, and finally on outside sources.[20] Outside sources can include friends, neighbors, or paid help. Caring for somebody with a chronic, progressive disease is not without its difficulties. A study on the spouse caregivers of heart failure patients found that the experience was both burdensome and stressful.[21] If we are to optimize the care of these patients, an awareness of the caregivers' needs is imperative.

Heart Failure Caregivers

When looking at the population of heart failure patients and their caregivers, they are as diverse as any other group. The age range is broad, and the ethnic, social, and economic backgrounds are likewise varied. However, one characteristic that is increasingly defining of this population is that it is getting older. Most persons with heart failure are more than 70 years old. Many, therefore, have other medical problems in addition to heart failure and as a cohort are frailer than ever. Their spouses, if living, are also old and often ill themselves. Some patients with severe heart failure are actually the "healthier" spouse and are providing care for another in the home.[18] So, caregiver issues among the heart failure population are often very complex and challenging. The impact of caregiving on the caregiver and their needs for support will vary on the basis of many factors.

Effects of Caregiving

Awareness has increased in the past couple of decades about the significant roles that families play in providing care for individuals in need. Research studies on the nature and the effects of family caregiving have flourished in recent years. This abundance of literature on caregiving testifies to its importance to health care professionals and to the impact it is having on patients, families, and communities. Family caregiving has been identified as the "silent arm of the current healthcare delivery system."[22] An impaired elder's ability to remain in the community and not be institutionalized is determined more by characteristics of the caregiver than by any other factor.[23,24] The financial impact of preventing institutionalization, in addition to the obvious benefits to the patient and family, is significant. It has been estimated that caregivers of the frail elderly save the federal government from $9 billion to $17 billion each year.[25] Some, however, challenge the assumption that family caregiving is "free."

> The tremendous amount of time and work that goes into caregiving is neither publicly nor economically valued. It is not counted in the calculations of the national economy, but is considered a labor of love and duty. Home caregiving is less costly than

institutional care only because it is assigned no monetary value.[22(p472)]

Despite the strain on caregivers, keeping the elderly living in their own homes in the community does have positive social and psychologic effects on elders and their families, encouraging them to be as independent as possible despite their disabilities.[26] According to the framework described earlier by Kerns,[2] a supportive family can influence the chronic disease process by helping chronically ill patients adhere to treatment regimens and can reduce levels of depression and anxiety in chronically ill individuals. Therefore, in the heart failure population, adequate family care and support should improve outcomes and decrease hospitalizations. If the strain of caregiving renders family members ill or unable to continue their care, patients' health and well-being will be affected. All health care professionals, therefore, have a vested interest in supporting family caregiving and promoting the health and independence of patients and their caregivers. Research on caregivers of heart failure patients in particular is sparse, but much can be learned from studies of caregivers of different populations.

The negative effects of caregiving are well documented. Extreme stress, strain, and burden among family caregivers is common.[21,24,27–32] Caregiver burden is the common variable of interest in the caregiving literature and has been explored as a multidimensional construct that includes time dependence, developmental, physical, social, and emotional burden.[28] Time dependence burden comes from the time demands that caregiving activities place on a caregiver. This time burden affects the other levels of burden experienced.

Developmental burden is the feeling of not being developmentally on time with respect to peers or where one would like to be. Spouse caregivers experience more developmental burden because their expectations for this time in their lives are changed as a result of the illness.[28] Adult children experience less developmental burden, but many feel that their own lives are "on-hold" while caring for an ill parent.[22]

Physical burden is well documented because caregiving has been found to take a significant toll on one's health.[33] There is a tendency for caregivers to ignore their own health needs and concentrate on the care recipient only.[34] One-third of admissions to a respite program were directly related to the health of the caregiver.[34] Caregivers in poor health also seem to experience more burden[35–40] and depression.[28,41,42]

Socially, caregivers experience decreased social and recreational involvement and financial difficulties. Caregivers sometimes have to quit work and lose their social network of friends and activities. Caregiving also can affect family dynamics by changing the balance of power in a family or marriage.[43] Role changes occur that cause internal conflict for many. A qualitative study on caregivers for the elderly found that the acknowledgment of a change in the relationship between the caregiver and care recipient was the turning point in the caregiver facing a new reality.[44] Marriage relationships can lose their reciprocity when one spouse is caring for another. Spouse caregivers may have to give up the vision of their ideal future together and realize that their relationship and plans have been altered.[44] Adult children have to relinquish their view of their parent as the protector and nurturer when they themselves must take on these roles.

Emotional burden is probably the most cited effect of caregiving. Emotional responses include anger, insecurity, loneliness, loss, isolation, resentment, depression, and bitterness.[43] Isolation and loneliness stem from less time for social contacts and few people who truly understand the caregiver's struggles. If the caregiver is caring for a spouse with cognitive impairments, this isolation and loneliness is substantial because they have lost their primary friend and confidant. Anger and resentment are common because the caregiver feels overwhelmed by the increased responsibilities and their own unmet personal needs. Depression scores have been reported as much as two to three times greater in caregivers than in noncaregivers.[45]

Negative consequences, however, are not the only outcomes that have emerged from caregiver research. Potential benefits of caregiving have been noted by many.[31,46] A qualitative study on caring for elderly relatives identified the paradoxical experiences of caregivers.[44] These caregivers expressed feelings of great personal loss as they confronted the reality of a change in the relationship between themselves and the sick elder. But, they also struggled to find meaning in the experience that resulted in a positive redefinition of self, feelings of self-worth, and an awareness to care for their own needs. Other research also supports the notion that caregiving can be appraised as stressful and beneficial at the same time.[38]

The consequences of the negative impact of caregiving include institutionalization of the ill person, role changes, psychiatric and physical morbidity of the caregiver, and less than adequate care or neglect of the care recipient. Although predictors of institutionalization are not clear, some evidence exists demonstrating that caregivers' increased feelings of burden precede nursing home placement.[24] Diminishing these negative effects and promoting the positive ones are necessary to optimize the quality of life of the heart failure patient and his or her family or caregiver. Recent research has been focused on what factors mitigate the negative effects of caregiving and lead to more effective coping.

Mitigating the Negative Effects of Caregiving

Two factors emerge repeatedly from the literature as lessening the negative effects of caregiving: (1) social support and (2) internal resources or hardiness. Social support has been found to have a buffering effect on the stress process.[47–49] This "social support hypothesis" suggests that people manage better when faced with stressful life conditions if they have social support. Applied to the transactional model of family functioning,[2] social support is a resource that the family considers when appraising their ability to respond successfully to the illness or stress. Some research on the stress of caregiving supports this hypothesis.[30,41,50,51] An inverse relationship has been found between a large informal helping network and burden.[52] Another

study found that when the caregiving responsibilities are shared among family members, the strain or burden is less.[50] The caregiver's "satisfaction" with the social support, rather than the actual presence or amount of support, seems to be the key to decreasing caregiver burden.[30,41] There is also some evidence that the neediest caregivers may receive the least tangible assistance, which suggests that something besides need stimulates social support from family and friends.[53]

Other research has identified internal resources of caregivers and families that may enhance family well-being and mitigate some negative effects of caregiving.[50] These internal resources may be defined as problem-solving ability, a sense of mastery, and the perception that changes can be managed.[50] This concept has also been labeled "hardiness" and is defined as a multidimensional attribute comprising challenge, commitment, and control.[54] It is speculated that persons with high levels of hardiness may be able to handle the stresses of caregiving better than persons with lower levels of hardiness. In the transactional model of family functioning,[2] hardiness would be considered a resource (similar to social support, although it is internal) that a family would appraise as helping them respond successfully to the stress of illness. A study of caregivers of cancer patients found that those with high family hardiness were less likely to appraise their situation negatively and more likely to perceive caregiving as challenging and beneficial.[36] Another study found that caregivers who are committed to and challenged by the caregiving situation (ie, those with hardiness) have enhanced energy, greater ego strength, and more positive feelings about their own self-care.[55] Perceived "control" over their own lives helped mitigate the negative emotions of caregiving and increased life satisfaction of wives of spinal cord–injured patients.[56] A study on caregivers of the frail elderly found that internal resourcefulness (defined as the skills to deal with negative internal experiences) significantly predicted changes in dysphoric affect over time.[57] Individuals with a greater belief in their own resourcefulness showed decreased negative affect over time. Both social support and internal resources were found to buffer the relationship between caregiver strains and well-being in another study of caregivers of the frail elderly.[50]

Although it is evident that caregivers of heart failure patients are at risk of having negative effects from the caregiving experience, social support and hardiness appear to mitigate the negative effects. These factors should be kept in mind when planning interventions to support caregivers.

Interventions To Support Caregivers

Given the varied responses to caregiving, what can health care providers do to support caregivers and promote the best responses to caregiving? Awareness and recognition is the first step. Health care professionals should assess the caregiver's coping and level of burden with each interaction and intervene as necessary. Unfortunately, even though there is an abundance of research describing caregiver burden and its correlates, little is documented about the effectiveness of interventions aimed at decreasing caregiver burden. From the research just cited, we can infer that interventions aimed at increasing caregivers' perceptions of social support and increasing their internal resources should decrease burden.

Key aspects of social support for caregivers of heart failure patients are emotional and tangible support. Caregivers undoubtedly need both types of support to deal with the effects of this illness. One study found that the support network for older adults did not expand in response to deteriorating health, but rather their present support network expanded their scope of assistance.[58] This indicates that older adults may have difficulty recruiting new support services and that as their needs increase, their present support system may get overwhelmed. Caregivers need to be encouraged to mobilize both informal and formal support for themselves. Many people feel a sense of pride over their independence and have difficulty asking for assistance from friends or other family members. A health professional is in a good position to counsel caregivers about the need to ask for help, talk through their hesitancies, and assist them in identifying people who might be interested in helping. In addition to family, friends, and neighbors, have them examine the organizations in which the patient has been involved where volunteers may be available (eg, churches, service organizations, social groups). As patient needs increase, informal assistance by family, friends, and volunteers may need to be supplemented with more formal assistance.[19] Skilled home health care and custodial/homemaker care are often needed and usually warranted for elderly patients and caregivers. Hospice care is a very supportive service that is often overlooked but very appropriate for end-stage heart failure patients who prefer to be managed at home. Respite care, or time away from caregiving, can also be very helpful and may include getting 24-hour care in the home or short-term placement in a nursing facility. Table 14–1 lists some resources for heart failure patients and their caregivers.

Health care workers themselves can be a form of support for caregivers. Visiting nurses have been cited by caregivers as being successful in providing needed counseling and supportive listening.[43] Simply validating caregivers' feelings and paying attention to the needs of the caregiver separately from the patient's needs can be effective in decreasing their stress and increasing their sense of support.[43] Although intensive and focused interventions for patients and families have shown more promise than general support groups,[43] caregiver support groups have proven helpful.[22] One of the most valuable aspects of one caregiver support program was reported as an opportunity for socializing with people with similar problems.[22] Caregivers reported they felt support and camaraderie with people who "were in the same boat" that was missing from their contacts with friends and family who were not in caregiving roles. Caregivers in the support group also learned to take care of their own needs without feeling guilty.

Interventions should also be aimed at increasing caregivers' internal resources or hardiness. The at-

Table 14–1 Patient and Caregiver Resources

Resource	Services Provided	Reimbursement Source	Eligibility
Skilled home health care	Home visits by RN, social workers, physical therapy, and home health aide, to assess and monitor medical and social needs and intervene. Care is short-term.	Medicare, Medicare HMOs, Medicaid, almost all insurances	MD ordered and medically necessary. Patient must be "homebound."
Hospice	Same as skilled home health care but focus is on palliative care and symptom management. Care is long-term.	Medicare, Medicare HMOs, Medicaid, most insurances	Prognosis < 6 mo; NYHA Class IV.
Custodial home care	Assist with ADLs, home-making, companionship, etc.	Usually private pay. Long-term care insurance. Some communities may have special grants/funding to provide.	No specific requirements.
Respite care	Relief for a family caregiver in the home, or short-term stay in nursing facility.	Usually private pay. Some insurances. Hospice programs. Some communities may have special grants/funding to provide.	Family caregiver has been providing care for patient.
Adult day care	Community day care for adults.	Usually private pay. Some communities may have special grants/funding to provide.	Varies.
Home-delivered meals	Delivery of meals to home, usually 1–2 meals/day, 5–7 days/wk.	Usually private pay but cost is minimal. Some communities may have special grants/funding to provide.	Varies. Usually need to be > 65 years or disabled.
Area Agency on Aging	Referral source for senior and caregiver resources.	No cost, federal/state funded.	Information available to public, no requirements.

tribute of hardiness is not a personality trait but rather a quality that can be learned. Control seems to be a recurrent theme of hardiness. Being in control and feeling like they can master their environments seems to empower caregivers and improve their ability to engage in self-care.[55] Information and counseling should be aimed at increasing this sense of control. Giving caregivers choices in treatment options and giving them more responsibility for monitoring symptoms and adjusting care accordingly is important in increasing their control and sense of mastery. This can be accomplished by giving the heart failure caregiver the responsibility for adjusting diuretic doses according to weight and symptoms. Recognition from the health care team of the good job that the caregiver is doing reinforces these feelings of mastery and enhances self-worth. Counseling should include assisting the caregiver to identify family strengths, their own internal strengths, coping techniques, problem-solving ability, and commitment.

Caregivers also need honest and accurate information from health care providers about disease process, treatment, and prognosis. Heart failure patients and their caregivers need to understand the illness trajectory for heart failure. They need to be given clear expectations and anticipatory guidance. For instance, caregivers need to understand that fatigue is a very real symptom of heart failure and that a patient's inability to contribute to his or her own care has a physical basis and is not laziness. The eventual decline of heart failure patients needs to be explained so caregivers can have realistic expectations and make plans for more assistance in the future. The more information caregivers are armed with regarding disease management and illness progression, the more in control and competent they will feel as caregivers.

Home Management of Heart Failure

For the most part, persons with heart failure reside in their own homes. A study of 1,176 persons discharged from an acute care hospital with a primary diagnosis of congestive heart failure (CHF) found that 79% of them returned to home.[59] It is imperative then that efforts to optimally manage these patients reach the place where it really matters...the home.

The home care needs of this population are enormous. As outlined in previous chapters, heart failure is pernicious in its nature, complex in its treatment, and characterized by episodic exacerbations and progressive decline. This makes management very challenging for clinicians, patients, and their families. High hospital readmission rates are well documented and are probably related to the characteristics of the disease, as well as to problems with inadequate home care and issues of noncompliance. Some have estimated that up to 50% of hospital readmissions of the chronically ill elderly population can be attributed to lack of adequate support services at home.[60] Even though pharmaceutical management is pivotal in control of heart failure, medication compliance is poor.[61] Studies show that the average number of medications a heart failure patient takes daily is anywhere between 7 and 8.6.[17,61] A medication compliance evaluation for 7,247 elderly CHF patients found that only 10% of the patients filled enough of their CHF medication prescriptions to have the correct amount for a year.[61] The average patient had enough drug for only two thirds of a year. Diet compliance is more difficult to study but is probably as significant a problem.

With the increased age of the heart failure population, patients have more comorbidities and are frailer. One study of CHF patients using home health services found that they had an average of almost three additional diagnoses in addition to CHF, and their functional status was quite poor.[17] The major functional limitations were in endurance (95%), dyspnea (87%), and ambulation (67%). Seventy percent of this small sample ($n = 40$) used safety or rehabilitation equipment, and most needed assistance with medication management, bathing, and dressing. Of concern is the fact that the availability of caregivers decreased with the increasing age of the patient in this sample. This suggests that those patients who are most needful may be lacking in support.

Studies looking at the status of heart failure patients after recent hospitalization are not any more encouraging. One study found that for 40% of CHF patients discharged home from the hospital, one or more components of the discharge plan were not implemented as planned, and negative consequences usually resulted.[60] A qualitative study found that 2 weeks after hospital discharge for CHF, patients described their home situation as "tentative" and characterized by ups and downs associated with managing the illness, caregiver issues, and quality of life challenges.[18] Even though these patients had received instruction during their hospitalization, they were not certain how to incorporate these principles into their home environments. Medications were one of the primary causes of uncertainty for this group, and they expressed a desire for more information about their medications. Patients who have difficulty with self-medication administration have been found to have higher hospital readmission rates.[62]

It appears that education that takes place in the hospital setting is frequently ineffective, because patients are too ill and their stays are too short to adequately learn.[63] The learning needs, however, are unmistakable. A study of 41 patients hospitalized with CHF found that 97% could not define CHF correctly, and almost 60% could not identify all their medications.[64] Seventy-five percent weighed themselves less than weekly. Once home, many patients report difficulty getting to groups or clinics for teaching because of fatigue, mobility, or transportation problems.[63] As new approaches in managing this population are developing, the use of home assessment and visiting should be seriously considered.

There is something powerful about visiting a patient's home that makes any other setting seem so much less effective in really assessing what is going on with a patient and family.

> The home is where a family's values are expressed. It is in the home that people can be themselves. The history of the family—its story, its joys and sorrows, its memories and aspirations—are there on the walls. What one can learn in the home is often of real practical value. For this reason assessment in the home is different from assessment in the office or the hospital. Instead of asking about activities of daily living, we see patients in their own bedroom, bathroom, and kitchen, climbing their own stairs, and so on. When we review the medications, we can assemble them all—including those from the bathroom cabinet, by the bedside or on the kitchen table. We can sense for ourselves either the peace or tension in the home. We can meet with the family on their own ground, where they are most likely to express their feelings. In the home the patient can be in control of his or her own care, and this can be a powerful influence on healing.[65(p430)]

Home assessment of a heart failure patient can be very valuable. The living environment can be assessed for cleanliness, organization, and air quality. A safe home environment is important in preventing falls and injuries for this population. A fall resulting in a fracture could be life threatening for a heart failure patient. On a home visit, safety hazards can be identified and recommendations made to make the home safer. A home visit also gives the health care provider insight into the amount of social support and financial resources available. Patients and families sometimes present their home situations as more supportive than they actually are.[60] A visit can help assess how much assistance the patient actually receives and the adequacy of this assistance. The dynamics of the family can be observed firsthand for patterns that lead to adaptation or maladaptation. The stress on the caregiver and needs for support are usually much more apparent on a visit to the home.

Most importantly for this population, a home visit gives the professional insight into the patient and family's ability to self-manage their heart failure. The refrigerator and cupboards can be assessed for diet understanding and compliance. The organization and knowledge of medications can be evaluated. The presence of a scale and the patient's ability to stand on it and visualize the weight can be assessed.

Interventions in the home setting are also likely to be more effective than in other settings.[66] In the home setting, patients are usually less acutely ill and are less anxious than they are in a hospital or other setting.[67] Teaching about diet and medications is bound to be more effective in the patient's own kitchen and with his or her own prescriptions in front of him or her. Barriers to noncompliance can be identified and solved together. Practical strategies to conserve energy and increase independence can be suggested to patients and caregivers.[66] Emotional and psychologic support to both patients and families can also be provided on a more personal level in the home setting.

In efforts to decrease hospitalizations and improve quality of life and functional status at home, intensive interventions are becoming more common in the home setting. These interventions include administration of both intravenous diuretics and positive inotropic agents. Intravenous diuretics can be given safely and can prevent the need for hospitalization because symptoms of fluid overload can be treated promptly at home.[68] The use of positive inotropic therapy (dobutamine and milrinone) in the home is more controversial. Some studies have suggested the benefits of this therapy for some patients.[69,70] The use of dobutamine and milrinone for at least 4 consecutive weeks was found to improve functional status and decrease hospital readmissions, length of stay, and cost of care for a small sample of patients with advanced heart failure.[69] However, problems with tachyphylaxis and increased morbidity and mortality rates have been documented and have prevented extensive use in the home setting. One study suggests that intermittent, rather than continuous, administration of inotropes may result in less deleterious effects and more satisfactory outcomes.[70] However, because of the concerns about toxicity and the lack of evidence supporting the efficacy of positive inotropic therapy, it is currently not recommended in the treatment of heart failure in the home setting.[71] If any intensive interventions such as intravenous diuretics or inotropes are considered for home use, it is imperative that patients have supportive and competent caregivers and proper professional support in the home.

Home health care has traditionally been the avenue of providing home care to heart failure patients and has been effective in managing this population.[59,72,73] A study of 1,176 patients discharged from a hospital with a primary diagnosis of CHF found that those receiving home health services (26% of the sample) were readmitted with CHF significantly less often within 90 days than those not receiving home health care.[59] This relationship was not significant at 14 days, indi-

cating that early readmissions may be related to factors such as premature discharge that home care cannot impact. At another institution, cross-training hospital nurses to provide "intensive home management" for heart failure patients was effective in reducing readmission rates.[72] Including home health care as part of a coordinated program of hospital and outpatient care led to positive outcomes in another CHF population.[73] Case management models that use specially trained cardiac nurses, critical paths, and variance monitoring tools are being used for heart failure patients in home care to try to improve outcomes even more.[74] Unfortunately, outcomes research in home health care is sparse, and little is known about what interventions actually have an impact on outcomes for the heart failure population. More attention is needed in this arena to support the current role of home health care in management of chronic illness and to demonstrate that these services may need to be expanded rather than curtailed as our recent government policy has mandated.[75]

The challenge that remains is how to integrate optimum home management of heart failure patients within disease management programs. Many successful heart failure programs have included some type of home visiting. Some have included it as an integral part of the program,[68] whereas others used home visiting as needed.[76–78] To successfully manage this difficult population, the value of home visiting should not be ignored. Every heart failure management program should include at least one professional visit to the home for a thorough home assessment. This would contribute valuable information to the team about the support system, barriers to compliance, and the functional status of the patient. Ongoing intervention in the home for instruction, monitoring, and support may hold the most promise at successfully managing this population.

CONCLUSION

Transitioning the care of the heart failure patient to the family is complex and challenging. Health care professionals need to be aware of the family's role in the health of a patient and the impact of the illness on the family and caregiver and identify ways to maintain the optimum health of both the patient and family. Interdisci-

plinary approaches with patients and families in both the home and outpatient settings have the most potential for achieving positive outcomes for heart failure patients and their families.

REFERENCES

1. Baker LC. Critical issues in family theory in family medicine research. In: Ramsey CN, ed. *Family Systems in Medicine*. New York: Guilford Press; 1989:150–163.

2. Kerns RD. Family assessment and intervention. In: Nicassio PM, Smith TW, eds. *Managing Chronic Illness, A Biopsychosocial Perspective*. Washington, DC: American Psychological Association; 1995:207–244.

3. Kerns RD, Weiss LH. Family influences on the course of chronic illness: A cognitive-behavioral transactional model. *Ann Behav Med*. 1994;16:116–121.

4. Turk DC, Kerns RD. The family in health and illness. In: Turk DC, Kerns RD, eds. *Health, Illness, and Families: A Life-span Perspective*. New York: John Wiley & Sons, Inc.; 1985:1–22.

5. Patterson JM. A family stress model: The family adjustment and adaptation response. In: Ramsey CN, ed. *Family Systems in Medicine*. New York: Guilford Press; 1989:95–118.

6. Reiss D. Families and their paradigms: An ecologic approach to understanding the family in its social world. In: Ramsey CN, ed. *Family Systems in Medicine*. New York: Guilford Press; 1989:119–134.

7. Steidl JH, Finkelstein FO, Wexler JP, et al. Medical condition, adherence to treatment regimens, and family functioning. *Arch Gen Psychiat*. 1980;37:1025–1027.

8. MacLean D, Lo R. The non-insulin-dependent diabetic: success and failure in compliance. *Aust J Adv Nurs*. 1998;15:33–42.

9. Levine DM, Green LW, Deeds SG, Chwalow J, Russell RP, Finlay J. Health education for hypertensive patients. *JAMA*. 1979;241(16):1700–1703.

10. Morisky DE, Levine DM, Green LW, Shapiro S, Russell RP, Smith CR. Five-year blood pressure control and mortality following health education for hypertensive patients. *Am J Public Health*. 1983;73:153–162.

11. Becker LA. Family systems and compliance with medical regimen. In: Ramsey CN, ed. *Family Systems in Medicine*. New York: Guilford Press; 1989:416–431.

12. Flor J, Kerns RD, Turk DC. The role of spouse reinforcement, perceived pain, and activity levels of chronic pain patients. *J Psychosom Res*. 1987;31:251–259.

13. Kerns RD, Haythornthwaite J, Southwick S, Giller EL. The role of marital interaction in chronic pain and depressive symptom severity. *J Psychosom Res*. 1990;34:401–408.

14. Romano JM, Turner JA, Friedman LS, et al. Sequential analysis of chronic pain behaviors and spouse responses. *J Consult Clin Psychol*. 1992;60:777–782.

15. Riegel BJ, Dracup KA. Does overprotection cause cardiac invalidism after acute myocardial infarction? *Heart Lung*. 1992;21:529–535.

16. Kerns RD, Turk DC. Depression and chronic pain: The mediating role of the spouse. *J Marriage Fam*. 1984;46:845–852.

17. Anderson MA, Pena RA, Helms LB. Home care utilization by congestive heart failure patients: A pilot study. *Public Health Nurs*. 1998;15:146–162.

18. Lough MA. Ongoing work of older adults at home after hospitalization. *J Adv Nurs*. 1996;23:804–809.

19. Friedman MM. Social support sources among older women with heart failure: continuity versus loss over time. *Res Nurs Health*. 1997;20:319–327.

20. Payne ME, Lubkin IM. Family caregivers. In: Lubkin IM, ed. *Chronic Illness: Impact and Interventions*. Boston: Jones & Bartlett Publishers; 1995:261–284.

21. Karmilovich SE. Burden and stress associated with spousal caregiving for individuals with heart failure. *Prog Cardiovasc Nurs*. 1994;9:33–38.

22. Kleffel D. Lives on hold: Evaluation of a caregivers' support program. *Home Healthcare Nurse*. 1998;16:465–472.

23. Soldo BJ, Myllyluoma J. Caregivers who live with dependent elderly. *Gerontologist*. 1983;23:605–611.

24. Zarit S, Todd PA, Zarit JM. Subjective burden of husbands and wives as caregivers: A longitudinal study. *Gerontologist*. 1986;26:260–266.

25. Vitaliano PP. Commentary. *J Fam Pract*. 1990;30:437–440.

26. Bunting SM. Stress on caregivers of the elderly. *Adv Nurs Sci*. 1989;11(2):63–73.

27. Cantor MH. Strain among caregivers: A study of experience in the U.S. *Gerontologist*. 1983;23:597–604.

28. Caserta MS, Lund DA, Wright SD. Exploring the caregiver burden inventory: Further evidence for a multidimensional view of burden. *Int J Aging Hum Dev*. 1996;43(1):21–34.

29. Coughlan AK, Humphrey M. Presenile stroke: Long-term outcome for patients and their families. *Rheumatol Rehabil*. 1982;21:115–122.

30. George LK, Gwyther LP. Caregiver well-being: A multidimensional examination of family caregivers of demented adults. *Gerontologist.* 1986;26:253–259.

31. Horowitz A. Family caregiving to the frail elderly. In M. D. Lawton & G. Maddox (Eds.), *Annual Review of Gerontology and Geriatrics.* (Vol. 5) . New York: Springer Publishing Co.; 1985:194–246.

32. Jones DA, Vetter NJ. A survey of those who care for the elderly at home: Their problems and their needs. *Soc Sci Med.* 1984;20:993–999.

33. Brocklehurst JC, Morris P, Andrews K, Richards B, Laycock P. Social effects of stroke. *Soc Sci Med.* 1981;15a:35–39.

34. Gaynor SE. The long haul: The effects of home care on caregivers. *Image: J Nurs Scholarship.* 1990;22(4):208–212.

35. Cafferata EL, Stone R. The caregiving role: Dimensions of burden and benefits. *Comp Gerontol: Clin Lab Sci.* 1989;(3 Suppl):57–69.

36. Carey PJ, Oberst MT, McCubbin MA, Hughes SH. Appraisal and caregiving burden in family members caring for patients receiving chemotherapy. *Oncol Nurs Forum.* 1991;18:1341–1348.

37. Lawton MP, Moss M, Kleban MH. Glicksman A, Roving M. A two-factor model of caregiving appraisal and psychological well-being. *J Gerontol.* 1991;46(4):181–189.

38. O'Connor PM. *Appraisal of Stress among Caregivers of Stroke Victims.* San Diego, CA: San Diego State University; 1992. Unpublished master's thesis.

39. Pratt C, Wright S, Schmall V. Burden, coping, and health status: A comparison of family caregivers to community dwelling and institutionalized Alzheimer's patients. *J Gerontol Social Work.* 1987;11:99–112.

40. Pruchno RA, Resch NC. Husbands and wives as caregivers: Antecedents of depression and burden. *Gerontologist.* 1989;29:159–165.

41. Scannell A. *Caregivers' Adaptation to Stroke: Long-Term Effects.* Portland, OR: Portland State University; 1988. Unpublished doctoral dissertation.

42. Tompkins CA, Schulz R, Ray MT. Post-stroke depression in primary support persons: Predicting those at risk. *J Consult Clin Psychol.* 1988;56:502–508.

43. Holicky R. Caring for the caregivers: The hidden victims of illness and disability. *Rehabil Nurs.* 1996;21(5):247–252.

44. Langner SR. Finding meaning in caring for elderly relatives: loss and personal growth. *Holistic Nurs Pract.* 1995;9(3):75–84.

45. Schulz R, Tompkins CA, Rau MT. A longitudinal study of the psychological impact of stroke on primary support persons. *Psychol Aging.* 1988;3:131–141.

46. Montenko AK. The frustrations, gratifications, and well-being of dementia caregivers. *Gerontologist.* 1989;29:166–172.

47. Cobb S. Social support as a moderator of life stress. *Psychosom Med.* 1976;38:300–314.

48. Dean A, Lin N. The stress-buffering role of social support. *J Nerv Ment Dis.* 1977;169:403–417.

49. Schaefer C, Coyne JC, Lazarus R. The health related functions of social support. *J Behav Med.* 1981;4:381–405.

50. Fink SV. The influence of family resources and family demands on the strains and well-being of caregiving families. *Nurs Res.* 1995;44(3):139–146.

51. Schulz R, Tompkins C, Wood D, Decker S. The social psychology of caregiving: The physical and psychological costs of providing support to the disabled. *J Appl Psychol.* 1987;17:401–428.

52. Zarit S, Reever K, Bach-Peterson J. Relatives of the impaired elderly: Correlates of feelings of burden. *Gerontologist.* 1980;20:649–655.

53. Clipp EC, George LK. Caregiver needs and patterns of social support. *J Gerontol.* 1990;45(3):S102–S111.

54. Pollock SE, Duffy ME. The health-related hardiness scale: development and psychometric analysis. *Nurs Res.* 1990;39:218–222.

55. Schott-Baer D, Fisher L, Gregory C. Dependent care, caregiver burden, hardiness, and self-care agency of caregivers. *Can Nurs.* 1995;18:299–305.

56. Decker SD, Schultz R, Wood D. Determinants of well-being in primary caregivers of spinal cord injured persons. *Rehabil Nurs.* 1989;14:6–8.

57. Fingerman KL, Gallagher-Thompson D, Lovett S, Rose J. Internal resourcefulness, task demands, coping, and dysphoric affect among caregivers of the frail elderly. *International J Aging Hum Dev.* 1996;42(3):229–248.

58. Stoller E, Pugliesi K. Size and effectiveness of informal helping networks: A panel study of older people in the community. *J Health Social Behav.* 1991;32:180–191.

59. Martens KH, Mellor S. A study of the relationship between home care services and hospital readmission of patients with congestive heart failure. *Home Healthcare Nurse.* 1997;15:123–129.

60. Proctor EK, Morrow-Howell N, Kaplan SJ. Implementation of discharge plans for chronically ill elders discharged home. *Health Social Work.* 1997;21(1):30–40.

61. Monane M, Bohn RL, Gurwitz JH, Glynn RJ, Avorn J. Noncompliance with congestive heart failure therapy in the elderly. *Arch Intern Med.* 1994;154: 433–437.

62. Blaylock A, Cason CL. Discharge planning: predicting patients' needs. *J Gerontol Nurs.* 1992;18 (7):5–10.

63. Harrison MB, Toman C, Logan J. Hospital to home: Evidence-based education for CHF. *Can Nurse.* 1998;94(2):36–42.

64. Bushnell FK. Self-care teaching for congestive heart failure patients. *J Gerontol Nurs.* 1992;Oct:27–32.

65. McWhinney IR. The doctor, the patient, and the home: Returning to our roots. *J Am Board Fam Pract.* 1997;10:430–435.

66. Sherman A. Critical care management of the heart failure patient in the home. *Crit Care Nurs Q.* 1995;18:77–87.

67. Green K. *Home Care Survival Guide.* Philadelphia: Lippincott-Raven Publishers; 1998.

68. Kornowski R, Zeeli D, Averbuch M, et al. Intensive home-care surveillance prevents hospitalization and improves morbidity rates among elderly patients with severe congestive heart failure. *Am Heart J.* 1995;129:762–766.

69. Harjai KJ, Mehra MR, Ventura HO, et al. Home inotropic therapy in advanced heart failure: Cost analysis and clinical outcomes. *Chest.* 1997;112:1298–1303.

70. Cesario D, Clark J, Maisel A. Beneficial effects of intermittent home administration of the inotrope/vasodilator milrinone in patients with end-stage congestive heart failure: A preliminary study. *Am Heart J.* 1998;135:121–129.

71. Packer M, Cohn JN and the Steering Committee and Membership of the Advisory Council to Improve Outcomes Nationwide in Heart Failure. Consensus Recommendations for the Management of Chronic Heart Failure. *Am J Cardiol.* 1999;83(2A):9A–38A.

72. Donlevy JA, Pietruch BL. The connection delivery model: Care across the continuum. *Nurs Manage.* 1996;27(5):34–35.

73. Venner GH, Seelbinder JS. Team management of congestive heart failure across the continuum. *J Cardiovasc Nurs.* 1996;10(2):71–84.

74. Huggins CM, Phillips CY. Using case management with clinical plans to improve patient outcomes. *Home Healthcare Nurse.* 1998;16:15–20.

75. Harris MD. The impact of the Balanced Budget Act of 1997 on Home Healthcare Agencies and Nurses. *Home Healthcare Nurse.* 1998;16:435–437.

76. Fonarow GC, Stevenson LW, Walden JA, et al. Impact of a comprehensive heart failure management program on hospital readmission and functional status of patients with advanced heart failure. *J Am Coll Cardiol.* 1997;30:725–732.

77. McCarthy R. CHF program reduces readmissions, raises revenue. *Drug Benefit Trends.* 1997;9(11):24–26.

78. Rich MW, Beckham V, Wittenberg C, Leven CL, Freedland KE, Carney RM. A multidisciplinary intervention to prevent the readmission of elderly patients with congestive heart failure. *N Engl J Med.* 1995;333:1190–1195.

PART VI

Improving Personal and Societal Outcomes with New Care Delivery Models

CHAPTER 15

Outcomes Measurement in Heart Failure

*Christi Deaton, Derek V. Exner, Eleanor B. Schron,
Barbara Riegel, and Suzanne Prevost*

Health care providers of all disciplines and specialties are expected to document outcomes associated with the care they provide. This expectation is particularly relevant in the care of heart failure patients. As the most costly health care problem in the United States and the most common diagnosis among hospitalized elders, heart failure immediately becomes a high priority target for outcomes measurement and management.[1,2] Recent successes of several new care delivery models, like those discussed elsewhere in this book, increase the incentive to evaluate heart failure outcomes and to implement systems to improve those outcomes.[3]

Heart failure therapies can be expected to achieve a wide variety of outcomes. End points such as survival or the need for heart transplantation are invariably assessed in outcomes research and provide important information to clinicians and patients alike. However, these measures do not necessarily provide information on what is considered most important to many patients—the capacity of the intervention to restore an individual to as normal a life as possible.[4,5] Therefore, other measures, such as health-related quality of life (HRQL) have become important end points in cardiovascular research.[6–8]

This chapter addresses the measurement of various outcomes of importance in the heart failure population. The chapter begins with an overview of important measurement issues that are applicable to study design and the choice of individual instruments (eg, reliability, validity). Instruments that can be used to assess HRQL as it is discussed in Chapter 2 are described and critiqued. Issues related to the economic measurement of resource use are discussed next. Then, important processes affecting heart failure outcomes (ie, knowledge, self-care, compliance, and caregiver burden) are discussed, and measurement instruments are suggested. Finally, some broader issues surrounding outcomes measurement (eg, quality of care) are discussed briefly. The emphasis of this chapter is on practical issues of measurement.

INITIAL CONSIDERATIONS IN OUTCOMES MEASUREMENT

The initial critical steps in outcomes measurement are conceptual and operational (Exhibit 15–1). These steps are discussed in general and then in depth as they relate to the measurement of various outcomes.

Conceptual Considerations

Clarify Purpose

Important initial work in outcomes measurement is conceptual. An essential first step in the process is to clarify the purpose for engaging in outcomes measurement. The purpose or reason may vary from a desire to engage in research, a need to evaluate the results of a particular program or change in practice, or the need to change practice and improve patient outcomes. A request for data on specific outcomes may come

Exhibit 15–1 Initial Critical Steps in Outcomes Measurement

I. Conceptualization	II. Operationalization
Clarify purpose	Define measures for conceptual variables
Determine approach	Decide on data sources
Develop conceptual framework	Determine level of aggregation for variables
Define goals and objectives	Develop plan for data management

from outside entities such as third-party payers or accrediting agencies. Reasons may be grouped as Kane[9] did, noting that outcomes measurement is undertaken for three basic reasons: to make (or influence) market decisions, to provide accountability, or to improve the knowledgebase in health care. Clarification of purpose helps to define the approach and scope of the endeavor.

Determine Approach

The second step is to determine the approach on the basis of the purpose of the project and resources that are available. Jennings[10] classifies outcomes measurement as outcomes research, outcomes evaluation, and outcomes management based on the purpose to be accomplished. *Outcomes research* refers to controlled, empirical assessments of the effect of a given product, technology, process, or intervention on patient, provider, or organizational outcomes. Clinical research and clinical trials are synonyms for outcomes research. *Outcomes evaluation* is a process of monitoring and/or measuring clinical or financial data related to the outcome goals of specific providers, patient groups, or institutions. Program evaluation is used synonymously with outcomes evaluation in this chapter. Finally, *outcomes management* is used to refer to the systematic improvement of outcomes by acting on information gained from outcomes evaluation, often using the strategies of continuous process improvement. Table 15–1 provides a comparison of these three approaches. Examples of each are shown in Table 15–2. Outcomes research usually requires more resources of money and time than the other two approaches, and the ability to write a research proposal is a skill that takes time to develop. Outcomes measurement

activities are fruitful areas for collaboration between clinicians and researchers, with each contributing expertise and skills. Outcomes evaluation and management are responsive to the needs of providers and institutions.

Develop Conceptual Framework

Another consideration is developing a conceptual framework for measuring outcomes. Although some investigators believe that working from a conceptual framework is what delineates outcomes research from outcomes evaluation or management, all efforts in outcomes measurement potentially benefit from this type of framework.[9] At its most basic, the conceptual framework indicates what is believed to cause the outcome.[9] For outcomes research, the conceptual framework should be well thought out, formalized, and based on a thorough review of the literature and the investigator's previous research. The framework should be a map or model of the expected relationship between the intervention and the outcomes, with identification of salient variables and relationships among variables specified.[9]

Define Goals and Objectives

Outcomes evaluation and outcomes management activities may be carried out within a less precise framework, but there is still the concept that a particular "intervention" (although it may be broadly defined as a program, practice, or organization) affects patient outcomes. The goal for these activities may not be to completely isolate or understand the important components or variables and how they relate to each other and contribute to patient outcomes but to measure and achieve the outcomes. Precision in measurement remains important if outcomes are to be believed.

Table 15–1 Comparison of Three Approaches to Heart Failure Outcomes Measurements

Features	Outcomes Research	Outcomes Evaluation	Outcomes Management
Similar to	Traditional research	Quality assurance	Continuous process improvement
Methods	Controlled trials *or* secondary analysis of large databases	Descriptive Often use medical record audits	Pre-experimental or quasi-experimental
Timing	Prospective or retrospective Several months to years in length	Usually retrospective Weeks to months	Prospective or retrospective Months to 1 or 2 years
Consent	Depends on method Informed consent for controlled trials	Rarely involves informed consent	May or may not use informed consent procedures
Typical interventions	Pharmacologic or precisely defined process	May be absent	Case/care management Structured HF protocols or programs
Instruments	Established, validated instruments	Investigator-developed audit tools	Standard economic measures and investigator-developed tools
Outcome focus	Mortality, quality of life	May evaluate adherence to standards (or processes) as an outcome	Often focused on costs or other economic issues
Analysis	Descriptive, inferential, and advanced procedures	Descriptive	Descriptive with basic comparisons
Published in	Peer-reviewed, research journals	Clinical journals	Publications focusing on care management and/or cost-effectiveness
Advantages	Generalizable, replicable	Identifies opportunities for improvement	Action-oriented, mirrors current practice
Disadvantages	Time-consuming, expensive	Limited to individual settings	Difficult to reproduce because of lack of controlled interventions and measures

Table 15–2 Examples of Outcomes Research, Outcomes Evaluation, and Outcomes Management in Heart Failure

Reference	Sample	Method	Intervention/ Independent Variable	Outcome
Outcomes Research in Heart Failure				
Dries, et al, 1999	5719 white 800 African-American patients from controlled trial	Secondary data analysis from the SOLVD trials	Ethnicity	Mortality rates were significantly higher for African-Americans than whites in both the prevention and treatment groups.
Packer, et al, 1996	1094 patients with chronic heart failure	RCT, study terminated early because of dramatic differences	Cavedilol vs placebo (in addition to background therapy digoxin, diuretics)	Treatment group had significantly lower mortality, heart failure progression, and CV hospitalizations.
Rogers, et al[55]	5025 patients with left ventricular dysfunction	RCT with 2-year follow-up	Enalapril vs placebo	Significant improvements in ADLs, general health perception, general life satisfaction, productivity.
Outcomes Evaluation in Heart Failure				
Bennett, et al, 1999	207 patients with heart failure as a discharge diagnosis	Medical and financial record review	Admissions caused by sodium retention vs other factors	Mean cost of hospitalization for all heart failure discharges = $12,400. Mean cost for admissions related to sodium retention = $9,050; all others = $16,723
Morrison & Beckwith, 1998	50 heart failure patients randomly selected from 1996 discharges	Medical and financial record review	Description of a single group, single setting	Basic descriptive data (eg, % and means) for multiple variables: demographics, vital signs, LOS, cost, health knowledge, availability of a caregiver.
Outcomes Management in Heart Failure				
Cunningham & Loucke, 1998	Heart failure patients admitted to home care agency in 1997 (N not noted)	Retrospective and prospective monitoring of readmission and patient satisfaction rates	"Heart at Home Program" (critical path, interdisciplinary team, staff, and patient education)	Heart failure readmissions decreased from 20% to 3%; patient satisfaction remained at 100%.
Lazarre & Ax, 1997	34 heart failure patients admitted to home care after acute exacerbation	Prospective monitoring of hospital readmissions	"Cardiac specialty" home care program	30-day hospital readmission rate—2.94%, 90-day readmission rate—8.8% (authors cite national trends as comparison).
Lasater, 1996	All patients admitted with heart failure or cardiomyopathy after 1993 (N not noted)	Retrospective and prospective monitoring of LOS and readmissions	Nurse-managed heart failure clinic	Readmissions decreased from 25.6% to 21.9%, LOS decreased from 7.3 to 5.7 days 6 months after implementation

N, sample size; LOS, length of stay; RCT, randomized controlled trial; CV, cardiovascular; ADL, activities of daily living.

Operational Issues

Operationalization means translating conceptual variables into empirical variables that can be measured. In other words, if investigators and providers want to improve patients' HRQL (conceptual variable), for example, they will measure this by changes in the score on a HRQL instrument (measured variable). Instruments chosen must be reliable, valid, and responsive or sensitive to clinically significant changes. These characteristics are discussed later in this chapter.

Operationalization also includes the steps of determining sources of data for measurable variables, such as claims databases, medical records, or self-administered questionnaires.[11] Level of aggregation of the data must be decided. That is, will ejection fraction (EF) be treated as a continuous variable (eg, 35%), or will patients be grouped into categories by preset parameters for EF (eg, "normal")?

Data Management

For outcomes research, a detailed plan for data management is needed. The plan includes operationalization of variables as discussed previously, rationale for the instruments and measures chosen, description of data collection and verification methods, description of training for persons involved in data collection, and a thorough discussion of data analysis. When more than one person is collecting data, interrater reliability for specific measures needs to be determined before the start of data collection. As an example, if more than one person is determining patients' New York Heart Association (NYHA) functional class, the two raters need to be trained and evaluated to ensure that they would give the same functional class level to the same patient.

Outcomes evaluation frequently relies on existing data sources (such as claims databases or medical records) rather than creating new databases. If all data come from an automated source such as a hospital or clinic claims database, then output from some queries (eg, a request for mean and median lengths of stay for patients with a primary diagnosis of heart failure in the past 6 months) can be retrieved and incorporated into a report without additional manipulation. Issues surrounding the retrieval and use of automated financial data are discussed later in this chapter.

If data are abstracted from the medical record, entry into a database will facilitate aggregation of the data. A spreadsheet program or one of many software programs specifically designed for data handling can be used to create a data file. The complexity of data collection, organization and entry into a file or database, verification, and analysis can be overwhelming to anyone without prior experience. Development of a feasible plan for data management is recommended before beginning outcomes evaluation. Talking through the issues of data management with someone with previous experience (eg, statistician, clinical researcher) is useful.

Managing Expectations

A final consideration before embarking on the journey into outcomes measurement is to assess expectations. Although important information can be and often is found as a result of outcomes measurement, there are limitations and sometimes disappointment related to the influence of findings. In general, it can be difficult to link process to outcome, because the process of care is invariably complex and composed of multiple parts provided by multiple people. Identifying the essential elements of the process associated with good outcomes (so that these can be duplicated in other settings) can be a daunting task. A poor outcome may not indicate what needs to be done differently because the outcomes of care may be due to many things, only some of which are under the clinician's control.[9]

SELECTING APPROPRIATE INSTRUMENTS FOR OUTCOMES MEASUREMENT

Instruments appropriate for outcomes measurement are valid (measuring what it is designed to measure) and reliable (providing consistent results on repeat administrations). Analogous to a game of darts, validity is synonymous with a dart landing on or near to the bullseye, whereas reliability corresponds to all of the darts landing in the same or a similar location. Although a detailed review of the assessment of validity and reliability is beyond the scope of this chapter, a brief overview of each is discussed to facilitate an understanding of the strengths and weaknesses of the instruments described later. Comprehensive discussions of these issues can be found in other sources.[12,13]

Validity

For an instrument to be valid its results should correlate with objective measures (criterion validity) or with self-report data using established instruments (construct validity). Moreover, the instrument must also be able to discriminate between individual characteristics and other unrelated characteristics such as height or hair color (discriminant validity).[14] Because of the subjective nature of some variables, criterion validity is an important means of assessing how well the instrument measures the intended outcome. For example, an instrument that evaluates functional status should correlate with exercise capacity (eg, 6-minute walk time, exercise treadmill performance, maximal oxygen consumption).[15-19] However, such "gold standards" are not available for determining the usefulness of instruments that measure other subjective variables such as perceived shortness of breath (symptoms). In these instances, the results obtained with the test instrument should positively correlate with other measurement methods (eg, a structured interview or a separate, valid assessment tool).

Reliability

Another key factor in instrument accuracy is its consistency in measuring a phenomenon in the same individual at two or more closely related time points *(test–retest reliability)* or in measuring a consistent concept throughout *(internal consistency)*.[20] For an instrument to provide meaningful data over time, it must have high reliability (>.70 at a minimum). This is particularly important in cases in which the investigator is interested in detecting serial changes over time with a therapy or therapeutic strategy.[21,22]

Practical Issues of Measurement

A major goal in outcomes measurement is to assess the outcome independent of comorbid illness and illness intensity.[23] Thus, the tool(s) used must have a sufficient capacity to detect subtle changes (sensitivity) yet not label clinically unimportant ones as significant (specificity). Although some contend that comprehensive outcome assessment necessitates the use of a large number of generic and disease-specific assessment tools in a clinical practice or clinical research setting, a select group of instruments is considered adequate because of issues of patient burden, investigator time, and cost.[23]

Another practical issue relates to questionnaire administration. The accuracy of the information obtained depends on the proper administration of instruments. For example, it is vital to this process that the research team recognize the importance of subjective measures (eg, HRQL) with interviewer training and ongoing quality assurance.[24,25] To ensure data accuracy, the investigators must assign collection of self-report data the same priority as other research information, such as EF or medication use. Further, the importance of adequate training of interviewers cannot be overstated. Adequate training of interviewers and adherence to a set protocol are essential to the collection of useful data. The protocol should include instructions on the wording of questions and attention to both verbal and nonverbal aspects of the exchange between interviewer and interviewee. Likewise, monitoring of the data that has been collected and ongoing review of these data are essential.

Missing or incomplete HRQL data is a common problem in heart failure studies. In fact, some studies have reported that as much as 75% of the HRQL data were incomplete (ie, 25% complete).[26] Missing data can create substantial problems with respect to the analysis and interpretation of results. When evaluating the influence of missing data, one must attempt to discriminate between data missing at random (uninformative) and data missing as a result of the treatment or perhaps even the choice of a research assistant (informative). For example, if small amounts of data are lost in both the intervention group and the usual care group because of waning participant interest or commitment, the results obtained by analyzing the remaining data are likely to be accurate. If, however, missing data result from the therapy being tested (patient withdrawal because of side effects or death) or the discomfort of the research assistant in asking about sexual activity, for example, the remaining data are unlikely to be representative or accurate. Unfortunately, most often it is not possible to determine whether losses are informative or uninformative. Therefore, prevention is important; extra effort should be devoted to ensuring that complete data are collected, especially when subjective variables such as HRQL are being measured. When more data are missing than present, as in the preceding example, the data set probably should not be used.

If missing data cannot be avoided, the analysis of data sets with significant amounts of missing data will be complex. One approach to dealing with this problem is to impute the data during analysis. This technique might involve substituting an individual's most recent value on the instrument, the average of several prior values for that individual, or the average value for patients in that group for that time period. Although these approaches might be appropriate estimations, they might also grossly misrepresent the true value if the individual did not complete the questionnaire because he or she was too ill. Although one might consider imputing an extreme value in these cases (worst possible value), the person might have been feeling extremely well and died suddenly from an arrhythmic event. In fact, there might be little relationship between symptoms, for example, and the risk of death at a particular time. Thus, other methods have been proposed. One approach is to analyze data from only patients who survive to a certain time point (eg, 6 months of follow-up). Although this technique offers a more reliable estimate of the difference between groups, it may result in the loss of a large amount of data. Further, this approach fails to deal with other missing data (ie, patient surviving but missing data). Thus, a variety of statistical methods have

been proposed to overcome these obstacles. These include the use of generalized estimating equation (GEE) models designed to evaluate serial changes in individual responses rather than population averages and other methods. An indepth review of the use of GEE models and contemporary statistical approaches for analyzing longitudinal data was recently published.[27]

Finally, an acceptable assessment tool must not only be sensitive or responsive but also able to detect changes at both the lower and upper ends of the spectrum being evaluated (ie, free of ceiling and floor effects, respectively). The absence of a ceiling effect ensures that individuals at higher levels of functioning are able to demonstrate further improvement, whereas the absence of a floor effect allows the identification of deterioration in persons at lower levels of a variable. These features are essential in outcomes measurement, where a change (improvement or deterioration) over time is an important outcome. The points discussed in this section are summarized in Exhibit 15–2.

MEASURING HEALTH-RELATED QUALITY OF LIFE

The most common focus of outcomes measurement is patient outcomes, which is a natural progression from clinicians' concentration on patient care. HRQL is a commonly assessed outcome in heart failure research, and one that can be particularly challenging for researchers. For this reason, and because of the importance of this outcome, a detailed discussion of instruments and measurement issues surrounding HRQL is provided.

As argued in Chapter 2, HRQL is a dynamic, multidimensional outcome that captures many of the variables that clinicians have traditionally valued. Few authors agree on a definition of HRQL, but for this discussion, we are using the conceptual model of Wilson and Cleary.[28] They define HRQL as health status and view it as a continuum of increasingly complex patient outcomes: biologic/physiologic factors, symptoms, functioning, general health perceptions, and overall well-being or quality of life (Figure 15–

Exhibit 15–2 Checklist for Identifying and Selecting Outcome Measures

---

Identifying measures
1. What is the variable to be measured?
2. How would you define the variable in your own words?
3. List categories and names of potential instruments
4. Review examples of instruments in the appropriate categories
   4.1 Did the instrument author view the variable as you defined it in No. 2?

Selecting outcome measures
5. What is the reliability coefficient(s)? (>.7 adequate)
   5.1 Published by the instrument author
   5.2 Published by other instrument users
6. What types of validity have been demonstrated for this instrument? (face and/or content validity indicate only preliminary testing has been conducted)
7. How sensitive is the instrument in terms of ability to detect subtle levels of the variable of interest?
   7.1 Examine the rating scale; yes/no answers are less sensitive than scaled (eg, 1–5) items
   7.2 Has it been shown to be usable in both extremely well (ceiling effects) and extremely ill populations (floor effects)?
8. Use in your sample:
   8.1 Has the instrument been used in your type of population?
   8.2 How long does it take to administer? Is this too much subject burden in relation to patient illness?
   8.3 Was it designed to be used in the way you want to use it (ie, by telephone, by interview, by self-report)?
   8.4 How many data collectors will be administering the instrument? Should interrater reliability be tested?
9. After selecting an instrument, pilot test it with a small sample of patients ($n = 10$)
   9.1 If you are testing an intervention, retest the instrument after the intervention to make sure that it is able to detect change

Source: Author.

---

1). Causal relationships are proposed between adjacent levels, although these relationships have not been explicitly tested in the setting of heart failure. Although biologic/physiologic factors are vital in evaluating the efficacy of a therapeutic strategy, higher levels of HRQL are essential to understanding how effective therapeutic strategies are in terms of their influence on the daily lives of patients.[29–31] Interestingly, the higher one moves on the continuum from biologic/physiologic factors to overall well-being the more difficult it is to demonstrate a difference in these outcomes. For this reason, we devote much of this chapter to issues of measurement in HRQL.

The measurement of HRQL provides a means of assessing the impact of an illness, a therapeutic strategy, and/or other illnesses on an individual's well-being[24,31] and may provide information on prognosis.[32] Comprehensive assessments incorporate all the dimensions on the HRQL continuum (ie, biologic/physiologic factors, symptoms, functioning, and health perceptions), as well as overall self-perceived sense of well-being, regardless of health[33,34] (see Figure 15–1). Some readers may believe that it is difficult to separate the domains of HRQL, but investigators have shown that patients distinguish among the various concepts. For example, Smith and colleagues[35] conducted a meta-analysis of HRQL research and demonstrated that patients make a distinction between quality of life or overall well-being and health perceptions.

Generic measures of HRQL are often used because use of such measures allows direct comparison of one population with another (eg, persons with heart failure versus persons with cancer). Disease-specific measures are used more commonly in heart failure research, however. A number of valid measures of HRQL have been developed as described later. Each instrument was assessed in terms of the Wilson and Cleary HRQL framework (see Figure 15–1) and placed at the highest level possible. That is, if an instrument measures symptoms and functional class, it was placed at functional class—a higher level—in the following discussion. It was diffi-

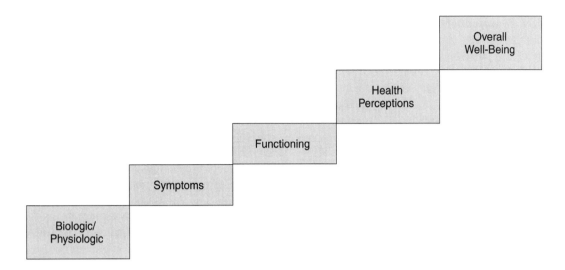

Figure 15–1 Graphic representation of the major concepts in health-related quality of life as described by Wilson and Cleary.[28]

cult to classify these instruments within the Wilson and Cleary HRQL framework, and some readers may rightfully disagree with the classification presented here. Instrument users are encouraged to assess their chosen instruments carefully and come to their own decisions about where these instruments fit in the HRQL continuum. A detailed review of the validation of these instruments is beyond the scope of this chapter, so the reader is referred to an in-depth review and discussion of these issues that was recently published.[36] The following section begins with overall well-being and proceeds throughout the continuum (ie, health perceptions, functioning, symptoms, biologic/physiologic outcomes).

Overall Well-Being

Minnesota Living with Heart Failure Questionnaire

The Minnesota Living with Heart Failure (LIhFE or MLHF) questionnaire is classified as a disease-specific measure. The LIhFE was placed in the overall well-being category be-

cause it is designed to evaluate patient perceptions of the effects of heart failure on physical, psychologic, and socioeconomic aspects of daily life. The LIhFE includes items on the functional status of heart failure patients (walking, climbing stairs, doing errands, working around the house, engaging in recreational activities), rest, and specific symptoms (fatigue, sleeping problems, shortness of breath, peripheral edema). In addition, it assesses issues related to earning a living, medical costs, side effects, hospitalizations, sexual activities, diet, worry, concentration, and symptoms of depression. These later components may be thought of as overall well-being.[37] The LIhFE is a 21-item questionnaire with responses to each question (ranging from "no," "very little," to "very much") and is scored (from 0–5) to provide a final score from 0 to 105. Higher scores indicate greater impairment.

The reproducibility and construct validity of the LIhFE have been demonstrated by the instrument authors. Highly reproducible results are obtained on repeat administrations and good correlation of LIhFE scores with other measures of components of HRQL (eg, NYHA classification, a measure of functional status) has been obtained.[38] Past studies have demonstrated a poor correlation between LIhFE scores and both EF and exercise time, as might be expected with a measure of perceptions.[21] However, changes in LIhFE scores have been demonstrated to correlate well with assessments of dyspnea and fatigue.[37,39] Because the reliability and validity of the LIhFE appear sound and it seems to be sensitive to changes in treatment, this instrument has been and continues to be used in a large number of clinical trials throughout the world.[36,37,40–45]

Quality of Life Questionnaire in Severe Heart Failure

Another disease-specific instrument measuring overall well-being is the Quality of Life Questionnaire in Severe Heart Failure, developed by Wiklund and colleagues.[46] The authors developed a 26-item questionnaire to assess symptom impact, physical functioning, and life satisfaction in heart failure. Responses to physical activities are quantified using a Likert-type scale similar to that used in the LIhFE questionnaire, whereas a visual analog scale is used to measure social and emotional aspects of life satisfaction. This instrument has been demonstrated to have excellent repeatability and content validity, correlating well with appropriate domains of the Sickness Impact Profile and other instruments.[46] Given the availability of other more broadly used instruments such as the LIhFE and CHF questionnaires (discussed later), the Quality of Life Questionnaire in Severe Heart Failure is used relatively less commonly.[26,47]

Medical Outcomes Short Form Questionnaires

The Medical Outcomes Short Form-36 Item Questionnaire (SF-36) is a self-administered generic well-being measure that evaluates self-perceived physical and emotional well-being.[48,49] Specifically, the SF-36 evaluates types and levels of daily activities; social interaction; the availability of help and support; and limitations in physical, usual role, or social activities because of health or emotional problems. It also quantifies bodily pain, assesses general health

perceptions, and measures vitality (energy and fatigue) and general mental health (psychologic distress and well-being). Four of the SF-36 subscales measure physical functioning, and four others evaluate the influence of the disease or treatment on an individual's mental well-being. The subscales can be reduced to a summary measure, a Physical Component Summary (PCS), and a Mental Component Summary (MCS) score.[49] Although the SF-36 is a popular measure of overall well-being, it does not address some important aspects of morbidity related to heart failure, such as the ability to sleep.[50] Further, generic measures are typically not as sensitive to changing condition as disease-specific measures.

The SF-36 has been demonstrated to be internally consistent in patients with both physical and mental illness[51] and reliably identifies limitations over a broad range of disease.[52] Moreover, the physical and mental health subscales appear to be relatively specific to medical and psychiatric disorders, respectively.[52] The internal consistency, reliability and validity of the SF-36 have been documented.[12,53] Serial assessments provide reliable information on physical functioning and mental well-being (>0.8), and good correlation between the SF-36 and other instruments has been demonstrated.[12] The SF-36 has been used in a number of large cardiovascular studies[54–56] and continues to be used in ongoing research.[57]

An abbreviated version of the SF-36, the Short Form-12 Item Questionnaire (SF-12) is a self-administered questionnaire that includes selected questions from the SF-36. Like the SF-36, the SF-12 evaluates self-perceived physical functioning and mental well-being[58] but takes even less than the 10 to 15 minutes required to complete the SF-36. Although the SF-12 appears to provide information similar to the SF-36,[59] the relative usefulness of the SF-12 versus the SF-36 in persons with cardiovascular disease has not been fully evaluated. However, initial studies suggest that the SF-12 and SF-36 provide similar information in patients with heart failure (ie, similar physical and mental component summary scores).[59] However, the SF-12 may be less sensitive at detecting changes in physical functioning in patients with heart failure compared with specific heart failure questionnaires.[60] Thus, consideration should be given to combining the SF-36 or SF-12 with a disease-specific measure or a direct measure of the variable of interest.[61]

Sickness Impact Profile

Bergner and colleagues[62,63] developed the Sickness Impact Profile (SIP) to evaluate changes in a person's behavior caused by illness. The SIP is a broadly applicable assessment tool that measures a variety of health outcomes, including serial changes in well-being over time. The SIP was developed from a review of the literature and the opinions of professional and lay people[64]; the purpose is to assess the impact of illness on a patient's daily activities, feelings, and attitudes.[62] The final version of the SIP contains 136 items that assess 12 categories of function.[63] Respondents check only those items that describe them on a given day. Higher scores indicate poorer health. SIP categories may be scored separately or aggregated into two-dimension scores, physical and psychosocial. Physical dimensions include ambulation, mobility, and body care/movement.[65] Psychosocial dimensions include social interaction, alertness behavior, emotional behavior, and communication.[65]

Interview-administration of the SIP tends to be somewhat more reliable (0.97) than self-administration (0.87).[64] However, both methods of administration are acceptable.[64] Further, although the reproducibility of individual items is relatively low (0.5), the reproducibility of category scores is high (0.82).[65] The SIP has been demonstrated to be internally consistent and valid. It correlates well with clinician assessment of limitation, functional capacity measures, and other health indices.[65] However, the SIP appears to be relatively insensitive in detecting small differences in dyspnea.[66] Further, some studies have suggested that the SIP appears to be less able to detect smaller changes in physical functioning compared with the SF-36 and other instruments,[67] but others have failed to confirm this observation.[68] The SIP offers a comprehensive means of assessing well-being,

although its relatively long length and the availability of other instruments that may be more responsive have resulted in limited use of the SIP in cardiovascular clinical trials.[69,70]

Quality of Life Index

The Quality of Life Index (QL-Index) was developed by Ferrans and Powers to measure well-being in both healthy and ill individuals.[71–73] It is a self-administered questionnaire that consists of two sections: satisfaction with various domains of life and the importance of that domain to the individual.[71] Both sections of the general QL-Index have 32 items that assess the following areas: health care, physical health and functioning, marriage, family, friends, stress, standard of living, occupation, education, leisure, future retirement, peace of mind, personal faith, life goals, personal appearance, self-acceptance, general happiness, and general satisfaction. The cardiac version includes four additional questions that deal with specific aspects of physical and emotional functioning of patients with cardiac disease.[72] Six-point Likert-type scales are used to categorize responses to each item in the satisfaction (very satisfied to very dissatisfied) and importance (very important to very unimportant) sections.

Six response categories maximize discrimination and reliability.[71] Final scores are determined by adjusting satisfaction responses by the values obtained from the importance section. Larger QL-Index scores reflect superior well-being. Internal consistency and reliability of the cardiac version of the QL-Index have been demonstrated.[54,74–76] The content validity, criterion validity, and reliability (>0.8) of the QL-Index have been evaluated in both healthy and ill populations. The results obtained using the QL-Index correspond well with other measures of well-being and satisfaction over the short term.[71] The QL-Index has been used and continues to be used in a number of cardiovascular clinical trials.[8,72,75–77]

Health Perception

The term "health perception" refers to personal beliefs and evaluations of general health status and where people see themselves along a continuum of well to unwell, healthy to unhealthy. These perceptions differ from other measures of health in that they are subjective and general rather than focused specifically on one component of health (ie, physical, mental, or social health). Health perception has been demonstrated repeatedly to be a significant predictor of mortality and health care resource use, even after controlling for clinical factors that influence these perceptions.[78-80]

The most common method of assessing health perception is through self-report responses to general questions like: "For your age, in general, would you say your health is excellent, good, fair, poor, or bad?" Objective measures of health status are not adequate surrogate measures of health perception. Health perceptions are purely subjective and verifiability is irrelevant.

The Health Perceptions Questionnaire

For those desiring a more comprehensive measure of health perceptions, the Health Perceptions Questionnaire[81] should be considered. The Health Perceptions Questionnaire is a self-report of perceptions of past, present, and future health, resistance to illness, and attitudes toward sickness. The 33 items are scored using a 5-point Likert-type response and grouped into six subscales. Both individual subscale scores and an overall score can be obtained. Reliability and validity of the questionnaire have been demonstrated repeatedly in large population studies. Reliability was slightly lower in low socioeconomic groups.[82] Convergent validity has been demonstrated. Test–retest reliability is surprisingly stable over 1 to 3 years. McDowell and Newell[83] note that this high stability over time suggests that the Health Perceptions Questionnaire may be more suitable as a measure of trait than an outcome that changes over time. For this reason, investigators involved in testing the effects of an intervention may be better advised to use the single-item measure described previously.

Functioning

The assessment of functioning quantifies the effects of impairment on an individual's ability to perform physical, mental, and social activities of daily life in a relatively objective fashion. Both physical and cognitive functioning are discussed in this section. Leidy specifies four dimensions of physical functional status: functional capacity, performance, reserve, and capacity utilization.[84,85] Functional performance refers to the day-to-day physical activities that people do in the normal course of their lives; this dimension is the most pertinent in terms of HRQL. Leidy and colleagues[86] argue that the primary HRQL domain affected by heart failure treatment is the performance of daily activities. A number of methods for assessing physical functioning are available, including simple scales, detailed questionnaires, and direct assessment of exercise capacity. The measures of functioning commonly used with heart failure patients are described in the following.

Physical Functioning

New York Heart Association (NYHA) Functional Classification. The NYHA functional classification was introduced in the 1920s and updated most recently in 1994 to provide the clinician with a simple method of quantifying functional capacity. Although the NYHA classification remains a common way to classify the severity of heart failure and to determine a participant's eligibility for clinical trials,[87-89] it lacks responsiveness, the ability to detect small yet clinically important changes in functional status.[90] Users refer to it as a measure of the heart's functional capacity (not the patient's), illness severity, symptoms in general and angina in particular, quality of life, functional status, cardiac disability, and cardiac disease.[91] Interrater reliability is rarely addressed in the trials using this measure and cannot be assumed with such a subjective measure. Furthermore, the NYHA functional classification does not have widespread use in other settings. Despite these major limitations, the NYHA classification remains the standard against which other measures are compared. It is almost uniformly collected and reported in published studies.

Canadian Cardiovascular Society Functional Classification. The Canadian Cardiovascular Society (CCS) functional classification was introduced in the 1970s as a simple method for rating the severity of angina.[92] The CCS classification has had broad acceptance for classifying the severity of functional disability from angina and has also been used to categorize symptoms from heart failure.[93] However, the CCS classification is limited by poor interrater reliability[94] and a lack of responsiveness.[95] Obviously, many of the same issues found with the clinically based NYHA classification are also evident in the CCS.

Specific Activity Scale. The Specific Activity Scale (SAS) was developed as a simple, noninvasive method of determining cardiovascular functional status on the basis of the maximal amount of activity an individual can perform.[96] Activities are grouped by the amount of exertion required, specifically by the number of metabolic equivalents (METS) associated with each activity. One MET equals 3.5 mL of oxygen uptake per kilogram body weight, the amount of energy expended while standing quietly. The SAS has been demonstrated to be a valid assessment tool[96] and has been used to assess functional status in clinical trials.[97] The SAS is limited by the fact that the activities sampled are distinctively outpatient (eg, Can you make a bed?). When interviewing hospitalized patients, the researcher must ask patients about their *theoretical* ability to perform the activity. Of course, any such prediction is associated with significant measurement error because of issues of recall accuracy. The SAS has also been criticized for being of limited value in less affluent populations. For example, the SAS categorizes functional status on the basis of the ability or inability to "weed a garden," "play golf," or "ride a bicycle." Although other, common, activities such as walking various distances are included in the SAS, the questions in this measure of physical functioning may be less applicable in some populations.

Functional Status Questionnaire. The Functional Status Questionnaire (FSQ) is a brief, self-administered tool used to screen for disability and to monitor changes in functional status

among ambulatory patients.[98] The FSQ assesses physical, psychologic, and social role functioning and can easily be scored by computer in a practitioner's office. The FSQ has 34 items that yield six single-item scores and six summary scores. Scores are standardized on a scale of 0 to 100, with higher scores indicating better function. A one-page summary report is generated detailing areas of possible concern. Unlike other measures of functional status, the FSQ is not designed to compare individual patients, or groups of patients, to others but to provide serial information on individual patients over time.[99] The FSQ appears to provide an accurate assessment of individual cardiovascular functional status and serial changes in functional status[100] and therefore is useful in clinical practice, but has a limited role in clinical research.

Duke Activity Status Instrument. The Duke Activity Status Instrument (DASI) was developed in 1989 by Hlatky and colleagues[101] as a brief, self-administered questionnaire to measure functional status and some additional aspects of HRQL in persons with cardiac disease. It was constructed from the SAS[96] and other validated physical activity[34,102–106] and nonphysical activity questionnaires.[107,108] The preliminary DASI addressed physical activity, personal care, ambulation, household tasks, sexual function, and recreational activities. Results of the preliminary DASI were compared with graded upright bicycle testing with peak oxygen consumption assessment. Stepwise regression analysis was used to identify items that correlated best with peak oxygen uptake. Final inclusion or exclusion of items was done, ensuring that a range of types and levels of activities was included; 12 activities, weighted by the level of intensity, are incorporated. These activities represent personal care, ambulation, household tasks, sexual function, and recreational spheres. Larger scores indicate higher functional status.

The DASI has been demonstrated to have a stronger correlation with peak oxygen uptake (r = 0.81), than the Canadian Cardiovascular Society functional classification system (r = 0.58) or Specific Activity Scale (r = 0.67) functional class scores. Thus, the DASI is a responsive tool for assessing functional status over a range of cardiovascular illness severity.[109,110] Moreover, when direct patient data cannot be obtained, a surrogate response form—the DASI-SRF—is an appropriate alternative,[111] although this surrogate form does not assess sexual functioning.

Heart Condition Assessment Questionnaire. The Heart Condition Assessment (HCA) is an 11-item, disease-specific measure using a modified Likert-type scale. The tool was developed to evaluate the ability of heart failure patients to walk, climb stairs, do errands, work around the house, engage in recreational activities, rest, and be free of sleeping problems and shortness of breath.[112] The HCA was used in some earlier studies[112,113] but has largely been abandoned because it provides little supplemental information to the LIhFE questionnaire (Jay N. Cohn, personal communication, 1999).

Cognitive Functioning

Cognitive dysfunction, although difficult to define, generally concerns problems that may also be associated with normal aging such as mild declines in recall and memory, concentration, or reasoning. Cognitive deficits in patients with heart failure may influence HRQL[114] and determine whether patients participate in outpatient care.[115]

Clinicians have used measures of mental status and cognitive functioning to evaluate patients for many years. These measures are now increasingly used in epidemiologic studies and clinical research to assess the natural history of cognitive decline, to study an individual's ability to live independently, and to evaluate the influence of treatment on cognitive status. In addition, cognitive testing may be needed to exclude reversible factors such as the effects of medications, depression, and metabolic or nutritional deficiencies.[116,117] There are numerous cognitive screening questionnaires, diagnostic instruments, and neuropsychologic tests; a few of the commonly used tools are highlighted here.

Mini-Mental State Examination. The Mini-Mental State Examination (MMSE) is used to screen for cognitive function, not to diagnose dementia, and therefore is useful in the general heart failure population. The MMSE is an 11-item questionnaire administered by clinical personnel after brief training. It provides information about orientation to time and place, recall ability, short-term memory, and arithmetic ability.[118] The maximum (worst) score is 30; at 23/24, an individual is recommended for further assessment. Some authors suggest a lower cut point (eg, 17/18) for those with less education.[119] The MMSE has been modified for use with hospitalized patients, people with hearing impairments,[120] and numerous languages.[12] A standardized version, the Standardized MMSE, has expanded guidelines for administration and scoring with improved intraclass interrater reliability (MMSE 0.69—standardized version 0.92).

The MMSE is currently being used in the Mode Selection Trial (MOST), a clinical trial designed to evaluate outcomes in more than 2,000 patients with sinus node dysfunction randomly assigned to pacemaker therapy (dual-chamber, rate-modulated pacing vs single-chamber ventricular pacing).[121] Heart failure requiring hospitalization is a secondary end point of the study. Mental status is measured primarily to identify patients who are not competent to participate in the well-being interviews, and secondarily as an outcome because improved cardiovascular function may influence cognitive function. Patients are not included in the well-being assessment if they have a MMSE score of <17. The MMSE is also being used in the Atrial Fibrillation Follow-up Investigation of Rhythm Management (AFFIRM) trial, which is evaluating rate versus rhythm control strategies in more than 4,000 patients with atrial fibrillation. In that trial, the MMSE is being used as part of the HRQL assessment.

Clock Drawing Test. The Clock Drawing Test was introduced in the early 1900s to identify disturbances of visuospatial skills, shown to be an early sign of dementia.[12] The person is asked to either draw a clock, draw the hands of a clock to illustrate specific times, or to read marks on a clock. There are various ways to score a clock drawing test, with reliability ranging from fair to good. The clock drawing test may be used among various culture and language groups but will require standard instructions and scoring system if it is to be used as a screening test in research. The MOST and AFFIRM studies, described previously, administer the Clock Drawing Test as part of the examination.

Symptoms

Heart failure is a clinical syndrome that is most visible in its effects on patient symptoms, and relief of symptoms is a paramount goal of the care of these patients. The most frequently assessed symptoms are physical ones, related to impaired cardiac function, such as dyspnea and fatigue. Symptoms can be characterized by frequency and duration of occurrence, intensity or severity, and their impact on activities.[122] Clinicians usually ask patients about their symptoms as a way of evaluating response to therapy.

In the research setting, patient responses regarding symptom frequency and severity are used commonly as outcomes. For example, in a recent randomized clinical trial of the effect of the drug fosinopril, symptoms of dyspnea, fatigue, peripheral edema, and paroxysmal nocturnal dyspnea were categorized by severity (method not specified) at the start of the trial. The percentage of patients with improvement or worsening of these symptoms was compared between the drug and placebo arms as a trial outcome.[123]

Because symptoms are subjective, patient report is the usual and best method of data collection. Patients may be asked to rate common symptoms by frequency and bothersomeness of the symptom. Frequencies may be the actual number of times in an average day that the symptom is experienced, or the patient may be asked to choose among descriptors such as "never, seldom, somewhat often, frequently". A Likert-type scale with both numbers and descriptors might be used to help the patient characterize the distress associated with the symptom. *Visual analog scales* have also been used with specific symptoms such as dyspnea to help patients characterize the intensity of the sensa-

tion or degree of difficulty in breathing.[124] Most dyspnea scales have been developed for and validated with patients with chronic lung disease but are sometimes used in studies of heart failure patients.[125]

Instruments used in the measurement of functional status and overall well-being are frequently focused on the effect that symptoms have on patient activities and the amount of exertion required to elicit symptoms. For this reason, investigators commonly confuse instruments or methods used to collect other variables in the HRQL framework with symptom measures. For example, the *NYHA functional classification* is considered by many clinicians to be a measure of symptom severity, but it was developed as a measure of physical functioning.[122] Also, many of the overall well-being instruments measure severity and impact of symptoms and correlate highly with specific measures of dyspnea and fatigue. For example, the *Chronic Heart Failure Questionnaire*[126] has subscales for dyspnea and fatigue and is responsive to changes in these symptoms. The *Minnesota Living with Heart Failure Questionnaire*[38] not only focuses on patient perceptions of the effects of heart failure on aspects of daily life (often related to limitations imposed by symptoms) but also includes items assessing specific symptoms (fatigue, sleeping problems, shortness of breath, peripheral edema, difficulty concentrating). The instruments described in the following section are fairly pure measures of symptoms, although it is difficult to separate this concept from functioning.

Yale Scale

The Yale scale, a disease-specific measure, may be viewed as a measure of heart failure symptoms, although it incorporates information on the activity that results in dyspnea/fatigue, the intensity of the activity, and the individual's functional capacity.[127] Its accuracy has been demonstrated in terms of both criterion validity and repeatability. Good correlation between dyspnea scores and 12-minute walking distance has been reported, along with high interrater agreement.[128] Although the Yale scale appears to be useful for assessing the influence of dyspnea and fatigue on functional status in persons with heart failure, it is used less frequently than the LIhFE questionnaire or other more comprehensive HRQL instruments.

Chronic Heart Failure Questionnaire

Guyatt and colleagues[129] developed the disease-specific Chronic Heart Failure (CHF) questionnaire to assess specific aspects of HRQL of relevance to patients with heart failure.[130] A large number of initial items was generated from the literature, consultation with health care providers and patients, and honed to 16 items relating to three subscales: self-perceived dyspnea, fatigue, and emotional function. The questions are scored using a Likert-type scale ranging from 1 (worst) to 7 (best). Given its construction, the CHF questionnaire is particularly responsive to changes in dyspnea and fatigue. For example, patients are asked to choose five activities associated with dyspnea that they do frequently and that are most important to them. The degree of dyspnea is then serially assessed with regard to these activities.

The criterion and content validity of the CHF questionnaire have been demonstrated.[130] Changes in scores have been demonstrated to closely correlate with both objective measures of functional capacity (eg, 6-minute walk test) and with other assessments that are influenced by dyspnea severity (eg, NYHA class and SAS score).[130] The CHF questionnaire has also been used in a number of clinical trials[126,131] and appears to be particularly useful in assessing serial changes in dyspnea and physical limitations caused by symptoms in patients with heart failure.[36]

Biologic and Physiologic Functioning

Biologic and physiologic functions represent the most basic level of HRQL, according to the Wilson and Cleary model. Parameters such as these are assessed as part of the evaluation of the patient's physical health and disease status and are primarily concerned with the function of cells, organs, and organ systems.[28] These measures range from assessments done as part of the history and physical examination (Exhibit 15–3)

to more complex measures requiring biochemical analysis of blood samples and technologic evaluations of cardiac function. The measures used in heart failure research depend on the goals of the intervention and, to some extent, anticipated effects of therapy.

Commonly used physiologic and biologic measures include noninvasive and invasive measures of left ventricular function and hemodynamic parameters, objective measurement of functional capacity, and blood chemistry analyses.[132–134] Table 15–3 lists commonly used measures. Because neurohormonal activation is instrumental in the progression of ventricular deterioration[135,136] and a target of medical therapy, investigators are measuring neurohormonal factors such as brain natriuretic peptide and tumor necrosing factor-".[132,133,137] The usefulness of neurohormonal and hemodynamic measures as outcomes and their relationships with other outcomes have not been clearly demonstrated, and they are not recommended as routine outcome measures.[122]

Packer noted that using physiologic and biologic measures as outcomes of therapeutic efficacy has conceptual and methodologic limitations and provides only an incomplete picture of a highly complex and multifaceted pathophysiologic state.[138] Changes in physiologic measures do not necessarily correlate with changes in clinical or functional status or in the patient's subjective sense of well-being. A needed area of research is to determine the relationships among

---

Exhibit 15–3 Clinical Measures Useful in Heart Failure Patients

Clinical assessment
- Heart rate and rhythm
- Blood pressure/pulse pressure
- Pulmonary crackles
- Peripheral edema
- Jugular venous distention
- Body weight
- Chest radiography

Table 15–3 Physiologic and Biologic Measures Useful in Heart Failure Patients

Measures	*Instruments*
Left ventricular ejection fraction	Transesophageal or transthoracic echocardiography Radionuclide ventriculography Contrast ventriculography
Ventricular chamber size/geometry	Transesophageal or transthoracic echocardiography Radionuclide ventriculography
Hemodynamic parameters (ventricular filling pressures, cardiac index, stroke volume, pulmonary artery pressures, derived values such as systemic vascular resistance)	Right heart catheterization Pulmonary artery catheter
Detailed functional capacity (maximal or peak oxygen uptake, anaerobic threshold, exercise duration and intensity)	Graded treadmill test Bicycle exercise test Respiratory gas exchange
Blood chemistry analysis (serum sodium, norepinephrine, blood urea nitrogen, creatinine, brain natriuretic peptide, tumor necrosis factor-α)	Laboratory analyses of blood samples
Heart rhythm, heart rate variability	Electrocardiogram, Holter monitor, signal-averaged electrocardiogram, electrophysiology studies
Exercise capacity	Exercise treadmill test Bicycle ergometric test 6-minute walk test

physiologic, biologic, clinical, and patient-perceived outcomes.

MEASURING FINANCIAL OUTCOMES

Resource Use

Heart failure is recognized as the major contributor to Medicare expenditures.[139] Therefore, economic analyses are becoming increasingly common in the evaluation of heart failure programs. Three common types of economic analyses are cost-identification, cost-benefit, and cost-effectiveness analyses.[140] Cost-identification is used to identify the lowest cost of differ-

ent treatment strategies with the goal of finding the least expensive approach. Cost-benefit analyses value health in monetary units. These two methods are purely financial in perspective, whereas cost-effectiveness analyses include a value index (eg, a health utilities index) in which the clinical benefits of a service are weighed against the cost of providing the service. The interested reader is referred to other sources.[141,142] Cost-effectiveness analyses capture the values of health care providers who are motivated by providing altruistic benefit; however, businesses spurred by the bottom line are interested primarily in the return on investment.[143] Such differences in goals demonstrate the importance of specifying the perspective from which a study was conducted.

A full discussion of economic analysis methods is beyond the scope of this chapter. The reader interested in this topic is referred to other excellent and classic discussions.[140,143] This next section of the chapter is devoted to practical issues in the measurement of resource use such as automated financial data, charges versus costs, and measurement of unplanned readmissions.

The measurement of acute care or hospital use is problematic for two reasons. First, the information available from the finance department of a hospital is designed to maximize reimbursement, not to facilitate outcomes measurement. Second, the definitions used to assess resource utilization are rarely articulated in published studies, so it can be assumed that researchers are "comparing apples and oranges." That is, without clearly stated decision rules and definitions, it is difficult to compare the outcomes obtained by one investigator with those of another. This section attempts to clarify some of those issues.

Risk Adjustment

An important issue to consider when measuring resource use is risk adjustment, described by Kane[9] as an effort to create a level playing field. Risk adjustment is an attempt to correct for differences among patients so that the effect of an intervention on outcomes can be appropriately assessed. For example, if the outcome is distance walked by patients with heart failure during a 6-minute walk test, severity of disease, age, comorbid conditions, age-related changes in gait stability, and rheumatoid arthritis can affect ability to walk and need to be adjusted or controlled in analyses. In outcomes research, randomization and statistical methods are used for risk adjustment. In outcomes evaluation, risk adjustment is not always done, or patients may be grouped by one major variable such as age or functional class.

Charges/Costs

Hospitals charge patients and their insurers for clinical activity. These charges are *proxies* for clinical events and do not always accurately reflect clinical occurrences, however. For ex-

ample, a heart failure patient may be charged for a multidose vial of furosemide for diuresis, which would show up on the financial record as a single unit. In situations like this, it is impossible to ascertain how much, if any, diuretic was received by the patient. Another example is the bundling of services and inclusion of nursing as part of the hospital room rate. If the unit manager were asked how much the care provided to that patient costs, he or she would have difficulty tracing the actual activities of staff from the charges available from the finance department. Realities such as this demonstrate that the relationship between charges and the true cost of patient care is extremely difficult to identify. Therefore, it is essential to recognize that charges obtained from the finance department are not the same as the costs associated with patient care. Clinical investigators use a variety of solutions for this problem.

One solution to the charge/cost dilemma is the use of a standardized ratio between charges and costs. For example, costs may be estimated as approximately 65% of the amount charged.[143] If only charges are available, the best solution is to consult with the finance department to estimate the cost to charge ratio that should be used to estimate the cost of care at a particular institution during a particular year because the ratio may change each fiscal year. When calculating costs in this manner, the ratio used and rationale for its choice must be clearly articulated so that the reader is aware of exactly how the costs were calculated.

Another solution is the use of direct cost data rather than charges. Hospital bills are routinely divided into categories such as total charges, reimbursement, direct fixed and variable costs, support costs, total costs, and profit and loss. Direct variable costs reflect the resource consumption associated with the treatment of the patient, whereas direct fixed costs typically cover overhead or the associated costs of running the business.[143] Automated financial databases such as Transition Systems Inc. use direct variable costs in their software. Again, it is essential that researchers clearly state the manner in which cost was estimated when reporting results.

Length of Stay

Length of stay is another commonly used outcomes measure. As with the measurement of costs, length of stay (LOS) appears straightforward but has hidden complexities that make measurement challenging. Length of stay for heart failure has decreased consistently nationwide, as has LOS for most diagnostic categories. Frequently, however, heart failure patients are discharged to a transitional care unit (TCU) or a skilled nursing facility (SNF) if they are unable to be discharged home. That is, the TCU or SNF has taken the place of an acute care hospital unit. Further complicating matters, some patients move from the hospital to the TCU or SNF and back again. Is this one long LOS or was the patient discharged and readmitted? Should a direct admission to a SNF and discharge home again be counted as an "admission"?

A recent survey of six heart failure clinical researchers from throughout the North American continent revealed some consensus on how to deal with these measurement issues (B. Riegel, personal communication, January, 2000). Discharge from acute care is typically considered to be the end of a hospitalization episode even when the patient is transferred to TCU or SNF. Readmission to acute care from TCU or SNF is identified as a different admission. Such a readmission may be indicative of a problem that cannot be handled in a nonacute setting, similar to readmission to a critical care unit once discharged to an acute care unit. Everyone surveyed agreed that it was important to be able to distinguish levels of care, so a separate category was advocated for coding. Use of a separate category would allow investigators to report in-hospital days, TCU, and/or SNF days and incidences of transition among the facilities without discharge home. The final category, if high, may be an indicator that hospital LOS is too short. Therefore, the reason for transfer to TCU or SNF rather than home should be captured along with the duration and cost of care, because these admissions represent additional health care costs and potential cost shifting. Cost shifting is an important issue in the measurement of resource use. It is conceivable that a decrease in acute care resources (eg, hospital days) could increase the need to visit a physician after hospital discharge. This issue is discussed later in this section.

Analyzing the cost of care when the setting changes is quite challenging because these events represent a nonnegative random variable. One expert in cost-effectiveness analysis advocated a log transformation of the data (G. Nichol, personal communication, January, 2000). Others use the data on TCU or SNF admissions as a covariate in analyses (D. Moser, personal communication, January, 2000).

A final issue in the measurement of LOS relates to the comparison group. When investigators use historical controls from an institution for comparison of the outcomes achieved by their heart failure program, program effectiveness is commonly overestimated. The reason for this inaccuracy is that LOS has been decreasing naturally for decades. If annual LOS for a particular diagnosis at one hospital is examined, significant declines will almost uniformly be observed, even without a change in care. For this reason, a concurrent comparison group, preferably one chosen at random from the same setting, is essential if one wants to claim effectiveness of an intervention. Alternately, national norms can be used for comparison.[144] Use of historical control groups should be avoided.

Unplanned Resource Utilization

Heart failure clinical researchers routinely monitor all-cause and heart failure hospital admissions, days from hospital discharge to first readmission, and the frequency of multiple admissions. Consistency in the definition of these variables is essential if outcomes are to be compared across programs and organizations. Hospital admission rates are calculated as the number of hospitalizations during the study period divided by the sample.[145–148] Patient readmission rates are calculated as the percentage of patients admitted at least once during the study period divided by the sample.[149] Timing of data collection on these variables begins after the index admission and does not include that index admission.

Categorization of admissions as "unplanned" or "planned" requires the expertise of a clinician with expertise in heart failure. Coded data available from administrative databases are helpful but not sufficient to categorize the reason for a hospital admission or the course of events during hospitalization. Some investigators code admissions as (1) a heart failure admission, (2) other cardiac admission, or (3) other (noncardiac) admission. Some code admissions as elective or nonelective; most heart failure admissions are nonelective. Still others code admissions as (1) related to the index hospitalization, (2) related to a comorbid condition identified at the index admission, or (3) a new health problem.[150] Coding software programs are oriented around diagnostic-related groupings (DRGs) and reimbursement potential. Therefore, coded data cannot be depended on to provide a clear and unbiased picture of a hospital admission.

DRG codes are assigned at hospital discharge on the basis of principal and secondary diagnoses, procedures, complications, and comorbidities.[151] This method of assigning DRG codes can lead to inaccuracies because the codes are chosen on the basis of reimbursement potential. For example, given the opportunity, DRG 483 ("tracheostomy except for face, mouth, and neck diagnosis") will be used preferentially rather than DRG 127 ("heart failure") because reimbursement is better for DRG 483. In this way, the true course of events during hospitalization is often masked. It is also important to note that the reason for hospital admission is replaced in the administrative database by the reason at hospital discharge. The discharge diagnosis is colored by the course of events during the hospitalization period.

Another problem with relying on clinical data from administrative databases is that coding practices are not uniform among coders or hospitals.[152] These variable coding practices often result in missing and discrepant data. Another factor that contributes to the potential for error is the need for the people who code charts for billing (ie, coders) to rely on physician documentation. Coders have specialized training in medical coding, but they are rarely clinicians and may not appreciate indirect references to secondary conditions. Therefore, comorbidities that are not related to the discharge diagnosis or are not clearly documented in the medical record often are missed.[153]

As mentioned previously, when hospitalizations are decreased, costs may be shifted to the outpatient setting. Little data are available on this issue. One issue complicating the process of getting such data is the fact that data on physician visits are extremely difficult to capture with any accuracy. Practice patterns vary widely among physicians; some encourage patients to return weekly for blood pressure monitoring, whereas others ask patients to purchase a cuff and call in measurements. Other costs that need to be captured when assessing cost shifting include personal costs of both patients and caregivers (eg, parking, medications, lost days of work). Systems to collect these data require effort and energy that heart failure patients may not have.

Statistical analysis of resource use variables is problematic because of the abundance of zero (0) data points (eg, no readmission). Correction of a highly positively skewed distribution can be done by logarithmic and inverse transformations, although normality is difficult to achieve. Similarity of conclusions should be tested with both transformed and untransformed data. It should be noted that use of transformed data results in a new metric that may be difficult to interpret.

MEASURING PROCESSES THAT INFLUENCE OUTCOMES

Much of this chapter has addressed the measurement of HRQL because of its importance to clinicians and issues related to the measurement of resource use because of its importance to administrators funding heart failure programs. In this next section of the chapter, other variables addressed in research and commonly believed to influence outcomes are addressed: knowledge, self-care, behaviors such as treatment compliance, and caregiver burden.

Knowledge, Self-Care, and Behavior

Most clinicians working with heart failure patients believe that an improvement in outcomes depends on patients' abilities to care for themselves and manage aspects of their condition.[154] Self-management is a term that is used widely and often interchangeably with self-care.[155] One way in which self-management is discussed by clinicians refers to individual behaviors intended to maintain or improve health (such as diet and fluid restriction or taking medications) and prevent exacerbation. Because clinicians prescribe these behaviors, they are often defined in terms of patient compliance or adherence to the treatment regimen. Many educational programs focus on providing patients with the incentive, knowledge, and skills necessary to carry out these behaviors, and thus there is a need to measure knowledge, self-care abilities, and behavioral outcomes in heart failure research.

Patient knowledge about heart failure, their medications, and other information can be assessed using tests before and after educational interventions. Use of tests must be tempered with knowledge of individual patient literacy. Materials should be written at a fifth grade reading level or lower.[156] Skills can be measured by return demonstrations, such as having the patient and family member identify low-sodium foods among several choices or read food labels. Multiple methods have been used to assess patient adherence to treatment regimens: pill counts, bottle caps with computer chips that count each time the bottle is opened, activity monitors, and diet diaries. Patient self-report is frequently used. For example, the proportion of patients reporting that they adhere to some desired behavior (such as weighing themselves daily) from one time period to another may be reported.

Patients are also responsible for monitoring and responding to changes in their health status and symptoms. Self-management has been defined as a component of self-care involving cognitive decision making in response to heart failure signs and symptoms.[157] Riegel and colleagues[157] used cognitive theory to describe patients' decision-making process in chronic disease management and conceptualized four stages in the process: (1) recognizing that a change in signs or symptoms is related to heart failure, (2) evaluating the change, (3) implementing a selected treatment strategy, and (4) evaluating the effectiveness of treatment. The investigators developed the *Self-Management of Heart Failure Instrument* specifically to measure patient decision making in response to symptoms. The clinical instrument has six subscales: recognizing a change (in symptoms), evaluating the change, implementing a treatment, evaluating a treatment, ease of evaluation, and self-efficacy. Initial reliability analyses demonstrated adequate internal consistency for the subscales, and face validity was demonstrated in a sample of heart failure patients.

The process by which patients become expert in heart failure self-management is not clearly delineated.[158,159] Both adherence and decision making in response to symptoms are contextual and dynamic processes. Specific interventions that facilitate progression in self-management expertise need to be developed and tested as a part of clinical research.

Caregiver Outcomes

Living with and managing heart failure affects the patient's family and significant others, as well as the patient. Family supporters and caregivers provide important assistance with diet and fluid restrictions, medication compliance, recognition of signs and symptoms of worsening heart failure, and decision making in regard to symptoms and may prevent rehospitalization.[160] Therefore, it is essential that caregivers be included in educational and supportive interventions.[161] It should be noted that caregivers may not be members of a traditionally defined family. A useful definition of family in caregiving situations is a self-identified group of two or more individuals whose association is characterized by special terms, who may or may not be related by bloodlines or law, but who function in a way that they consider themselves to be family.[162]

Knowledge and skills as outcomes for family members can be assessed in the same way as described for patients. Other outcomes include caregiving burden, appraisal of the caregiving situation, and psychologic and physical well-being of the caregiver. Burden or strain refers to the financial, physical, and emotional effects of caring for a person with a disabling condition.[163] Burden or strain can also be conceptualized as the psychologic or physical distress resulting from the stress of caregiving.[164] Caregiver burden is an understudied area in research; Karmilovich[165] found that providing care for individuals with heart failure was burdensome and stressful for a sample of 41 spouse caregivers. More research is needed in this area.

Caregiver Burden

Several instruments to measure caregiving burden and strain have been developed. Zarit and Zarit[166] developed the *Burden Interview* (BI) as a composite measure to assess the stresses experienced by family caregivers of elderly and disabled persons. Although it can be used as part of an interview, caregivers themselves can also complete the 22 questions. A summary score is obtained by summing responses to all questions with higher scores indicating greater distress. Two subscales—personal strain and role strain—were identified with confirmatory factor analysis. Internal reliability of the total BI is high (Chronbach's α .88 and .91); subscale scores are adequate; personal strain α .80, role strain α .81. Validity was estimated by correlation with a single global rating of burden ($r = .71$), and with the Brief Symptom Inventory ($r = .41$).[166]

The *Caregiver Strain Index* (CSI) is a 13-item ordinal scale that measures caregiver strain as a result of providing various degrees of care to patients at home.[167] Internal consistency reliability coefficient for the scale was 0.86 in a study of 81 caregivers. Construct validity was obtained for patient characteristics, subjective perceptions of caretaking relationship, and emotional health of caregivers.[168] A summed score can be obtained,

although there has been criticism that the scale is multidimensional, and a total strain score is reductionistic.[163] A factor analysis of CSI scores from a study of 93 caregiver–care receiver dyads yielded four factor clusters. However, only factor 1 (called physical and emotional strains of caregiving) had the four or more items necessary to make up a subscale.[169]

Caregiving Appraisal

Caregiving appraisal, which includes both positive and negative aspects of caregivng has been assessed by the *Philadelphia Geriatric Center Caregiving Appraisal Scale* (PGCCAS) or the *Appraisal of Caregiving Scale* (ACS). The PGCCAS has 28 items and four dimensions: subjective burden, impact, mastery, and satisfaction.[170] Higher scores indicate more positive caregiving appraisal. Construct validity has been supported by factor analysis. In a study of 65 primary caregivers of functionally impaired older adults, Cronbach's α of the PGCCAS was .88.[170] Oberst et al[171] developed the ACS, a 53-item self-report instrument designed to measure the meaning of the illness-caregiving situation in terms of the intensity of four appraisal dimensions: harm/loss, threat, challenge, and benign. Six clinical experts determined content validity. The ACS was tested in a sample of 47 family caregivers providing care to adults receiving outpatient radiotherapy. Internal consistency of the subscales ranged from 0.72 to 0.91. High intercorrelation between harm/loss and threat may indicate that these subscales measure overlapping constructs.[171]

Caregiver Symptoms

Measures of caregiving burden and appraisal provide a perspective on the stress and resultant strain of the caregivers, but investigators have argued that measures of psychologic and physical symptoms and well-being should be incorporated into caregiver assessment as well.[163,164] Measures of fatigue and depression, such as the *Piper Fatigue Scale and Center for Epidemiological Studies Depression Scale* (CES-D), have been used for these purposes.[164,170] Hughes et al[172] evaluated the effect of caregiver burden on caregiver HRQL, using the *SF 36* to measure HRQL. In that study, caregiver burden was assessed with the *Montgomery Caregiver Burden Scale*, a 22-item instrument assessing objective and subjective burden. Findings suggested a direct effect of objective burden on caregiving HRQL, with greater impact on mental health than physical health outcomes.[172]

Careful consideration should be given to determining measures to use for family caregivers. The use of multiple measures of caregiver burden in the literature has been problematic in examining outcomes across studies (and in synthesizing findings). A measure of caregiving burden in conjunction with standard measures of depression, fatigue, or HRQL allows for comparisons across groups.

Quality of Care

The skill and knowledge of providers, the appropriate use of therapies, the quality of facilities, and other factors all influence the quality of care received.[173] Past studies have indicated that the knowledge and training of providers and adherence to nationally adopted guidelines have direct relationships to heart failure patient outcomes such as rehospitalization and death.[174] Thus, assessment of these areas has been used to improve the quality of care patients receive on an ongoing basis (ie, continuous quality improvement).

A substantial amount of research has shown a relationship between the knowledge and accreditation of providers and patient outcomes. For example, patients with a myocardial infarction (MI) who are treated by general internists and family practitioners have a significantly higher risk of dying after the MI compared with patients treated by cardiologists.[175,176] Presumably, the rate of subsequent heart failure after MI is also lower in patients treated by cardiologists, but this relationship has not been tested. The reasons for these differences are not entirely clear but may relate to the more frequent use of medications and procedures that have been shown to

reduce mortality after MI (eg, aspirin, β-blockers, and coronary revascularization procedures).[175] However, differences in illness severity among patients may be partially responsible for these differences.[176] Further, cardiologists have been shown to underprescribe proven heart failure therapies such as ACE inhibitors and β-blockers.[177] Thus, although knowledge and credentials are necessary to promote quality of care, other means of assuring quality are required.

Institutional volume with a particular type of problem also appears to be important in terms of quality of care. For example, elderly patients with acute MI admitted directly to hospitals with more experience in treating MI (ie, larger case volumes) are less likely to die in the initial 30 days after MI compared with patients admitted to low-volume hospitals, independent of illness severity.[178] Moreover, the availability of catheterization facilities and physician specialty do not appear responsible for these differences, but the experience of the health care team does. In support of this notion is evidence that physicians working in larger groups are more likely to prescribe aspirin and β-blockers after MI compared with similarly trained solo practitioners.[179]

It has recently been suggested that patients should be referred to high-volume hospitals to reduce morbidity and mortality from heart disease in the United States.[180] The realization that specialization improves care has important implications for outpatient and inpatient heart failure care. Perhaps if heart failure patients were grouped on one hospital unit and provided excellent education by the interdisciplinary team and thorough discharge planning during each encounter, outcomes would be improved in this large population of patients. The results of some studies have suggested that higher levels of nursing staffing are associated with better outcomes.[181,182] However, a major nursing shortage is projected, and retention of experienced hospital staff is problematic.[183] Further, staffing level is probably only part of this complex problem because hospitals have been reorganizing, downsizing, and restructuring for the past decade, and some argue that the hospital environment no longer supports professional development and leadership models.[184] Another factor complicating the picture is the regulatory changes facing health care providers. All of these changes and more have contributed to problems with quality of care.

Standards and Guidelines

The lack of standardized diagnostic and therapeutic approaches in the management of heart failure and other conditions has led to the development of guidelines. These guidelines, based primarily on the results of large randomized trials, aim to standardize the level of care patients receive. The Heart Failure Society of America (HFSA), Agency for HealthCare Research and Quality (AHRQ), formerly the Agency for HealthCare Policy and Research (AHCPR), the American Heart Association (AHA), the American College of Cardiology (ACC), and the Canadian Cardiovascular Society have all published guidelines for improving the care of patients with heart failure.[133,174,185,186] Further, a variety of approaches have been used to facilitate the adoption of practice guidelines for heart failure. For example, interactive, problem-based, small group workshops guided by local trained facilitators and experts appear to be an effective teaching tool and means of transferring guidelines into clinical practice.[187] The usefulness of these approaches is currently being assessed.[188]

SUGGESTIONS FOR FUTURE OUTCOMES MEASUREMENT IN HEART FAILURE

A decade or so ago, research in heart failure was relatively uncommon. Now there are journals devoted to heart failure research and practice. Cardiovascular clinicians, scientists, and hospital administrators are attentive to the reality that heart failure patients are growing in numbers, continue to use exorbitant amounts of health care resources, and live a poor quality of life. The opportunities for outcomes research, evaluation, and management are vast. Sources of resources to support heart failure outcomes measurement are shown in Exhibit 15–4.

It is difficult to suggest specific areas of emphasis when so little is known about what really causes heart failure and how to best manage it. However, in reference to the topics discussed in this chapter, a few areas are evident. First, many investigators are currently trying programs or packages of interventions for heart failure patients. As noted earlier, it is challenging to separate the components of these packages and identify what exactly contributes to observed improvements. Investigators are encouraged to choose a focused area of intervention and to refine it in repeated investigations aimed at teasing out the essential components. Different approaches should be tested simultaneously against each other using a consistent set of instruments. Only in this manner will we be able to determine what interventions actually improve outcomes.

When considering which outcomes to evaluate, a comprehensive approach is favored. Given the legitimate needs and interests of patients, health administrators, clinicians, and payers, it is no longer sufficient to measure a single outcome such as survival. In addition, the relationships among variables are complex, and another goal of outcomes research is to explain these relationships. As discussed previously, Wilson and Cleary[28] define a continuum of decreasingly complex patient outcomes: overall well-being, general health perceptions, functioning, symptoms, and biologic/physiologic factors. The proposed causal relationships within the continuum need to be tested in the setting of heart failure. Additional economic measures and the inclusion of the processes hypothesized to mediate or moderate outcomes will add to our body of knowledge.

Another observation is that few investigators have focused on cognitive dysfunction, although this factor is becoming increasingly recognized as important in heart failure. Research is needed into the causes, sequelae, and treatments of this important contributor to hospital admission.

Finally, as noted in several places throughout this book, few of the interventions currently being used in heart failure management truly improve HRQL. Perhaps the treatments are ad-

Exhibit 15–4 Resources to Support Heart Failure Outcomes Measurement

---

Web Sites

http://www.americanheart.org	American Heart Association with links to AHA statistics on Cardiovascular Diseases (including update for 2000)
http://www.ahrq.gov	Agency for Healthcare Research and Quality with links to the National Guideline Clearinghouse (includes >90 guidelines related to heart failure), Research activities—the AHRQ online newsletter, Medical Expenditure Panel Survey (MEPS) instruments and data, and the Healthcare Cost and Utilization Project (HCUP) data
http://www.cdc.gov/nchs	Center for Disease Control—National Center for Health Statistics
http://www.cochrane.org/	The Cochrane Collaboration—International collaborative groups who prepare, maintain, and promote the accessibility of systematic reviews of the effects of health care interventions to support evidence-based practice
http://www.dartmouth.edu/dms/cecs	Dartmouth Center for the Evaluative Clinical Sciences with links to the Dartmouth Atlas of Health Care and the Dartmouth Atlas of Cardiovascular Health Care
http://www.nhlbi.nih.gov	National Heart, Lung, and Blood Institute at the National Institute of Health
http://www,nlm.nih.gov	National Library of Medicine with links to MEDLINE and other library databases
http://www.cdc.gov/nchs	Center for Disease Control—National Center for Health Statistics
http://www.outcomes-trust.org	Medical Outcomes Trust—Supports outcomes measurement and evaluation through development and distribution of instruments

Books

American Health Consultants. *Congestive Heart Failure: The Disease State Management Resource.* Atlanta: American Health Consultants; 1997.

American Medical Association. *Clinical Process and Outcomes Measurement Directory.* Chicago: American Medical Association Publishing; 1999.

American Medical Association. *Outcomes Research Resource Guide: A Survey of Current Activities.* Chicago: American Medical Association Publishing; 1998.

Bowling A. *Measuring Disease.* Buckingham: Open University Press; 1995.

Bowling A. *Measuring Health: A Review of Quality of Life Measurement Scales. 2nd ed.* Buckingham: Open University Press; 1997.

Dartmouth Center for the Evaluative Clinical Sciences Staff. *The Dartmouth Atlas of Cardiovascular Health Care.* Oxford University Press; 2000.

Dittmar S, Gresham G. *Functional Assessment and Outcome Measures for the Rehabilitation Health Professional.* Gaithersburg, MD: Aspen; 1997.

Faulkner & Gray. *Medical Outcomes & Guidelines Sourcebook.* New York: Faulkner & Gray; 1999.

Lorig K, Stewart A, Ritter P, Gonzalez V, Laurent D, Lynch J. *Outcomes Measures for Health Education and Other Health Care Interventions.* Thousand Oaks, CA: Sage Publications; 1996.

Medical Outcomes Trust. *SourcePages.* Boston: Medical Outcomes Trust; 1999.

equate and the measurement instruments are not. Or, it is quite possible that the interventions prolong life but fail to improve HRQL. This reality needs to be acknowledged and addressed in future research.

Using outcomes wisely requires having a clear understanding of the problem and a concise statement of the question being asked. A hypothesis regarding what factors are likely to influence the answer keeps the investigator focused. What makes this model different from that used by other scientists, however, is that outcomes research is still largely a clinical undertaking with a clinical model of causation at its heart.

REFERENCES

1. O'Connell JB, Bristow MR. Economic impact of heart failure in the United States: Time for a different approach. *J Heart Lung Transplant.* 1993;13:S107.

2. Massie BM, Shah NB. The heart failure epidemic. *Curr Opin Cardiol.* 1996;11:221–226.

3. Massie BM, Shah NB. Evolving trends in the epidemiologic factors of heart failure: Rationale for preventive strategies and comprehensive disease management. *Am Heart J.* 1997;133:703–712.

4. Buchanan A, Tan RS. Congestive heart failure in elderly patients. The treatment goal is improved quality, not quantity, of life. *Postgrad Med.* 1997;102:207–208, 211–215.

5. Cluff LE. Chronic disease, function and the quality of care. *J Chronic Dis.* 1981;34:299–304.

6. Hlatky MA, Rogers WJ, Johnstone I, et al. Medical care costs and quality of life after randomization to coronary angioplasty or coronary bypass surgery. Bypass Angioplasty Revascularization Investigation (BARI) Investigators. *N Engl J Med.* 1997;336:92–99.

7. Cohn JN, Goldstein SO, Greenberg BH, et al. A dose-dependent increase in mortality with vesnarinone among patients with severe heart failure. Vesnarinone Trial Investigators. *N Engl J Med.* 1998;339:1810–1816.

8. The antiarrhythmics versus Implantable defibrillators (AVID) Investigators. A comparison of antiarrhythmic-drug therapy with implantable defibrillators in patients resuscitated from near-fatal ventricular arrhythmias. *N Engl J Med.* 1997;337:1576–1583.

9. Kane RL. Approaching the outcomes question. In: Kane RL, ed. *Understanding Health Care Outcomes Research.* Gaithersburg, MD: Aspen; 1997:1–15.

10. Jennings BM. The hazards of outcomes management. *J Outcomes Manage.* 1997;4:18–23.

11. Frytak J. Measurement. In: Kane RL, ed. *Understanding Health Care Outcomes Research.* Gaithersburg, MD: Aspen; 1997.

12. McDowell I, Newell C. The theoretical and technical foundations of health measurement. In: McDowell I, Newell C, eds. *Measuring Health: A Guide to Rating Scales and Questionnaires.* 2nd ed. New York: Oxford University Press; 1996:29–42.

13. Juniper EF, Guyatt GH, Jaeschke R. How to develop and validate a health-related quality of life instrument. In: Spilker B, ed. *Quality of Life and Pharmacoeconomics in Clinical Trials.* 2nd ed. Philadelphia: Lippincott-Raven; 1996:49–56.

14. Muldoon MF, Barger SD, Flory JD, Manuck SB. What are quality of life measurements measuring. *BMJ.* 1998;316:542–545.

15. Swedberg K. Exercise testing in heart failure. A critical review. *Drugs.* 1994;47:14–24.

16. Guyatt GH, Sullivan MJ, Thompson PJ, et al. The 6-minute walk: a new measure of exercise capacity in patients with chronic heart failure. *Can Med Assoc J.* 1985;132:919–923.

17. Astrand PO. Quantification of exercise capability and evaluation of physical capacity in man. *Prog Cardiovasc Dis.* 1976;19:51–67.

18. Bittner V, Weiner DH, Yusuf S, et al. Prediction of mortality and morbidity with a 6-minute walk test in patients with left ventricular dysfunction. *JAMA.* 1993;270:1702–1707.

19. Wilson JR, Schwartz JS, Sutton MS, et al. Prognosis in severe heart failure: relation to hemodynamic measurements and ventricular ectopic activity. *J Am Coll Cardiol.* 1983;2:403–410.

20. Pedhazur EJ, Schmelkin LP. *Measurement, Design, and Analysis: An Integrated Approach.* 1st ed. Hillsdale, NJ: Lawrence Erlbaum Associates, Inc.; 1991:819.

21. Kubo SH, Gollub S, Bourge R, et al. Beneficial effects of pimobendan on exercise tolerance and quality of life in patients with heart failure. Results of a multicenter trial. *Circulation.* 1992;85:942–949.

22. Bubien RS, Knotts-Dolson SM, Plumb VJ, Kay GN. Effect of radiofrequency catheter ablation on health-related quality of life and activities of daily living in patients with recurrent arrhythmias. *Circulation.* 1996;94:1585–1591.

23. Ellwood PM. Shattuck lecture-outcomes management. A technology of patient experience. *N Engl J Med.* 1988;318:1549–1556.

24. Guyatt GH, Feeny DH, Patrick DL. Measuring health-related quality of life. *Ann Intern Med.* 1993;118:622–629.

25. Schron EB, Shumaker SA. The integration of health quality of life in clinical research: Experience from cardiovascular clinical trials. *Prog Cardiovasc Nurs.* 1992;7:21–28.

26. Wiklund I, Waagstein F, Swedberg K, Hjalmarsson A. Quality of life on treatment with metoprolol in dilated cardiomyopathy: results from the MDC trial. *Cardiovasc Drugs Ther.* 1996;10:361–368.

27. Albert PS. Longitudinal data analysis (repeated measures) in clinical trials. *Stat Med.* 1999;18:1707–1732.

28. Wilson IB, Cleary PD. Linking clinical variables with health-related quality of life. A conceptual model of patient outcomes. *JAMA.* 1995;27:59–65.

29. Dracup K, Walden JA, Stevenson LW, Brecht ML. Quality of life in patients with advanced heart failure. *J Heart Lung Transplant.* 1992;11:273–279.

30. McMurray J, Davie A. The Pharmacoeconomics of ACE inhibitors in chronic heart failure. *Pharmacoeconomics.* 1996;9:188–197.

31. Wenger NK, Mattson ME, Furberg CD, Elinson J. Assessment of quality of life in clinical trials of cardiovascular therapies. *Am J Cardiol.* 1984;54:908–913.

32. Konstam V, Salem D, Pouleur H, et al. Baseline quality of life as a predictor of mortality and hospitalization in 5,025 patients with congestive heart failure. SOLVD Investigators. Studies of Left Ventricular Dysfunction Investigators. *Am J Cardiol.* 1996;78:890–895.

33. Ware JE, Jr. Scales for measuring general health perceptions. *Health Serv Res.* 1976;11:396–415.

34. Stewart AL, Greenfield S, Hays RD, et al. Functional status and well-being of patients with chronic conditions. Results from the Medical Outcomes Study. *JAMA.* 1989;262:907–913.

35. Smith KW, Avis NE, Assmann SF. Distinguishing between quality of life and health status in quality of life research: A meta-analysis. *Qual Life Res.* 1999;8:447–459.

36. Berry C, McMurray J. A review of quality-of-life evaluations in patients with congestive heart failure. *Pharmacoeconomics.* 1999;16:247–271.

37. Rector TS, Kubo SH, Cohn JN. Validity of the Minnesota Living with Heart Failure questionnaire as a measure of therapeutic response to enalapril or placebo. *Am J Cardiol.* 1993;71:1106–1107.

38. Rector TS, Cohn JN. Assessment of patient outcome with the Minnesota Living with Heart Failure questionnaire: reliability and validity during a randomized, double-blinded, placebo-controlled trial of pimobendan. Pimobendan Multicenter Research Group. *Am Heart J.* 1992;124:1017–1025.

39. Wilson JR, Rayos G, Yeoh TK, Gothard P, Bak K. Dissociation between exertional symptoms and circulatory function in patients with heart failure. *Circulation.* 1995;92:47–53.

40. Cohn JN, Fowler MB, Bristow MR, et al. Safety and efficacy of carvedilol in severe heart failure. The U.S. Carvedilol Heart Failure Study Group. *J Card Fail.* 1997;3:173–179.

41. Briancon S, Alla F, Mejat E, et al. Measurement of functional inability and quality of life in cardiac failure. Transcultural adaptation and validation of the Goldman, Minnesota and Duke questionnaires. *Arch Mal Coeur Vaiss.* 1997;90:1577–1585.

42. Gras D, Mabo P, Tang T, et al. Multisite pacing as supplemental treatment of congestive heart failure: preliminary results of the Medtronic Inc. InSync Study. *Pacing Clin Electrophysiol.* 1998;21:2249–2255.

43. Auricchio A, Stellbrink C, Sack S, et al. The Pacing Therapies for Congestive Heart Failure (PATH-CHF) study: rationale, design, and endpoints of a prospective randomized multicenter study. *Am J Cardiol.* 1999;83:130D–135D.

44. Belardinelli R, Georgiou D, Cianci G, Purcaro A. Randomized, controlled trial of long-term moderate exercise training in chronic heart failure- Effects on functional capacity, quality of life, and clinical outcome. *Circulation.* 1999;99:1173–1182.

45. Elkayam U, Johnson JV, Shotan A, et al. Double-blinded, placebo-controlled study to evaluate the effect of organic nitrates in patients with chronic heart failure treated with angiotensin-converting enzyme inhibition. *Circulation.* 1999;99:2652–2657.

46. Wiklund I, Lindvall K, Swedberg K, Zupkis RV. Self-assessment of quality of life in severe heart failure. An instrument for clinical use. *Scand J Psychol.* 1987;28:220–225.

47. Gundersen T, Wiklund I, Swedberg K, et al. Effects of 12 weeks of ramipril treatment on the quality of life in patients with moderate congestive heart failure: results of a placebo-controlled trial. *Cardiovasc Drugs Ther.* 1995;9:589–594.

48. Tarlov AR, Ware JE, Jr., Greenfield S, Nelson E, Zubkoff M. The medical outcomes study: an application of methods for monitoring the results of medical care. *JAMA.* 1989;262:925–930.

49. Ware JE, Jr., Gandek B, Kosinski M, et al. The equivalence of SF-36 summary health scores estimated using standard and country-specific algorithms in 10 countries: results from the IQOLA Project. *J Clin Epidemiol.* 1998;51:1167–1170.

50. Garratt AM, Ruta DA, Abdalla MI, Buckingham JK, Russell IT. The SF-36 health survey questionnaire: an outcome measure suitable for routine use within the NHS. *BMJ.* 1993;306:1440–1444.

51. McHorney CA, Ware JE, Jr., Rogers W, Raczek AE, Lu JF. The validity and relative precision of MOS short- and long-form health status scales and Dartmouth COOP charts. Results from the Medical Outcomes Study. *Med Care.* 1992;30:MS253–MS265.

52. McHorney CA, Ware JE, Jr., Raczek AE. The MOS 36-item Short Form Health Survey (SF-36): II. Psychometric and clinical tests of validity in measuring physical and mental health constructs. *Med Care.* 1993;31:247–263.

53. McHorney CA, Ware JE, Jr., Lu JFR, et al. The MOS 36-item Short Form Health Survey (SF-36): III. Tests of data quality, scaling assumptions, and reliability across diverse patient groups. *Med Care.* 1994;32:40–66.

54. Mori-Brooks M, et al. Quality of Life at Baseline—Is assessment after randomization valid. *Med Care.* 1998;36:1515–1519.

55. Rogers WJ, Johnstone DE, Yusuf S, et al. Quality of Life among 5,025 patients with left ventricular dysfunction randomized between placebo and enalapril: The studies of Left Ventricular Dysfunction. *J Am Coll Cardiol.* 1994;23:393–400.

56. Wiklund I, Gorkin L, Pawitan Y, et al. Methods for assessing quality of life in the Cardiac Arrhythmia Suppression Trial (CAST). *Qual Life Res.* 1992;1:187–201.

57. The Planning and Steering Committees of the AFFIRM Study for the NHLBI AFFIRM Investigators. Atrial Fibrillation Follow-up Investigation of Rhythm Management—The AFFIRM study design. *Am J Cardiol.* 1997;79:1198–1202.

58. Bessette L, Sangha O, Kuntz KM, et al. Comparative responsiveness of generic versus disease-specific and weighted versus unweighted health status measures in carpal tunnel syndrome. *Med Care.* 1998;36:491–502.

59. Jenkinson C, Layte R, Jenkinson D, et al. A shorter form health survey: can the SF-12 replicate results from the SF-36 in longitudinal studies. *J Public Health Med.* 1997;19:179–186.

60. Ni H, Nauman DJ, Burgess D, Wise K. Comparison of SF-12 and Minnesota Living with Heart Failure Questionnaire regarding their sensitivities to the effect of program interventions on restoring quality of life [abstract]. *Heart Failure Soc.* 1998;212.

61. Jenkinson C, Jenkinson D, Shepperd S, Layte R, Petersen S. Evaluation of treatment for congestive heart failure in patients aged 60 years and older using generic measures of health status (SF-36 and COOP charts). *Age Ageing.* 1997;26:7–13.

62. Bergner M, Bobbitt RA, Kressel S, Pollard WE, Gilson BS, Morris JR. The sickness impact profile: conceptual formulation and methodology for the development of a health status measure. *Int J Health Serv.* 1976;6:393–415.

63. Bergner M. The Sickness Impact Profile (SIP). In: Wenger NK, Mattson ME, Furberg CD, Elinson J, eds. *Assessment of Quality of Life in Clinical Trials of Cardiovascular Therapy.* Greenwich, CT: Le Jacq Communications, Inc.; 1984:787–805.

64. McDowell I, Newell C. The Sickness Impact Profile. In: McDowell I, Newell C, eds. *Measuring Health: A Guide to Rating Scales and Questionnaires.* 2nd ed. New York: Oxford University Press; 1996:431–438.

65. Bergner M, Bobbitt RA, Carter WB, Gilson BS. The Sickness Impact Profile: development and final revision of a health status measure. *Med Care.* 1981;19:787–805.

66. Jones PW. Quality of life measurement for patients with diseases of the airways. *Thorax.* 1991;46:676–682.

67. Rothman ML, Hedrick S, Inui T. The Sickness Impact Profile as a measure of the health status of noncognitively impaired nursing home residents. *Med Care.* 1989;27:S157–S167.

68. Liang MH, Fossel AH, Larson MG. Comparisons of five health status instruments for orthopedic evaluation. *Med Care.* 1990;28:632–642.

69. Rector TS. Usefulness of OPC-8212, a quinolone derivative, for chronic congestive heart failure in patients with ischaemic heart disease or idiopathic dilated cardiomyopathy. *Am J Cardiol.* 1991;68:1203–1210.

70. Bulpitt CJ, Fletcher AE, Dossenger L, et al. Quality of life in chronic heart failure: cilazapril and captopril versus placebo. *Heart.* 1998;79:593–598.

71. Ferrans CE, Powers MJ. Quality of Life Index: development and psychometric properties. *Adv Nurs Sci.* 1985;8:15–24.

72. Ferrans CE. Conceptualization of quality of life in cardiovascular research. *Prog Cardiovasc Nurs.* 1992;7:2–6.

73. Ferrans CE, Powers MJ. Psychometric assessment of the Quality of Life Index. *Res Nurs Health.* 1992;15:29–38.

74. Sharpe N, Doughty R. Epidemiology of heart failure and ventricular dysfunction. *Lancet.* 1998;352:SI3–S70.

75. Arteaga WJ, Windle JR. The quality of life of patients with life-threatening arrhythmias. *Arch Intern Med.* 1995;155:2086–2091.

76. Brooks MM, Gorkin L, Schron EB, Wiklund I, Campion J, Ledingham RB. Moricizine and quality of life in the Cardiac Arrhythmia Suppression Trial II (CAST II). *Control Clin Trials.* 1994;15:437–449.

77. Schron EB, Exner DV, Yao Q, et al. Quality of life in the Antiarrhythmics Versus Implantable Defibrillators (AVID) Trial: Influence of treatment assignment, adverse symptoms and defibrillator shocks. *J Am Coll Cardiol.* 2000;35(2):153A. (abstract).

78. Connelly JE, Philbrick JT, Smith GR, Kaiser KL, Wymer A. Health perceptions of primary care patients and the influence on health care utilization. *Med Care.* 1989;27:S99–S109.

79. Idler EL. Self-assessed health and mortality: A review of studies. In: Maes S, Leventhal H, Johnston M, eds. *International Review of Health Psychology.* New York: John Wiley & Sons Ltd.; 1992.

80. Idler EL, Kasl S. Health perceptions and survival: Do global evaluations of health status really predict mortality? *J Gerontol.* 1991;46:S55–S65.

81. Ware JE Jr. Scales for measuring general health perceptions. *Health Services Res.* 1976;11:396–415.

82. Ware JE Jr, Davies-Avery A, Donald CA. Conceptualization and measurement of health for adults in the Health Insurance Study: Vol. V. General health perceptions. Santa Monica, CA: Rand Corporation; 1978.

83. McDowell I, Newell C. *Measuring Health.* New York: Oxford University Press; 1996:523.

84. Leidy NK. Functional status and the forward progress of merry-go-rounds: Toward a coherent analytical framework. *Nurs Res.* 1994;43:196–202.

85. Leidy NK. Psychometric properties of the functional performance inventory in patients with chronic obstructive pulmonary disease. *Nurs Res.* 1999;48:20–28.

86. Leidy NK, Rentz AM, Zyczynski TM. Evaluating health-related quality-of-life outcomes in patients with congestive heart failure: A review of recent randomised controlled trials. *Pharmacoeconomics.* 1999;15:19–46.

87. The SOLVD Investigators. Effect of enalapril on survival in patients with reduced left ventricular ejection fractions and congestive heart failure. *N Engl J Med.* 1991;325:293–302.

88. Dunselman PH, Kuntze CE, van Bruggen A, et al. Value of New York Heart Association classification, radionuclide ventriculography, and cardiopulmonary exercise tests for selection of patients for congestive heart failure studies. *Am Heart J.* 1988;116:1475–1482.

89. Singh SN, Fletcher RD, Fisher SG, et al. Amiodarone in patients with congestive heart failure and asymptomatic ventricular arrhythmia. Survival Trial of Antiarrhythmic Therapy in Congestive Heart Failure. *N Engl J Med.* 1995;333:77–82.

90. Ganiats TG, Browner DK, Dittrich HC. Comparison of Quality of Well-being scale and NYHA functional status classification in patients with atrial fibrillation. *Am Heart J.* 1998;135:819–824.

91. Bennett J, Riegel B, Nichols J. *Uses and Misuses of the New York Heart Association Classification.* In press.

92. Campeau L. Grading of angina pectoris [letter]. *Circulation.* 1976;54:522–523.

93. Doval HC, Nul DR, Grancelli HO, Perrone SV, Bortman GR, Curiel R. Randomised trial of low-dose amiodarone in severe congestive heart failure. Grupo de Estudio de la Sobrevida en la Insuficiencia Cardiaca en Argentina. *Lancet.* 1994;344:493–498.

94. Kong WH, Llewellyn-Thomas H, Naylor CD. The internal logic of the Canadian Cardiovascular Society scale for grading angina pectoris: a first appraisal. *Can J Cardiol.* 1992;8:947–953.

95. Cox J, Naylor CD. The Canadian Cardiovascular Society grading scale for angina pectoris: is it time for refinements. *Ann Intern Med.* 1992;117:677–683.

96. Goldman L, Hashimoto B, Cook EF, Loscalzo A. Comparative reproducibility and validity of systems for assessing cardiovascular functional class: advantages of a new specific activity scale. *Circulation.* 1981;64:1227–1234.

97. Lamas GA, Orav EJ, Stambler BS, et al. Quality of life and clinical outcomes in elderly patients treated with ventricular pacing as compared with dual-chamber pacing. Pacemaker Selection in the Elderly Investigators. *N Engl J Med.* 1998;338:1097–1104.

98. Jette AM, Davies AR, Cleary PD, et al. The Functional Status Questionnaire: reliability and validity when used in primary care. *J Gen Intern Med.* 1986;1:143–147.

99. Rubenstein LV, Calkins DR, Young RT, et al. Improving patient function: a randomized trial of functional disability screening. *Ann Intern Med.* 1989;111:836–842.

100. Tedesco C, Manning S, Lindsay R, Alexander C, Owen R, Smucker ML. Functional assessment of elderly patients after percutaneous aortic balloon valvuloplasty: New York Heart Association classification versus functional status questionnaire. *Heart Lung.* 1990;19:118–125.

101. Hlatky MA, Boineau RE, Higginbotham MB, et al. A brief self-administered questionnaire to determine functional capacity (the Duke Activity Status Index). *Am J Cardiol.* 1989;64:651–654.

102. Reiff GG, Montoye HJ, Remington RD, Napier JA, Metzner HL, Epstein FH. Assessment of physical activity by questionnaire and interview. *J Sports Med Phys Fitness.* 1967;7:135–142.

103. Taylor HL, Jacobs DRJ, Schucker B, Knudsen J, Leon AS, Debacker G. A questionnaire for the assessment of leisure time physical activities. *J Chronic Dis.* 1978;31:741–755.

104. Paffenbarger RS Jr., Wing AL, Hyde RT. Physical activity as an index of heart attack risk in college alumni. *Am J Epidemiol.* 1978;108:161–175.

105. Kannel WB, Sorlie P. Some health benefits of physical activity. The Framingham Study. *Arch Intern Med.* 1979;139:857–861.

106. Brook RH, Ware JE Jr., Davies-Avery A, et al. Overview of adult health measures fielded in Rand's health insurance study. *Med Care.* 1979;17:III–X.

107. Nelson CL, Herndon JE, Mark DB, Pryor DB, Califf RM, Hlatky MA. Relation of clinical and angiographic factors to functional capacity as measured by the Duke Activity Status Index. *Am J Cardiol*. 1991;68:973–975.

108. Alonso J, Permanyer-Miralda G, Cascant P, Brotons C, Prieto L, Soler-Soler J. Measuring functional status of chronic coronary patients. Reliability, validity and responsiveness to clinical change of the reduced version of the Duke Activity Status Index (DASI). *Eur Heart J*. 1997;18:414–419.

109. Mark DB, Lam LC, Lee KL, et al. Identification of patients with coronary disease at high risk for loss of employment. A prospective validation study. *Circulation*. 1992;86.

110. Mark DB, Naylor CD, Hlatky MA, et al. Use of medical resources and quality of life after acute myocardial infarction in Canada and the United States. *N Engl J Med*. 1994;331:1130–1135.

111. Von Dras DD, Siegler IC, Williams RB, Clapp-Channing N, Haney TL, Mark DB. Surrogate assessment of coronary artery disease patients' functional capacity. *Soc Sci Med*. 1997;44.

112. Rector TS, Johnson G, Dunkman WB, et al. Evaluation by patients with heart failure of the effects of enalapril compared with hydralazine plus isosorbide dinitrate on quality of life. V-HeFT II. The V-HeFT VA Cooperative Studies Group. *Circulation*. 1993;87:V171–V177.

113. Hertzeanu HL, Shemesh J, Aron LA, et al. Ventricular arrhythmias in rehabilitated and nonrehabilitated post-myocardial infarction patients with left ventricular dysfunction. *Am J Cardiol*. 1993;71:24–27.

114. Sauve MJ, Bennett S. Unrecognized cognitive deficits in chronic heart failure: The pilot [abstract]. *Circulation*. 1999;100:#1312.

115. Fagerberg B, Ekman I, Skoog I. Cognitive impairment in elderly patients with chronic heart failure: occurrence and clinical implications [abstract]. *Circulation*. 1999;100:#1316.

116. Webster B. Recognition and treatment of dementing disorders in the elderly. *Clin Geriatr*. 1999;2:61–68.

117. Borland C, Amadi A, Murphy P, Shallcross T. Biochemical and clinical correlates of diuretic therapy in the elderly. *Age Ageing*. 1986;15:357–363.

118. Folstein MF, Folstein SE, McHugh PR. "Mini-Mental State": a practical method for grading the cognitive state of patients for the clinician. *J Psychiat Res*. 1975;12:189–198.

119. Murden RA, McRae TD, Kaner S, et al. Mini-Mental State Exam scores vary with education in blacks and whites. *J Am Geriatr Soc*. 1991;39:149–155.

120. Uhlmann RF, Larson EB. Effect of education on the Mini-Mental State Examination as a screening test for dementia. *J Am Geriatr Soc*. 1991;39:876–880.

121. Lamas GA, Lee K, Sweeney M, Leon A, Yee R, Ellenbogen K, Greer S, Wilber D, Silverman R, Marinchak R, Bernstein R, Mittleman RS, Lieberman EH, Sullivan C, Zom L, Flaker G, Schron E, Orav EJ, Goldman L. The Mode selection trial (MOST) in sinus node dysfunction: Design, rationale, and baseline characteristics of the first 100 patients. *Am Heart J*. 2000;140: in press.

122. Packer M, Cohn JN. Consensus recommendations for the management of chronic heart failure. *Am J Cardiol*. 1999;83:3A–79A.

123. Shettigar U, Hare T, Gelperin K, Ilgenfritz JP, Deitchman D, Blumenthal M. Effects of fosinopril on exercise tolerance, symptoms, and clinical outcomes in patients with decompensated heart failure. *CHF*. 1999;5:27–34.

124. Subratty AH, Manraj M, Baligadoo S. A new visual analogue scale for assessment of dyspneoea in congestive heart failure. *Int J Clin Pharmacol Ther*. 1994;32:259–261.

125. Gorkin L, Norvell NK, Rosen RC, et al. Assessment of quality of life as observed from the baseline data of the studies of left ventricular dysfunction (SOLVD) trial quality-of-life substudy. *Am J Cardiol*. 1993;71:1069–1073.

126. Guyatt GH, Sullivan MJ, Fallen EL, et al. A controlled trial of digoxin in congestive heart failure. *Am J Cardiol*. 1988;61:371–375.

127. Feinstein AR, Fisher MB, Pigeon JG. Changes in dyspnea-fatigue ratings as indicators of quality of life in the treatment of congestive heart failure. *Am J Cardiol*. 1989;64:50–55.

128. Mahler DA, Weinberg DH, Wells CK, Feinstein AR. The measurement of dyspnea. Contents, interobserver agreement, and physiologic correlates of two new clinical indexes. *Chest*. 1984;85:751–758.

129. Guyatt GH, Nogradi S, Halcrow S, Singer J, Sullivan MJ, Fallen EL. Development and testing of a new measure of health status for clinical trials in heart failure. *J Gen Intern Med*. 1989;4:101–107.

130. Guyatt GH. Measurement of health-related quality of life in heart failure. *J Am Coll Cardiol*. 1993;22:185A–191A.

131. O'Keeffe ST, Lye M, Donnellan C, Carmichael DN. Reproducibility and responsiveness of quality of life assessment and six minute walk test in elderly heart failure patients. *Heart*. 1998;80:377–382.

132. Gheorghiade M, Cody RJ, Francis GS, McKenna WJ, Young JB, Bonow RO. Current medical therapy for advanced heart failure. *Heart Lung*. 2000;29:16–32.

133. Packer M, Cohn JN. Consensus recommendations for the management of chronic heart failure. *Am J Cardiol*. 1999;83:3A–79A.

134. Pitt B, Zannad F, Remme WJ, et al. The effect of spironolactone on morbidity and mortality in patients with severe heart failure. Randomized Aldactone Evaluation Study Investigators. *N Engl J Med*. 1999;341:709–717.

135. McKelvie RS, Benedict CR, Yusuf S. Prevention of congestive heart failure and management of asymptomatic left ventricular dysfunction. *BMJ.* 1999;318:1400–1402.

136. Moser DK. Pathophysiology of heart failure update: The role of neurohormonal activation in the progression of heart failure. *AACN Clin Issues.* 1998;9:157–171.

137. McKelvie RS, Benedict CR, Yusuf S. Prevention of congestive heart failure and management of asymptomatic left ventricular dysfunction. *BMJ.* 1999;318:1400–1402.

138. Packer M. How should we judge the clinical efficacy of drug therapy in patients with chronic congestive heart failure? The insights of six blind men. *J Am Coll Cardiol.* 1987;9:433–438.

139. O'Connell JB. The economic burden of heart failure. *Clin Cardiol.* 2000;23:III-6–III-10.

140. Eisenberg JM. Clinical economics: A guide to the economic analysis of clinical practices. *JAMA.* 1989;262:2879–2886.

141. Torrance GW. Utility approach to measuring health-related quality of life. *J Chron Dis.* 1987;40:593–600.

142. Torrance GW. Social preferences for health states: An empirical evaluation of three measurement techniques. *Socio-Economic Planning Sci.* 1976;10:129–136.

143. Gold MR, Siegel JE, Russell LB, Weinstein MC. Cost-effectiveness in health and medicine. New York: Oxford University Press; 1996.

144. Rich MW. Heart failure disease management: A critical review. *J Card Fail.* 1999;5:64–75.

145. Rich MW, Beckham V, Wittenberg C, Leven CL, Freedland KE, Carney RM. A multidisciplinary intervention to prevent the readmission of elderly patients with congestive heart failure. *N Engl J Med.* 1995;333:1190–1195.

146. Fonarow GC, Stevenson LW, Walden JA, et al. Impact of a comprehensive heart failure management program on hospital readmissions and functional status of patients with advanced heart failure. *J Am Coll Cardiol.* 1997;30:725–732.

147. Shah NB, Der E, Ruggerio C, Heidenreich PA, Massie BM. Prevention of hospitalizations for heart failure with an interactive home monitoring program. *Am Heart J.* 1998;135:373–378.

148. West J, Miller NH, Parker KM, et al. A comprehensive management system for heart failure improves clinical outcomes and reduces medical resource utilization. *Am J Cardiol.* 1997;79:58–63.

149. Vinson JM, Rich MW, Sperry JC, Shah AS, McNamara T. Early readmission of elderly patients with CHF. *J Am Geriatr Soc.* 1990;38:1290–1295.

150. Naylor M, Brooten D, Jones R, Lavizzo-Mourey R, Mezey M, Pauly M. Comprehensive discharge planning for the hospitalized elderly. A randomized clinical trial. *Ann Intern Med.* 1994;120:999–1006.

151. Averill RF. *DRGs: Diagnosis related groups: Definitions manual.* New Haven, CT: Health System International; 1986.

152. Brandt M. Roles of health information managers and coders in patient-focused care. *J Am Health Information Management Assoc.* 1993;64:68–70.

153. Palmer L. A case of coding controversy. *J Am Health Information Management Assoc.* 1995;66:43–44.

154. Glasgow RE, Fisher EB, Anderson BJ, et al. Behavioral science in diabetes: Contributions and opportunities. *Diabetes Care.* 1999;22:832–843.

155. Gantz SB. Self-care: Perspectives from six disciplines. *Holistic Nurs Pract.* 1990;4:1–12.

156. Kirsch IS. Adult Literacy in America: A First Look at the Results of the National Adult Literacy Survey. Upland, PA: Diane Publishing Co; 1993:143.

157. Riegel B, Carlson B, Glaser D. Development and testing of a clinical tool measuring self-management of heart failure. *Heart Lung.* 2000;29:4–12.

158. Russell CK, Paterson BL, Thorne SE, Gregory DM. An exploration of data collection strategies for research on self care decision-making. *14th Annual Southern Nursing Research Society Conference;* 2000.

159. Thorne SE, Paterson BL, Russell CK. Researching expertise in self care decision-making: The state of the art and directions for the future. *14th Annual Southern Nursing Research Society Conference;* 2000.

160. Happ MB, Naylor MD, Roe-Prior P. Factors contributing to rehospitalization of elderly patients with heart failure. *J Cardiovasc Nurs.* 1997;11:75–84.

161. Lough MA. Ongoing work of older adults at home after hospitalization. *J Adv Nur.* 1996;23:804–809.

162. Whall A. The family as a unit of care in nursing: A historical review. *Public Health Nurs.* 1986;3:240–249.

163. George LK, Gwyther LP. Caregiver well-being: A multidimensional examination of family caregivers of demented adults. *Gerontologist.* 1986;26:253–259.

164. Clark PC. Effect of individual and family hardiness on the stress of caregivers of older adults (Doctoral dissertation, University of Rochester, 1998). *Dissertation Abstracts International: Section B: the Sciences & Engineering.* 59;1045.

165. Karmilovich SE. Burden and stress associated with spousal caregiving for individuals with heart failure. *Progr Cardiovasc Nurs.* 1994;9:33–38.

166. Zarit SH, Zarit JM. The memory and behavior problems checklist and the burden interview. Pennsylvania: Gerontology Center, Pennsylvania State University; 1990.

167. Robinson BC. Validation of the caregiver strain index. *J Gerontol.* 1983;38:344–348.

168. Ferrell BR, Rhiner M. Measuring family outcomes. In: Frank-Stromberg M, Olsen SJ, eds. *Instruments for Clinical Health-Care Research.* Boston: Jones & Bartlett; 1997:319–328.

169. Marchi-Jones S, Murphy JF, Rousseau P. Caring for the caregivers. *J Gerontol Nurs*. 1996;22:7–13.

170. Schwartz KA, Roberts BL. Social support and strain of family caregivers of older adults. *Holist Nurs Pract*. 2000;14:77–90.

171. Oberst MT, Thomas SE, Gass KA, Ward SE. Caregiving demands and appraisal of stress among family caregivers. *Cancer Nurs*. 1989;12:209–215.

172. Hughes SL, Giobbie-Hurder A, Weaver FM, Kubal JD, Henderson W. Relationship between caregiver burden and health-related quality of life. *Gerontologist*. 1999;39:534–545.

173. Sheldon TA. Quality: link with effectiveness. *Qual Health Care*. 1994;3:41–45.

174. Konstam MA, Dracup K, Baker DW, et al. *Heart Failure: Evaluation and Care of Patients with Left-Ventricular Systolic Dysfunction*. Washington, DC: Agency for Health Care Policy and Research; 1994.

175. Jollis JG, DeLong ER, Peterson ED, et al. Outcome of acute myocardial infarction according to the specialty of the admitting physician. *N Engl J Med*. 1996;335:1880–1887.

176. Frances CD, Go AS, Dauterman KW, et al. Outcome following acute myocardial infarction: are differences among physician specialties the result of quality of care or case mix? *Arch Intern Med*. 1999;159:1429–1436.

177. Young JB, Weiner DH, Yusuf S, et al. Patterns of medication use in patients with heart failure: A report from the registry of studies of left ventricular dysfunction (SOLVD). *South Med J*. 1995;88:514–523.

178. Thiemann DR, Coresh J, Oetgen WJ, Powe NR. The association between hospital volume and survival after acute myocardial infarction in elderly patients. *N Engl J Med*. 1999;340:1640–1648.

179. Chen J, Radford MJ, Wang Y, Krumholz HM. Physician characteristics and variation in treatment of acute myocardial infarction. *J Am Coll Cardiol*. 2000;35.

180. Dudley RA, Johansen KL, Brand R, et al. Selective referral to high-volume hospitals: estimating potentially avoidable deaths. *JAMA*. 2000;283:1159–1166.

181. American Nurses Association. *Implementing Nursing's Report Card: A Study of RN Staffing, Length of Stay and Patient Outcomes*. Washington, DC: American Nurses Publishing; 1997:1–32.

182. Aiken LH, Sloane EM, Lake ET, Sochalski J, Weber AL. Organization and outcomes of inpatient AIDS care. *Med Care*. 1999;37(8):760–772.

183. Association of Nurse Executives. Executive summary: Nurse staffing survey. 1999.

184. Aiken L, Patrician P. Measuring organizational traits of hospitals: The revised nursing work index. *Nurs Res*. 49(3);146–153.

185. The American College of Cardiology/American Heart Association Task Force on Practice Guidelines. Guidelines for the evaluation and management of heart failure. Report of the American College of Cardiology/American Heart Association Task Force on Practice Guidelines (Committee on Evaluation and Management of Heart Failure). *J Am Coll Cardiol*. 1995;26(5):1376–1398.

186. Johnstone DE, Abdulla A, Arnold JM, et al. Diagnosis and management of heart failure. Canadian Cardiovascular Society. *Can J Cardiol*. 1994;10:613–631, 635–654.

187. Simpson RJ Jr., Sueta CA, Boccuzzi SJ, et al. Performance assessment model for guideline-recommended pharmacotherapy in the secondary prevention of coronary artery disease and treatment of left ventricular dysfunction. *Am J Cardiol*. 1997;80:53H–56H.

188. O'Connor GT, Plume SK, Olmstead EM, et al. A regional intervention to improve the hospital mortality associated with coronary artery bypass graft surgery. The Northern New England Cardiovascular Disease Study Group. *JAMA*. 1996;20:841–846.

CHAPTER 16

Heart Failure Disease Management Models

Barbara Riegel and Barbara LePetri

Disease management (DM) is an imprecise, vague term used in modern health care. The purpose of this chapter is to define DM and to categorize and describe the various approaches currently in use with heart failure patients. Guidelines for setting up a DM program are provided. The following chapters will explore, in detail, the specific approaches currently in use.

DEFINITION

The term "disease management" was not accepted as an MeSH heading in the professional medical literature until 1997. Before 1997, articles on DM were indexed under managed care programs or patient care planning. Associated terms included financial management, risk management, self-care, integrated advanced information management systems, and total quality management. Together, these terms suggest that the phrase DM is being used to describe a system of patient care used in areas of the country where managed care penetration has motivated the health care industry to control its financial risk. This conclusion is supported by the descriptor from the National Library of Medicine in which DM is defined as "a broad approach to appropriate coordination of the entire disease treatment process that often involves shifting away from more expensive inpatient and acute care to areas such as preventive medicine, patient counseling and education, and outpatient care. This concept includes implications of appropriate versus in-

appropriate therapy on the overall cost and clinical outcome of a particular disease."

Some published definitions of DM are provided in Exhibit 16–1 with the intention of providing the reader with a clearer understanding of this vague concept. Themes evident from published definitions suggest that DM is an appropriate term for those clinical programs that are comprehensive, integrated, and aimed at improving the quality of care provided to populations of patients rather than individuals (Exhibit 16–2). True DM programs address *structure, population*, and *disease*. That is, a defining characteristic of DM is that the structure of care delivery is improved for a group of patients with a particular disease. When efforts are made to organize care in this manner, attributes of the group of patients with the disease and the setting in which care is provided drive the arrangement, similar to the architectural caveat: "Form follows function."

Bernard cautions that programs reporting one individual element such as a treatment guideline are not sufficiently comprehensive to be called DM.[1] In addition, drug company marketing tools, physician education seminars, patient compliance programs, and capitation or risk-sharing endeavors are not sufficient to denote a true DM program. For example, a recently published description of a patient education intervention in which patients were mailed a variety of brochures cannot be called true DM, although it was represented as such.[2] Another study in which educational mailings were augmented by

Exhibit 16–1 Definitions of Disease Management

Bernard: Disease management is "a comprehensive integrated system for managing patients . . . by using best practices, clinical practice improvement information technology, and other resources and tools to reduce overall cost and improve measurable outcomes in the quality of care."[1(p48)]

Zitter: Disease management is ". . . a comprehensive integrated approach to care and reimbursement based fundamentally on the natural course of a disease, with treatment designed to address the illness with maximum effectiveness and efficiency."[65(p70)]

Coons: "Disease management targets populations with a specific condition and involves the implementation of coordinated, comprehensive interventions that will improve the clinical, humanistic, and economic outcomes associated with the management of that condition."[66(p1323)]

Ellrodt et al: "Disease management is an approach to patient care that emphasizes coordinated, comprehensive care along the continuum of disease and across health care delivery systems."[67(p1687)]

Exhibit 16–2 Disease Management Criteria

- Disease specific
- Multifactorial therapy
- Patients are involved in the care (ie, patient education)
- Reinforcement of information
- Involves changes in how the care is structured
- Reorganization of practice systems and provider roles
- Increased access to expertise
- Measurement of outcomes

phone calls from nurses reminding patients to comply with therapeutic recommendations also was not included in this review.[3] Both of these interventions lacked the comprehensiveness of true DM. The subsequent chapters in this section will demonstrate that the isolated elements listed by Bernard are often components of a comprehensive DM program, but alone they probably are insufficient to significantly improve the care of patients with heart failure.

EVOLUTION OF DISEASE MANAGEMENT

The rush into DM as we know it today was begun by the pharmaceutical industry.[4] Managed care organizations were the first to embrace the concept because of their economic risk structure. In such organizations, coverage for outpatient and inpatient care is combined into a single insurance premium, and physicians accept at least partial financial risk for keeping their subscribers healthy and out of the hospital.[5] Hospital resource use accounts for approximately 40% or more of the total expenses in a managed care plan, so a DM program designed to decrease hospital admissions and days in the hospital is financially attractive to the organization.[6]

The predecessors of DM were critical pathways and guidelines. Over the past decade, acute care facilities have implemented critical pathways with enthusiasm as a means of limiting resource use and promoting early hospital discharge.[7] It is now recognized, however, that critical pathways alone will not save money unless systems are in place to avoid rehospitalization.[8] Clinical guidelines continue to proliferate, but data are beginning to demonstrate that guidelines alone are not sufficient to change practice radically.[9] For this reason, institutions, medical groups, and individual providers have embraced the comprehensive approaches of DM.

Models of Disease Management

Reports of DM programs for heart failure patients are proliferating in the literature. These programs, by definition, are multifactorial and therefore are difficult to replicate. What they all have in common, however, is a transition from "traditional heart failure care" (Figure 16–1) to "emerging heart failure care" (Figure 16–2).[10] Traditional

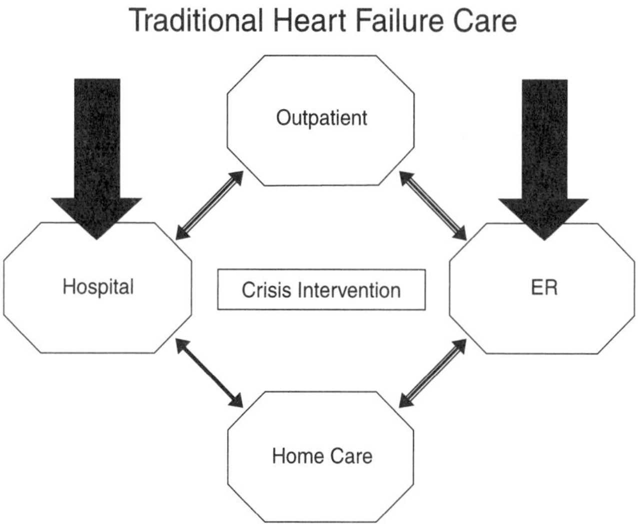

Traditional Heart Failure Care

Figure 16–1 Model of traditional heart failure care with an emphasis on crisis intervention. Patients care for themselves at home until they are so symptomatic that they enter the hospital, often through the emergency department. Home care may be provided after discharge but rarely are heart failure patients followed intensely once home in an attempt to prevent decompensation.

care is characterized as crisis intervention with a heavy emphasis on use of the hospital and the emergency department. Emerging care models provide aggressive care in the hospital, home, and clinic. Many models bridge the inpatient and outpatient settings or "continuum of care."

Because the DM programs being used are all different, we propose a classification scheme that could facilitate comparison among the various models being used. Few others have attempted to classify DM approaches into distinct categories. Moser categorized the approaches as (1) specialty heart failure clinics, (2) specialty care that extends to the home, and (3) increased access to primary care.[11] We chose a different classification scheme arranged around the primary provider(s) of the DM intervention, because the treatments themselves are very similar (eg, patient education, continuing contact, consistency of care), regardless of the location of care. Although few of the published descriptions fit nicely into these categories, no matter how broadly defined, we chose the following classification scheme:

- Multidisciplinary models
- Case management models
- Clinic models

These categories represent a beginning attempt to structure the current proliferation of interventions; these groupings may be revised in the future. Refer to subsequent chapters for a detailed description of the populations studied, the specific interventions used, and the outcomes achieved with these various approaches.

To identify published descriptions of DM programs for review, the English-language literature was searched for research and clinical reports using the MEDLINE database. Search terms used included heart failure, disease management, and therapy. The abstracts of potential articles were reviewed to determine whether a comprehensive approach to patient management was used. The reference lists of all the articles obtained using that method were searched for additional reports. Review articles published by other authors were reviewed as well to ensure that no relevant articles were omitted. The litera-

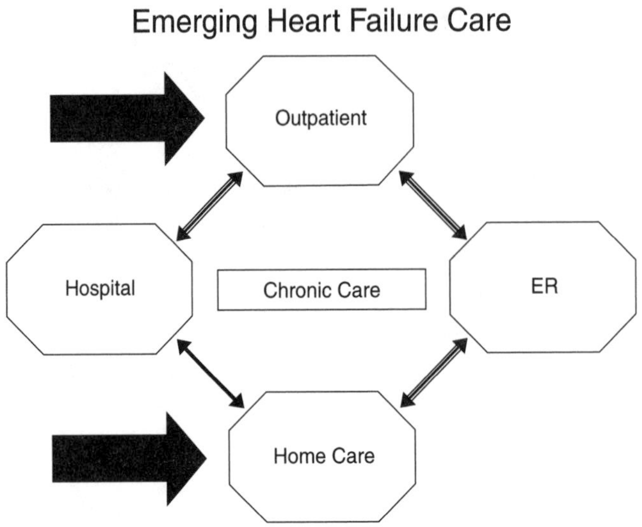

Emerging Heart Failure Care

Figure 16–2 The emerging model of heart failure care in which acute care (ie, hospital and emergency department services) is minimized through an emphasis on chronic care provided to patients in their homes.

ture review process was repeated at three different intervals in the course of manuscript preparation. It should be noted that many articles other than the ones discussed in this chapter were located using these methods. Those eliminated from this discussion were reports that did not fit the definition of true DM, as presented earlier in this chapter. Some clinical descriptions are included if few other reports were available, but clinical trials with a concurrent comparison group were chosen preferentially.

Multidisciplinary Approach

The multidisciplinary approach to DM is defined as "a holistic approach adapted to each patient's unique set of medical, psychosocial, behavioral, and financial circumstances."[12(p64)] The approach typically involves nurses, physicians, dietitians, social workers, and pharmacists, as well as others (eg, discharge planners, pastors, cardiac rehabilitation staff, exercise physiologists) collaborating to provide care across the natural course of the disease. The gap between hospitalization, other health care delivery systems (eg, skilled nursing facilities, hospice), and home is

bridged by a team of individuals knowledgeable about heart failure and committed to patient care. Each of these programs offers a different solution to a unique set of local and environmental challenges and patient characteristics.

The first report of a multidisciplinary DM program for heart faiulre patients was published by Rich and colleagues in 1993 and 1995.[13,14] Since that time, five more groups have described systems of care for heart failure patients that are similar.[15–19] In the program designed by Rich and colleagues,[13,14] nurses, physician gerontologists, social workers, and dietitians collaborated to provide care during hospitalization and follow-up after discharge. The program designed by Riegel and colleagues[17] was similar but with the addition of pharmacists and later exercise physiologists and cardiac rehabilitation staff to the multidisciplinary team. Staff members who have been included in the teams have been cardiac rehabilitation staff,[15,18] as well as laboratory personnel and discharge planners.[18]

The multidisciplinary programs are similar in their focus on continuity, education, and reinforcement that is continued into the home after hospital discharge. The stated goal of Rich et al,[14] Chapman and Torpy,[16] and Knox and Mischke[18] was to increase treatment compliance; Gattis and colleagues[19] focused their intervention specifically on medication compliance. Riegel and colleagues[17] sought to improve patient self-care abilities. Services provided by the various teams to achieve these goals included medication review, simplification, and optimization; discharge planning; use of standardized treatment protocols and pathways; availability of research protocols; home care; inotropic infusions in the home or emergency department; emotional support; patient education; exercise prescription; scales when needed; symptom monitoring; and support groups.

The investigators in this category have demonstrated a 30%–44%[14,16] reduction in general all-cause admissions and a decrease in heart failure admissions of 56%.[14] Event rates (eg, deaths) were significantly lower in the sample studied by Gattis et al.[19] Hospital days have been shown to decline 17%–25%.[13,16] Riegel and colleagues[20] did not demonstrate a treatment effect by group, but in a secondary analysis they found a 68% reduction in acute care costs in functional class II patients. Functional class III and IV heart failure patients benefited from the multidisciplinary DM approach if they were elderly and had moderate levels of comorbidity. Interestingly, class I heart failure patients in the intervention group experienced a 288% *increase* in costs after 6 months and overall quality of life *declined* compared with the usual care group. Other investigators have shown that the quality of life of patients enrolled in these programs increases.[14] These studies are discussed in more detail in the next chapter.

Case Management Models

In case management approaches to DM, patients are monitored intensely by an individual after they are discharged from an acute care facility. Monitoring is typically done by telephone or community outreach (ie, home visits). Nurses are the primary case managers for heart failure patients. Three reports of nurse case management models have been published[21–23]; a fourth

and fifth are in process (Macko M., personal communication, 1998).[24] Other disciplines are being hired as case managers as well. Varma and colleagues[25] reported the results of a program in which heart failure patients were managed by pharmacists. Social workers are being hired as case managers for other patient populations, especially those requiring coordination of services rather than intense clinical monitoring and disease-specific patient education. An interesting model of case management by physicians was published by Kornowski et al.[26] Internists visited patients with severe heart failure at home at weekly intervals. Stewart and colleagues[27] reported an interesting approach in which a nurse and a pharmacist made a single home visit. Monitoring by caregivers was encouraged for patients demonstrating noncompliance, and/or they were referred to a community pharmacist for continued monitoring.

The focus of clinical case management is typically intense, frequent, individualized education on essential skills such as maintaining a low-sodium diet, setting up systems to enhance medication compliance, and improving symptom monitoring ability. Other services include home visits, medication modifications, provision of weekly medication distribution systems and reminder cards, and newsletters for patients. In programs that include home visits,[26–28] physical examination and intravenous drug therapy may be included. The approach used by Macko[28] is entirely home-based without a telephone-monitoring component. Nurses visit patients and families in the home to assess them physically and continue the educational process. Three of these groups[25,27,28] included a scientifically sound assessment of their community outreach models of case management; three observational reports support this approach as well.[29–31] Numerous anecdotal reports of success have been published in industry newsletters also.

An interesting component of the intervention provided by West et al[22] was the inclusion of behavioral interventions based on social learning theory.[32,33] Baseline self-efficacy ratings regarding self-management skills were used to guide the nursing intervention. Self-efficacy or one's perceived ability to perform a specific skill or achieve a particular goal has been shown to predict subsequent performance.[34] Self-efficacy can be modified through a variety of strategies intended to increase self-confidence (eg, role-modeling, persuasion).[33]

The case managers are in a unique position to offer a valuable care-coordination service. Because they are in frequent contact with the patients, case managers are ideal coordinators of communication with the other providers. For example, West and colleagues[22] described a system in which the nurses and physicians collaborated closely and talked frequently to plan care for individual patients. Other programs are better described as parallel systems in which case managers send routine updates but only contact physicians when there is a specific need or a problem.[24,28] For example, Roglieri and colleagues[21] used an automated telephone questionnaire during their weekly telephone calls. The results of this standardized survey were provided routinely to physicians when patients were stable, but physicians were notified immediately when there were problems. The internist case managers referred, in the study by Kornowski et al, the patients to their usual physician for urgent problems; there was no mention of ongoing collaboration between physicians in that study.[26]

These case management programs have decreased general all-cause hospital admissions by 60%–74%[22,23] and heart failure admissions 50%–87%.[22,28] Length of hospital stay,[21,23,26] hospitalization costs,[23,28] and clinic and emergency department visits[22,27] have declined significantly as well. Functional status has been shown to improve.[22,23,25,26,28] Further, intervention effects have been shown to be maintained at 18 months' follow-up.[35]

Clinic Models

Clinic models are typically outpatient settings organized and run by cardiologists with special expertise in heart failure. The emphasis in these clinics is on in-depth laboratory and diagnostic assessment of the cause of the heart failure (eg, echocardiography, exercise testing). An optimal medication regimen is prescribed, and the results of these approaches are carefully monitored. One version of the clinic model is the nurse-run clinic coordinated by advanced practice nurses using standard protocols to manage medication regimens.[36,37]

It should be noted that an assumption of the clinic model is that patients are sufficiently mobile to visit the clinic as needed. This is not always the case with heart failure patients, however, as Ekman and colleagues[38] demonstrated. Their patient population, which was elderly and had predominately severe heart failure, reported that they did not have the strength to travel to the clinic. This observation should make us question our traditional models of requiring that patients travel to us.

Eight reports of clinic DM models have been published.[36–43] These clinics typically include intense follow-up by a cardiologist or nurse practitioner, repeated testing as needed, standardized treatment protocols, aggressive treatment of modifiable causes of heart failure (eg, coronary artery disease, hypertension, ethanol abuse), patient education by nurses with reinforcement, and home visits as needed. An innovation of the clinic model is the inclusion of instruction in self-management of a flexible diuretic regimen based on daily weights.[39,41]

Four of the descriptions of the clinic approach included outcome data with comparison with a control group.[39–42] The clinic model decreased total hospital admissions 44%–85%[39,40] and heart failure admissions 69%–86%.[40,41] Mean time to readmission was significantly longer in the intervention group (141 days) than the control group (106 days) in the study by Cline and colleagues.[42] Emergency department visits declined 100% in one study.[41] Functional status improved significantly in three studies.[39–41] One-year survival did not differ between the groups in the one study that examined this outcome.[42]

Critique of the Published Research

Differences in Models of Care

Our conclusion, on the basis of this brief overview, is that DM appears to be an effective approach to improving outcomes in this challenging patient group. It is important to recognize, however, that DM programs have not been uniformly effective in other patient populations.[44,45] Further, the optimal timing, intensity, and duration of DM is not yet known. The ideal patient population for DM appears to be the high-risk patient, but more data are needed to substantiate this belief.[20,21,46]

Methodologic approaches abound in the published evaluations. For example, few of these studies have used randomized controlled designs; the apparently greater benefit of the clinics over multidisciplinary teams and case management may be the result of spurious inflation of the magnitude of the impact caused by pre–post comparisons. It is believed that in most cases, the magnitude of impact will be less for a randomized controlled study when its results are compared with those obtained from a pre–post within-subjects design. However, it should be noted that two recently published studies failed to demonstrate that well-conducted observational studies overestimated treatment effects when the same interventions were tested in randomized controlled trials.[47,48] The approaches (ie, multidisciplinary team, case management, clinic) also have not been formally compared in a rigorous trial. In fact, all models of DM might be equally effective if they provide equal intensity of resources and follow-up.

A study from Weinberger and colleagues[49] supports the premise that outcomes may be a function of the intensity of the treatment provided. Medical inpatients, including heart failure patients, were randomly assigned to a control group or an intervention group that received discharge planning, a primary care physician hospital visit, and assistance with follow-up appointment scheduling before hospital discharge. After discharge, a nurse telephoned 87% of patients and spent, on average, 5.7 minutes per call. Half of the patients received an appointment reminder. This intervention, which was weak in intensity, increased rather than decreased admissions and days in the hospital compared with the control group. It should be noted that Rich[12] argues that this intervention does not fit the criteria for DM because it was not population focused and disease specific. Rather, it was aimed only at improving the structure of care delivery by increasing access.

It is difficult to compare the published studies. Each DM program currently in the literature is unique, so it is difficult to identify components that contribute to effectiveness of the care. One common thread across models seems to be the inclusion of patient education and reinforcement. Moser[11] argues that another common trait is the inclusion of care that is directed/managed or coordinated/assisted by an advanced practice nurse (ie, a clinical nurse specialist or a nurse practitioner). Contact with a health care professional is facilitated in all the DM models, and patients are encouraged to call if they detect early signs or symptoms of deterioration. In addition, many of the predominately outpatient programs include a method of bridging the inpatient and outpatient settings.[39] Clearly, our attempt to classify intervention approaches is arbitrary and open for discussion.

Differences in Patients Studied

Not only are the DM approaches different, but the patient populations studied in the various models are also quite different. For example, in the multidisciplinary model from Riegel and colleagues,[17] the mean age of the patient population served was 73 years, whereas the mean age of the patients in the Fonarow et al[39] study was 52 years. It remains unclear whether the clinic intervention of Fonarow and colleagues is superior to the multidisciplinary DM model of Riegel and colleagues[20] or if younger patients do better, regardless of the model of DM provided.

The degree of left ventricular dysfunction also varies in the studies. Some investigators have included only those heart failure patients with severely compromised systolic function,[40] whereas others[14,17,24] have included patients with both preserved left ventricular function (eg, diastolic heart failure) and those with poorly preserved systolic function. Left ventricular dysfunction may be an important factor to consider when designing DM programs for heart failure patients because mortality is known to be higher in patients with left ventricular dysfunction. Hospital admissions, however, are no different regardless of the cause of heart failure.[50] Therefore, it is reasonable to assume that patients with all levels of left ventricular dysfunction could benefit from DM if the outcome of interest is hospital admission but not if decreases in mortality are sought.

Whether other patient characteristics can be used to predict responsiveness to a DM intervention is still unknown. Riegel and colleagues[20] included any patient admitted with a primary clinical diagnosis of heart failure, regardless of ejection fraction. Six months of a multidisciplinary DM intervention demonstrated the best results in patients who were functionally compromised, had other illnesses, and were elderly. These results suggest that targeting symptomatic and/or elderly patients may yield a heart failure patient group that will benefit from DM. It has been suggested that education is more salient to patients who are symptomatic.[51] Learning principles specify that adults absorb information more readily when they perceive it as relevant to their lives.[52] Perhaps patients who are symptomatic are more ready to learn about ways to better care for themselves than patients who are not symptomatic. More research aimed at identifying the ideal patient population for specific types of DM is needed.

It should be noted that exclusion criteria greatly limit the generalizability of all the studies conducted to date. For example, Ekman and associates[38] screened 1,058 elderly heart failure patients, but only 158 (15%) met study criteria. The primary reason for exclusion was communication problems including dysphasia and disability (27%). Riegel and colleagues[20] screened 1,069 heart failure patients and excluded 829 (77%); only 23% were eligible for the study. The primary reasons for exclusion were confusion or cognitive deficits (23%), inability to communicate in English (21%), severe renal failure requiring dialysis (17%), and discharge to a long-term care facility rather than home (13%). There is a large percentage of the heart failure patient population that is not being reached by existing DM programs.

Differences in Study Methods

Another issue making it difficult to compare the published research is the diversity in data collected and the manner in which the data from each study were analyzed and reported. For example, some have compared the admission rates obtained during their intervention period to historical rates at the same institution.[21,22,26] Rich[12] notes that this process inflates estimates of treatment effectiveness because it ignores the fact that the treatment of heart failure has improved nationwide[53] since the publication of the heart failure guidelines in 1994.[54] An improvement in outcomes may simply be a reflection of better care rather than the DM intervention. Rich[12] advocates comparing the observed readmission rates with expected readmission rates (eg, Krumholz et al[55] found, in data published in 1997, that 44% of heart failure patients were readmitted annually). Only one investigative team used this approach.[18]

A better technique was used by some investigators who compared their outcomes with a concurrent[28] or matched[20] sample of similar individuals. Others used patients as their own controls and compared readmission rates before and after receipt of the intervention.[16,39–41] This technique ignores the natural history of the disease and probably underestimates the effectiveness of the treatment because an increased frequency of readmissions is expected as the disease progresses. It may also overestimate treatment effectiveness if the patients in the DM intervention were selected because they were extremely ill. In this case, we expect patients to be readmitted within the next few months, so any intervention appears beneficial in a selected patient population. Selection bias also can be introduced by differential group mortality.[56] If more patients die in the treatment group than in the control group, quality of life may look better in the treatment group because those who were most ill and feeling the worst have died. These problems can be avoided by the use of a true random sample.

A variety of unique analysis problems was identified in various studies. For example, Chapman and Torpy[16] compared outcomes from a 12-month period before treatment to those obtained during an average of 16 months after treatment. Using a longer time period for the posttreatment analysis probably underestimates treatment effectiveness by allowing more time for readmissions unless the results are prorated. Some investigators appear to have compared admissions in the pretreatment period to all-cause admissions in the follow-up period. This technique underestimates the effectiveness of their intervention because all-cause admissions are expected to be higher than the subset of admissions. Others have used unpaired *t* tests to assess a single group of subjects over time. This error can deflate findings by decreasing the precision in measurement they could have obtained by controlling the effect of individual subject differences in a paired analysis.[57]

Although the data presented in this chapter suggest that the clinic models may have better cost outcomes than other approaches, this conclusion must be tempered by study differences. Few of the studies have used similar clinical approaches, intensity has varied widely, the patient groups studied differ markedly, few investigators have analyzed their data in comparable ways, and fewer still have used research methods that control threats to internal validity (ie, randomization). No one has simultaneously compared treatments with each other. The true effectiveness of the DM models used to date remains unknown at this time.

DESIGNING A DISEASE MANAGEMENT PROGRAM

The designers of a DM program are reminded to keep the key components of DM in mind. Specifically, a good DM program focuses on a particular patient population that is costly and common (eg, heart failure, diabetes mellitus, chronic obstructive pulmonary disease). Care is individualized on the basis of patient needs and designed to accommodate the natural course of the disease and to achieve specific outcomes. The clinical program—often led by a nurse case manager—must be designed to support rather than interfere with the physician–patient relationship. The case manager must be able to maneuver the wide variety of care providers and benefit designs currently in place.[58] No effective DM program is stagnant. Rather, a continuous

quality improvement process is used to refine the program as new information is obtained.[56] This new information should be available from a versatile, accessible database containing both clinical and financial information.

Effective programs integrate the services provided, improve the structure of care delivery, provide comprehensive care, and incorporate best practices (eg, clinical guidelines) identified through the literature and the experiences of others. In an interesting mathematical analysis of the joint contributions of various DM components, Sonnenberg et al[59] documented a reduction in overall treatment success, despite the inclusion of individually successful treatment components, when aspects of the program were missed. Patient noncompliance, for example, could contribute to missing components (eg, angiotensin-converting enzyme inhibitor use). They argue for "redundancy provided by parallel subsystems" to maximize DM treatment effectiveness.

The process of setting up a DM program involves several steps (see Exhibit 16–3). First, re-

---

Exhibit 16–3 Summary of Steps Involved in Setting up a Successful Disease Management Program

1. Review organizational financial reports to identify the patient groups responsible for most of the health care resource use.
2. Assess your target patient population.
3. Decide what outcomes you want to achieve.
4. Obtain institutional commitment for the plans to develop a disease management program.
5. Coordinate meetings of the major stakeholders.
6. Learn from the experience of others.
7. Consider including case management, home care, support groups, education, and consultation with a variety of experts.
8. Plan to collect and analyze data that will allow you to evaluate your program.
9. Write a procedure manual describing the manner in which your disease management program has evolved.

view organizational financial reports listing the patient groups responsible for most admissions, visits, and/or costs for a particular time period. You will probably note that the diseases heart failure and chronic obstructive lung disease are among the 10 major reasons for hospital admission or clinic visit. When institutional and provider reimbursement were fee-for-service, there was no motivation to limit use of resources, and these patients were welcomed because they filled the beds or schedule. In areas with high managed care penetration, repeated hospital admissions and visits are not reimbursed well. When patients are readmitted within 30 days of discharge, this event is flagged by reimbursing organizations as an indicator of a potential quality problem, so minimizing this common scenario is an effective maneuver, regardless of the level of managed care penetration in your area of the country. This is the evidence that administration will require when you get to step four in the process.

Second, assess your target population. Know the typical age, race, socioeconomic status, ethnic and cultural characteristics of your patients. For example, if you work at a rural hospital on an American Indian reservation, your DM program will look different from one instituted at an urban heart transplant referral center. A common error has been to build a DM model around the traditional clinic when the patient population to be served is elderly and does not drive. Such patients will be difficult to access with the frequency and intensity that a good DM program needs. Ekman et al[38] found that the need for home assistance was the major predictor of failure to seek care. Having identified reasons such as this in your patient population, interventions can be designed to address these specific problems.

Third, decide what you want to affect in addition to improved patient quality of life, reduced hospitalizations, and/or emergency department visits. Explore the causes of poor outcomes. For example, two of the reasons for hospitalization identified by Vinson and colleagues[60] were inadequate social support and failure of the patient to seek medical attention. Bennett and colleagues[61] identified patient compliance as a major factor in

hospital readmission. If you know the factors that are problematic for your patients or the reasons why they are being readmitted, you can design your interventions around those factors and measure your processes of care and your outcomes.

Fourth, obtain institutional commitment for the planned DM program. This commitment is essential to the viability of the program during the early stages when the return on investment is low. The initial planning will require that staff be able to attend meetings and training sessions. If management is not committed to the program, key individuals will not be given the time to attend meetings and progress will be slowed. Financial resources may also be needed if you are required to pay for consultation with the organizers of other successful DM programs or if published resources must be purchased.

Fifth, coordinate meetings of those individuals with a stake in the program (eg, cardiologists, primary care physicians, inpatient dietary, social work, pharmacy and/or nursing staff, outpatient services such as home care, cardiac rehabilitation, financial representatives). If you have individuals dedicated to maintaining clinical databases and/or conducting clinical research at your organization, involve those persons early in the process so that systems are set in place to obtain and evaluate outcome data on your program. Some key stakeholders will not be able to attend meetings, so other methods of communication and soliciting input are essential. Consider sending letters to all the physicians, writing an article for internal publications, attending meetings where you are given the opportunity to give a short update on your efforts to design and implement a DM program. Make sure that no one is embarrassed by a lack of awareness of your efforts. That embarrassment may make that individual unsupportive or even vindictive at the expense of your efforts.

At this point it is realistic to warn the reader that physician resistance to organized DM programs is common. A recent Request for Proposals from the Health Care Financing Administration (HCFA) of the Department of Health and Human Services noted that organizers of DM projects have experienced low levels of physician enthusiasm.[62] This has also been our experience. The resistance appears to derive from a basic distrust of organized systems of care, a phenomenon that is not surprising considering recent changes in physician reimbursement and esteem from society. Another source of resistance is a misconception that care provided by others (ie, a case manager or a multidisciplinary team) will deteriorate into a dramatic increase in home care visits, physician telephone calls, and burden. For this reason, we strongly recommend that a physician champion on the planning team be asked to represent the program to her or his colleagues. The choice of this individual is key; she or he must be someone with good communication skills, enthusiasm for the effort, time to commit to the project, and the respect of colleagues. Honesty with the physicians about what the program is and what it is not and specific information about the time expected of the physician to make the program a success is essential. Listening to potential concerns of the physicians is helpful in problem solving and in assuaging their concerns.

Sixth in the process of beginning a DM program is to learn from the experience of others. If there is a successful DM program in your area, call someone there and ask if you can visit the program, attend meetings, and learn from their experiences. Search the published literature for descriptions of successful DM programs. Study descriptions of the natural course of the disease (ie, disease etiology, common unstable periods, expected length of life, usual age groups). Is your patient population different in any way? Design your program to be sensitive to your specific patient population, as well as the disease. For example, requiring frequent clinic visits of an elderly, ill patient population may be unrealistic and doomed to failure unless you have systems in place to transport patients who are unable to drive. Be open-minded to all descriptions of best practices, knowing that the solution you decide on for your institution will be uniquely suited to the particular strengths and weaknesses of your setting. No two snowflakes are exactly the same. Bring the information on best practices to the group meetings and discuss which

ideas might work best. Try various options and let the program evolve naturally, keeping the organizational mission and specific requirements from administration, stakeholders, and physicians in mind for direction. It is essential to monitor the program so that if there are pieces that are not working they can be identified and changed.

In our experience, communication is the key to a successful DM program. The heart failure disease management program at Sharp HealthCare in San Diego, California, was launched in January 1996 after about 18 months of planning. We were personally and institutionally new at DM, and the initial steps of the process, as described earlier, required more time than anticipated. Also, our search for grant funding for a formal evaluation of the program delayed initiation of the program for a year. Once we received a commitment of grant funding, we moved forward rapidly into the planning and implementation phases. Communication has been key to our progress. The clinical DM team continued to meet every 2 weeks for more than 2 years to monitor the program, plan patient activities, and solve problems. We spent the first 2 months just trying to refine communication systems so that we could notify each other rapidly when we learned of a heart failure patient admission (ie, pager, e-mail, facsimile). San Diego is an advanced managed care market, and patients are typically discharged from the hospital quite rapidly. Currently, we continue to write articles for internal publications, attend physician and administration meetings to discuss our progress and outcomes, and present at internal and external forums (eg, inservices, administrative meetings, quality symposia, research conferences). The clinical staff members continue to meet monthly.

Seventh, the actual process of care you put in place will be unique, but common themes include many of the following: case management by telephone after discharge (ie, telemanagement), home care, support groups, newsletters, education in a variety of forms, and consultation with a variety of experts (eg, dietitian, exercise physiologist, pharmacist, gerontologist, social worker, discharge planner). Interesting lessons were learned from prior unsuccessful DM programs and noted in the HCFA Request for Proposals.[63] These lessons included the need for:

- A focused intervention that is based on careful consideration of the problem to be addressed, the content to be taught, and the necessary frequency of contact based on differing levels of illness severity.
- Expertise in case management. Sufficient training and continuing education are essential, especially when working with a complex diagnosis such as heart failure.

Although the stakeholders may need to see financial outcomes and patient benefit, the clinical team implementing the program will be pleased to focus on clinical practice. This result, combined with the satisfaction gained from collaboration and team bonding, provided much of the enthusiasm that has kept the Sharp HealthCare multidisciplinary team motivated over time.

Eighth, data are essential to allow you to continually evaluate your program. Outcomes commonly monitored include health care resource use such as admissions and days in the hospital and office visits. These data are available from financial databases and, ideally, should be severity adjusted. If you have a clinical database, it should contain information that will allow you to track complications and perhaps adherence to care standards (eg, angiotensin-converting enzyme inhibitor therapy). This information is most useful as a covariate in outcome analyses along with severity of illness. That is, if you see changes in health care resource use, you will want to ask whether such changes were a function of your DM program, widespread changes in pharmaceutical therapy caused by the availability of a new medication, or regional changes in managed care and reimbursement patterns. Some clinical databases include information on variables such as functional status, an important outcome in heart failure.

Quality of life is another outcome variable that is frequently monitored by outcomes researchers. This information is rarely collected routinely, although it probably should be because it is useful in accreditation and national benchmarking efforts. You will probably need to put systems in place to obtain this information directly from patients. Our experience has been that verbal self-report (ie, interview) yields better data than that obtained by sending mailed questionnaires. This is probably related to patient age, lack of experience with questionnaires in the elderly population, subject burden caused by illness, low literacy rates among the US population, and poor comprehension among individuals who speak English as a second language.

Patient satisfaction is also commonly measured as an outcome of DM programs. It is advisable to collect data on this variable for the reasons cited earlier, as well as marketing efforts within the institution. Patient satisfaction is a common outcome measure in large organizations, so systems may be in place to capture this outcome. It is important to ensure that the instruments used to collect these data are sufficiently sensitive and appropriately focused to detect changes in your patient population from your DM program. For example, many patient satisfaction surveys ask about satisfaction with food, equipment functioning (eg, the television), and staff politeness. These are not outcomes that will change as a result of your DM program.

Physician satisfaction is another important outcome measure. If you have planned your DM program to assist and support the physician, his or her satisfaction should increase. If, however, you have pitted the patient or the case manager against the physician, you will see the result in your physician satisfaction surveys. Remember that DM is a process and therefore is not stagnant. You will want to use the results of your outcome measures to monitor your program and continuously improve it.

Ninth, after you get your program developed, write it down so that others can follow it if the program leaders leave or shift their focus of responsibility. Having done this, it will probably be useful when someone else hears about your program and wants to replicate it.

Final words of advice are drawn from a recent health care business publication describing models of care for cardiovascular disease.[64] The leaders of DM programs across the United States were interviewed to obtain their descriptions of best practices for cardiovascular patients. At the end of each interview, the interviewees were asked to give "Words of Advice." This sage advice is summarized here:

- Advance planning is important.
- Be inclusive; if others want to participate, include them and their contributions.
- Don't wait for the "perfect" time to begin your program.
- Don't spread yourself too thin; there are probably a handful of clinical areas where you can make an impact.
- The best clinical practice will be the best business practice. Administrators with long-term success in mind rather than short-term financial goals will spend money on prevention and education to avoid spending money later on treatment.
- Do not give up if your DM program does not flow smoothly initially. Find another way. Make a commitment to stay the course of the process.
- Think of DM as a partnership with the provider or plan. Agree on performance measures and sharing of data.
- Build collaborative relationships with the patients, caregivers, and physicians. The goal is for the patients and caregivers to become managing partners in their own health care.

REFERENCES

1. Bernard S. Disease management: Pharmaceutical industry perspective. *Pharmacy Executive.* 1995:48–50.

2. Serzner S, Miyaji M, Jeffords J. Congestive heart failure disease management study: A patient education intervention. *Congestive Heart Failure.* 1998;4:23–28.

3. Shah NB, Der E, Ruggerio C, Heidenreich PA, Massie BM. Prevention of hospitalizations for heart failure with an interactive home monitoring program. *Am Heart J.* 1998;135:373–378.

4. Bodenheimer T. Disease management—promises and pitfalls. *N Engl J Med.* 1999;340:1202–1205.

5. MacLeod GK. An overview of managed health care. In: Kongstvedt PR, ed. *The Managed Health Care Handbook.* 2nd ed. Rockville, MD: Aspen; 1993:3–11.

6. Kongstvedt PR. Controlling hospital utilization. In: Kongstvedt PR, ed. *The Managed Health Care Handbook.* 2nd ed. Rockville, MD: Aspen; 1993:102–115.

7. Kegel LM. Case management, critical pathways, and myocardial infarction. *Crit Care Nurs.* 1996;16:97–112.

8. Committee TG. The rising tide: Emergence of a new competitive standard in health care. Washington, DC: The Advisory Board Company; 1996.

9. Rhew DC, Riedinger MS, Sandhu M, Bowers C, Greengold N, Weingarten SR. A prospective, multicenter study of a pneumonia practice guideline. *Chest.* 1998;114:115–120.

10. Mehra MR. Changing climate in heart failure. *Cardiovasc Reviews Reports* 1998;4:15–22.

11. Moser DK. Expert management of heart failure: Optimal health care delivery programs. *Annu Rev Nurs Res.* 2000;18:91–126.

12. Rich MW. Heart failure disease management: A critical review. *J Card Fail.* 1999;5:64–75.

13. Rich MW, Vinson JM, Sperry JC, et al. Prevention of readmissions in elderly patients with CHF. Results of a prospective, randomized pilot study. *J Gen Intern Med.* 1993;8:585–590.

14. Rich MW, Beckham V, Wittenberg C, Leven CL, Freedland KE, Carney RM. A multidisciplinary intervention to prevent the readmission of elderly patients with congestive heart failure. *N Engl J Med.* 1995;333:1190–1195.

15. Block L, Fredericks LA, Wilker J. The design and implementation of a disease management program for congestive heart failure at a community hospital. *Congestive Heart Failure.* 1997:3:22–37.

16. Chapman DB, Torpy J. Development of a heart failure center: A medical center and cardiology practice join forces to improve care and reduce costs. *Am J Managed Care.* 1997;3:431–437.

17. Riegel B, Thomason T, Carlson B, et al. Implementation of a multidisciplinary disease management program for heart failure patients. *Congestive Heart Failure.* 1999;5:164–170.

18. Knox D, Mischke K. Implementing a congestive heart failure disease management program to decrease length of stay and cost. *J Cardiovasc Nurs.* 1999;14:55–74.

19. Gattis WA, Hasselblad V, Whellan DJ, O'Connor CM. Reduction in heart failure events by the addition of a clinical pharmacist to the heart failure management team: Results of the Pharmacist in Heart Failure Assessment Recommendation and Monitoring (PHARM) Study. *Arch Intern Med.* 1999; 159(16):1939–1945.

20. Riegel B, Carlson B, Glaser D, Hoagland P. Which heart failure patients respond best to a multidisciplinary disease management approach? *J Cardiac Fail.* In press.

21. Roglieri JL, Futterman R, McDonough KL, et al. Disease management interventions to improve outcomes in congestive heart failure. *Am J Managed Care*. 1997;3:1831–1839.

22. West J, Miller NH, Parker KM, et al. A comprehensive management system for heart failure improves clinical outcomes and reduces medical resource utilization. *Am J Cardiol*. 1997;79:58–63.

23. Tilney CK, Whiting SB, Horrar JL, Perkins BD, Vance RP, Reeves JD. Improved clinical and financial outcomes associated with a comprehensive congestive heart failure program. *Dis Management*. 1998;1:175–183.

24. Riegel B, Carlson B, Unger A, Kopp Z, LePetri B. *Effect of a Computer-Driven Nurse Case Management Telephone Intervention on Resource Use in Chronic Heart Failure Patients*. Amsterdam, Holland: European Society of Cardiology; 2000.

25. Varma S, McElnay JC, Hughes CM, Passmore AP, Varma M. Pharmaceutical care of patients with congestive heart failure: Interventions and outcomes. *Pharmacotherapy*. 1999;19:860–869.

26. Kornowski R, Zeeli D, Averbuch M, et al. Intensive home-care surveillance prevents hospitalization and improves morbidity rates among elderly patients with severe congestive heart failure. *Am Heart J*. 1995;129:762–766.

27. Stewart S, Pearson S, Horowitz JD. Effects of a home-based intervention among patients with congestive heart failure discharged from acute hospital care. *Arch Intern Med*. 1998;158:1067–1072.

28. Macko MJ. Evaluation of cost and hospitalization outcomes from a community case management program serving heart failure clients. *J Cardiac Failure*. 1998;4, 59.

29. Dennis LI, Blue CL, Stahl SM, Benge ME, Carol CJ. The relationship between hospital readmissions of Medicare beneficiaries with chronic illness and home care nursing interventions. *Home Healthcare Nurse*. 1996;14:303–309.

30. Martens KH, Mellor SD. A study of the relationship between home care services and hospital readmissions of patients with congestive heart failure. *Home Healthcare Nurse*. 1997;15:123–129.

31. Lasater M. The effect of a nurse-managed CHF clinic on patient readmission and length of stay. *Home Healthcare Nurse*. 1996;14:351–356.

32. Bandura A. Self-efficacy: Toward a unifying theory of behavioral change. *Psychol Rev*. 1977;84:191–215.

33. Bandura A. Self-efficacy mechanism in human agency. *Am Psychologist*. 1982;37:122–147.

34. Johnson JL, Budz B, Mackay M, Miller C. Evaluation of a nurse-delivered smoking cessation intervention for hospitalized patients with cardiac disease. *Heart Lung*. 1999;28:55–64.

35. Stewart S, Vandenbroek AJ, Pearson S, Horowitz JD. Prolonged beneficial effects of a home-based intervention on unplanned readmissions and mortality among patients with congestive heart failure. *Arch Intern Med*. 1999;159:257–261.

36. Cintron G, Bigas C, Linares E, Aranda JM, Hernandez E. Nurse practitioner role in a chronic congestive heart failure clinic: In-hospital time, costs, and patient satisfaction. *Heart Lung*. 1983;12:237–240.

37. Brass-Mynderse N. Disease management for chronic congestive heart failure. *J Cardiovasc Nurs*. 1996;11: 54–62.

38. Ekman I, Andersson B, Ehnforst M, Matejka G, Persson B, Fagerberg B. Feasibility of a nurse-monitored, outpatient-care programme for elderly patients with moderate-to-severe chronic heart failure. *Eur Heart J*. 1998; 19:1254–1260.

39. Fonarow GC, Stevenson LW, Walden JA, et al. Impact of a comprehensive heart failure management program on hospital readmissions and functional status of patients with advanced heart failure. *J Am Coll Cardiol*. 1997;30:725–732.

40. Hanumanthu S, Butler J, Chomsky D, Davis S, Wilson JR. Effect of a heart failure program on hospitalization frequency and exercise tolerance. *Circulation*. 1997;96:2842–2848.

41. Smith LE, Fabbri SA, Pai R, Ferry D, Heywood JT. Symptomatic improvement and reduced hospitalization for patients attending a cardiomyopathy clinic. *Clin Cardiol*. 1997;20:949–954.

42. Cline CMJ, Israelsson BYA, Willenheimer RB, Broms K, Erhardt LR. Cost effective management programme for heart failure reduces hospitalisation. *Heart*. 1998;80:442–446.

43. McAlister FA, Teo KK, Taher M, et al. Insights into the contemporary epidemiology and outpatient management of congestive heart failure. *Am Heart J*. 1999;138:87–94.

44. Bailey WC, Kohler CL, Richards JM, et al. Asthma self-management: Do patient education programs always have an impact? *Arch Intern Med*. 1999;159:2422–2428.

45. Harris LE, Luft FC, Rudy DW, Kesterson JC, Tierney WM. Effects of multidisciplinary case management in patients with chronic renal insufficiency. *Am J Med*. 1998;105:464–471.

46. Naylor MD, Brooten D, Campbell R, et al. Comprehensive discharge planning and home follow-up of hospitalized elders: A randomized clinical trial. *JAMA*. 1999;281:613–620.

47. Benson K, Hart AJ. A comparison of observational studies and randomized, controlled trials. *N Engl J Med*. 2000;342:1878–1886.

48. Concato J, Shah N, Horwitz RI. Randomized, controlled trials, observational studies, and the hierarchy of research designs. *N Engl J Med*. 2000; 342:1887–1892.

49. Weinberger M, Oddone EZ, Henderson WG for the Veterans' Affairs Cooperative Study Group on Primary Care and Hospital Readmission. Does increased access to primary care reduce hospital readmissions? *N Engl J Med*. 1996;334:1441–1447.

50. Massie BM, Shah NB. Evolving trends in the epidemiologic factors of heart failure: Rationale for preventive strategies and comprehensive disease management. *Am Heart J*. 1997;133:703–712.

51. Whitman NI. Health status. In: Boyd M, Graham BA, Gleit CJ, Whitman NI, eds. *Health Teaching in Nursing Practice: A Professional Model*. 3rd ed. Stamford, CT: Appleton & Lange; 1998:109–122.

52. Whitman NI. Age-related factors influencing selection of teaching strategies. In: Boyd M, Graham BA, Gleit CJ, Whitman NI, eds. *Health Teaching in Nursing Practice: A Professional Model*. 3rd ed. Stamford, CT: Appleton & Lange; 1998:229–252.

53. Rich MW, Brooks K, Luther P. Temporal trends in pharmacotherapy for congestive heart failure at an academic medical center: 1990–1995. *Am Heart J*. 1998;135:367–372.

54. Research AHCP. Heart failure: Evaluation and care of patients with left-ventricular systolic dysfunction. Washington, DC: National Institutes of Health; 1994.

55. Krumholz HM, Parent EM, Tu N, et al. Readmission after hospitalization for CHF among Medicare beneficiaries. *Arch Intern Med*. 1997;157:99–104.

56. Schulman KA, Mark DB, Califf RM. Outcomes and costs within a disease management program for advanced congestive heart failure. *Am Heart J*. 1998;135:S285–S292.

57. Pedhazur EJ, Schmelkin PL. *Measurement, Design, and Analysis: An Integrated Approach*. Hillsdale, NJ: Lawrence Erlbaum Associates; 1991.

58. Summers KH. Measuring and monitoring outcomes of disease management programs. *Clin Ther*. 1996;18:1341–1348.

59. Sonnenberg A, Inadomi JM, Bauerfeind P. Reliability block diagrams to model disease management. *Med Decision Making*. 1999;19:180–185.

60. Vinson JM, Rich MW, Sperry JC, Shah AS, McNamara T. Early readmission of elderly patients with CHF. *J Am Geriatr Soc*. 1990;38:1290–1295.

61. Bennett SJ, Huster GA, Baker SL, et al. Characterization of the precipitants of hospitalization for heart failure decompensation. *Am J Crit Care*. 1998;7:168–174.

62. Department of Health and Human Services. *Medicare Program: Notice for the Solicitation for Proposals for a Case Management Demonstration Project Focused on Congestive Heart Failure or Diabetes Mellitus*. Washington DC: Federal Register; 1998:1–9.

63. Health Care Financing Administration. *Medicare Program: Notice for the Solicitation for Proposals for a Case Management Demonstration Project Focused on Congestive Heart Failure or Diabetes Mellitus*. Washington, DC: Federal Register; 1998:32015–32019.

64. Anonymous. Models of care for cardiovascular disease. *Models Care*. 1998:1(3)1–28.

65. Zitter M. Disease management: a new approach to health care. *Medical Interface*. August;7:70–72 and 75–76.

66. Coons SJ. Disease management: Definitions and exploration of issues. *Clin Ther*. 1996;18:1321–1326.

67. Ellrodt G, Cook DJ, Lee J, Cho M, Hunt D, Weingarten S. Evidence-based disease management. *JAMA*. 1997;278:1687–1692.

CHAPTER 17

Community Case Management Models of Heart Failure Care

Debra K. Moser, Marlene J. Macko, F. Kevin Hackett, and Maggie Roush Hutchins

The effective, efficient management of patients with heart failure is one of the most important challenges facing clinicians and health care systems today. Patients with heart failure consume a disproportionately high percentage of the health care dollar because of repeated periods of decompensation that frequently require hospitalization. Innovative health care delivery programs, such as community case management (CCM), can offer new options that optimize the care of these individuals, improve outcomes, and are cost-effective.

Case management, as defined by the Individual Case Management Association and the Case Management Society of America, is a collaborative process in which the nurse or other health care provider "assesses, plans, implements, coordinates, monitors and evaluates options and services to meet an individual's health needs through communication and..." use of "...available resources to promote quality, cost-effective outcomes."[1] Case management can occur in a variety of settings and across settings. CCM is a distinct form of case management in which care is provided throughout the care continuum but primarily occurs in the patient's home. Thus, in contrast to hospital-based case managers, community case managers do most of their assessment, planning, and evaluation in the patient's home.

The use of CCM has increased in the United States, primarily in response to the need to effectively manage and provide services for high-risk patient populations.[2] These high-risk yet histori-cally underserved individuals are excellent targets for CCM because although they represent a minority of clients, they consume most of the health care costs. CCM programs typically provide home visits from an experienced nurse for chronically ill individuals who are at risk for repeated rehospitalizations to assist them to appropriately manage their condition. Assessments, education, support, communication with physicians, and links to appropriate community resources are components of most CCM programs. In addition, a less tangible component, the caring, long-term relationship that is formed between the case manager and the client, has been shown to be crucial in the success of CCM programs.[3]

CCM delivered to a homogeneous patient population has been demonstrated to be effective in decreasing rehospitalizations, hospital length of stay, and health care costs for patients with a variety of chronic illnesses including heart failure.[4] A growing body of evidence in heart failure indicates that other outcomes are improved substantially by the use of CCM.[5–12] The purpose of this chapter is to provide an overview of heart failure CCM programs. In addition, one successful heart failure CCM program is described in detail.

RATIONALE FOR HEART FAILURE COMMUNITY CASE MANAGEMENT

Most heart failure patients are elderly.[13–15] Elders have repeated exacerbations of heart failure and have the highest hospital admission rates of all adult patient groups.[16–18] Elders with heart failure commonly have characteristics that make them more vulnerable to repeated exacerbations of failure. These characteristics include the following: multiple comorbidities, polypharmacy, economic difficulties, social isolation or other social problems, depression and other psychologic problems, impaired functional capacity with limited mobility, and impaired sensory functions.[5,11,16,18–21] To reduce rehospitalizations and associated health care costs and improve quality of life, these characteristics must be addressed. CCM is an effective model for dealing with them, and some evidence indicates that it may be more effective than other new heart failure health care delivery models that are not home based.[19]

Home-based CCM programs may be the superior choice for managing elderly patients or younger patients with similar limitations for a number of reasons. As Ekman and associates[19] point out, the target population for specialized heart failure care may be exactly the one unable to come to outpatient heart failure clinics or other outpatient services because multiple comorbidities, impaired functional capacity, excessive fatigue, and other factors make these patients unable to seek care routinely outside the home. Home-based CCM also is useful because many problems associated with noncompliance do not emerge or are not evident until the patient returns home and are then detected best or only in the home setting.[21] Furthermore, in the home setting, problems associated with lack of social support are more evident and in addition to detecting these, the nurse providing care can be an important source of social support.[22]

Additional reasons that home-based CCM programs are appropriate for patients with heart failure include enhanced patient education and counseling effectiveness in the home setting. Traditional thinking holds that intensive education and counseling regarding the posthospital regimen for heart failure patients should be given before the patient is discharged. However, with decreasing length of hospital stay, earlier discharge of sicker patients, and inadequate personnel resources to provide other than cursory

education, this ideal is rarely realized. Subsequently, most patients do not receive adequate education and counseling about most aspects of heart failure care.[23–25]

Even when patients do receive education, the reality is that the hospital environment is not ideal for learning and retaining information.[26,27] Because of a combination of patient anxiety, poor concentration, inadequate teaching methods, and inability of patients to "practice" what they are taught, patient retention of information is uniformly poor. Physician office-based education has many of the same issues, including lack of time for adequate education. By addressing these issues, CCM programs offer several advantages.[28] First, the nurse making the home visit can obtain a realistic assessment of the patient's education, level of understanding, and other resources. Second, impediments to learning or adoption of learned material can be assessed more readily and accurately and more easily overcome. Third, family members or other caregivers are more likely to be available and receptive to education and counseling. Fourth, anxiety is decreased in the home, setting the stage for substantially better learning and recall. Fifth, the nurse making the home visit has the time and expertise to provide detailed information and to reinforce the information at later visits. Finally, difficulties getting to an office, which are particularly troublesome for elderly patients with chronic diseases, are eliminated.[19,28] This is important because to be effective, education and counseling must take place over a period of many visits.[26,27]

Following patients at home after hospital discharge offers other advantages. The time of transition from hospital to home is one of marked vulnerability for elderly patients with heart failure.[29] Once home, patients typically express considerable uncertainty about their prescribed regimen[21] and about the meaning of symptoms and frustration about perceived inaccessibility of health care providers to answer questions.[30] Emotional problems peak after discharge and are not routinely assessed or well managed in the office setting.[29] Home-based patient follow-up allows assessment and intervention for these issues in a nonthreatening environment, in which patients and their families often feel freer to express their concerns and are more open to suggestions for change.[28,29]

TESTED HEART FAILURE COMMUNITY CASE MANAGEMENT PROGRAMS

Most patients with heart failure are still treated traditionally using health care delivery models in which episodic acute care is delivered during periods of exacerbation of heart failure with little systematic follow-up. What follow-up occurs after hospital discharge usually consists of a few short physician office visits in which there is little time to address the multiple and complex medical, behavioral, psychosocial, environmental, and financial issues that complicate the care of patients with heart failure. Recognition that these aspects of traditional care delivery must be changed to improve heart failure outcomes, coupled with the increasing incidence, prevalence, and economic costs of heart failure,[31] have prompted calls for a change from our current treatment patterns to comprehensive, integrated heart failure specialty care patterns.[14]

The variety of alternative heart failure health care delivery models that have been tested can be categorized as multidisciplinary disease management programs,[32–34] outpatient heart failure clinics,[35–39] telephonic case management,[40,41] and the focus of this chapter, CCM.[6–9,11,12] Although each of the models has some components in common with CCM, the CCM programs are distinguished from the other types of programs in that care delivery is based almost entirely in the home.

The research literature on heart failure CCM programs has grown in recent years, and these programs have demonstrated a positive impact on patient and health care resource utilization outcomes.[6–9,11,12] There is considerable variability in the operationalization of CCM in the various programs. Although some CCM programs include inpatient components and increased access to health care providers, patients do not go to a clinic or other outpatient setting to receive care, rather the health care provider comes to them. Tested CCM programs are summarized in Table 17–1.

The first heart failure disease management program that can be categorized as CCM was conducted by Kornowski and associates in Israel.[6] These investigators reported outcomes from their intensive home care program in 42 elderly (57% men; mean age, 78 ± 8 years) New York Heart Association (NYHA) Class III or IV heart failure patients. In this program, an internal medicine physician and nurse conducted weekly home visits. At each visit, patients' conditions were assessed, medications were reviewed and any necessary changes made, laboratory tests were done, and intravenous diuretics were given if needed. The team was available for extra home visits if needed, and patients could call with problems. To ensure continuity, each physician was responsible for the same patients during follow-up.

To determine the impact of the intervention, hospitalizations and length of stay for the period 12 months after the intervention were compared with those 12 months before the intervention. After receiving the intervention, patients demonstrated a 62% reduction in the number of subsequent total rehospitalizations and a 77% reduction in associated hospital days. Hospitalizations for cardiovascular causes were reduced by 72% and associated hospital days by 83%. In addition, after the intervention, patients experienced a significant improvement in functional status as assessed by a physician assessment of patients' ability to perform daily activities.

Stewart and associates[7,8,12] have conducted two studies of home-based interventions in Australia. In the first, a nurse and pharmacist team provided care for 97 elderly heart failure patients (49% men; mean age, 75 years).[7] Patients were randomly assigned to either a home-based nurse–pharmacist intervention plus usual care or to usual care alone. Patients were identified for the study during their hospitalization for exacerbation of heart failure. The program consisted of an inpatient educational visit from the nurse, followed by one home visit within a week of discharge from the pharmacist and nurse. The purpose of this visit was to assess patients'

Table 17–1 Tested Heart Failure Community Case Management Programs

Reference	Patients (n; sample NYHA classification if available; sample age)	Study Design	Program and Components	Program Outcomes*
Kornowski et al, 1995	• 42; NYHA III–IV; mean age 78 ± 8 years	Within subjects' comparison of preintervention and postintervention outcomes with follow-up of 12 months	• Home care by physician and nurse • Study conducted in Israel • Weekly home visits by physician and nurse • Physical examination • Medication review • Change in medication if needed • Intravenous diuretic therapy as needed • Increased availability of physician (extra visits if needed)	• 62% reduction in total rehospitalizations with 77% reduction in hospital days • 72% reduction in cardiovascular rehospitalizations with 83% reduction in hospital days • 50% of patients never hospitalized during follow-up period • Improvement in functional status
Stewart et al, 1998	• 97; NYHA II 49%, III 43%, IV 4%; mean age 75 years	Randomized controlled trial with follow-up of 6 months	• Nurse and pharmacist home-based assessment, education, and counseling • Study conducted in Australia • Before hospital discharge, patient education and counseling from nurse about complying with treatment regimen and reporting signs of worsening heart failure • Home visit 1 week after hospital discharge by nurse and pharmacist • Pharmacist assessed knowledge about medications and extent of compliance • For those with low knowledge or compliance, remedial counseling, daily medication reminders, medication box given, incremental monitoring by caregivers, medication information and cards, referral to community pharmacist for more regular review • Nurse assessed signs of clinical deterioration and adverse drug effects	• 42% fewer unplanned admissions • 43% fewer hospital days

continues

Table 17–1 continued

Reference	Patients (n; sample NYHA classification if available; sample age)	Study Design	Program and Components	Program Outcomes*
Stewart et al, 1999	• 97; NYHA II 49%, III 43%, IV 4%; mean age 75 years	Randomized controlled trial, follow-up of Stewart et al, 1998 at 18 months	• Nurse and pharmacist home-based assessment, education, and counseling • Study conducted in Australia • Pre-hospital patient education and counseling from nurse about complying with treatment regimen and reporting signs of worsening heart failure • Home visit 1 week after hospital discharge by nurse and pharmacist • Pharmacist assessed knowledge about medications and extent of compliance • For those with low knowledge or compliance, remedial counseling, daily medication reminders, medication box given, incremental monitoring by caregivers, medication information and cards, referral to community pharmacist for more regular review • Nurse assessed signs of clinical deterioration and adverse drug effects	• Fewer unplanned readmissions • Lower length of hospital stay • Fewer out-of-hospital deaths • Lower hospital costs

continues

Table 17–1 continued

Reference	Patients (n; sample NYHA classification if available; sample age)	Study Design	Program and Components	Program Outcomes*
Macko 1998	• 80; mean age 70 ± 13 years	Intervention group compared to usual care group (not randomly assigned) after 6 months' follow-up	• Nurse home-based assessment, education, and counseling • Study conducted in the United States • Comprehensive education and counseling about pharmacologic and nonpharmacologic therapy • Behavioral strategies to improve compliance • Frequent long-term follow-up in the home • Patient access to health care providers as needed • Attention to social, environmental, financial, behavioral problems • Coordination of social and health care services	• 50% fewer heart failure admissions in intervention group • Fewer multiple heart failure admissions in intervention group • Hospitalization costs 50% lower (even after cost of the intervention) in the intervention group
Naylor et al, 1999	• 363 (60 heart failure); mean age 75 years	Randomized controlled trial with 6 months' follow-up	• Comprehensive discharge planning and home follow-up from advanced practice nurses • Study conducted in the United States • Program designed specifically for elders at risk for poor outcomes after discharge • Sample not limited to heart failure patients and included those with other common medical and surgical problems • Individualized patient management with physician collaboration • Assessments and individualized intervention to assist patients and caregivers to problem solve	• Intervention group less likely to be readmitted than control group (37.1% vs 20.3%) • Fewer intervention group patients had multiple admissions • Time to first readmission was longer in the intervention group • Total Medicare reimbursements in intervention group were one half those of control group • No differences in functional status, depression, or patient satisfaction • Intervention effective in heart failure patients but less so than in other patient groups *continues*

Table 17–1 continued

Reference	Patients (n; sample NYHA classification if available; sample age)	Study Design	Program and Components	Program Outcomes*
Stewart et al, 1999	• 200; NYHA class II 45%; III 45%; IV 10%; mean age 76 years	Randomized controlled trial with 6 months' follow-up	• Nurse home-based assessment and education and counseling • Study conducted in Australia • Structured home visit 7–14 days after discharge • Assessment of patient compliance and understanding of regimen • Strategies to improve compliance • Communication with physician • Flexible diuretic regimen prescription is appropriate • Access to nurse for subsequent problems	• 40% reduction in number of primary end points (unplanned readmission plus out-of-hospital death) in intervention group compared with usual care • More intervention group patients remained event free • Lower total hospital-based costs in the intervention versus usual care group • Improved quality of life across follow-up in both groups with greater improvement at 3 months in intervention vs usual care groups

*Results are statistically significant unless otherwise indicated.
NYHA, New York Heart Association functional class.

knowledge of their medication regimen, compliance with that regimen (by pill count), and to evaluate patients' physical status. Patients who had poor knowledge or poor compliance received further counseling, a daily reminder routine, pillbox that contained 1 week's medications, incremental monitoring by caregivers, medication information and reminder card, and referral to a community pharmacist for additional attention. The nurse–pharmacist team collaborated with patients' primary physicians and gave them an update on their patients' status after the home visit. After 6 months of follow-up and compared with the usual care group, patients in the intervention group experienced 42% fewer hospitalizations and hospital days and had lower hospital costs, although the latter did not reach statistical significance.

Many studies of newer heart failure health care delivery methods include relatively short-term follow-ups of 6 months or less. To determine the long-term impact of the intervention described previously,[7] Stewart and associates[8] extended follow-up of the original cohort for a total of 18 months. After 18-months follow-up, patients in the intervention group experienced fewer out-of-hospital deaths and unplanned readmissions and required fewer days of hospitalization and emergency department (ED) visits than usual care patients. As a result, the cost of hospital care was significantly lower for patients in the intervention group, even taking into account the cost of the home-based intervention.

In the second study by Stewart and associates,[12] a randomized controlled trial was again used. An intervention similar to the one described previously was tested in a different cohort of 200 heart failure patients (62% men; mean age, 76 years). In contrast to the first intervention tested by this group, this intervention was delivered by the nurse and not a nurse–pharmacist team. In addition, several important outcomes were added. After 6 months' follow-up, significantly more intervention-than-usual-care patients remained event-free, 40% fewer primary end points (readmissions and out-of-hospital deaths) occurred in the intervention group, and hospital costs were lower by nearly half in

the intervention group. Quality of life improved in both groups over time, although it improved more quickly in the intervention group.

In a study of the impact of discharge planning and home care delivered by advanced practice nurses, Naylor and associates[11] randomly assigned 363 patients with common medical or surgical problems, including heart failure ($n = 60$), to one of two groups, a control or intervention group. To be included in the study, patients needed to exhibit at least one of several criteria that are associated with poorer outcomes after hospital discharge: age 80 or older, inadequate social support available, active, chronic comorbidities, history of depression, functional disability, multiple hospitalizations in prior 6 months, hospitalization within prior 30 days, history of noncompliance, or fair to poor self-perception of own health. The mean age of patients enrolled was 75 years, there were equal numbers of women and men enrolled, and the sample was ethnically diverse. The intervention consisted of comprehensive discharge planning and home follow-up designed specially to address problems of high-risk elders. On the basis of patient, family/caregiver, and environmental assessments an individualized plan for education and counseling, validation of learning, and coordination of home services was developed. Both patients and family/caregivers were targeted for intervention. On discharge, all patients were visited within 48 hours and again at 7 to 10 days after discharge by the advanced practice nurse. The number of home visits was not limited, and visits were scheduled on the basis of individual patient and family needs.

Outcomes that were tracked in the study included readmissions, time to first admission, costs, functional status, depression, and patient satisfaction. After 6 months, patients in the intervention had significantly fewer rehospitalizations, longer time to first readmission, and decreased costs of care compared with the control group. No differences were found between the intervention and usual care groups in functional status, depression, or patient satisfaction. Although effective in heart failure patients, the intervention was not as powerful in those patients as it was in patients without heart failure. This finding highlights the increased vulnerability of heart failure patients after hospital discharge.

A final example of CCM in its classic form is the study by Macko[9] of a program started at a Midwest community hospital in the early 1990s to address the high rehospitalization rates and unreimbursed costs seen for heart failure patients. This program demonstrated positive outcomes similar to those seen for the previous programs and is described in the following section.

AN IN-DEPTH VIEW AND OUTCOMES OF ONE HEART FAILURE COMMUNITY CASE MANAGEMENT PROGRAM

Program Development and Implementation

At Mount Carmel Health in Columbus, Ohio, CCM is used as an approach to optimization of the care of four groups of patients at risk for repeated rehospitalizations or high health care resource utilization: diabetes, renal failure, chronic lung diseases, and heart failure. The first community nurse case manager for heart failure was hired in November 1993. The impetus for this was the disturbing health care system heart failure statistics. Readmission rates and length of stay for heart failure patients were high, and the health care system was losing money on each heart failure admission. Therefore, the community nurse case manager for heart failure was hired to work within the system to develop a CCM program that would decrease the number of readmissions for heart failure. The steps taken to implement the Mount Carmel CCM program are appropriate steps for any institution working to develop a similar program.

The first step to setting up the CCM program was a review of the current literature on CCM programs. At the time this program was set up, there were no published examples of heart failure CCM programs on which to pattern the program. Although not a heart failure CCM program, the St. Mary's Carondelet Community Case Management program, in Tucson, Arizona, was very successful and well represented in the literature.[4,42] As a result, the Mount Carmel CCM program was patterned after the Carondelet program by alteration of their general guidelines to meet local needs.

In preparing to establish the heart failure CCM program, the community nurse case manager underwent an extensive 6-week orientation process. The purpose of this orientation was to enhance the nurse's existing expertise in heart failure by adding orientation experiences in community nursing. In starting the program and in subsequent years as new nurses were hired, it was believed that it was more important to begin with a nurse with heart failure expertise and to supplement this vital clinical expertise with community nursing skills. Thus, during orientation, the community nurse case manager received education on community services and resources and clinical experience with home care, hospice, and social work teams. Time with home care and hospice gave the nurse opportunities to learn useful practices needed in the CCM of patients with heart failure. It also allowed the nurse to learn the policies of the different areas and to ease client transfer between the areas. Orientation with social workers was critical for the community nurse case manager to learn about the multitude of community resources available. It also helped the nurse to make needed contacts with local social workers who could provide assistance with complex patient situations.

Also stressed in the community nurse case manager's orientation was development of expert assessment skills. In addition, the nurse spent time with physicians from each of the major cardiology groups in the health system. This promoted physician acceptance of the program, as well as assisted in development of an understanding of specific physician practices. The community nurse case manager used this time with physicians to work with them to sharpen cardiovascular assessment skills, such as heart tone auscultation and jugular vein distention evaluation. It is a philosophy of the Mount Carmel CCM program that because assessment is such a vital component of CCM, the community nurse case manager's assessment skills should be at the expert level. Furthermore, because the physician would be unable, in most cases, to confirm the nurse's assessment and would be making therapy changes on the basis of that assessment, he or she needed confidence in the nurse's ability. If physicians did not trust the nurse's assessments, they would be unlikely to make the appropriate treatment changes to alter a potentially adverse outcome for the client.

Another important component of the nurse's orientation was development of communication skills. The community nurse case manager must be able to communicate effectively with people from varying backgrounds, including ethnically diverse patients and family members, individuals with varying levels of literacy, other nurses, social workers, pharmacists, and physicians. Classes and conferences on communication skills were therefore included in the orientation process.

At the same time the community nurse case manager was gaining the necessary expertise for heart failure CCM, policies and documentation procedures were developed. Admission criteria for the program were set up and included the following: (1) diagnosis of heart failure; (2) two or more hospital admissions for heart failure in the previous year; (3) not receiving other nursing services, such as home care or hospice; and (4) live within a 30-minute drive of either of the two community hospitals. This last criterion was included to allow more efficient use of the community nurse case manager's time because initially this program included only one nurse. During the review of the literature, it was found that confusion and duplication of services could occur if more than one nursing service provided care; therefore, the restriction about other nursing services was included.

The Program

The Mount Carmel CCM program has been active for more than 6 years. Several more case managers have been hired since the program's inception. Experience with the needs of CCM patients has reinforced the need to provide extensive orientation for community nurse case managers that focuses on provision of commu-

nity nursing skills and builds on existing cardiovascular nursing expertise (Exhibit 17–1). A typical caseload for each community nurse case manager is 35 to 40 active patients with an additional portfolio of inactive patients who may call for assistance or questions at any time and some of whom may be on the schedule for calls from the nurse. Currently, community nurse case managers are paid by the institution and services are not reimbursed by third-party payers. The estimated cost of the program is an average of $80.00 per visit, based on the nurse's salary, mileage, materials, and cellular phone charges.

One goal of the CCM program is to improve continuity. To this end, the community nurse case manager identifies patients during a hospitalization, visits them while they are still hospitalized, prepares them for discharge, and then provides care in the home after discharge. Patients are referred to the program directly from physicians, hospital social workers, and registered nurses during the patient's hospitalization or occasionally as outpatients from physician of-

---

Exhibit 17–1 Recommended Skills and Training for Heart Failure Community Nurse Case Managers

- Registered nurse with at least 3–5 years of cardiovascular nursing experience and preferably cardiac critical care nursing experience
- Orientation to community and social services
- Education about latest heart failure innovations, pharmacologic and nonpharmacologic care, evaluation of literature for utilization of research innovations, and best practices for patient and family/caregiver education and counseling
- Advanced physical assessment training
- Time with cardiologists to learn practice patterns and learn and demonstrate assessment skills
- Orientation regarding legal issues related to delivering care in home
- Orientation with experienced, successful community nurse case manager

fices. To facilitate referral of appropriate patients, the community nurse case manager periodically meets with and sends letters to these groups of health care providers to update them about the program and its impact. Once in the heart failure CCM program, although patients receive care primarily from the community nurse case manager, they remain under the care of their primary physicians and any specialist physicians.

The CCM program follows recommendations of consensus guidelines for the nonpharmacologic management of heart failure.[43–46] In addition, the program addresses the common reasons for heart failure rehospitalizations (eg, noncompliance with medication or diet and sodium overload, inadequate discharge follow-up, failed social support systems, and failure to obtain medical assistance when symptoms increase). Because family and/or caregiver support is thought to be fundamental to patient compliance, the program is targeted to both patients and their families or caregivers.

In the heart failure CCM program, the community nurse case manager provides in-home patient assessment, social and environmental evaluation, evaluation of wishes and counseling regarding resuscitation and advance directives, patient and family member/caregiver education and counseling, a link to other health care providers as needed, access to appropriate community services, long-term follow-up, and emotional support to clients. Nursing care is guided by the use of care maps, which are based on the NYHA's functional class. They were designed to be a flexible guideline, not an unbending rule for care delivery. Focused, intensive education and counseling are a major focus of the heart failure CCM program, and specific education components included in the program are outlined in Exhibit 17–2.

Because noncompliance with drug therapy is a major contributor to exacerbations of failure, multiple tactics are used to assist patients to comply with the prescribed plan. Some factors associated with higher risk of hospitalization caused by noncompliance include poor recall of the medical regimen, greater number of medica-

Exhibit 17–2 Patient and Family/Caregiver Education and Counseling Components of the Mount Carmel Community Case Management Program

- Education about the prescribed pharmacologic medications prescribed and clarification of entire prescribed pharmacologic regimen including what to do with old medications and previously prescribed medications dosages, reasons for each, common possible side effects and what to do about them, importance of following the regimen
- Dietary sodium restriction
- Alcohol and fluid restriction (if indicated)
- Self-assessment and early recognition of symptoms heralding an increase or exacerbation of failure and appropriate response
- Daily weight instruction and what to do about weight changes
- Activity recommendations and strategies to meet patient activity goals
- Promotion of strategies to enhance patient problem solving
- Promotion of strategies to enhance compliance to recommended therapy
- Individual goal setting and plan development for achieving goals
- How to effectively communicate with health care providers to become effective partners in care

tions prescribed, and concerns over medication costs.[21,47] Thus strategies to address these are used in the program and include written schedules and use of pillboxes that contain boxes for multiple doses each day. The community nurse case manager provides each patient with a pillbox and instructions on how to fill it. The nurse also assists patients with financial concerns that impede compliance with drug therapy to secure lower-cost medications through appropriate programs. In addition, a medication schedule is worked out with the patient and family that has the least adverse effect on sleep and daily activities.[48]

Similarly, because dietary sodium indiscretion is common, multiple tactics to improve compliance are used.[49,50] Patients' existing eating habits are taken into account as the nurse assists the patient to adapt preferred foods. Plans are developed to help patients eat out or to assist them to make appropriate choices when eating convenience foods that are usually very high in sodium content.

Other components of the program that enhance compliance are ability of patients to ask frequent questions of the nurse in a low-stress environment and the knowledge that they have access to a health-care professional who can assist them with problem solving.[51] A major strength of the program is that it promotes patient problem-solving and self-management skills. Another strength of the program is that it is individualized, based on patient and family needs. The community nurse case manager assists patients to determine their barriers to compliance or adoption of changes and works with them to overcome these.[41,52]

The community nurse case manager provides patients with a booklet called "Living with Heart Failure"[53] that discusses in simple, understandable language the symptoms of heart failure; symptoms indicating a need for action; typical heart failure drugs, effects, any side effects to watch for, and the importance of following the prescribed regimen; importance of the low-sodium diet and how to follow one; and activity recommendations. In addition, patients receive a booklet, "How to Eat a Low Sodium Diet," with detailed material on the sodium content of a large variety of foods, including packaged, prepared, restaurant, and fast food. Both of these booklets reinforce teaching by the nurse and enhance retention of material.

Initially, the community nurse case manager visits patients in their homes from one to three times a week depending on the client's needs. The first visit always occurs within 1 to 3 days of hospital discharge. The first visit occurs so early after discharge because the early postdischarge days are a time of high vulnerability for patients. Even though they may have received explicit discharge instructions, once home even 1 day, many patients do not understand the specifics of their treatment plan including how and which

medications to take, what diet to follow, what symptoms to watch for, how to monitor weights, and when to next visit their physician.[21] However, to avoid overwhelming the patient, limited material is covered in the first visit. Instead, the community nurse case manager concentrates on developing the seeds of a long-term trusting relationship. In addition, the nurse focuses on medication teaching and ensuring that patients understand their medication regimen. The community nurse case manager concentrates on medications during this initial visit based on data from the CCM program that 38% of patients do not take their medications as prescribed immediately on returning home even though they have written discharge instructions. These data are further supported by published data demonstrating that the incidence of medication noncompliance and inadequate medication knowledge are extremely high in patients just released from a hospitalization despite medication education before discharge.[21] In this initial and all subsequent visits, the principles of flexibility and dependence on individual patient needs guide the community nurse case manager's approach.

Although the schedule for visits and content to be covered is flexible depending on patient need, the following basic schedule adequately serves most patients. As described earlier, all patients are visited within 1 to 3 days of hospital discharge. Some patients will receive a second visit if necessary the first week or two after discharge. Patients then receive weekly visits for the next month, biweekly visits for the following month, monthly visits for the next 2 months for particularly high-risk patients, and then a monthly call for the next 2 months. A typical patient schedule for a high-risk patient with content is presented in Table 17–2. However, on average, patients do well with seven or less visits and phone follow-up as needed.

The community nurse case manager is available by beeper 7 days a week from 8:00 AM to 8:00 PM. If an emergency situation occurs at another time, the client is instructed to call the emergency squad, their physician, or a nurse hotline that is sponsored by the corporate system. The client is advised to assess the severity

Table 17–2 Content of Mount Carmel Heart Failure Community Case Management Program

Contact	Content
Visit 1	• Patient and home assessment with appropriate referrals to community services (eg, "Meals on Wheels") as needed • Assess patient and family understanding of condition and treatment • Elicit patient and family concerns and provide support • Medication review and strategies to increase compliance • Important symptoms and what to do about them • Daily weights teaching • Give "Living with Heart Failure" booklet
Visit 2	• Patient and home assessment • Ask about problems or questions/assist with problem solving • Determine patient goals • Review previous information • Review patient daily weights since last visit • Begin 2-g sodium diet teaching and give "How To Eat a Low Sodium Diet" booklet • Medication review
Visit 3	• Patient assessment • Ask about problems or questions/assist with problem solving • As appropriate, discuss wishes regarding resuscitation and advance directives • Continue diet teaching and explore strategies for success • Discuss activity issues (including sexual activity) and exercise goals • Review weights, symptoms, and medications
Visit 4	• Patient assessment • Ask about problems or questions/assist with problem solving • Discuss diet, activity issues, and, if needed, guidelines for alcohol use • Review weights, symptoms, and medications
Visit 5	• Patient assessment • Ask about problems or questions/assist with problem solving • Discuss common patient and family emotional issues • Discuss influenza and pneumococcal vaccination recommendations • Review weights, symptoms, and medications
Visit 6	• Patient assessment • Ask about problems or questions/assist with problem solving • Review weights, symptoms, and medications
Visit 7	• Patient assessment • Ask about problems or questions/assist with problem solving • Assess progress toward activity, diet, and other goals • Review weights, symptoms, and medications
Visit 8	• Patient assessment • Ask about problems or questions/assist with problem solving • Review weights, symptoms, and medications

continues

Table 17–2 continued

Contact	Content
Visit 9	• Patient assessment • Ask about problems or questions/assist with problem solving • Review weights, symptoms, and medications
Call 1	• Review weights, symptoms, medications • Ask about questions or other concerns • Ask about compliance with medications, diet, other life-style changes
Call 2	• Review weights, symptoms, medications • Ask about questions or other concerns • Ask about compliance with medications, diet, other life-style changes

of his or her symptoms to determine where the call should be placed.

Program Outcomes

A variety of outcome measures are used to evaluate the program on an ongoing basis. The number of hospital readmissions for heart failure and all causes, length of stay, and total costs for admissions are measured every 6 months, as are the number of ED visits and associated costs. Over the 6 years that the program has been in place, our outcomes have remained positive. At each 6-month evaluation, hospital readmissions for heart failure are reduced by 70% to 80% compared with a comparable period before the patient was enrolled in CCM. Total costs for hospital readmissions are reduced by 50% to 60%. ED visits and associated costs also have been consistently reduced. Patient and physician satisfaction is measured on a yearly basis using mailed surveys. Patients and physicians consistently rate their satisfaction with the program as very high.

In addition to the routine 6-month outcome measures, the original community nurse case manager completed a study in which the impact of the program on 1-year rehospitalization rates and costs was examined.[9] Patients eligible for the study were those who had two or more hospitalizations for heart failure in the prior 12 months; were discharged home; were not receiv-

ing home care, hospice care, or cardiac rehabilitation; and who lived within a 30-minute drive of either hospital. For the study, 80 patients (40% women; mean age, 70 ± 13 years; mean left ventricular ejection fraction 30% ± 15%) were recruited from two community hospitals in the Mount Carmel system in central Ohio; 34 served as a control group and received usual care, and 46 received usual care plus CCM.

No differences were found in baseline sociodemographic or clinical (including age; discharge medications, including use of angiotensin-converting enzyme inhibitors, diuretics, digoxin or β-blockers; cardiology consult; NYHA class; ejection fraction; cause of heart failure; or number of previous heart failure admissions) characteristics between the two groups. Compared with control group patients, patients who received the CCM program had significantly fewer rehospitalizations for heart failure and for all other causes. In the intervention group, 22% of patients were admitted with heart failure during follow-up versus 44% in the control group ($p < 0.05$), and there were fewer multiple heart failure admissions in the intervention group ($p < 0.05$). Hospitalization costs for the CCM program group also were significantly lower by 50% ($p < 0.05$) than those for the control group, even after the costs of the program (materials, nurses' salaries, travel costs, phone costs) were included.

Summary and Critique

In each of these studies the CCM approach tested produced positive outcomes. Patients receiving care in CCM programs experienced significantly fewer total and heart failure rehospitalizations, fewer hospital days when hospitalized, improved quality of life, and lower health care costs. Most studies falling under the category of CCM are randomized controlled trials.[7,8,11–12] Only one study in this group was a preintervention, postintervention comparison.[6] This strengthens the credibility of the conclusion that CCM programs do reduce significantly rehospitalizations and associated costs and allows us to draw realistic conclusions about the magnitude of impact that one can expect from them.

Generalizability, a problem in the heart failure disease management literature in general,[54] was relatively good in this group of studies. All these studies enrolled women and most of them enrolled nearly equal numbers of men and women (range, 40% to 50% women). The mean age of patients in this group of studies was greater than 70 years, more closely reflecting the true demographic of heart failure in the community than many studies. There was considerable ethnic diversity among the patients enrolled in this group of studies, particularly the study by Naylor and associates[11]; however, generalizability of findings to patients in the United States may be limited in the studies conducted in Israel[6] and Australia.[7,8,12] Although all studies excluded heart failure patients who were sent to nursing homes or other institutions after hospital discharge and who were cognitively impaired, enrollment of patients who might not be able to come to a clinic or other outpatient setting considerably increases generalizability because these patients more accurately reflect the reality of heart failure in the community.

Translating the results of CCM research into practice given the realities of heart failure in the community is challenging. Another factor that contributes to this difficulty is determining which of the many different components used in each of the CCM programs is essential to make the program successful. Compounding this difficulty is the lack of studies comparing the effectiveness of each of the components. There was considerable diversity in this group of programs, although each one has components that clearly are identifiable as CCM. Lacking appropriate comparisons, it seems prudent at this time to examine each of the studies for common components that likely contribute to the program's success. Common components among the approaches include the following: (1) comprehensive care that always included patient follow-up in the home; (2) collaborative care that was nonetheless largely under the direction of a nurse; (3) optimization of medical therapy and/or attention to improving compliance to prescribed medications; (4) increased patient access to health care providers; and (5) vigilant patient follow-up.

Pitfalls of CCM and Other Considerations

Program Costs

Although CCM programs demonstrate positive outcomes, any balanced presentation of CCM should include discussion of the pitfalls and potential problems associated with CCM. One major concern is the cost of these programs. Although a direct cost comparison has never been done, CCM programs are probably the most costly of the specialty heart failure disease management strategies because nurses usually manage smaller caseloads than is possible in the other models of care. For example, the per patient cost for the Mount Carmel program is approximately twice the cost per patient of Riegel and associates'[53] multidisciplinary disease management program of $330.00. Although these costs are offset by savings of health care resource utilization dollars related to decreased hospital readmissions,[9,11,12] these savings are rarely directly returned to the department in which the CCM program is housed because of budgeting patterns in many institutions. Thus, CCM programs are often perceived as being very expensive by their parent institutions. Further compounding this problem is difficulty securing reimbursement for CCM services. Changing federal policy regarding reimbursement of advanced practice nurses and the approval of proposals, by some insurance companies, from institutions for reimbursement that document the cost-effectiveness of their program may begin to resolve this issue.

Appropriate Patient Referral

CCM is not appropriate for all heart failure patients. Given the personnel and time commitment for CCM, it seems practical to limit CCM services to those patients at higher risk for rehospitalizations. On the basis of the eligibility requirements of the CCM studies reviewed, higher risk can be operationalized as presence of one or more of the following: older age, presence of multiple comorbidities, one or more hospitalizations in the previous 6 to 12 months for heart failure or multiple hospitalizations for any reason, lack of or inadequate social support, moderate–severe functional impairment, history of noncompliance, or depression.

Building Patient Independence

CCM is usually characterized by multiple home visits at which the nurse attempts to form a trusting relationship in which the patient feels free to seek advice and counseling. Ultimately the nurse works to empower the patient to take an active role in his or her own care. Sometimes, however, this relationship can degenerate into one in which the patient becomes dependent on the nurse. Nurses can inadvertently foster such dependence by encouraging the patient to call with every problem and by solving problems for patients without teaching them how to problem solve. A related problem is potential difficulty making the decision to discharge the patient from active service and to stop home visits. When a long-term relationship develops between patient and nurse, it is sometimes quite difficult to terminate the relationship. However, moving the patient to inactive status should be viewed in a positive light and communicated as such to the patient, thus moving the patient to a higher level of independence and self-responsibility for management of his or her own condition.

At the other end of the spectrum are problems with patients who refuse services because they do not want health care providers to come into their homes. Although the number of patients who actually refuse services for this reason is relatively small (less than 10% in the Mount Carmel system), it is a consideration in setting up a CCM program.

CCM vs Home Health Care

One question that arises on examination of CCM programs and the nurses who manage patients within them is how these programs and nurses are different from home health care services and home health nurses. Some argue that there is no need to develop CCM programs when heart failure patients who need home services could simply be referred to existing home health services. Several points argue against this stance, and explanation of them demonstrates the distinct differences between CCM and home health.

For home health nurses, the number of visits allowed for a given patient is regulated by third-party payers, whereas nurses operating in heart failure CCM or home-based programs are not bound by such regulations and can independently determine the number of visits needed by a patient.[11] Home health nurses are usually generalists with bachelor's degrees, whereas most CCM managers are specialists with master's degrees. Most home health nurses do not have the time for extended interventions and do not have the expertise related to heart failure pharmacologic and nonpharmacologic therapy or behavioral strategies to improve compliance. Home health nurses usually interact less with patients' physicians and other health care providers. As a consequence, the interventions used by CCM nurses are generally more individualized and characterized by a greater degree of heart failure–specific clinical expertise, communication and counseling proficiency, and collaboration with other health care providers.[11]

Home health services also are limited by regulatory guidelines to patients who are homebound with so-called skilled nursing needs such as dressing changes or intravenous therapy. Specialized education and counseling does not fall under the rubric of "skilled" nursing needs, and thus many heart failure patients are not eligible for home health services. Unlike CCM nurses, home health nurses do not perform discharge planning nor visit their patients when they are hospitalized. Home health nurses generally do not follow patients after their discharge from home health services, whereas many CCM programs continue follow-up of their inactive patients.

Although a few chart audit studies of home health services have demonstrated improved outcomes for heart failure patients as a result of home health services, these studies were retrospective in nature and lacked adequate controls.[55,56] There are no direct comparison studies of patient outcomes between home health care and CCM. However in Naylor and associates' study[11] of comprehensive discharge planning and home follow-up, outcomes were compared between patients who received home visits from visiting nurses versus those who received home visits from the intervention advanced practice nurses. One in two patients in the usual care group who were visited by visiting nurses were rehospitalized, whereas only one in five patients in the intervention group visited by advanced practice nurses were rehospitalized. These data demonstrate that it is not the home visit alone that improves outcomes, but rather the specialized content and focus of the visit.

CONCLUSION

CCM has been criticized by some as too expensive, too labor intensive, and too complex to be of practical value in optimal patient management. However, complex problems sometimes require complex solutions. Existing evidence suggests that when applied to appropriate high-risk patient populations notable for disproportionately high health care resource utilization, CCM is cost-efficient and effective.[6–9,11,12,57] The lack of studies comparing different heart failure health care delivery models makes it impossible to determine at this time whether CCM is more or less effective than other models such as heart failure clinics, multidisciplinary disease management, or telephonic case management. Investigators are challenged to compare these approaches in the future.

REFERENCES

1. Case Management Society of America. CMSA proposes standards of practice. *Case Manager*. 1994;5:60–75.

2. Lamb G. Conceptual and methodological issues in nurse case management research. *Adv Nurs Sci*. 1992;15(2):16–24.

3. Newman MA. Theory of the nurse–client partnership. In: Cohen CL, ed. *Nurse Case Management in the 21st Century*. St. Louis, MO: Mosby; 1996.

4. Ethridge P. A nursing HMO: Carondelet St. Mary's experience. *Nurs Manag*. 1991;22(7):22–27.

5. Rich MW. Heart failure disease management: A critical review. *J Card Fail*. 1999;5:64–75.

6. Kornowski R, Zeeli D, Averbuch M, et al. Intensive home-care surveillance prevents hospitalization and improves morbidity rates among elderly patients with severe congestive heart failure. *Am Heart J*. 1995;129:762–766.

7. Stewart S, Pearson S, Horowitz JD. Effects of a home-based intervention among patients with congestive heart failure discharged from acute hospital care. *Arch Intern Med*. 1998;158:1067–1072.

8. Stewart S, Vandenbroek AJ, Pearson S, Horowitz JD. Prolonged beneficial effects of a home-based intervention on unplanned readmissions and mortality among patients with congestive heart failure. *Arch Intern Med*. 1999;159:257–261.

9. Macko MJ. Evaluation of cost and hospitalization outcomes from a community case management program serving heart failure clients. *J Card Fail*. 1998;4:59.

10. Boling PA. The value of targeted case management during transitional care. *JAMA*. 1999;281:656–657.

11. Naylor MD, Brooten D, Campbell R, et al. Comprehensive discharge planning and home follow-up of hospitalized elders. *JAMA*. 1999;281:613–620.

12. Stewart S, Marley JE, Horowitz JD. Effects of a multidisciplinary, home-based intervention on unplanned readmission and survival among patients with chronic congestive heart failure: a randomized controlled study. *Lancet*. 1999;354:1077–1083.

13. American Heart Association. *Heart and Stroke 2000 Statistical Update*. Dallas, TX: AHA; 1999.

14. O'Connell JB, Bristow MR. Economic impact of heart failure in the United States: Time for a different approach. *J Heart Lung Transplant.* 1993;13:S107–S112.

15. Haldeman GA, Croft JB, Giles Wh, Rashidee A. Hospitalization of patients with heart failure: National Hospital Discharge Survey, 1985–1995. *Am Heart J.* 1999;137:352–360.

16. Vinson JM, Rich MW, Sperry JC, et al. Early readmission of elderly patients with congestive heart failure. *J Am Geriatr Soc.* 1990;38:1290–1295.

17. Lenfant C. Report of the task force on research in heart failure. *Circulation.* 1994;90:1118–1123.

18. Happ MB, Naylor MD, Roe-Prior P. Factors contributing to rehospitalization for elderly patients with heart failure. *J Cardiovasc Nurs.* 1997;11(4):75–84.

19. Ekman I, Andersson B, Ehnfors M, Matejka G, Persson B, Fagerberg B. Feasibility of a nurse-monitored, outpatient programme for elderly patients with moderate-to-severe, chronic heart failure. *Eur Heart J.* 1998;19:1254–1260.

20. Jaarsma T. Readmission of older heart failure patients. *Prog Cardiovasc Nurs.* 1996;11:15–20,48.

21. Stewart S, Pearson S. Uncovering a multitude of sins: medication management in the home post acute hospitalisation among the chronically ill. *Aust N Z J Med.* 1999;29:220–227.

22. Moser DK. Social support and cardiac recovery. *J Cardiovasc Nurs.* 1994;9(1):27–36.

23. Krumholz HM, Wang Y, Parent EM, Mockalis J, Petrillo M, Radford MJ. Quality of care for elderly patients hospitalized with heart failure. *Arch Intern Med.* 1997;157:2242–2247.

24. McDermott MM, Feinglass J, Lee P, et al. Heart failure between 1986 and 1994: Temporal trends in drug-prescribing practices, hospital admissions, and survival at an academic medical center. *Am Heart J.* 1997;134: 901–909.

25. Ashton CM, Kuykendall DH, Johnson ML, Wray NP, Wu L. The association between the quality of inpatient care and early readmission. *Ann Intern Med.* 1995;122:415–421.

26. Cimprich B. A perspective on attention and patient education. *J Adv Nurs.* 1992;14:39–51.

27. Oberst MT. Perspectives on research in patient teaching. *Nurs Clinic North Am.* 1989;24:621–627.

28. Anderson MA, Pena RA, Helms LB. Home care utilization by congestive heart failure patients. *Public Health Nurs.* 1998;15:146–162.

29. Lough MA. Ongoing work of older adults at home after hospital. *J Adv Nurs.* 1996;23:804–809.

30. Moser DK., Dracup KA, Marsden C. Needs of recovering cardiac patients and their spouses: Compared views. *Int J Nurs Studies.* 1993;30:105–114.

31. Croft JB, Giles WH, Pollard RA, Casper ML, Anda RF, Livengood JR. National trends in the initial hospitalization for heart failure. *J Am Geriatr Soc.* 1997;45:227–275.

32. Rich MW, Beckham V, Wittenberg C, Leven CL, Freedland KE, Carney RM. A multidisciplinary intervention to prevent readmission of elderly patients with congestive heart failure. *N Engl J Med.* 1995;333:1190–1195.

33. Rich MW, Vinson JM, Sperry JC, et al. Prevention of readmission in elderly patients with congestive heart failure: Results of a prospective, randomized pilot study. *J Gen Intern Med.* 1993;8:585–590.

34. Riegel B, Carlson B, Glaser S, Hoaglund P. Which heart failure patients respond best to a multidisciplinary disease management approach. *J Cardiol Fail.* In press.

35. Cintron G, Bigas C, Linares E, Aranda JM, Hernandez E. Nurse practitioner role in a chronic congestive heart failure clinic: In-hospital time, costs, and patient satisfaction. *Heart Lung.* 1983;12:237–240.

36. Fonarow GG, Stevenson LW, Walden JA, et al. Impact of a comprehensive heart failure management program on hospital readmission and functional status of patients with advanced heart failure. *J Am Coll Cardiol.* 1997;30:725–732.

37. Hanumanthu S, Butler J, Chomsky D, Davis S, Wilson JR. Effects of a heart failure program on hospitalization frequency and exercise tolerance. *Circulation.* 1997;96:2842–2848.

38. Cline CMJ, Israelsson BYA, Willenheimer RB, Broms K, Erhardt LR. Cost effective management programme for heart failure reduces rehospitalisation. *Heart.* 1998;80:442–446.

39. Smith LE, Fabbri SA, Pai R, Ferry D, Heywood JT. Symptomatic improvement and reduced hospitalization for patients attending a cardiomyopathy clinic. *Clin Cardiol.* 1997;20:949–954.

40. West JA, Miller NH, Parker KM, et al. A comprehensive management system for heart failure improves clinical outcomes and reduces medical resources. *Am J Cardiol.* 1997;79:58–63.

41. Shah NB, Der E, Ruggerio C, Heidenreich PA, Massie BM. Prevention of hospitalizations for heart failure with an interactive home monitoring program. *Am Heart J.* 1998;135:373–378.

42. Michaels C. Carondelet St. Mary's nursing enterprise. *Nurs Clin North Am.* 1992;27(1):77–85.

43. American College of Cardiology/American Heart Association Task Force on Practice Guidelines. Guidelines for the evaluation and management of heart failure. *Circulation.* 1995;92:2764–2784.

44. Konstam M, Dracup K, Baker D, et al. *Heart Failure: Evaluation and Care of Patients with Left-Ventricular Systolic Dysfunction.* Clinical Practice Guideline No.

11. AHCPR Publication No. 94–0612. Rockville, MD: Agency for Health Care Policy and Research, Public Health Services, U.S. Department of Health and Human Services; 1994.

45. Packer M, Cohn JN on behalf of the Steering Committee and Membership of the Advisory Council to Improve Outcomes Nationwide in Heart Failure. Consensus recommendations for the management of chronic heart failure. *Am J Cardiol.* 1999;83:2A–38A.

46. Heart Failure Society of America. Heart Failure Society of America (HFSA) practice guidelines. HFSA Guidelines for the management of patients with heart failure due to left ventricular systolic dysfunction—pharmacological approaches. *J Card Fail.* 1999;5:357–382.

47. Col A, Fanale JE, Kronholm P. The role of medication noncompliance and adverse drug reactions in hospitalizations of the elderly. *Arch Intern Med.* 1990;150:841–845.

48. Dracup K, Baker DW, Dunbar SB, et al. Management of heart failure. II. Counseling, education, and lifestyle modification. *JAMA.* 1994;272:1442–1446.

49. Dunbar SB, Jacobson LH, Deaton C. Heart failure: strategies to enhance patient self-management. *AACN Clin Issues Crit Care.* 1998;9:244–256.

50. Wagner EH, Austin BT, VonKorff M. Organizing care for patients with chronic illness. *Milbank Q.* 1996;74:511–543.

51. DiMatteo MR, Sherbourne CD, Hays RD, et al. Physicians' characteristics influence patients' adherence to medical treatment: results from the medical outcomes study. *Health Psychol.* 1993;12(2):93–99.

52. Bennett SJ, Milgron LB, Champion V, Huster GA. Beliefs about medication and dietary compliance in people with heart failure: an instrument development study. *Heart Lung.* 1997;26:273–279.

53. Riegel B, Thomason T, Carlson B, et al. Implementation of a multidisciplinary disease management program for heart failure patients. *Congestive Heart Failure.* 1999;5:164–170.

54. Moser DK. Expert management of heart failure: optimal health care delivery programs. *Ann Rev Nurs Res.* 2000;18:91–126.

55. Martens KH, Mellor SD A study of the relationship between home care services and hospital readmission of patients with congestive heart failure. *Home Healthcare Nurse.* 1997;15:123–129.

56. Dennis LI, Blue CL, Stahl SM, Benge ME, Shaw CJ. The relationship between hospital readmissions of Medicare beneficiaries with chronic illnesses and home care nursing interventions. *Home Healthcare Nurse.* 1996;14:303–309.

57. Rich MW, Nease RF. Cost-effectiveness analysis in clinical practice. The case of heart failure. *Arch Intern Med.* 1999;159:1690–1700.

CHAPTER 18

The Clinic Model of Heart Failure Care

Gregg C. Fonarow, Julie Walden Creaser, and Nancy Livingston

Heart failure is a major health care problem that consumes significant medical and financial resources. Heart failure is the most common and expensive discharge diagnosis among hospitalized patients age 65 years and older.[1–4] Declining quality of life is an almost universal phenomenon in these patients. In 1995, epidemiologic data revealed that heart failure as a primary or secondary diagnosis accounted for nearly 2.5 million hospital admissions per year in the United States.[5] With alarming hospitalization rates, declining quality of life, significant morbidity, and high mortality rates among patients with heart failure, it has become obvious that there are opportunities for improvements in the inpatient and outpatient management of heart failure.

Care for patients with chronic heart failure ideally integrates inpatient and outpatient health care delivery with the goal of reducing symptoms, improving functional capacity, decreasing the need for hospitalization, and prolonging life. There is, however, marked variation in the management of patients with heart failure.[6,7] Many overburdened primary care and cardiology practices have not fully integrated the treatment recommendations from randomized clinical trials and practice guidelines into routine clinical practice. Lack of familiarity with medications and doses for heart failure or concern regarding potential side effects may lead to underutilization of beneficial therapies such as angiotensin-converting enzyme (ACE) inhibitors, β-blockers, and aldosterone antagonists.

Education of patients and family members regarding nonpharmacologic therapies such as diet and exercise requires staff time, commitment, and expertise. Close tracking of relevant clinical and laboratory data by health care providers may not be practical except for groups of patients with similar diagnoses. Concentrated heart failure programs provide more focused care that could improve patient outcome and decrease hospitalizations, thus decreasing costs.

On the basis of early reports of success with heart failure clinics, there is a growing recognition of the role these programs can play in improving the management of patients with heart failure. In 1994, the Cardiology Preeminence Roundtable published results of an assessment of heart failure patient management.[8] The Roundtable suggested strategies to reduce total health care costs and hospital readmissions for patients with heart failure. A primary recommendation for improvement was the development of a heart failure clinic model that integrates care directed by advanced practice nurses and physicians.

The general aims of heart failure programs are to successfully influence clinical outcomes such as rehospitalization rates, patients' functional status, quality of life, patient satisfaction, and medical costs. Heart failure clinics are well suited to meet these aims. There are several components of heart failure clinics frequently highlighted as being important to improving outcomes, including:

- Optimization of medical therapy
- A flexible diuretic regimen
- Heart failure education for both inpatients and outpatients
- Hospital discharge planning
- Increased outpatient access to health care professionals
- Long-term follow-up of patients[5]

Probably the most distinctive and unique components in this model of care are optimization of the medication regimen and flexible diuretic dosing, so these aspects are described in some detail later in this chapter.

Recently a number of heart failure programs centered around the heart failure clinic model have developed with slightly different management emphasis, outcome focus, and utilization of health care team members.[9–16] These programs are summarized in Table 18–1. This chapter will review the key components of a heart failure clinic, typical patient management and educational approaches, and the impact that such programs can have on heart failure patient outcomes.

COMPONENTS OF A HEART FAILURE CLINIC

Heart failure clinics are organized in a variety of ways. Some of the most successful clinics are organized as a combination of a clinic and a multidisciplinary team approach. This combination of approaches makes it challenging to distinguish outcomes that are attributable to the various components of care. In the clinic model, cardiologists with expertise in heart failure evaluate and manage patients in conjunction with advanced practice nurses. The advanced practice nurses may have training as either clinical nurse specialists or nurse practitioners. If a multidisciplinary team is not involved, the advanced practice nurse provides patient education, dietary counseling, social support assessment, review of medications, exercise counseling, discharge planning, and ongoing assessment of clinical stability.[15] Other programs that combine the clinic model with a multidisciplinary approach incorporate dietitians, pharma-

cists, and medical social workers to provide these functions or augment the services provided by the advanced practice nurses. Some programs provide home health nursing or refer to outside home nursing agencies.

Many heart failure clinic programs are designed to encounter patients when they are first hospitalized with heart failure. An initial hospitalization for heart failure presents opportunities to begin optimization of medical therapy and provide intensive patient education. The readmission rate for heart failure has been reported to be as high as 28% to 52% within 90 days.[17,18] Deficiencies in heart failure inpatient care as defined by explicit process criteria are associated with higher rehospitalization rates and increased death rates after hospital discharge.[19] Members of the heart failure clinic, specifically the advanced practice nurse, can work in conjunction with inpatient physicians and nurses to develop pathways to expedite patient care and begin the education process.

The transition from inpatient hospitalization to outpatient management is a critical period where medication errors frequently are made. Educating patients as to how their medical regimen has been altered during hospitalization poses a challenge, especially if left to busy hospital staff. The heart failure advanced practice nurse can provide this education in a comprehensive fashion by reviewing what new medications are now in the regimen and creating a simplified medication schedule for the patient. Involving the heart failure clinic team members in the inpatient setting improves continuity of care and creates a situation that should minimize medication errors and improves care, because these health care providers will be the ones following and tracking patients on an outpatient basis.

Heart failure clinics may be hospital or outpatient practice based with regard to their organizational and financial structure. Many heart failure clinics have developed in conjunction with heart transplantation programs or were organized to conduct research and clinical trials in heart failure management.[5] The components that are integrated into the heart failure clinic are illustrated below with an overview of the process of patient evaluation, management, and education.

Table 18–1 Studies of Heart Failure Clinic Programs

Reference	Sample	Study Design	Intervention	Components of Intervention	Outcomes*
Cintron et al, 1983[9]	• *n* = 15, NYHA III–IV, mean age 65 years • Puerto Rico	Within subjects preintervention, postintervention comparison	Heart failure clinic staffed with nurse practitioners	• Nurse practitioner managed • Frequent follow-up by clinic visits • Education reinforced at each visit: medication, weight control, diet • Assessment of home situation • Family support • Increased availability of nurse practitioner ("walk-ins" encouraged) • Cardiologist consultation for unstable patients	• 60% reduction in rehospitalizations • 85% reduction in hospital days • Reduction in total medical costs of $8009 per patient
Lasater, 1996[10]	• *n* = 41 • United States	Within subjects preintervention, postintervention comparison	Heart failure clinic staffed by advanced practice nurses	• Four weekly visits with an experienced hospital staff nurse • Direct access to physician consultation, social worker, dietitian • Patient education regarding diuretic regimen and importance of daily weights • Scales provided as needed • Diuretics adjusted on basis at physical assessment • Medication compliance monitored • Assistance with financial constraints	• 4% decrease in readmission rate • Mean hospital length of stay decreased 1.6 days • Increased knowledge of medical regimen demonstrated at 1 yr
Hanumanthu et al, 1997[11]	• *n* = 134, NYHA not indicated, mean age 52 ± 12 yr	Within subjects preintervention, postintervention comparison	Physician-directed, nurse-coordinated comprehensive heart failure clinic	• Heart failure/transplant physician-directed • Nurse coordinators assisted with inpatient and outpatient management • Team exclusively managed heart failure patients • Optimization of medical therapy • Periodic meetings with home health care agency and hospice program to integrate care	• 53% reduction in annual hospitalization rate • 63% reduction in heart failure rehospitalizations • Increased peak V_{O_2}

continues

Table 18–1 continued

Reference	Sample	Study Design	Intervention	Components of Intervention	Outcomes*
Fonarow et al, 1997[16]	• n = 214, NYHA III and IV, mean age 52 ± 10 years • United States	Within subjects preintervention, postintervention comparison	Heart failure cardiologist directed, advanced practice nurse, follow-up, comprehensive inpatient and outpatient management program	• Heart failure cardiologist directed • Follow-up by heart failure cardiologist, advanced practice nurse, and referring physician • Optimization of drug therapy in hospital and during follow-up • Comprehensive patient and family/caregiver education by heart failure clinical nurse specialist about daily weights and flexible diuretic regimen, diet, medications, smoking and alcohol abstinence, home exercise instruction, warning signs of worsening heart failure, and prognosis • Weekly follow-up at heart failure clinic until stable with education reinforced • Phone follow-up after medication changes and if indicated	• 89% reduction in rehospitalizations • Improvement in functional status • Lower costs
Smith et al, 1997[12]	• n = 21, mean NYHA 2.6 ± 0.5, mean age 61 years • United States	Within subjects preintervention, postintervention comparison	Physician or nurse practitioner comprehensive care in heart failure clinic	• Care provided by physician or nurse practitioner • Optimization of medical therapy • Identification and management of etiology of heart failure • Patient education about diet, medications, compliance, daily weights and flexible diuretic regimen, alcohol abstinence • Nurse practitioner available by phone • Increased access to clinic (without appointment) for worsening symptoms or medication needs	• 86% reduction in heart failure hospitalizations • Improved quality of life • Improved functional status • More patients on optimal medications and doses

continues

Table 18–1 continued

Reference	Sample	Study Design	Intervention	Components of Intervention	Outcomes*
Cline et al, 1998[13]	• *n* = 190, Mean NYHA 2.6 ± 0.7, mean age 75.6 ± 5.3 years • Sweden	Randomized control trial	Nurse-directed outpatient clinic	• Before hospital discharge, patient and family education about heart failure and pharmacologic and nonpharmacologic aspects of its treatment • Medication organizer given • Patients receive guidelines for self-management of diuretics • One-hour information visits for patient and family at home after discharge • Easy access to a nurse-directed outpatient clinic with one prescheduled visit at 8 months; nurses available by phone and could see patients at short notice • Encouragement to contact nurses at clinic for any problems or questions or concerns	• Time to first admission 33% longer in intervention group • 59% increase in number of days hospitalized compared to 12-month period before start of study in control group versus no increase in intervention group • 36% fewer hospitalizations in intervention group (but nonsignificant at *p* = .08) • Trend toward mean annual reduction in health care costs (*p* = .07)
Paul, 2000[14]	• *n* = 15 • Mean age 62 years • United States	Within subjects preintervention, postintervention comparison	Nurse coordinated multidisciplinary team in an outpatient heart failure clinic	• Patients seen by a cardiologist, advanced practice nurse, and clinical pharmacist at each visit • Access to a dietitian and social worker if needed • Increased access to advanced practice nurse (walk-ins) • Advanced practice nurse telephoned regularly to assess patient status, reinforce teaching, and change medications • Intravenous diuretics administered in clinic by the advanced practice nurse	• Hospital admissions decreased (mean 2.4/patient to 1.3/patient) • Hospital days decreased (10.1 days/patient to 5.1 days/patient) • Mean length of stay, hospital charges, number of emergency medical center visits decreased but failed to reach statistical significance

continues

Table 18–1 continued

Reference	Sample	Study Design	Intervention	Components of Intervention	Outcomes*
Dahl & Penque, 2000[15]	• *n* = 1,192 nonrandomized patients (583 before program, 609 after program initiated) • Pretreatment group mean age 72 years • Posttreatment group mean age 75 years • United States	Posttest only design with nonequivalent groups	Advanced practice nurse-directed inpatient heart failure program	• Advanced practice nurse-coordinated inpatient care • Intensive patient education • Heart failure medical orders reviewed with primary physician in reference to clinical guidelines • Multidisciplinary services as needed • Home health care plan • High-risk patients telephoned after discharge	• 36% reduction in hospital deaths • Increased ACE inhibitor use • Decreased 90 day heart failure readmission rates (14.6% to 8.4%) • Shorter length of hospital stay (6.1 days to 5.3 days/patient)

*Results are statistically significant unless otherwise indicated.
ACE, angiotensin-converting enzyme; NYHA, New York Heart Association functional class

HEART FAILURE PATIENT EVALUATION

Patients referred to a heart failure clinic usually undergo a detailed evaluation. Both the cardiologist and advanced practice nurse obtain a comprehensive history and review available medical records. The goal is to define the cause of the patient's heart failure, identify contributing causes and comorbidities, review treatments and responses, and define the patients' current physiologic state. Physical examination by the cardiologist together with the advanced practice nurse takes place on the initial visit and each subsequent visit with close assessment of volume status and documentation of physical findings. Diagnostic testing is reviewed and the need for further testing assessed. Evaluation of left ventricular function by echocardiography is indicated, if it has not yet been performed or assessed in the prior year. Functional status is not only assessed by self-report, but frequently by cardiopulmonary exercise testing or the 6-minute walk test. The physician–advanced practice nurse team also evaluates the patient's understanding of his or her disease and compliance history with medications, diet, and fluids. An important part of the evaluation is to determine whether there is a reversible cause of heart failure, such as coronary artery disease with significant ischemia and/or hibernating myocardium or uncorrected valvular heart disease. Such patients could potentially benefit from surgical therapies such as revascularization or valve replacement. For patients with severe symptoms and/or a high risk of mortality, heart transplantation is considered.

Each patient is assessed for risk of sudden death. Patients undergo 24-hour Holter monitoring to screen for significant ventricular arrhythmias. Those with a history of syncope, history of malignant ventricular arrhythmia, or ischemic cardiomyopathy and left ventricular ejection fraction (LVEF) < 0.35 with nonsustained ventricular tachycardia, are referred for electrophysiologic testing. Patients with prior history of cardiac arrest, sustained ventricular tachycardia, syncope, or who are inducible on electrophysiologic testing are treated with an implantable cardioverter-defibrillator, unless contraindications exist.

After initial assessment, the cardiologist and advanced practice nurse devise a medical and nonpharmacologic treatment plan collaboratively. Patients receive detailed information regarding the nature and severity of their disease, warning signs of worsened heart failure, medications and potential side effects, and the short-term and long-term follow-up plans. Arrangements are made for further testing, additional patient education, and medical follow-up. The assessment and treatment plans are also communicated to other physicians who may be involved in the patient's care.

HEART FAILURE PATIENT MANAGEMENT

Heart failure clinics have the potential to improve the use and dosing of beneficial medical therapies. There is marked practice variation in the management of patients with heart failure.[6,7] This variation is often the result of a failure of clinicians to incorporate the advances in clinical management that are supported by clinical trials. Despite several multicenter randomized trials demonstrating that the use of ACE inhibitors reduces hospitalizations, improves functional status, and prolongs life in patients with heart failure, ACE inhibitors are prescribed for less than half the patients with symptomatic heart failure in many practice settings.[20] Additional therapies for heart failure such as β-blockers and aldosterone antagonists are slow to be integrated into the care of patients in conventional practice settings.[21] Calcium channel blockers are not indicated but continue to be prescribed.

A standardized approach to pharmacologic therapy for patients with heart failure may improve patient outcomes if it results in greater use of beneficial therapies available and reduces use of therapies that are detrimental. Heart failure clinics frequently incorporate such a standardized approach. Evidence-based heart failure therapies are initiated as described in detail in heart failure clinical guidelines.[22] Treatment regimens are updated when new information from clinical trials becomes available. There is a greater focus on ensuring initiation of evidence-based therapies; researchers have documented increased use of therapies such as ACE inhibitors and β-blockers in heart failure clinics.[5] The advanced practice nurse and/or pharmacist are available to discuss the indications and potential side effects of these medications with patients and their family members.

Many heart failure medications require titration over time and careful monitoring of patients' clinical responses. ACE inhibitors are initiated at lower starting doses, and the dose is titrated upward over time. Monitoring of serum potassium, BUN, and creatinine during initiation and titration of heart failure medications allows early identification of potential abnormalities before they are manifested clinically. β-Blockers are initiated at low doses in stabilized patients with New York Heart Association (NYHA) Class II to IV heart failure, with up-titration occurring at 2- to 4-week intervals.[21] Patients may require three to five titration steps before target doses are achieved. To enhance the safety of initiation of β-adrenergic blocking therapy, patients are closely monitored for signs of volume overload and bradycardia.[21] During initiation of the aldosterone antagonist, spironolactone, in patients with NYHA Class II to IV heart failure, adjustment of other diuretic dosing and potassium supplementation may be necessary. In addition, patients will require close monitoring of renal function and serum potassium levels.

Heart failure centers are organized to track closely patients' medications and dosing regimens, thus facilitating the titration of multiple medications and ensuring appropriate laboratory testing. Medications that can result in complications or that can worsen outcome in patients with heart failure such as nonsteroidal anti-inflammatory disease agents (NSAIDs) can be avoided.[21] Potential drug interactions, for example the effect of amiodarone on digoxin levels, may more readily be recognized and addressed prospectively by the heart failure clinic team.

Tracking patients' symptoms, functional status, weights, medications, compliance, labora-

tory monitoring, and diagnostic tests poses a major challenge. Conventional clinical practices are rarely organized to provide this type of monitoring. Heart failure clinics use a variety of tracking methods to closely follow patients. For example, specialized tracking sheets and computerized monitoring programs can track patients' weights, NYHA functional class, medications and doses, diagnostic parameters such as LVEF, degree of mitral regurgitation, left ventricular end diastolic dimension, and laboratory values (ie, serum sodium, potassium, BUN, and creatinine). These tracking programs make trends easy to follow, and significant changes can be readily identified. With close monitoring, changes in a patient's condition can be identified early and alterations in management made *before* the patient has deteriorated to the point of requiring hospitalization.

Patients with heart failure and atrial fibrillation, left ventricular thrombus, or prior systemic embolization require systemic anticoagulation, unless contraindications exist.[23] The advanced practice nurse, following standardized protocols, can monitor anticoagulation status quite effectively.[23] Approximately two thirds of patients with heart failure also have coronary artery disease, and many of these patients would benefit from lipid management and other secondary prevention measures.[24] Many studies have shown lipid-lowering medications are underused in conventional practice settings, with only 10%–20% of patients with coronary artery disease at goal for low-density lipoprotein (LDL) cholesterol.[20] With initiation and titration of lipid-lowering medications, most patients can achieve National Cholesterol Education Program goals of an LDL cholesterol of <100 mg/dL.

THE UCLA HEART FAILURE PROGRAM EXPERIENCE

The concentrated care and expertise typically found in a heart failure clinic improves subjective outcomes, decreases hospitalizations, and decreases total medical costs. One of the first organized heart failure clinics began at the University of California, Los Angeles (UCLA) Medical Center. At UCLA, the comprehensive heart failure management program incorporates a systematic approach to drug therapy; extensive patient education about diet, exercise, self-monitoring with weights, and the flexible diuretic regimen; and regular contact between the patient and the heart failure team. Patients are evaluated and managed by a heart failure specialty cardiologist in conjunction with advanced practice nurses who have specialized heart failure training.

Patients referred to the UCLA heart failure clinic are initially assessed for possible eligibility for transplantation, including right heart catheterization to determine pulmonary pressures. Patients with a pulmonary artery wedge pressure >20 mm Hg or cardiac index < 2.2 L/min-m^2 have the catheter left in place for further vasodilator and diuretic therapy. Nitroprusside is frequently used as the initial therapy, as described previously in transplant candidates.[25] Medications are adjusted to achieve a pulmonary artery wedge pressure of 15 mm Hg and systemic vascular resistance of 1,000 to 1,200 dynes-sec-cm^{-5}, while maintaining systolic blood pressure of 80 mm Hg. Unless patients develop acute decompensation, hemodynamic monitoring is performed in an intermediate "step-down" unit with a lower nursing ratio and daily cost than standard intensive care unit beds. Oral ACE inhibitors are initiated or reinitiated and titrated to match the hemodynamics achieved on intravenous therapy or to "target" doses. Oral nitrates such as isosorbide dinitrate are added if filling pressures remained elevated on the ACE inhibitor or for angina.[26] Hydralazine is used in a small percentage of patients, in whom additional vasodilation appears to be needed or in whom the ACE inhibitor is not tolerated.

Patients are followed by the heart failure cardiologist and advanced practice nurse in conjunction with their referring physician(s). Phone calls are made by the advanced practice nurses within 3 days of hospital discharge and weekly thereafter during the initial month after discharge and less often after stability is demonstrated. Patients are seen twice a month at the heart failure center until criteria for clinical stability are met.[27] During those visits, patients are interviewed regarding symptoms and examined for any signs of fluid retention. The patient education program, described later, is reinforced during each visit, and the weight charts and exercise program are carefully reviewed by the advanced practice nurse and cardiologist. Diuretic regimens are adjusted for frequent weight gain or physical examination signs of volume overload or when postural hypotension or low jugular venous pressure suggests excessive diuresis. The ACE inhibitor doses prescribed at discharge typically are well tolerated and rarely require adjustment either for symptomatic hypotension or for changes in renal function.

At 6 months, patients undergo detailed reassessment with review of all hospitalizations, determination of NYHA class, and repeat cardiopulmonary exercise testing. Patients previously put on the transplant list who demonstrate a major improvement in exercise performance, defined as an increase in peak oxygen uptake 2 mL/kg/min to 12 mL/kg/min and who also meet criteria for clinical stability, are taken off the transplant list.[28]

The regimen of loop diuretics is adjusted to achieve and then maintain the patient's daily weight to within 2 pounds of the weight at which optimal hemodynamics were achieved. Metolazone is added if necessary but in general is reserved for intermittent use. Digoxin is continued in all patients who previously have been receiving digoxin and initiated in patients without relative contraindications such as conduction system disease or fluctuating renal dysfunction. First-generation calcium channel blockers are discontinued as are nonsteroidal anti-inflammatory agents. Anticoagulation with warfarin is prescribed for patients with atrial fibrillation, previous embolic events, or a mobile intracardiac thrombus observed on echocardiogram.[23] Patients with atrial fibrillation or high-grade nonsustained ventricular tachycardia receive low-dose amiodarone (200 mg/day) using varied loading protocols. Type I antiarrhythmic agents prescribed for nonsustained ventricular tachycardia or atrial fibrillation are generally discontinued.

Patients and their family members receive comprehensive education taught individually by one of the heart failure advanced practice nurses. The verbal instruction is reinforced with a heart failure patient education booklet provided to each patient. A flexible diuretic regimen is used. Dietary guidelines include a 2 g sodium restriction and a 2 L fluid restriction. Complete abstinence from smoking and alcohol are emphasized. A home-based walking exercise regimen is prescribed. Patients and families are also advised of their uncertain prognosis and the risk of sudden death. They are given detailed instruction regarding warning symptoms of worsening heart failure or other complications such as arrhythmias or embolic events. The details of this education are described in the following sections.

PATIENT TEACHING

In the ideal circumstance, all patients are given both written and verbal instruction on diet and alcohol, fluid restriction, daily weights, flexible diuretic regimen, exercise, warning signs of worsening heart failure, and compliance.[22] The effectiveness of patient education is enhanced by including family members and/or significant others in the teaching sessions. At each follow-up visit, a detailed set of written guidelines is provided, patient understanding is reviewed, and compliance is assessed.

Diet, Smoking, and Alcohol

Because volume overload is a major contributor to patients' symptoms and a frequent cause of hospitalization, dietary salt restriction is emphasized. A sodium-restricted diet (usually a 2-g sodium diet) is prescribed.[29] Specific instructions include the need to avoid adding salt to food, how to read food labels for sodium content, and cooking tips with fresh foods. When formal dietary consultation with a registered dietitian is available, the dietitian provides more detailed instruction on the sodium-restricted diet in conjunction with information about a low-fat, low-cholesterol, and/or diabetic diet, when indicated.

The importance of alcohol and smoking abstinence are emphasized, and patients are closely monitored for adherence. Ingestion of alcohol is

contraindicated for any patient with alcoholic cardiomyopathy.[22] Alcohol is also discouraged for any patient with decreased left ventricular function, although randomized studies on this topic are lacking.

Fluid Restriction

Although the exact amount of fluid restriction and which patients would benefit most from this restriction have not been well studied, fluid restriction is generally recommended for heart failure patients. The rationale for the restriction is based on the need to reduce fluid retention for patients with advanced heart failure. Heart failure patients are told to restrict their fluid intake to 2 quarts daily.[22] Patients are instructed to record and measure the amount of liquids they ingest daily for 1 or 2 weeks to familiarize themselves with the restriction. In addition, patients are taught to include the water content of foods such as citrus fruits and melons and to restrict their liquid intake further if they consume large amounts of these fruits. Recorded intake measurements are reviewed during follow-up visits to promote success. Oral intake measurements and daily weight are compared to identify possible patterns and correlations between weight gain and fluid intake.

Daily Weights

Close monitoring of volume status is essential, and daily weights have been shown to be an efficient way of tracking volume status.[22] Home weight tracking sheets are provided to encourage the measurement and recording of daily morning weights. Patients are instructed to weigh each morning, at the same time, with the same amount of clothing (for example, in the morning after they have urinated, but before they eat breakfast). Weight charts are reviewed at each clinic visit. Active involvement in weight monitoring helps patients identify when they have consumed too much salt or fluid, missed diuretic doses, or when their underlying condition has worsened. Patients are educated that gaining 2 pounds overnight or 3 to 4 pounds in a week is abnormal and may be the earliest sign of fluid retention. Some heart failure clinics have used computerized scales that will transmit the daily weight information back to the heart failure clinic.[5]

Flexible Diuretic Regimen

At the early signs of volume overload, patients are instructed to adjust their diuretic dose.[5] It is well recognized that salt and fluid intake, as well as absorption of diuretics, can vary daily. Not all patients are capable of adjusting their own diuretics, but many are. Patients who have a creatinine level >2.5 mg/dL, lack a good understanding of how and when to make changes in the diuretic regimen, have demonstrated poor compliance previously, or are already on a high diuretic maintenance dose are not candidates for such instruction. Instead, diuretics are adjusted under the direct guidance of the advanced practice nurse and physician. When 2 pounds are gained overnight or 3 to 4 pounds are gained in a week, patients are instructed to double the dose of their loop diuretic. Patients who require more than 100 to 160 mg of furosemide (Lasix) twice a day are often prescribed metolazone (Zaroxolyn), as a "booster" diuretic to further enhance diuresis. Patients are usually instructed to take an extra dose of potassium whenever they double their diuretic dose and/or take metolazone. Once the patient returns to a dry weight, she or he is instructed to resume the usual diuretic dose. Daily use of metolazone has been associated with increased mortality, so its daily use is avoided.[22] When adjustments are made in the diuretic dosage, clinical laboratory screening is obtained to monitor serum electrolytes and renal function. Some heart failure programs provide for the administration of outpatient intravenous diuretics as a way of facilitating diuresis in patients who have stopped responding to high dose oral diuretics.

Exercise

In years past, persons with heart failure were advised to avoid exercise. There is a growing level of evidence that aerobic exercise is safe and potentially beneficial in patients with heart failure.[30] As described elsewhere in this book, exercise appears to prevent the progression of heart disease by improving endothelial function, enhancing peripheral responses, and decreasing neurohormonal activation. Exercise training has been found to improve exercise capacity and reduce symptoms, which can improve overall quality of life.[30] Exercise has not been shown to increase mortality in patients with heart failure, although a number of ongoing or planned clinical trials are seeking to validate this understanding.

Formal cardiac rehabilitation is included in many heart failure clinic programs.[5] Insurance coverage can pose a significant barrier, however, because heart failure is not yet considered a covered indication for cardiac rehabilitation by many health care providers. Home-based exercise regimens are used by other heart failure clinics.[5] At the UCLA clinic, patients are instructed to warm up for 5 to 10 minutes, and then walk 5 to 10 minutes at a slow pace. A 5- to 10-minute cool down is prescribed. As the fitness level increases, the length of exercise time can increase. Ultimately, patients are given a goal to perform some form of aerobic exercise 6 to 7 days a week. Once they can comfortably walk 30 minutes a day, patients are asked to incorporate other aerobic activities such as jogging, biking, or swimming. Patients are taught how to take their pulse so they can monitor heart rate during exercise, which allows them to track their exercise/activity progress. They are given a list of warning signs and things they should avoid such as isometric exercise and the lifting of weights greater than 10 lb. If cardiopulmonary exercise testing has been performed, then specific heart rate targets are provided on the basis of the heart rate achieved at anaerobic threshold and peak exercise.

Medication Compliance

Promoting patient compliance with the medical regimen is a major focus for clinicians in a heart failure clinic because it is a key determinate of clinical outcomes.[22] Noncompliance has been described in 54% of patients with heart failure[17] and was implicated in 53% of readmissions in a group of elderly patients with heart failure.[18] Educational programs aimed at improving compliance have been shown to be effective for heart failure[31] and other chronic illnesses.[32]

Patients and families are taught the importance of knowing about their medications—not just the names—but the doses, frequency, potential side effects, and long-term benefits to be expected on the basis of clinical research trials. Compliance is enhanced with medication sheets and heart failure clinic medication logs.[33] Patients are provided with a written medication card for carrying in their wallets. The card contains a current and updated medication list and other essential information such as physician and emergency contact phone numbers.

Another tactic used to facilitate compliance is simplifying the medication regimen and controlling costs. If a pharmacist is part of the heart failure clinic team, this may help to control costs and to facilitate identification of drug interactions, optimize medication dosing, address formulary issues, and educate patients about potential side effects. A number of important psychosocial and financial issues are faced by patients with a chronic disease such as heart failure, and these issues can have an impact on patient compliance.[33] Social service evaluation, financial counseling, and psychologic counseling services are made available to patients and their caregivers to further address these issues.

EVALUATION OF OUTCOMES

The study population at the UCLA Medical Center in which this approach was validated consisted of patients with severe heart failure who were referred between 1991 and 1994 to the Ahmanson-UCLA Cardiomyopathy Center as potential candidates for heart transplantation.[16] All patients included in this study had NYHA Class III or IV heart failure and symptoms for at least 6 months before referral. This analysis was confined to patients who were determined to be candidates for transplantation. That is, they had sufficient indications for transplantation without contraindications[34] and were discharged to await

heart transplantation on an elective basis. At the time of referral, patients underwent a detailed initial assessment, as described previously, including review of all available medical records. The number of hospitalizations, precipitating symptoms, and admission diagnoses for all hospitalizations in the 6 months before referral were determined by patient interview and confirmed by review of the discharge summaries.

During the study period, 394 patients were referred and considered appropriate for full evaluation for transplantation. Of these, 127 were rejected after evaluation because of contraindications, and 29 were determined to be too well or to have a potentially reversible cause of cardiomyopathy. Of the remaining 236 accepted candidates, 22 (9.3%) could not be stabilized for discharge and required urgent status transplantation during the initial hospitalization, leaving 214 accepted candidates who were discharged home. Baseline characteristics for the 214 study patients included LVEF 0.21 ± 0.07 and heart failure symptom duration 18 ± 29 months (all at least 6 months). Peak oxygen uptake within 6 weeks of referral was 11.0 ± 4.0 mL/kg/min. ACE inhibitors had been prescribed before referral in 165 patients (77.1%) at an average dose of 95 ± 120 mg captopril equivalence. The patient's referring physician was an internist or family physician in 12.1% of patients and a cardiologist in 87.8%. During therapy with vasodilators and diuretics, pulmonary artery wedge pressure fell by 36%, right atrial pressure by 38%, and systemic vascular resistance by 31%, whereas cardiac index increased by 24% (all $P < .001$ compared with baseline). Average net diuresis was 4.2 ± 4.6 L. Redesign of the medical regimen included initiation of an ACE inhibitor in an additional 18% of patients, for a total of 95% of patients on an ACE inhibitor. Compared with the time of referral, the mean daily dose of ACE inhibitor in patients receiving one increased by 98% before discharge. During the period of the study reported in the following, β-adrenergic receptor antagonists were not considered standard of care. No investigational agents were used.

During reassessment at 6 months, patients had significant improvement in subjective and objective indices of functional status. NYHA Class improved significantly for the 179 patients alive without transplantation at 6 months ($P < .001$), with 48.6% of patients reclassified as Class I or II. The improvement remained significant ($P < .01$) even when the 35 patients dying or undergoing transplantation were included and ranked as Class IV for reassessment. Repeat cardiopulmonary exercise testing was available in 121 of the 179 patients (68%), and oxygen consumption increased from 11.0 ± 3.6 to 15.2 ± 4.4 mL/kg/min ($P < .001$), demonstrating comparable improvement in anaerobic threshold. On the basis of improved exercise capacity and demonstrated clinical stability, 30% of patients were removed from the active transplant list with subsequent 18-month survival of 92% without death or relisting for transplantation, as described previously for a small cohort of similar patients.[28]

The improved functional status of these patients was reflected in the decreased hospitalization rate after referral. In the 6 months before referral, 429 hospitalizations for heart failure occurred in the study population. In the 6 months after discharge as transplant candidates, there were 63 hospitalizations, an 85% reduction. Although only admissions attributed directly to heart failure were included from the prereferral period, all 63 rehospitalizations after referral were included as potentially related to the redesign of therapy. During the 6 months of follow-up, only 25.7% of the 214 patients required any hospitalization compared with 91.6% in the prior 6 months. Of the nine deaths, six occurred suddenly, two were attributed to pump failure, and one was noncardiac. Actuarial survival was 95.8% at 6 months, with 89.2% of patients without death or urgent transplantation.

The average cost of rehospitalization at UCLA was $9,178 (range, $2,890–$38,930), comparable to estimates previously published by O'Connell and Bristow.[35] Using this average to compute costs, for the whole group, the cost of rehospitalization after referral was estimated to be $578,000 compared with $3,937,000 before referral. Hospitalization costs are considered to dominate overall costs of heart failure. Therefore, no attempt was made to track the total outpatient costs shared between the heart failure center and referring physicians, but these have been estimated in previous literature to be about $4,238 per patient per year.[36] The additional burden of these candidates constituted half of a full-time equivalent heart failure advanced practice nurse, or about $490 per patient for the 6 months. Further management costs included office administration for the coordination of communication between the heart failure team, referring physicians, and visiting nurses. These costs are hard to isolate for transplant candidates within the much larger volume of an active regional heart failure program. Any outpatient costs, however, were dwarfed by the costs of rehospitalization, which were reduced by approximately $15,700 per patient over the 6 months after referral.

The study demonstrated that clinical improvement that follows referral to a comprehensive heart failure clinic translated into a major improvement in patients' clinical and functional status, with reductions in hospitalization rates and the cost of heart failure care. Several other heart failure clinics have shown savings also (see Table 18–1). Many of these studies have used a pre and post design similar to the one used in this study, although one used a randomized prospective design with a concurrent control group and also demonstrated savings. The studies are consistent overall in that significant reductions in hospitalization rates have been demonstrated when the heart failure clinic model is compared with usual care.

ANALYSIS OF VARIABLES THAT MAY INFLUENCE OUTCOMES

The clinical studies reviewed in this chapter demonstrate that provision of heart failure specialty care using the heart failure clinic model can have a significant and favorable impact on patient outcomes. The design of these studies does not isolate the discrete contributions of the many program components and patient care interventions, each of which could have variable degrees of influence on patient outcomes. Many of these components of care are provided at relatively low marginal cost by heart failure clinics so determining the individual impact of each variable may not be that essential, with the net effect being so favorable.

Increased use of appropriate heart failure medications is one of the variables that may contribute to the improved outcomes of patients managed in a heart failure clinic. As mentioned previously, medical therapies that have been demonstrated by major clinical trials to be effective in heart failure have been found to be underused outside of heart failure clinics.[36,37] The number of patients referred to the heart failure clinic on ACE inhibitors was variable, as other authors have found (Table 18–1). There are multiple reasons why heart failure patients are not treated with ACE inhibitors. Often, concerns about side effects and the impact ACE inhibitors may have on blood pressure limit the use of these medications. Many investigators have shown that patients managed in a heart failure clinic are more likely to be treated with ACE inhibitors and more likely to be treated with a higher, more effective, dose.[5] In the UCLA study, there was an increase from 77% to 95% in ACE inhibitor use. In addition, patients taking ACE inhibitors had an increase of 98% in average daily dose equivalents, which may have been a major component in clinical improvement.[38] Both the SOLVD trial of mild to moderate heart failure and the CONSENSUS trial of severe heart failure showed a decrease in hospitalization rates with ACE inhibitor therapy.[39,40]

Since this study was conducted, major new therapies have been added to the armamentarium of the heart failure specialist. The addition of β-adrenergic blocking agents to patients' medical regimens has been shown to reduce hospitalizations by 10% to 32%.[41] In the RALES trial, aldosterone blockade with spironolactone significantly reduced the risk of hospitalization in patients with Class III and IV heart failure.[42] Increased use of these medications in patients followed in a heart failure clinic can be expected to improve rehospitalization rates as well as survival.

Improved volume status management and early adjustment of the diuretic regimen is another variable that is likely to contribute to the reduced hospitalization rate seen in heart failure clinics. There is limited information regarding the optimal dosing of diuretics,[43] but heart failure clinics often dose diuretics to maintain a dry weight determined through physical examination done by clinicians with extensive heart failure management experience. Further outpatient modifications of the diuretic regimen are made during clinic assessment at follow-up visits, with the specific goal being freedom from congestion as assessed by absence of orthopnea, edema, or ascites and jugular venous pressure.

The vigilant instruction provided to patients and families may help to decrease the rate of noncompliance, which, in turn, may improve the ability of the medical regimen to influence outcomes. Another possibility is that the newer treatments such as exercise are incorporated into the care program at a specialty clinic. For example, although exercise/activity is routinely recommended at most heart failure clinics, many patients in general practices continue to receive specific instructions to avoid exercise and stress. Lack of activity contributes to the deconditioning and sense of helplessness that often accompanies advanced heart failure. In addition to improving patients' attitudes and feeling of self-worth, exercise has been shown to improve functional capacity and decrease symptoms.[44] There may be additional long-term benefits resulting from improvement of autonomic balance.[45]

It is not possible to isolate the specific impact of continuity of care that is provided by the heart failure clinic team. It appears, however, that care provided on a routine basis rather than that triggered by symptoms of deterioration is a key predictor of outcome in this chronically ill patient population. Continuity of care after hospital discharge allows the clinicians to build a strong and trusting relationship that facilitates assessment of subtle changes in signs and symptoms.

OUTCOMES MEASUREMENT

Rehospitalization represents a useful outcome for analysis in studies of the effectiveness of heart failure clinics because it reflects both the frequency of clinical decompensation and the major cost component for the syndrome. Explicit process criteria have demonstrated rehospitalization rates to be influenced by the quality of care for heart failure.[46] In the studies summarized in the table and elsewhere, the major cause of rehospitalization is typically heart failure decompensation. Hospitalization rates noted in various heart failure populations before referral usually reflect the severity of patients' heart failure. In general hospital populations, 30%–58%

of heart failure patients are rehospitalized during the 3 to 6 months after discharge, with higher rates seen in the elderly.[47,48]

Referral to a heart failure clinic has been associated with increased functional capacity and clinical stability, as well. For patients with advanced heart failure who are transplant candidates, the improvement in clinical status often leads to delayed or avoided cardiac transplantation. In studies that assessed the influence of a heart failure clinic on medical costs, most investigators showed substantial reductions. Increased costs associated with the cost of providing care have been offset by the reduction in hospitalizations.

In the UCLA study, the cost of inpatient care was reduced by approximately half during the 6 months after referral, even if the initial hospitalization at the time of referral was included as part of postreferral care. It should be emphasized that the cost of the initial referral hospitalization is lower than the cost of urgent hospitalizations for decompensation. This is an important point because it is often assumed that heart failure therapy of the intensity provided by a heart failure clinic is more expensive than other heart failure admissions. The lower inpatient medical costs for patients followed by heart failure clinic staff reflects an economy of scale resulting from an organized approach to optimization of therapy before discharge. At UCLA, heart failure patients are admitted to the intermediate care unit rather than a critical care unit for elective hemodynamic monitoring, which lowers the cost.

It has been estimated that routine outpatient care for advanced heart failure costs about $4,238 per patient per year.[35] We argue that the cost of providing care in a heart failure clinic is not significantly more than routine care, and the financial rewards of providing such care offset the expense. For example, although the salary and benefits for a heart failure advanced practice nurse vary greatly between regions, an average salary may be estimated at $50,000 to $60,000 plus benefits. Most advanced practice nurses can carry a standard caseload of 100 to 150 patients with NYHA Class III to IV heart failure. These costs, when distributed among patients, do not approach the cost of a single hospitalization for heart failure.

CONCLUSION

The number of patients with NYHA Class III to IV heart failure has been estimated to be between 400,000 and 800,000. These patients account for almost 1,000,000 hospitalizations yearly. At an average cost of $9,000 per hospitalization, approximately $9 billion or $11,000 to $22,000 per patient is spent annually on hospitalizations alone for NYHA Class III and IV heart failure. If the hospitalization rate could be decreased by half, this would represent a $4.5 billion reduction in costs to the American public. Improved clinical status and decreased hospitalizations have now been shown for patients with heart failure cared for in a heart failure clinic. Heart failure patients with persistent moderate or severe symptoms are best managed in such a specialty setting. Patients with milder heart failure also appear to benefit from the comprehensive approach to patient management provided by a heart failure clinic. With the cost and complexity of heart failure patient care, the heart failure clinic is ideally suited to provide care that improves patient outcomes at substantially lower total medical costs.

REFERENCES

1. Brass-Mynderse N. Disease management for chronic congestive heart failure. *J Cardiovasc Nurs.* 1996;1(1): 54–62.

2. Schulman K, Mark D, Califf R. Outcomes and costs within a disease management program for advanced congestive heart failure. *Am Heart J.* 1998;135(6): S285–S292.

3. Lowe J, Candlish P, Henry D, Wlodarcyk J, Heller R, Fletcher P. Management and outcomes of congestive heart failure: A prospective study of hospitalized patients. *Med J Aust.* 1998;168:115–118.

4. American Heart Association. *2000 Heart and Stroke Statistical Update.* Dallas TX: American Heart Association; 1999.

5. Rich MW, Nease RF. Cost-effectiveness analysis in clinical practice: the case of heart failure. *Arch Intern Med.* 1999;159(15):1690–700.

6. Hlatky MA, Fleg JL, Hinton PC, Lakatta EG, Marcus FI. Physician practice in the management of congestive heart failure. *J Am Coll Cardiol.* 1986;8:966–970.

7. Fleg JL, Hinton PC, Lakatta EG, Marcus FI, Marcus FI. Physician practice in the management of congestive heart failure. *J Am Coll Cardiol.* 1986;8:966–970.

8. Advisory Board Company. Beyond Four Walls. *Cost Effectiveness Management of Chronic Congestive Heart Failure.* Washington DC: The Company; 1994.

9. Cintron G, Bigas C, Linares E, Aranda J, Hernandez E. Nurse practitioner role in a chronic congestive heart failure clinic: In hospital time, costs and patient satisfaction. *Heart Lung.* 1993;12(3):237–240.

10. Lasater M. The effect of a nurse managed CHF clinic on patient readmission and length of stay. *Home Healthcare Nurse.* 1996;14(5):351–356.

11. Hanumanthu S, Butler J, Chomsky D, Davis S, Wilson J. Effect of a heart failure program on hospitalization frequency and exercise tolerance. *Circulation.* 1997;96(9):2842–2848.

12. Smith L, Fabbri S, Pai R, Ferry D, Heywood T. Symptomatic improvement and reduced hospitalization for patients attending a cardiomyopathy clinic. *Clin Cardiol.* 1997;20:949–954.

13. Cline CM, Israelsson BY, Willenheimer RB, Broms K, Erhardt LR. Cost effective management program for heart failure reduces hospitalization. *Heart.* 1998;80:442–446.

14. Paul S. Impact of a nurse-managed heart failure clinic: a pilot study. *Am J Crit Care.* 2000;9(2):140–146.

15. Dahl J, Penque S. The effects of an advanced practice nurse-directed heart failure program. *The Nurse Practitioner.* 2000;25(3):61–77.

16. Fonarow GC, Stevenson LW, Walden JA, et al. Impact of a comprehensive heart failure management program on hospital readmission and functional status of patients with advanced heart failure. *J Am Coll Cardiol.* 1997;30(3):725–732.

17. Ghali JK, Kadakia S, Cooper R, Ferlinz J. Precipitating factors leading to decompensation of heart failure. Traits among urban blacks. *Arch Intern Med.* 1988;148:2013–2016.

18. Vinson JM, Rich MW, Sperry JC, Shah AS, McNamara T. Early readmission of elderly patients with congestive heart failure. *J Am Geriatr Soc.* 1990;38:1290–1295.

19. Kahn KL, Rogers WH, Rubenstein LV, Sherwood MJ, Reinisch EJ. Measuring quality of care with explicit process criteria before and after implementation of the DRG-based prospective payment system. *JAMA.* 1990;264(15):1969–1973.

20. Sueta CA, Chowdhury M, Boccuzzi SJ, Smith SCJ, Alexander CM. Analysis of the degree of undertreatment of hyperlipidemia and congestive heart failure secondary to coronary artery disease. *Am J Cardiol.* 1999;83:1303–1307.

21. Membership of the advisory council to improve outcomes nationwide in heart failure. Consensus recommendations for the management of chronic heart failure. *Am J Cardiol.* 1999;83:1A-38A.

22. Agency for Health Care Policy and Research. Heart failure: management of patients with left-ventricular systolic dysfunction. *Clinical Practice Guidelines Quick Reference Guide Clinics.* 1994;1–25.

23. Chiquette E, Amato MG, Bussey HI. Comparison of an anticoagulation clinic with usual medical care: anticoagulation control, patient outcomes, and health care costs. *Arch Intern Med.* 1998;158(15):1641–1647.

24. Gheorghiade M, Bonow RO. Chronic heart failure in the United States: a manifestation of coronary artery disease. *Circulation.* 1998;97(3):282–289.

25. Pierpont GL, Francis GS. Medical management of terminal cardiomyopathy. *J Heart Transplant.* 1982;2:18–27.

26. Fonarow GC, Chelimsky-Fallick C, Stevenson LW, et al. Effect of direct vasodilation with hydralazine versus angiotensin-converting enzyme inhibition with captopril on mortality in advanced heart failure: the Hy-C trial. *J Am Coll Cardiol.* 1992;19:842–850.

27. Stevenson LW. Tailored therapy before transplantation for treatment of advanced heart failure: effective use of vasodilators and diuretics. *J Heart Lung Transplant.* 1991;10:468–476.

28. Stevenson LW, Steimle AE, Fonarow G, et al. Improvement in exercise capacity of candidates awaiting heart transplantation. *J Am Coll Cardiol.* 1995;25:163–170.

29. Agency for Health Care Policy and Research. Public Health Service, U. S. Department of Health and Human Services. *Heart Failure Evaluation and Care of Patients with Left-ventricular Systolic Dysfunction.* Clinical practice guideline No. 11 (June 1994). AHCPR Publication No. 94–0612. Rockville, MD.

30. McKelvie R, Teo K, McCartny N, Humen D, Montague T, Yusuf S. Effects of exercise training in patients with congestive heart failure: A critical review. *J Am Coll Cardiol.* 1995; 25(3):789–796.

31. Rosenberg S. Patient education leads to better care for heart patients. *HSMHA Health Rep.* 1971;86:793–802.

32. Mullen PD, Green LW, Persinger GS. Clinical trials of patient education for chronic conditions: a comparative meta-analysis of intervention types. *Prev Med.* 1985;14:753–781.

33. Dracup K., Baker DW, Dunbar SB, Dacey RA, Brooks NH. Management of heart failure. II. Counseling, education, and lifestyle modifications. *JAMA.* 1994;272: 1442–1446.

34. Mudge GH, Goldstein S, Addonizio LJ, et al. 24th Bethesda conference: Cardiac transplantation. Task Force 3: Recipient guidelines/prioritization. *J Am Coll Cardiol.* 1993; 22:21–31.

35. O'Connell JB, Bristow MR. Economic impact of heart failure in the United States: time for a different approach. *J Heart Lung Transplant.* 1994;13:S107–S112.

36. Rajfer SI. Perspective of the pharmaceutical industry on the development of new drugs for heart failure. *J Am Coll Cardiol.* 93;22:198A–200A.

37. Edep ME, Shah NB, Tateo I, Massie BM. Differences in practice patterns in managing of heart failure patients between cardiologists, family practitioners and internists. *J Am Coll Cardiol.* 1996;27:367A.

38. Pouleur H, Rousseau MF, Oakley C, Ryden L. Difference in mortality between patients treated with captopril or enalapril in the Xamoterol in Severe Heart Failure Study. *Am J Cardiol.* 1991;68:71–74.

39. Effect of enalapril on survival in patients with reduced left ventricular ejection fractions and congestive heart failure. The SOLVD Investigators. *N Engl J Med.* 1991;325:293–302.

40. Effects of enalapril on mortality in severe congestive heart failure. Results of the Cooperative North Scandinavian Enalapril Survival Study (CONSENSUS). The CONSENSUS Trial Study Group. *N Engl J Med.* 1987;316:1429–1435.

41. Heidenreich PA, Lee TL, Massie MB. Effect of beta-blockage on mortality in patients with heart failure: A meta-analysis of randomized clinical trial. *J Am Coll Cardiol.* 1997;30:27–34.

42. Pitt B, Zannad F, Remme WJ, et al. The effect of spironolactone on morbidity and mortality in patients with severe heart failure. *N Engl J Med.* 1999;341(10): 709–717.

43. Baker DW, Konstam MA, Bottorff M, Pitt B. Management of heart failure. I. Pharmacologic treatment. *JAMA.* 1994;272:1361–1366.

44. McKelvie RS, Teo KK, McCartney N, Humen D, Montague T, Yusuf S. Effects of exercise training in patients with congestive heart failure: a critical review. *J Am Coll Cardiol.* 1995;25:789–796.

45. Coats AJ, Adamopoulos S, Radaelli A, et al. Controlled trial of physical training in chronic heart failure. Exercise performance, hemodynamics, ventilation, and autonomic function. *Circulation.* 1992;85:2119–2131.

46. Kahn KL, Rogers WH, Rubenstein LV, et al. Measuring quality of care with explicit process criteria before and after implementation of the DRG-based prospective payment system. *JAMA.* 1990;264:1969–1973.

47. Brophy JM, Deslauriers G, Boucher B, Rouleau JL. The hospital course and short term prognosis of patients presenting to the emergency room with decompensated congestive heart failure. *Can J Cardiol.* 1993;9:219–224.

48. Rich MW, Beckham V, Wittenberg C, Leven CL, Freedland KE, Carney RM. A multidisciplinary intervention to prevent the readmission of elderly patients with congestive heart failure. *N Engl J Med.* 1995;333:1190–1195.

CHAPTER 19

Telephonic Case Management Models of Heart Failure Care

Nancy Houston Miller and Jeffrey A. West

Over the past few years, new models of health care delivery have emerged to help patients and health care professionals better manage chronic conditions such as heart failure. The new models address many of the logistical barriers to effective care encountered by patients in the traditional model of a face-to-face visit. They also address many of the barriers encountered by health care professionals such as lack of time for counseling. Case management models often extend the care for patients with chronic heart failure from the hospital to the outpatient setting. Moreover, they usually incorporate some form of telephone follow-up or community outreach through home visits to help patients effectively manage their disease. The purpose of this chapter is to highlight the various case management models applied in clinical practice and to more fully describe one model developed and tested through the Stanford Cardiac Rehabilitation Program known as MULTIFIT.[1]

Historically, studies in the early 1980s demonstrated the value of communication technologies such as the telephone to facilitate education,[2,3] behavior change,[4,5] and surveillance of patients.[5,6] Telephone follow-up was used to increase patients' knowledge about coronary artery disease and self-care measures after hospitalization for an acute myocardial infarction or coronary artery bypass surgery.[2,3] In addition, the telephone served as a method to enhance patient compliance to exercise regimens and to facilitate surveillance during exercise sessions.[4,5] In the early 1990s, investigators extended this

early success with the telephone. Attempting to overcome some of the logistical difficulties of patients reaching a clinic setting in a randomized controlled trial, Wasson and colleagues[7] randomly allocated a group of elderly patients, one third of whom believed they were in failing health, to receive standard office visits at regular intervals (usual care) or to receive visits extended by 2 months with two telephone calls initiated by a physician or nurse practitioner in the intervening period. Patients lived an average of 47 miles from the clinic setting. They had multiple health problems including hypertension (53%), angina pectoris (32%), respiratory disease (23%), and degenerative arthritis (24%). At the end of 1 year patients assigned to receiving telephone care showed not only a reduction in utilization, including visits for all reasons, but also a significant decrease in rehospitalizations and length of stay. Savings were estimated at approximately $2,000 per patient. Furthermore, patients in the treatment group showed a higher degree of satisfaction compared with those assigned to usual care. Wasson and colleagues clearly showed that numerous benefits may be derived from seeking new approaches to the way in which care is delivered to patients.

AN OVERVIEW OF CASE MANAGEMENT MODELS

Various case management models extend the work of Wasson and colleagues in caring for patients with chronic heart failure. These models are highlighted in Table 19–1.[8–13] Most of the models have incorporated some form of face-to-face visit either in the clinic or home along with nurse-initiated telephone calls or call-in systems for patients and caregivers to use in the case of questions and emergency situations. One unique model[11] incorporated home visits by physicians in addition to the use of a nurse and physiotherapist to provide additional follow-up to patients.

Weinberger and associates[8] randomly allocated 1,396 patients with heart failure, diabetes, or chronic obstructive pulmonary disease to receive usual care or coordinated care that involved close follow-up by a primary care physician and a nurse beginning at hospital discharge and continuing through 6 months. During hospitalization, patients were assessed about educational issues, provided educational materials, and assigned a primary care physician who visited them within the 2 days before discharge to review discharge plans and medication regimens. Primary care follow-up appointments were scheduled by the nurse at discharge. After discharge, study nurses telephoned patients within 48 hours to ascertain difficulties with medications or medical regimens and to remind patients of their appointments. During the 6-month hospital discharge period, nurses spoke with patients by telephone on average 7.5 times; the average call lasted 5.7 minutes. In this study it was not specified whether telephone contact was initiated proactively by the nurses or in response to patients' calls with problems or concerns.

At 180 days, the readmission rate was higher in the intervention group than in those assigned to the usual care group (0.19 vs 0.14, $P = 0.005$). This greater readmission rate was apparent for all three conditions. The length of hospital stay was also longer (10.2 vs 8.8 days, $P = 0.041$). Overall patient satisfaction with care was higher in the intervention group than in the usual care group.

The investigators offer several potential explanations as to why a greater proportion of patients in the intervention group was readmitted. These include (1) systematizing primary care led to greater detection and treatment of previously undetected medical problems, (2) patients'

greater access to physicians may have improved communication leading to readmissions, and (3) a potentially sicker group of patients in the intervention group led to more use of inpatient services by this group compared with the 6 months before enrollment. Importantly, the investigators note the lack of disease-specific protocols designed to optimize the success of nurses involved in the management of their patients.

In a much smaller but similar study conducted in Europe by Ekman and colleagues,[9] no difference in the rate of rehospitalization or length of hospital stay was noted in elderly heart failure patients randomly allocated to a nurse-managed outpatient program incorporating telephone follow-up compared with those assigned to usual care. One week after discharge, patients were offered a clinic visit that included a relative or caregiver. Nurses' teaching focused on daily weights, medications, and early recognition of clinical warning signs and how to report a change in symptoms. Goals were set with the patient, and the frequency of visits was based on patient need. Nurses made follow-up telephone contacts with patients to discuss issues raised during clinic visits. For those who did not have regularly scheduled visits to the clinic, phone calls were made monthly. The median number of telephone contacts over the course of the 5 months was four. Investigators of this study chose to include only Class III and IV elderly patients. Only a minority (13%–17%) was eligible to participate in the program, because many were too sick to come to the clinic. At the end of 5 months the groups (intervention vs usual care) did not differ in the number of readmissions, mortality, or survival without readmission. As in the study by Weinberger et al, the lack of a difference in rehospitalization rates was ascribed to more highly structured care leading to detection of previously undetected problems and to better communication among medical care staff, patients, and caregivers.

In a small case-control study of 27 patients conducted through the Veteran's Affairs Medical Center in San Francisco, California, Shah and colleagues[10] showed the efficacy of a less intensive intervention in enhancing recovery in

Table 19–1 Case Management Model Programs

References	Patients	Intervention/Follow-up	Outcomes
Weinberger et al (1996)[8]	RCT—504 CHF (Class III/IV); 751 diabetic; 583 COPD (V.A. Pop)	• Visit and review of post-discharge needs by primary MD • Follow-up visit scheduled by nurse • Telephone follow-up with nurse (7.5 contacts) • Appointment reminders; missed visit protocol	At 6 months higher readmission rate in intervention vs control (0.19 vs 0.14 per month, $P = 0.005$) and rehospitalization days (10.2 vs 8.8, $P = 0.041$). Higher intervention satisfaction ($P < 0.001$) No difference in quality of life.
Ekman et al (1998)[9]	RCT—158 CHF; mean age = 80 yr; gender = 42% women	• Visit by nurse before discharge • Outpatient visit to nurse for education/counseling/goal setting (71%) • Telephone follow-up (median = 4 contacts)	At 5 months, no difference in readmission rates (0.5 vs 0.3), mortality, or survival without readmission.
Shah et al (1998)[10]	Sample—27 CHF clinic patients; mean age = 62 yr; gender = 100% men	• Mailings over 8 weeks re: CHF education • Digital sphygmomanometer, digital weight scale, and alphanumeric pager provided to patient by nurse. • Weekly calls by nurse • 24-hour telephone access to nurse	Mean participation = 8.5 mo. All-cause and CVD hospital days declined from 9.5 to 0.8 per patient year and 7.8 to 0.7 per patient year ($P < 0.05$). CVD hospitalization declined from 0.6 to 0.2 hospitalizations during monitoring ($P < 0.05$).
Kornowski et al (1995)[11]	Sample—48 CHF (Class III/IV); mean age = 78 yr; gender = 43% women	• Weekly home visits by physicians for education; review of meds, infusion therapy, and ordering of lab tests • On-call follow-up by nurse/physiotherapist as needed for paramedical support (IV injections, lab tests, etc.)	Mean total hospitalizations, CVD admissions, and all hospital days were reduced from year before to year during participation ($P < 0.0001$). Improvement in performance of daily activities.
Roglieri et al (1997)[12]	Sample—149 CHF program enrollees; mean age = 75 yr; gender = 41% women	• Single home visit by nurse for education and to provide self-management skills • Follow-up education materials mailed to patient • Weekly phone contacts by nurse including an automated telephone questionnaire resulting in MD notification if necessary	Length of stay was reduced by 82% ($P < 0.001$). An 83% reduction was seen in 90-day readmission rate. No readmissions were seen in the first 30 days.

continues

Table 19–1 Case Management Model Programs

References	Patients	Intervention/Follow-up	Outcomes
Stewart et al (1998)[13]	RCT—97 hospitalized CHF patients; mean age = 75 yr; gender = 50% women	• Single home visit by nurse and pharmacist to optimize medication management, identify early clinical deterioration, and intensify medical follow-up and caregiver vigilance. • Follow-up by pharmacist for additional intervention in noncompliant patients (52%).	At 6 months overall reduction in intervention group readmission (36 vs 63, $P = 0.3$) and fewer out-of-hospital deaths (1 vs 5; $P = 0.11$). Intervention patients also had fewer hospital days ($P = 0.5$) and total deaths ($P = 0.11$).

Rx = treatment; CHF = congestive heart failure; RCT = randomized controlled trial; VA = Veterans Administration; COPD = chronic obstructive pulmonary disease

patients with chronic heart failure. This pilot study included patient education materials, an automated reminder system for medications, and daily self-monitoring of weights and vital signs. Nurse case managers provided patients with a digital sphygmomanometer, digital weight scale, and an alphanumeric pager with instructions on how to operate these devices. The pager was used to transmit information to the patient about medication taking, weights, and measurement of blood pressure and heart rate. In addition to having 24-hour telephone access to the nurse to report any changes in weight or symptoms, patients were also called weekly by the nurse to obtain physiologic data. This information was transferred to a cardiologist on a monthly basis, and physicians were notified immediately by the nurse if there were signs of worsening symptoms, excessive weight gain, or changes in vital signs. Patients were contacted by the nurse within 24 hours of notification of the physician to determine whether the physician had contacted the patient.

In an 8.5-month average follow-up period, the rate of cardiovascular hospitalizations declined from 0.6 per patient year before the study to 0.2 per year during the monitoring period ($P < 0.05$). All cause and cardiovascular hospital days were also significantly reduced. The authors speculate that the differences were due to the nature of the patient population, which included Class II pa-

tients (40%), or to the behavior of the treating physicians. In the previous two studies reported, primary care physicians were ultimately responsible for care and appear to have opted to hospitalize patients at the first sign of clinical deterioration. In this study, patients were cared for primarily by practicing cardiologists who may have opted to adjust diuretic therapies immediately on notification of fluid retention without the need for hospitalization. Patient satisfaction with this type of automated reminder system and nurse-initiated telephone follow-up was quite high, especially in Class III and IV patients. Patients felt the reminder system also helped them to be more adherent to their medications.

Similar to the article by Shah, the final three studies reported in Table 19–1 show more promising outcomes than those noted by Weinberger and Ekman. They all offered different case management approaches ranging from physician visits[11] to multiple contacts by a nurse with automated telephone questions as part of the contact[12] to a single outpatient visit by a nurse and pharmacist. From these studies, it is apparent that no one case management model clearly shows superior outcomes in patients with heart failure. Moreover, limited information is detailed about the cost of providing interventions[14] and a more in-depth overview of the content of interventions and frequency of contact is needed. Finally, the large variations in the delivery of care require a greater understanding of which models are successful for the largest group of patients with chronic heart failure. Notwithstanding, some of the same limitations, a more in-depth overview of our case management model is provided.

THE STANFORD CARDIAC REHABILITATION PROGRAM EXPERIENCE

In a study funded by the Robert Wood Johnson Foundation we evaluated the feasibility and safety of a physician-supervised, nurse-mediated home-based system, known as MULTIFIT, that used the telephone as the primary means of communication. Guided by consensus-based guidelines for pharmacologic and dietary therapy,[15,16] nurse case managers enhanced pharmacologic and dietary adherence and monitored the clinical status of patients through frequent telephone contacts. This program was based on the success of MULTIFIT for cardiovascular risk reduction, which was evaluated in a randomized controlled study in five Kaiser Permanente Medical Care Centers in Northern California.[17] The success of the MULTIFIT system for cardiovascular risk reduction led to the dissemination of this program into clinical practice in all 18 medical care centers of the Kaiser Permanente system and numerous other regions of the country. Why was this system so successful for cardiovascular risk reduction? The MULTIFIT system was built on the basis of the outcomes of single intervention studies of cardiovascular risk factors.[4,5] The use of nurses as key health care professionals to provide interventions by telephone in the early 1980s resulted in success from the bond established between patient and nurse, individualization and tailoring of interventions, and the behavioral skills imparted to patients to help them self-manage their conditions.

The theoretical framework for the MULTIFIT system is based on social learning theory as developed by Bandura and the elements of health behavior change.[18,19] Assessments of the patients' perceived capabilities to adhere to a low-sodium diet and pharmacologic therapies, moni-

tor signs and symptoms of worsening heart failure, and carry out self-management skills such as the self-monitoring of daily weights form the basis for education and counseling. This education and counseling is conducted primarily by telephone. Elements of health behavior change known to be successful in clinical practice such as goal-setting, prompting, self-monitoring, positive reinforcement, and feedback were incorporated into the development of educational materials and telephone contacts by the nurse.[20] For example, patients were asked to self-monitor symptoms, weight, and exercise behaviors on a daily log that was mailed to nurses biweekly. Telephone contacts provided an opportunity for nurses to provide positive reinforcement for exercise adherence and monitoring functions.

The MULTIFIT system for heart failure was originally tested at the Kaiser Permanente Medical Care Center in Hayward, California. Fifty-one patients were followed for a mean of 138 ± 44 days.[1] These patients had been hospitalized in the preceding 12 months with a primary or secondary diagnosis of heart failure. To be involved in the study, patients had to meet both the clinical features of heart failure (dyspnea on exertion, orthopnea, paroxysmal nocturnal dyspnea, fatigue, or lower extremity swelling) and objective signs of left ventricular dysfunction by physical examination (elevated jugular venous pressure, pulmonary congestion, lower extremity edema) by chest X-ray (pulmonary congestion or cardiothoracic ratio 0.55) or imaging studies such as echocardiography (fractional shortening < 25%), radionuclide angiography or left ventricular angiography (both with left ventricular ejection fraction <40%). Exclusion criteria included acute myocardial infarction within 8 weeks; uncontrolled angina pectoris; hemodynamically significant valvular or myocardial obstructive diseases; comorbid conditions compromising prognosis such as metastatic lung disease, planned cardiac surgery, lack of a telephone, inability to speak English; or psychosocial reasons such as patient refusal, substance abuse, and psychiatric disorders. Overall, 18% of the 291 patients who were screened enrolled in the intervention.

The MULTIFIT intervention consisted of a single face-to-face visit with a nurse case manager followed by multiple telephone contacts with the same nurse over the course of 6 months. The initial face-to-face visit, which occurred within the first week after hospitalization, lasted approximately 1.5 hours. Patients were asked to return to the medical center for this visit and spouses were encouraged to attend. Before this visit, patients completed questionnaires related to quality of life (Medical Outcomes Study SF-36),[21] overall functional status (Duke Activity Status Index [DASI][22] and New York Heart Association [NYHA]),[23] self-efficacy measures, and a food-frequency tool for measurement of sodium intake, both developed by the investigators. Patients were asked to bring all medications they were taking including over-the-counter drugs to the visit. During the visit, nurses undertook a short history and physical examination that included clinical questions related to lifestyle behaviors and psychologic status and provided counseling about sodium restriction, medications, warning symptoms of worsening heart failure, and the self-monitoring of daily weights, symptoms, and exercise. Smoking cessation counseling provided to all smokers was based on previous work by the investigators.[24,25] Results of the self-efficacy measures helped to guide the nurses' counseling. Patients who reported low self-efficacy (confidence) regarding their ability to make specific changes in their behaviors (<70%) were provided additional counseling, which included methods to enhance overall efficacy such as verbal persuasion by the nurses.

Dietary counseling was supplemented by an expert system developed by our group, which originally measured only total fat consumption but was enhanced for sodium intake.[26] Upon completion of a 49-item daily sodium food frequency questionnaire, nurses input the data into a computer. Input requires only 1 to 2 minutes. During the visit, patients were provided with a computer-generated nutrition progress report that highlighted the key food items in the patients' diet that were high in sodium and visually displayed for them the total daily intake of so-dium in milligrams on a bar graph. The goal for daily dietary intake of sodium was < 2 g. Suggestions for making dietary changes were keyed to a 90-page dietary notebook highlighting total fat and sodium. Patients completed five additional food frequency questionnaires in the following 6 months. These reports allowed them to see changes in the course of their treatment. An example of the nutrition progress report mailed to patients is shown in Appendix 19–A.

Before the study, the physician investigators and nurses worked with the cardiologists within the medical center to develop treatment algorithms for pharmacologic therapy. These algorithms were based on consensus statements[15,16] and modified for medications approved for the formulary. The goals of the pharmacologic intervention were to optimize therapy with angiotensin-converting enzyme (ACE) inhibitors and isosorbide dinitrate/hydralazine therapy as identified by the consensus statements. In addition, algorithms were developed for the use of diuretics, digoxin, and potassium supplements. During the course of the initial patient visit, nurses evaluated the patients' medications, counseling them about the target goals of therapy, medication adherence, and medication interactions. Medications were transferred onto a large medication log where patients could make changes if asked to do so during telephone follow-up. Patients were provided specific medication handouts developed for this project. In addition, patients were given electronic medication caps and bottles that were used to measure their adherence to diuretics and ACE inhibitors. Patients were asked to use the monitors during the course of the 6 months of therapy.

During the initial visit, when patients were also oriented to daily self-monitoring of signs and symptoms, they were asked to record three variables: (1) daily weights, (2) any significant change in symptoms, and (3) the duration of daily exercise. Monitoring logs were mailed to the nurses at biweekly intervals. In addition, patients were provided a written card about how and when to access the appropriate medical personnel in case of a worsening of their medical condition. The program did not provide 24-hour surveillance but specified for patients how to access help after 5:00 PM.

The MULTIFIT program was designed to be a telephonic case management intervention with the goal of helping patients titrate medications, providing overall surveillance of dietary habits, medication adherence, symptoms, and the psychosocial aspects of recovery. Nurses involved in this study had at least 10 years' experience in cardiovascular nursing and were bachelor's or master's prepared. Their training consisted of 3 days of didactic lecture, role-playing and case study presentation about heart failure, telephone education and counseling, behavioral science, computer entry and retrieval, and study procedures. Ongoing biweekly staff meetings offered the opportunity for additional training and case consultation.

During the first 6 weeks of follow-up, nurses initiated weekly phone contacts to patients to titrate ACE inhibitor therapy or vasodilators and manipulate diuretics as needed. They followed prespecified questions during telephone contacts, asking patients about symptoms, daily weights, adherence to exercise, sodium restriction, and medication taking. Nurses also used the nutrition progress reports generated from food frequency questionnaires completed by patients at monthly intervals to counsel them about diet during telephone contacts. Patients were asked to return to the medical center at their convenience to obtain laboratory measures as needed for the titration of medications. They were also told to contact nurses by phone with any questions or in the case of a change in their condition.

Follow-up telephone contacts initiated by the nurse case managers occurred weekly for 6 weeks, biweekly through 2 months, and then monthly through 24 weeks. During the intervention period, patients received 13.2 scheduled telephone contacts, which averaged 21.4 minutes per call. In addition, patients initiated telephone contacts to nurses on average 1.7 ± 2.2 times. The appearance of a worsening symptom or sign such as a 3 lb weight gain over 2 to 3 days or an abnormal laboratory value increased the frequency of the nurses' phone contact. Nurses used treatment algorithms with established thresholds for emergent or urgent evaluation by primary care physicians.

During the time of the study, no attempt was made to alter the physician–patient relationship. Nurses contacted primary care physicians to obtain consent to add a medication or to apprise them of a worsening change in the patient's condition. Progress reports, in the form of letters, were also generated to physicians and faxed to their offices. In the absence of the primary care physician, a liaison cardiologist was available to the nurses by telephone to discuss difficult cases, most often involving patients with significant comorbidities.

In general, physicians were well satisfied with their patients' participation in the program. They were actively involved in the decision-making process when new heart failure medications were added to patient regimens. The most difficult task for the nurses early on was triaging patients back to their physicians for other medical problems not related to heart failure. Patients would often initiate calls to their nurse about medical concerns that were best handled by their physicians. When new systems of care are initiated, clarifying the roles of the nurse case managers and physicians is important for day-to-day management.

Outcomes of MULTIFIT

Of 291 patients screened for eligibility over 8 months, 51 patients met inclusion criteria. These 51 patients, mean age 66 ± 10, were followed in the MULTIFIT Program for a mean of 138 ± 44 days. Patients had an average of five comorbidities and 40% had poor functional status as evidenced by NYHA Class III or IV.[23] They were predominantly men (71%), Caucasian (80%), and married (77%). Eighty percent had been hospitalized with heart failure within the previous year. Among the 73% of patients who had an echocardiogram or left ventricular angiogram, left ventricular dysfunction was noted to be severely compromised in 84%.

Rehospitalization, emergency department visits, and utilization rates for general medical and cardiology visits are shown in Table 19–2. Medical resource utilization for both emergency

Table 19–2 Medical Resource Utilization (MULTIFIT Program, n = 51)

	Baseline (6 mo before Enrollment)	Follow-Up	P Value
General medical visits	3.9	3.0	0.03
Cardiology visits	1.6	1.1	.02
Emergency department visits for CHF	0.6	0.2	0.001
Total emergency room visits	1.5	0.7	0.001
	Baseline (12 mo before Enrollment)	Follow-Up	P Value
Hospitalization (CHF)	1.12	0.15	0.0001
Total hospitalizations	1.61	0.42	0.42

department and clinic visits was assessed by chart review. The hospitalization rate in the 12 months before enrollment was measured by use of administrative databases and chart review. When these 51 patients were normalized for variable follow-up and compared with the previous 6 to 12 months, significant declines were seen in the rate of emergency department visits, rehospitalizations for congestive heart failure and for any cause, and the rate of general internal medicine and cardiology visits.[1]

Functional state and symptom status also improved during the intervention. This was noted by a change in NYHA classification[23] and the Duke Activity Status Index,[22] measures of functional state (Figure 19–1). In addition, the percentage of patients achieving target doses of ACE inhibitor therapy increased from 45% to 83% and those taking target doses of hydralazine increased from 10% to 70%. Dietary sodium declined 38% from 3393 mg/day to 2088 mg/day, on average ($P < .0001$).

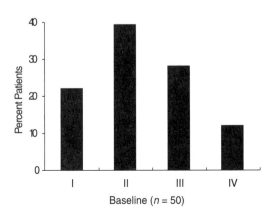

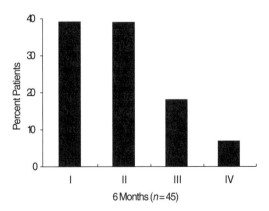

Figure 19–1 Change in NYHA classification (MULTIFIT program)

The MULTIFIT study also included a sub-study to examine the relationship between self-efficacy ratings and pharmacologic adherence. Adherence to pharmacologic agents was measured quantitatively using the Aprex Corporation Medication Event Memory System (MEMS). A high correlation between openings and pill-taking behavior has been demonstrated previously.[27] Of the 51 patients enrolled in the project, 43 patients (84%) were enrolled in the substudy. Eight patients declined enrollment because of their preference for weekly pill containers to organize their daily medications. Of the 43 patients enrolled, 41 and 33 patients received MEMS devices for diuretics (97% furosemide) and ACE inhibitors (68% lisinopril, 38% captopril), respectively. Analyzable data were obtained from MEMS devices in 29 patients taking diuretics (71%) and 22 patients taking ACE inhibitors (67%). Reasons for exclusion from analysis included: MEMS device damaged by patient (13%, $n = 3$); MEMS device not understood by patient and returned (9%, $n = 2$); MEMS device not returned (9%, $n = 2$); MEMS device used less than 60 days (9%, $n = 2$); incomplete analysis (9%, $n = 2$); and no data obtained from Aprex Corporation secondary to loss by the company (52%, $n = 12$).

Adherence rates were calculated using the rigorous definition of the percentage of days on which medications were taken on the prescribed dosing schedule divided by the total days of monitoring with the MEMS device. Cap openings within 15 minutes of a prior opening were filtered and not included in the total daily dose. Days when the patient was hospitalized were also censored. Monitoring began the day the patient received the device and ended on the day before the last day the patient was enrolled in the project or the last day the MEMS device was used by the patient.

Patients were monitored with MEMS devices for 144 ± 43 days. Adherence rates averaged 82% overall. Adherence rates for patients on diuretics averaged $85\% \pm 17\%$ and $78\% \pm 20\%$ for patients on ACE inhibitors.[28] No significant differences were noted between patients on lisinopril (twice per day) or captopril (three times per day) by unpaired t test ($P = .40$). More than 82% of patients taking diuretics had adherence rates greater than 75%; more than 68% of patients taking ACE inhibitors had adherence rates greater than 75%. Despite relatively complex regimens, the MEMS device revealed that patients treated in the MULTIFIT intervention and using the MEMS device achieved a high level of adherence to diuretic and ACE inhibitor therapy. However, lacking a control group, it is difficult to know whether this was an effect of the MULTIFIT treatment program or the device provided to patients.

The MULTIFIT system facilitates management of heart failure and other chronic diseases in a systematic way. It was highly successful in enhancing pharmacologic and dietary therapy, improving functional status, and reducing medical resource utilization in a group of patients with moderate to severe heart failure. Frequent telephone contact provided an alternative to managing patients in a clinic setting. Nurse managers have effectively worked with patients to titrate their medications without the need for a face-to-face contact. Well-developed algorithms for medication titration, formulated from national guidelines and tailored to the medical center, enhanced the success of nurses' management. Although the initial study outcomes were positive in one treatment center, the efficacy of the MULTIFIT system remains to be shown in a randomized, controlled study that is now underway in several medical centers in Northern California.

CONCLUSION

Numerous disease management models for the treatment of heart failure have been tested in both observational and randomized controlled trials.[8–13,29,30] Although many of these studies are small, they generally show promise for improving the outcomes of patients with heart failure.[31] Case management programs that employ nurses to provide systematic follow-up of patients through telephone contact are attractive because they alleviate the large logistical burden of patients' frequent clinic visits. Moreover, programs like MULTIFIT use a single type of caregiver, the registered nurse, to provide many of the functions performed by a multidisciplinary team in other models.[30] Over the long-term this approach may reduce costs of caring for patients with chronic diseases; however, at present this is not known. No trials simultaneously comparing telephonic case management with other styles of disease management have been conducted.

Many questions remain about the use of communication technologies such as telephone follow-up systems to manage patients with heart failure. For example, it is largely unknown whether systems that use automated voice recognition to question patients about daily weights and symptoms and that cue patients to take their medications appropriately may alleviate some of the burden nurses and others face when providing frequent phone interactions. Moreover, patient satisfaction with these systems needs further study. The frequency of phone contacts needed to provide education and help patients self-manage their condition has also not been fully studied. It is unclear how long a patient must remain in a system of care delivery to prevent the high utilization costs associated with heart failure. Further research from randomized controlled studies and the outcomes of programs that have been successfully implemented in clinical practice will certainly help to answer many of these questions. Finally, case management systems that use the telephone may become the standard of care if the outcomes of interest like death, nonfatal cardiovascular events, quality of life, and cost can be improved. Extension of these systems to other communication modalities like automated voice messaging with interactive voice response systems or the Internet may occur once the preceding issues have been clarified.

Many of the models developed for case management have also arisen out of academic medical centers. Whether employing expert multidisciplinary teams, or single caregivers, they have often provided interventions to only a select patient population. It remains unclear whether they may be broadly disseminated to a large proportion of patients with chronic heart failure. Holding promise, however, the greatest challenge remains in integrating case management with other models such as home health to ensure that patients are cared for from the onset of heart failure through the end of life.

REFERENCES

1. West JA, Miller NH, Parker KM, et al. A comprehensive management system for heart failure improves clinical outcomes and reduces medical resource utilization. *Am J Cardiol*. 1997;79:58–63.

2. Beckie T. A supportive-educative telephone program: Impact on knowledge and anxiety after coronary artery bypass graft surgery. *Heart Lung*. 1989;18:46–55.

3. Garding BS, Kerr JC, Bay K. Effectiveness of a program of information and support for myocardial infarction patients recovering at home. *Heart Lung*. 1988;17:355–362.

4. Miller NH, Haskell WL, Berra K, DeBusk RF. Home versus group exercise training for increasing functional capacity after myocardial infarction. *Circulation*. 1984;70:645–649.

5. DeBusk RF, Haskell WL, Miller NH, et al. Medically directed at-home rehabilitation soon after uncomplicated acute myocardial infarction: a new model for patient care. *Am J Cardiol*. 1985;55:251–257.

6. Nicklin WM. Postdischarge concerns of cardiac patients as presented via a telephone callback system. *Heart Lung*. 1986;15:268–272.

7. Wasson J, Gaudette C, Whaley F, Sauvigne A, Baribeau P, Welch G. Telephone care as a substitute for routine clinic follow-up. *JAMA*. 1992;267:1788–1793.

8. Weinberger M, Oddone EZ, Henderson WG for the Veterans Affairs Cooperative Study Group on Primary Care and Hospital Readmission. Does increased access to primary care reduce hospital readmissions? *N Engl J Med*. 1996;334:1441–1447.

9. Ekman I, Andersson B, Ehnforst M, Matejka G, Persson B, Fagerberg B. Feasibility of a nurse-monitored, outpatient-care programme for elderly patients with moderate-to-severe, chronic heart failure. *Eur Heart J*. 1998;19:1254–1260.

10. Shah NB, Der E, Ruggerio C, Heidenreich PA, Massie BM. Prevention of hospitalizations for heart failure with an interactive home monitoring program. *Am Heart J*. 1998;135:173–178.

11. Kornowski R, Zeeli D, Averbuch M, et al. Intensive home-care surveillance prevents hospitalization and improves morbidity rates among elderly patients with severe congestive heart failure. *Am Heart J*. 1995;129:762–766.

12. Roglieri J, Futterman R, McDonough K, et al. Disease management interventions to improve outcomes in congestive heart failure. *Am J Managed Care.* 1997;3:1831–1839.

13. Stewart S, Pearson S, Horowitz JD. Effects of a home-based intervention among patients with congestive heart failure discharged from acute hospital care. *Arch Intern Med.* 1998;158:1067–1072.

14. Philbin E. Comprehensive Multidisciplinary programs for the management of patients with congestive heart failure. *J Gen Intern Med.* 1999;14:130–137.

15. Williams JF, Bristow MR, Fowler MB, et al. Guidelines for the evaluation and management of heart failure. *Circulation.* 1995;92:2764–2784.

16. Konstam M, Dracup K, Baker DW, et al. *Heart Failure: Evaluation and Care of Patients with Left Ventricular Systolic Dysfunction.* Clinical Practice Guideline No. 11 (AHCPR publication No. 94–0612). Rockville, MD: Agency for Health Care Policy and Research, Public Health Service, U.S. Department of Health and Human Services; June 1994.

17. DeBusk RF, Houston Miller N, Superko HR, et al. A case-management system for coronary risk factor modification after acute myocardial infarction. *Ann Intern Med.* 1994;120:721–729.

18. Bandura A. *Social Learning Theory.* Englewood Cliffs, NJ: Prentice-Hall; 1977.

19. Miller NH, Taylor CB. *Lifestyle Management for Patients with Coronary Heart Disease.* Champaign, IL: Human Kinetics; 1995.

20. Miller NH, Warren D, Myers D. Home-based cardiac rehabilitation and lifestyle modification: The MULTIFIT model. *J Cardiovasc Nurs.* 1996;11(1):76–87.

21. Ware JE, Sherbourne CD. The MOS 36-item short-form health survey (SF-36): I. Conceptual framework and item selection. *Med Care.* 1992;30:473–483.

22. Hlatky MA, Boineau RE, Higginbotham MB, et al. A brief self-administered questionnaire to determine functional capacity (the Duke Activity Status Index). *Am J Cardiol.* 1989;64:651–654.

23. Criteria Committee for the New York Heart Association. Nomenclature and criteria for diagnosis. In: *Diseases of the Heart and Blood Vessels* (6th ed). Boston: Little, Brown; 1964:110–114.

24. Taylor CB, Houston Miller N, Killen JD, DeBusk RF. Smoking cessation after acute myocardial infarction: effects of a nurse-managed intervention. *Ann Intern Med.* 1990;113:118–123.

25. Houston Miller N, Smith PM, DeBusk RF, Sobel DS, Taylor CB. Smoking cessation in hospitalized patients. *Arch Intern Med.* 1997;157:409–415.

26. Clark M, Ghandour G, Houston Miller N, Taylor CB, Bandura A, DeBusk RF: Development and evaluation of a computer-based system for dietary management of hyperlipidemia. *J Am Diet Assoc.* 1997;97:146–150.

27. Cramer JA. How often is medication taken as prescribed? *JAMA.* 1989;261:3273–3237.

28. West JA, De Busk RF. Disease management systems for chronic cardiovascular diseases: Focus on heart failure. In RW Schrier, JD Baxter, VJ Dzau, AS Fauci (eds.) *Advances in Internal Medicine.* Vol. 46. St. Louis: Mosby, 2001.

29. Fonarow GC, Stevenson LW, Waden JA et al. Impact of a comprehensive heart failure management program on hospital readmission and functional status of patients with advanced heart failure. *J Am Coll Cardiol.* 1997;30:725–732.

30. Rich MW, Beckham V, Wittemberg C, Leven CL, Freedland KE, Carney RM. A multidisciplinary intervention to prevent the readmission of elderly patients with congestive heart failure. *N Engl J Med.* 1995;333:1190–1195.

31. Rich MW. Heart failure disease management: a critical review. *J Card Fail.* 1999;5:64–75.

Kaiser/Stanford Heart Failure Program Sodium Progress Report #2

Name_____ Date _____

It is critical to your health that you limit the amount of sodium you eat. Sodium from food can cause your body to retain fluid, which presents a serious threat to your health. You can help avoid this danger by reducing your sodium intake as much as possible.

We recommend a sodium limit for you of:

1000 to 2000 Milligrams per day

According to your recent Food Frequency Questionnaire, your level is close to your prescription. This is a significant improvement since your last report. This chart tracks the amount of sodium in the food you're eating as measured by your two recent Food Frequency Questionnaires.

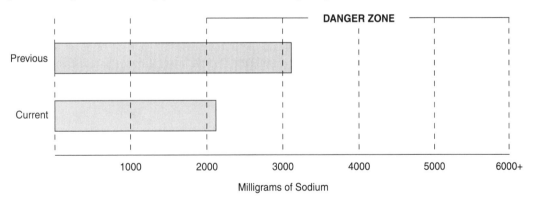

Congratulations! You have reduced your sodium intake since your last Sodium Progress Report. The foods that show the most improvement include:

- Donuts, cakes, pies, cookies

Keep up the good work with these food items!

You should continue to work on reducing your sodium intake until you reach your goal level. The following foods add extra sodium to your diet:

1. Pancakes or waffles
2. Sauce, gravy (including spaghetti sauce)

3. Ready-to-eat cereal
4. Canned vegetables or beans
5. Frozen peas, frozen lima beans

Here are some tips for reducing the amount of sodium you get from these foods.

Pancakes or waffles

A typical serving of pancakes or waffles usually contains 300–500 mg of sodium. Frozen brands contain even more. It's better to make your pancakes and waffles from scratch, with no added salt.

Sauce, gravy (including spaghetti sauce)

Almost all sauces and gravies are made with a generous amount of salt (at least 300–500 mg of sodium per serving). The best way to avoid sodium in sauces and gravies is to make them from scratch using fresh ingredients and herbs instead of salt. Spaghetti sauce is easily made from tomato paste (which is usually salt-free) mixed with an equal amount of water and plenty of herbs like parsley, oregano, and pepper.

Ready-to-eat cereal

Most cold cereals contain plenty of sodium (as much as 400 mg per cup of cereal). Cereals with no sodium at all include Shredded Wheat, Puffed Wheat, and Puffed Rice. Before buying any cereal, read the label to be sure it contains less than 100 mg of sodium per serving that you eat. (For example, if you eat 2 cups of cereal for breakfast, be sure the cereal you choose has less than 50 mg per cup.)

Canned vegetables or beans

Like most canned foods, vegetables and beans are put into cans with generous amounts of sodium (150–350 mg sodium per half cup of drained veggies!). Choose fresh, frozen, or salt-free versions instead.

Frozen peas, frozen lima beans

For some reason, salt is added to peas and lima beans when they are frozen—100 mg sodium per half cup. Other frozen vegetables are salt-free, as long as they are not frozen in sauce.

Remember . . .

Fresh unprocessed foods contain very little sodium: fresh meats, poultry, fish, fruits, vegetables, and grains. Other staples like milk, bread, and margarine are fine in moderation, even though they contain a bit more sodium.

CHAPTER 20

Multidisciplinary Disease Management Models of Heart Failure Care

Barbara Riegel and Michael W. Rich

Of the three models of disease management (DM) proposed in Chapter 16, the multidisciplinary model may be the most challenging to describe and measure. Such models are clearly effective, as others and we have demonstrated.[1-6] The attractiveness of these models, however, may also be their downfall in some situations. By definition, the model involves varied personnel from multiple disciplines and different departments who must coordinate their efforts to assist a patient group that is ill, typically elderly, often cognitively impaired, and rarely hospitalized for more than a few days. Future investigators will have the difficult task of attempting to identify which components of this multifaceted approach are most effective.

As argued in Chapter 16, published descriptions of heart failure programs are difficult to classify, but a schema based on three types (multidisciplinary team, case management, and clinic) has been proposed. Four published programs fit clearly into the multidisciplinary DM category defined as "a holistic approach adapted to each patient's unique set of medical, psychosocial, behavioral, and financial circumstances."[7(p 64)] Other published reports appear to be an amalgam of types (ie, clinic and multidisciplinary). In such situations, programs have been classified according to the predominant feature. For example, the program described by Fonarow and colleagues[8] is predominately a cardiologist-run heart failure clinic, although multiple disciplines contribute to the care provided. This and other programs are reviewed and analyzed in other chapters.

AN IN-DEPTH ANALYSIS OF EXISTING PROGRAMS

The focus of this chapter is in-depth analysis of published reports of multidisciplinary DM approaches for heart failure patients. The available information is summarized and analyzed in an attempt to provide guidance for future program designers (Table 20–1). Our hope is that such an examination will assist clinicians and investigators in linking the characteristics and intensity of the various interventions with the outcomes achieved. This should allow future developers of DM programs to tailor their interventions to meet the specific needs of their patients.

The Jewish Hospital of St. Louis Model

The first prospective randomized study of a multidisciplinary DM approach to heart failure was published by Rich and colleagues in 1993.[3] They tested the efficacy of a multifaceted intervention provided to an elderly (70 years of age or older) patient population with at least one of four risk factors for readmission on the basis of data from a previous analysis:

- Four or more prior hospitalizations for any reason within the preceding 5 years
- Prior history of heart failure
- Hypocholesterolemia (an indicator of cardiac cachexia)
- Right (not left) bundle-branch block on the admitting electrocardiogram

Table 20–1 Summary of the Published Reports of Multidisciplinary Disease Management Programs

Authors	Program Site	Definition of Population Included	Major Intervention Components	Nature and Frequency of Intervention	Staff
Rich et al, 1995[4]	Jewish Hospital of St. Louis, Missouri. Integrated health care system	70 years 1 risk factor for readmission	Intensive education, detailed analysis of medications, early discharge planning, enhanced follow-up	Daily hospital visits by multiple staff, home visit within 48 hours after discharge, 3 visits first week, home visits thereafter as needed for 90 days	Registered nurse, gerocardiologist, dietitian, social worker, home care nurse
Riegel et al[6]	Sharp HealthCare in San Diego, California. Integrated health care system	All heart failure patients except those confused, with primary renal failure, or discharged to a long-term nursing facility	Standardized education, social support, early discharge planning, postdischarge follow-up	In-hospital education by pharmacist and dietitian; after discharge, monthly support group, home care visits, and/or telemanagement for 6 mo	Registered nurses, pharmacists, dietitians, physicians, social workers
Block et al[1]	Atlanti-Care Medical Center, a small (120-bed) community hospital in Lynn, Massachusetts	In-patient, outpatient, and community members with heart failure	Education, communication, bridge from inpatient to outpatient care	Standardized admission orders and care map, inpatient teaching by case manager, exercise prescription, computerized database, communication with physicians, medical grand rounds, outpatient educational sessions, telemonitoring, community education	Cardiologist, nurse case manager, exercise specialist from cardiac rehabilitation, dietitian
Chapman and Torpy[2]	Joint program with Alegent/Immanuel Medical Center and Heart Consultants, PC, a private-practice cardiology group in Omaha, Nebraska	Not specified but 50% of first sample was functional Class III or IV, mean age 64.7 yr	Consistency of care, frequent follow-up to maintain stability and prevent acute decompensation	Standardized treatment protocols and forms, seen in clinic weekly and then every 6 weeks (15–20 times/yr), intense patient/spouse education, support groups, outpatient inotropic infusions, emergency department link, central computer database, home health care nursing	Cardiologists, registered nurses, dietitian, pharmacist, exercise rehabilitation, pastors, hospital volunteers

Patients with none of these risk factors were excluded from the study on the premise that they would be unlikely to benefit from a program designed to reduce hospital admissions.

The 3-month long intervention involved four key components: (1) intensive education, (2) a detailed analysis of medications, (3) early discharge planning, and (4) enhanced follow-up through home visits and telephone calls. The intervention was based on identification of several potentially correctable behavioral and social factors found to contribute to readmission in their prior research: noncompliance with medications or diet; inadequate patient education, discharge planning, or follow-up; and an insufficient social support system.[9] A nonpharmacologic, comprehensive, and intensive multidisciplinary DM intervention was developed to augment usual care. Each component of the approach is elaborated in the following narrative.

Individualized education was provided during hospitalization with daily visits by an experienced registered nurse with both cardiac and geriatric expertise. Patients were hospitalized an average of 4.8 days, allowing for repeated contacts, relationship building, and reinforcement. The educational content focused on heart failure diagnosis, symptoms, treatment, follow-up, and prognosis. All teaching was done using a booklet entitled, "Congestive Heart Failure: A Patient's Guide," developed by the team for use with elderly heart failure patients. A registered dietitian obtained a detailed dietary history from each patient and designed an individualized 1.5 to 2.0 g sodium diet, conforming to patient preferences as much as possible. The cardiac nurse taught and reinforced the diet during the daily visits. The importance of monitoring daily weights was emphasized repeatedly, and charts for noting the weights were provided. Home scales were provided if needed. Patients were instructed to call the physician or nurse if they had a change in their weight of 3 to 5 pounds.

The second major component of the intervention was a detailed medication analysis by a gerocardiologist with specific recommendations for reducing adverse effects and improving compliance. Unnecessary medications were eliminated, potential drug interactions were identified, and a simplified dosing schedule was recommended. The number of medications was typically reduced by 25% to 40%, and the regimen was consolidated to a no more than twice-a-day or three-times-a-day schedule. Reference medication cards were provided, as were medication schedules with drug names, dosages, and times. Potential side effects, especially serious ones requiring a call to the physician or nurse, were discussed. All teaching was reinforced repeatedly by the nurse.

The third aspect of the intervention was discharge planning by a social worker. Potential economic, social, and transportation problems were identified early in the admission and rectified by arranging for additional support to be provided after hospital discharge. The decisions and observations made during hospitalization (medication regimen changes, dietary restrictions, potential problems identified by the social worker) were summarized by the nurse case manager and communicated to a home health nurse responsible for postdischarge follow-up.

The final component of the intervention was enhanced follow-up. In all cases, the home care nurse visited the patient within 48 hours after hospital discharge to assess the home environment and to identify additional barriers to successful compliance with the treatment program. A physical examination was performed to assess physiologic stability. Compliance with medications, diet, activity, and weight monitoring was assessed. All teaching was reinforced. Three home visits were made in the first week; subsequent visit frequency was determined by federal home care regulations. The cardiac nurse who taught the patient in the hospital continued to contact the patient intermittently by telephone. The cardiac nurse also made home visits on an individualized, as-needed basis. The principal goals of follow-up were to reinforce patient teaching, to ensure compliance with medications and diet, and to identify recurrent symptoms that could be treated early before readmission was necessary.

Although the study intervention was generally well accepted by both physicians and patients, some physicians were resistant to what they perceived as "interference," and some patients found the frequency of contacts to be disruptive. In addition, some indigent patients did not have telephones, which hampered follow-up. Despite these challenges, overall compliance with the treatment program was excellent.

The effectiveness of the intervention was tested in a large, prospective randomized trial of 282 older heart failure patients.[4] The investigators found significant reductions in the number of heart failure readmissions (56.2% reduction; $P = 0.04$) and average days in the hospital (36.6% reduction; $P = 0.04$), and a nonsignificant increase in survival without readmission (19.6% increase; $P = 0.09$) during a 90-day follow-up period. Quality of life, as measured by the Chronic Heart Failure Questionnaire, improved to a significantly greater extent in the intervention group than in the control group ($P = 0.001$). During the 9-month period after discontinuation of the intervention, total readmissions were 11% lower ($P = NS$) and heart failure readmissions were 29% lower ($P = 0.08$) in the intervention group compared with the control group, suggesting that the beneficial effects of the intervention persisted for at least 1 year. The cost of the intervention was calculated as $216/patient in 1994 dollars. Two thirds of this cost was for nursing time, which averaged 7.2 hours per patient, and the remaining costs were for the provision of other services. Average total medical costs during the 90-day follow-up period were $460 lower for patients in the intervention group, reflecting the substantial reduction in readmission costs.

The Sharp HealthCare Model

Sharp HealthCare is the largest integrated health care system in Southern California, with five acute care hospitals, several affiliated physician groups, and a health maintenance organization. Health care providers from various disciplines began meeting in 1994 to design a multidisciplinary system of care that would meet the unique requirements of this system of hospitals. The program was implemented in early 1996.

A multidisciplinary team of nurses, pharmacists, dietitians, physicians, and social workers met weekly to structure existing support services and focus them on the heart failure population.[5] The intervention involved four key components: (1) standardized education, (2) social support, (3) early discharge planning, and (4) postdischarge follow-up through home visits and telephone calls. The design of the program was based on the published work of Rich and colleagues[3,4] but evolved to reflect the unique resources and patients at Sharp HealthCare. Each component of the intervention is elaborated in the following narrative.

To avoid confusion caused by conflicting patient education materials provided by different sources, standardized education was a major focus of the intervention. Information from patient education brochures used across the system of hospitals was gathered and integrated into a colorful binder entitled, "Living Successfully with Heart Failure." A three-ring binder was used so that it could be updated easily as new information became available (eg, efficacy of β-blockers). Weight charts were included. Team members visited patients in the hospital when possible and began diet and medication education using the binder. The team members continued education after hospital discharge through videotapes, quarterly newsletters, and short didactic presentations at monthly support group meetings. Individual discussions using the binder took place by phone, during home visits, and after support group sessions.

Social support was the second major component of the intervention. Support was provided in monthly support groups that integrated educational reinforcement with an opportunity for social interaction with other heart failure patients and caregivers. The monthly group meeting of 2 hours' duration was led by the social worker and attended by a member of each discipline. The format of the support group meeting was a brief educational offering followed by group discussion and individual time with team members. This provided an opportunity for patients to ask questions about their illness, diet, medications, or activity in the past month. Almost half of the patients in the intervention group attended one or more support group sessions (Table 20–2).

Table 20–2 Summary of the Intervention Received in the Sharp HealthCare Multidisciplinary Disease Management Program (*N* = 240)[6]

	Intervention Group (n = 120)	Usual Care Group (n = 120)
Average number of total contacts by team members	13.49	2.01
Received the educational binder	100%	0
Watched a heart failure video	34.2%	0.8%
Attended a support group	47.5%	6.7%
Received an inpatient pharmacist visit	42.5%	*
Assessed during hospitalization by the heart failure social worker	31.7%	*
Received an inpatient dietary visit	50.8%	*
Average number of case manager calls after discharge	5.62	0
Average number of home health generalist RN visits	4.29	1.93
Average number of home health specialty RN visits	3.27	0

*Not measured.
RN, registered nurse

Recently, the group meetings began to be broadcast on local cable television to access patients unable to travel to the meeting site.

Early discharge planning, the third major component of the intervention, was assumed by the medical social worker with some assistance from the home health liaison nurses. Assessment by the social worker focused on the current living situation and the resources available to the patient after discharge. Anticipated problems included living arrangements, economic status, cognitive abilities, social support, and physical challenges such as stairs in the home. Services (eg, Meals on Wheels), assistance with expenses (eg, Medi-Cal), and legal advice (eg, wills) were arranged as needed. Short-term counseling was provided by the social worker for those individuals having difficulty in adjusting to chronic illness.

The fourth component of the intervention was enhanced follow-up. A cadre of specialized cardiac home health registered nurses was trained in heart failure management and assigned to care for these patients whenever the physician requested home care. Home care was needed so that a nurse could assess physiologic stability and home safety, reinforce education, and set up

systems to promote medication compliance (eg, daily pillbox). The team recommended at least one home care visit for all heart failure patients, but that was not uniformly authorized and only 35% of patients in the intervention group received home care. Care was referred back to a registered nurse case manager when home visits were completed. The case manager typically called several times in the first month and monthly thereafter. The average number of calls was only 5.6 per patient over 6 months because the case manager did not call patients currently receiving home care. When no order for home care was obtained, telephonic case management began immediately after hospital discharge. The 6-month intervention was calculated to cost $330 in 1997 dollars.

Some challenges were encountered in program implementation. No additional staff members were hired to implement the program, so inpatient education was divided among the team members in addition to their usual responsibilities. The potential for lack of attention to these added responsibilities was a concern, but the staff was enthused about the program and made time to incorporate it into their routines. In addition, although pharmacists assessed the complexity of the medication regimen,[10] they lacked the authority to simplify the dosing pattern or add important medications (eg, angiotensin-converting enzyme [ACE] inhibitors). To overcome this barrier, physicians were contacted and relevant articles were placed on the chart by the pharmacists.

A prospective, quasi-experimental design was used to compare outcomes in patients assigned to the intervention group with a matched sample of patients enrolled into the control group. Patients were matched on functional status, comorbidity, and age. All patients admitted to a Sharp HealthCare hospital with a definitive diagnosis of heart failure were eligible to participate in the program unless self-care—the underlying philosophy of the program—was an unrealistic goal. For example, heart failure patients discharged to a long-term care facility were excluded because such facilities typically administer medications and prepare meals; self-care is rarely an option. For practical reasons related to data collection, patients with confusion, dementia, or major psychiatric illness were also excluded. The average age of the 240 patients in the study was 73 years. The sample was 55% women and almost half were married. Baseline functional status was Class I (22%), Class II (22%), Class III (43%), or Class IV (12%) as measured by the Specific Activity Scale.[11]

No differences in acute care resource use or quality of life were evident when the data were analyzed by group (intervention vs usual care), perhaps because an unselected group of all admitted heart failure patients was used. However, subgroup analyses based on the prospectively identified matching variables revealed that the program was effective in selected groups of patients. Total in-hospital costs were 68% lower in functional Class II patients in the intervention group compared with those in the usual care group. An actual direct cost savings of $3,476 per patient was achieved in this group of 54 individuals. In functional Class III patients, total costs were 11% ($289/patient) lower in the intervention group. Class IV patients receiving the intervention experienced a 30% decrease in hospital readmissions. Among Class III and IV pa-

tients, elderly individuals with other comorbid conditions benefited most from the multidisciplinary DM intervention.[6]

An additional important finding of the study was that Class I patients did not benefit from the intervention. Indeed, Class I patients in the intervention group experienced a marked increase in total acute care costs and heart failure costs and a decrease in overall quality of life. These observations suggest that a high-intensity intervention may be counterproductive in low-risk patients and that such patients may be better served by a less aggressive approach.

Other Multidisciplinary Models

Block and colleagues[1] expanded the multidisciplinary model by integrating it into a community hospital setting and combining inpatient and outpatient care even more thoroughly than either of the two programs described previously. The chief of cardiology, the nurse manager for the coronary care unit, a heart failure case manager, and the nurse director of outpatient cardiac rehabilitation collaborated to design a comprehensive system of care for heart failure patients. The "Success with Heart Failure" program was designed to promote collaboration with the primary care physician. Standardized hospital admission and discharge orders were developed. Intensive patient and family education was provided, including exercise prescription at hospital discharge. In the outpatient setting, education continued with cardiac rehabilitation, home care, and telemonitoring until patients were stable. No outcome data on the effectiveness of this program have yet been published.

Chapman and Torpy[2] described a multidisciplinary approach that improved the consistency of outpatient care through protocol-based practices. This example of multidisciplinary care was unique in that it evolved in an outpatient setting and later incorporated inpatient care; in most multidisciplinary models, care is initiated in the hospital. The clinicians provided aggressive, optimal drug therapy, frequent clinic visits, and intensive patient education and support to maximize compliance. The intervention cost an estimated $2,000 per year of care. Results from the first 67 patients enrolled in the program demonstrated a 30% decrease in hospital admissions, a 42% reduction in hospital days, and an average length of hospital stay that was almost a full day shorter (5.3 to 4.4 days) than in the year before the program began. The 67 patients were predominately men (66%), 64.7 years of age on average, and functionally compromised (50% Class III or IV, 47% Class II, 3% Class I).

The authors did not calculate their actual cost savings, but they note that an average heart failure hospital admission at their institution costs $9,000. They report 38 admissions in a comparison group of 67 patients before the program began; presumably these admissions cost them $342,000. After the program began, they had 27 admissions in the 67 patients receiving their intervention ($243,000). It appears that their program saved $99,000 or $1,478 per patient, an amount that would not have covered the cost of their program ($2,000/patient) unless the decrease in hospital days resulted in admissions that cost less than $9,000. No quality of life or patient satisfaction outcomes were reported.

ANALYSIS AND DIRECTIONS FOR FUTURE RESEARCH

The four programs described previously are similar in several ways. Each included the following characteristics: (1) multiple disciplines (eg, nurses, physicians, dietitians, social workers); (2) a bridge between inpatient and outpatient care settings; (3) contact with hospitalized patients that continued after hospital discharge; (4) repetition of patient education; and (5) a positive, encouraging approach designed to promote patient self-confidence. Nurse case management is also a common thread, although Chapman and Torpy do not appear to have used the nurse to coordinate individual care.[2] All the programs except Rich's included an exercise component as part of the intervention.

On the other hand, no two programs were identical, and each had unique features. On the basis of published accounts, it appears that only Block et al[1] included specific standards for inpatient care

(eg, heart failure admission and discharge orders). The Block team was the only one that used their database as a tool for disseminating clinical information to the primary care providers as a means to facilitate communication and avoid duplicative testing. Chapman and Torpy were the only ones to report the inclusion of inotropic infusions as a component of the program.[2] With the exception of Chapman and Torpy's intervention, all programs implemented to date appear to be cost-saving, with reduced hospital costs being sufficient to compensate for the cost of the intervention.

Much has been learned in the short interval during which disease management has been put into practice and tested. At this stage, however, many unanswered questions remain concerning the multidisciplinary approach. Specifically, research is needed to examine the intensity of the intervention in relation to clinically relevant outcomes. Intensity was measured by Rich et al as hours of time spent by the nurse (7.2 hours/patient, on average), who was the individual providing most of the intervention. Riegel and colleagues[6] measured intensity as the number of patient-team contacts (13.49 contacts per patient, on average), but they did not find a significant relationship between the number of contacts received and the outcomes achieved. Confounding variables such as disease severity, functional ability, comorbid conditions, age, and unmeasured personality characteristics probably overshadowed the relationship between treatment intensity and outcome. Another confounding factor is the lack of a clear standard for measuring the intensity of an intervention of this sort.

A second important area for future research is the identification of which components of the intervention are most effective from both the clinical and cost perspectives. All the interventions analyzed provided repetition of education, frequent contact, individualization of care, simplification of the treatment regimen, high-intensity care, consistency of staff and messages provided to patients, and coordination among care providers. In addition, all facets were provided by a staff with expertise in heart failure. Are specific treatment components essential, or is it the combination of interventions that is effective?

What is the incremental value of each component of the intervention? Although repetition seems key, at this point it is not possible to make any definitive statement about the vital threads underlying effective multidisciplinary DM. A clear definition of what constitutes multidisciplinary DM would facilitate research in this area.

A thorough analysis of the impact of specific interventions on patient behaviors could provide valuable insights into understanding the beneficial effects of multidisciplinary DM. If patients have learned to incorporate new information into their everyday lives, a continuing effect may be expected. If, however, patients have learned only to "comply" (ie, obey), an enduring treatment effect may not occur without continued reinforcement. Compliance itself may eventually lead to true behavioral change, however. Patients who comply with treatment recommendations may learn that the recommendation is effective and one worth continuing when rewarded with a decrease in symptoms. In this case, some treatment effects may persist. Further study of the factors that influence changes in health behaviors is needed to answer these important questions.

There may be other predictors of program success besides those alluded to previously. Experience suggests that situational factors are important contributors to success in programs such as these. One factor that appears to be extremely important is physician buy-in. Much of the multidisciplinary DM approach is made up of a packaging of existing support services. Because physicians are essential team members, services must support both patients and physicians. The intense patient education and follow-up provided by nurses and others can support physicians by reducing the time burden inherent in caring for patients with chronic illness. Another factor that appears to predict success is the culture of the institution where the program is implemented. Block et al,[1] for example, developed a program at a small community hospital. The culture of such a setting may be easier to influence than a large, multihospital system such as Sharp HealthCare. If future investigators can identify the contextual factors that contribute to success, it may be possible to develop interventions that can be more readily adapted to different environments.

Another important unresolved question relates to the duration of a DM intervention. Do we need to develop systems that provide intensive, continuing inpatient and outpatient care until the patient dies? Conversely, is it realistic to believe that we can work closely with patients for a relatively short interval (eg, weeks to a few months) and see sustained improvements in outcomes during long-term follow-up? A trial evaluating the impact of intervention duration on long-term outcomes would be helpful. Rich et al[4] demonstrated persistent effects for up to a year after a 3-month intervention. Stewart et al[12,13] found continuing effects on acute care resource use 18 months after a home-based intervention by a nurse and a pharmacist. Longitudinal data on treated and untreated cohorts would be a meaningful contribution to this literature.

Another important issue is the identification of patient groups that are most likely to benefit from a multidisciplinary DM program. The treatment effects demonstrated by Rich and colleagues[3,4] and by Chapman and Torpy[2] suggest that higher risk, sicker patient populations are the best candidates for such programs. This conclusion is supported by the data from Riegel and colleagues,[6] who demonstrated positive effects in functionally compromised heart failure patients but negative effects in functional class I patients. At this point we would not recommend an intensive intervention for relatively well heart failure patients. However, a modification of the intervention model may be suitable for this patient population.

A crucial therapeutic goal in heart failure patients is the prevention of disease progression during long-term follow-up, and future research efforts should be directed at the development of effective approaches for achieving this objective in functional Class I heart failure patients. Such patients might respond well to brief counseling or printed educational materials provided in person or by mail. Class I patients have few symptoms and may not perceive the need for change, so it may be helpful to target information delivery on the basis of their assessed stage of change. Prochaska and colleagues[14] have shown that people move from precontemplation to contemplation (ie, thinking about the need to change), to preparation, action, and maintenance when incorporating any change into their lives (eg, daily weights, low-sodium diet). They have also demonstrated that stage-specific educational materials are effective in helping individuals begin the process of change even when they are not yet ready to face the need for a change.[15] This approach has helped smokers, hypertensives, the sedentary, the obese, and others by helping them feel progress without confrontation. A similar approach may assist relatively well heart failure patients to begin to make changes that will ultimately enable them to delay disease progression and maintain a high quality of life.

The primary outcomes examined in the studies published to date have, for the most part, reflected acute care resource utilization (eg, admissions, days in the hospital, length of stay during an admission). Both Riegel[5,6] and Rich[4] measured quality of life, although the methods differed. Others have alluded to patient satisfaction, but no data have been reported.[2] As of this time, there are few data available to refute the belief that DM programs simply shift costs from acute care settings to physician offices. Opponents of DM argue that no true cost saving occurs because patients use exorbitant amounts of outpatient services to avoid the need for inpatient services. Results from Chapman and Torpy could be interpreted as supporting this viewpoint. Only Rich and colleagues included outpatient (ie, office visits and caregiver costs) as well as inpatient costs (ie, interventions, hospital care) in their analysis and demonstrated a decrease in overall, total costs.[4] Some cost-shifting

may occur, however, and additional data are needed to evaluate the effects of DM programs on total medical costs.

The effect of heart failure DM programs on long-term survival is currently unknown. However, improved compliance with ACE inhibitors and β-blockers could theoretically translate into improved survival. Recently, Stewart et al[13] reported a significant reduction in 18-month mortality among 97 heart failure patients randomly assigned to a home-based intervention or usual care. Similarly, Rich et al[4] reported a 25% lower 1-year mortality among patients randomly assigned to multidisciplinary DM, although this difference was not statistically significant. Clearly, additional research is needed on the effects of DM on long-term clinical outcomes, including mortality.

Perhaps the last question that needs to be addressed is whether multidisciplinary DM interventions are truly different from "good care" provided in the premanaged care days of old. Certainly, the structure differs from the era in which the physician provided all the education, counseling, problem solving, and follow-up. Is multidisciplinary DM any different in content? The most important difference we see is the synergy provided by team members coming together with their cumulative years of education and experience in different but related disciplines. Given the complexity of issues confronting heart failure patients, it is unrealistic to expect that any single individual can provide all the answers to all the patients' problems. However, through the coordinated efforts of a multidisciplinary team, virtually all issues and concerns can be managed effectively. Indeed, the capacity to deal with all problems may represent the essential strength of the multidisciplinary DM model.

REFERENCES

1. Block L, Fredricks LA, Wilker J. The design and implementation of a disease management program for congestive heart failure at a community hospital. *Congestive Heart Failure.* 1997;3:22–37.

2. Chapman DB, Torpy J. Development of a heart failure center: A medical center and cardiology practice join forces to improve care and reduce costs. *Am J Managed Care.* 1997;3:431–437.

3. Rich MW, Vinson JM, Sperry JC, et al. Prevention of readmissions in elderly patients with CHF. Results of a prospective, randomized pilot study. *J Gen Intern Med.* 1993;8:585–590.

4. Rich MW, Beckham V, Wittenberg C, Leven CL, Freedland KE, Carney RM. A multidisciplinary intervention to prevent the readmission of elderly patients with congestive heart failure. *N Engl J Med.* 1995;333:1190–1195.

5. Riegel B, Thomason T, Carlson, B, et al. Implementation of a multidisciplinary disease management program for heart failure patients. *Congestive Heart Failure.* 1999;5:164–170.

6. Riegel B, Carlson B, Glaser D, Hoagland P. Which heart failure patients respond best to a multidisciplinary disease management approach? *J Cardiol Fail.* In press.

7. Rich MW. Heart failure disease management: A critical review. *J Cardiac Fail.* 1999;5:64–75.

8. Fonarow GC, Stevenson LW, Walden JA, et al. Impact of a comprehensive heart failure management program on hospital readmissions and functional status of patients with advanced heart failure. *J Am Coll Cardiol.* 1997;30:725–732.

9. Vinson JM, Rich MW, Sperry JC, Shah AS, McNamara T. Early readmission of elderly patients with CHF. *J Am Geriatr Soc.* 1990;38:1290–1295.

10. Conn VS, Taylor SG, Kelley S. Medication regimen complexity and adherence among older adults. *Image.* 1991;23:231–235.

11. Goldman L, Hasimoto B, Cook EJ, Loscalzo A. Comparative reproducibility and validity of systems for assessing cardiovascular functional class: Advantages of a new specific activity scale. *Circulation.* 1981;64:1227–1234.

12. Stewart S, Pearson S, Horowitz JD. Effects of a home-based intervention among patients with congestive heart failure discharged from acute hospital care. *Arch Intern Med.* 1998;158:1067–1072.

13. Stewart S, Vandenbroek AJ, Pearson S, Horowitz JD. Prolonged beneficial effects of a home-based intervention on unplanned readmissions and mortality among patients with congestive heart failure. *Arch Intern Med.* 1999;159:257–261.

14. Prochaska JO, DeClemente CC, Norcross JC. In search of how people change: Applications to addictive behaviors. *Am Psychologist.* 1992;47:1102–1114.

15. Prochaska JO, Velicer WF, Rossi JS, et al. Stages of change and decisions balance for 12 problem behaviors. *Health Psychol.* 1994;13:39–46.

PART VII

Summary and the Future

CHAPTER 21

Summary and the Future of Heart Failure Care

Debra K. Moser and Barbara Riegel

The fact that heart failure is prevalent, costly, and expected to increase in incidence and prevalence should come as no surprise to the readers of this summary chapter. Each author of the preceding chapters has made these points convincingly, and they are covered in detail in Chapters 1 and 3. Only four additional details still are to be added to this dismal overview. First, the epidemic of heart failure can be expected to continue unabated. Second, the life expectancy of individuals with this diagnosis is currently quite poor, although some improvement can be anticipated. Third, quality of the life remaining after a heart failure diagnosis is increasingly poor for the individual. Fourth, the cooperation and involvement required of heart failure patients is extremely challenging for most. Each of these four points will be expanded upon briefly.

The epidemic of heart failure will continue. One reason for this is that people are living longer. Another reason is that the cardiology community has made great strides in the treatment of cardiovascular diseases in the past few decades. Age-adjusted death from cardiovascular disease has declined significantly since 1972.[1] Widespread use of thrombolytics, percutaneous transluminal coronary angioplasty, stents, and coronary artery bypass surgery has decreased the number of individuals dying with acute myocardial infarction. The problem is that cardiovascular disease is not declining—we are simply treating it better. Thus, patients with coronary heart disease, the primary cause of systolic dysfunction, are living long enough to develop heart failure. Further, hypertension, the primary cause of diastolic dysfunction, remains inadequately recognized and treated. Only 27% of the 50 million hypertensives in the United States have their blood pressures controlled to an adequate level (ie, < 140/90 mm Hg).[2] Obesity is becoming recognized as a national catastrophe; more than half of our population is overweight or obese.[3] Obesity is an independent risk factor for coronary heart disease and for diabetes mellitus, in itself a major risk factor for coronary heart disease.[4] Thus, with an aging population that is overweight, diabetic, and hypertensive, and a medical community increasingly adept at treating myocardial infarction, we can expect to see even more than the current 1 of 10 elders with heart failure in the future.

Currently, about half of the individuals diagnosed with heart failure can expect to die within 5 years. Specifically, in a recent community-based survey, 76% survived 1 year, and 35% were alive at 5 years.[5] The survival rate of such patients can be expected to improve in the coming years, however. Heart failure medical research has increased exponentially over the past 5 years. A decade ago, few colleagues were interested in heart failure. Now, many scientists are actively working in the field. The Heart Failure Society of America has a scientific journal, a practice journal, and an annual meeting that is growing in attendance. The tipping point was publication of the Agency for Health Care

Policy and Research (AHCPR) guidelines for systolic dysfunction,[6] publication of the Cardiology Preeminence Roundtable document, *Beyond Four Walls*,[7] and Rich and colleagues'[8] publication of the first randomized clinical trial of a heart failure disease management program. Since these mid-decade events, heart failure research has produced such miracles as β-blockers for heart failure[9] and spironolactone.[10] Spironolactone is now recognized as improving survival, even in the most functionally compromised heart failure patients, when added to a regimen of angiotensin-converting enzyme (ACE) inhibitor therapy, loop diuretic, and perhaps digoxin.[11] The cardiovascular surgeon's dream of implanting a pump off the shelf instead of a donor heart is closer to reality than ever before, with the vented electric left ventricular assist device.

Despite this exciting progress, the life of a person with heart failure becomes increasingly limited and uncomfortable as the illness progresses.[12–14] It appears that careful compliance with the treatment regimen may minimize symptoms, but for some patients, the lifestyle needed to control symptoms is too odious to tolerate. For others, the treatment itself is associated with an increase in symptoms (ie, hypotension, dizziness, fatigue, intermittent confusion, thirst).[15] Further, symptom control alone is not adequate to improve quality of life in heart failure patients.

The therapeutic regimen required to control symptoms is extremely challenging. Hemodynamic imbalance is responsible for most symptoms, hospital admissions, and costs. Pharmacologic therapy is the primary means of optimizing hemodynamics. However, drug therapy is not simple or benign. Patients usually take multiple medications. Such a regimen is confusing, expensive, and difficult to manage.[16,17] Early warning symptoms of hemodynamic imbalance often are subtle and difficult to recognize. Thus, the complex regimen of medications, dietary restrictions, self-monitoring requirements, and activity recommendations designed to control heart failure can seriously challenge these patients.

IMPROVING OUTCOMES

How effective are the various interventions available today in improving outcomes in persons with heart failure? Is there a magic bullet currently available? To answer these questions, a brief summary of the conclusions of our authors is provided below. Much of the discussion will center on the conceptual model of Wilson and Cleary, which was presented in Chapter 15 of this book. In that model, health-related quality of life (HRQL) is viewed as a continuum of biologic/physiologic factors, symptoms, functional status, health perceptions, and overall quality of life (Figure 21–1). Note that HRQL is that subset of quality of life that relates specifically to one's health and, thus, is the component that we, as health care providers, can influence. Each new step of the HRQL model represents an increasing level of complexity that builds on the prior step. In this book, although morbidity, mortality, and health care costs were discussed, quality of life was the outcome most commonly addressed in detail because it has received relatively little attention in other references and because it is emerging as an outcome of equal importance with morbidity and mortality.

Pharmacologic therapy is the mainstay of treatment for heart failure. Exner and Schron argued in Chapter 4 that therapy with ACE inhibitors, β-blockers, and spironolactone has been shown to improve survival. ACE inhibitors, β-blockers and digoxin decrease the need for rehospitalization. However, few of the pharmacologic therapies currently used significantly influence the higher, more complex and subjective components of HRQL (eg, health perceptions). Only modest improvements in HRQL have been observed in most of the large heart failure clinical trials. There appears to be little relationship between survival and HRQL, and some investigators have shown a decrease in HRQL with pharmacologic therapy. Only inotropic therapy has been found to improve overall quality of life significantly, and this therapy has been shown to decrease survival. Thus, although pharmacologic therapy is vital in the manage-

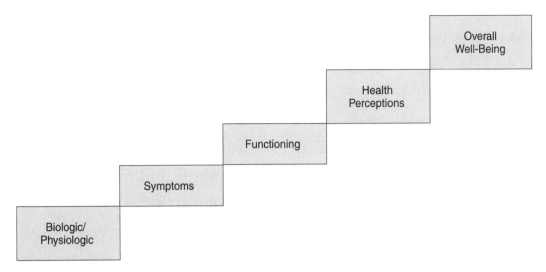

Figure 21–1 Graphic representation of the major concepts in health-related quality of life, as described by Wilson and Cleary.

ment of heart failure, it must be supplemented by other therapies if HRQL is to be improved.

Grady and colleagues, in Chapter 5, presented the surgical interventions most commonly employed in the management of patients with heart failure and discuss outcomes associated with their use. Revascularization and mitral valve repair improve ventricular function, symptoms, functional status, and quality of life in patients with heart failure. However, only a minority of patients with significant ventricular dysfunction has the requisite "hibernating" myocardium to make them eligible for surgical revascularization, and fewer yet have mitral valve problems amenable to surgical repair. Similarly, the use of the ventricular assist device as a bridge to transplant and cardiac transplantation improves quality of life, but the restricted supply of donor hearts severely limits the viability of these options for most patients with heart failure.

Nonpharmacologic, noninvasive therapies appear to hold the most promise for improving HRQL in persons with heart failure and to improve rehospitalization rates and decrease health care costs. These therapies include diet, exercise, cognitive/behavioral interventions, risk

factor modification, education aimed at improving self-care and treatment compliance, social support, or a combination of therapies packaged as "disease management." In Chapter 6, Moser and Dracup presented evidence that the largest gains to be made in the improvement of HRQL may be made with use of heart failure disease management programs, biobehavioral therapies, and exercise training. The success of these adjunctive therapies in addressing both quality of life and morbidity outcomes highlights the importance of expanding our definitions of appropriate heart failure therapy to include a balanced nonpharmacologic and pharmacologic approach.

A dietary sodium load may cause fluid overload and hemodynamic imbalance, the need for rehospitalization, and even death.[6,18] Bennett and colleagues, in Chapter 7, argued that diet and nutrition can make a significant impact on symptoms and functional status, midrange HRQL concepts. Conversely, symptoms and functional status influence a patient's appetite and ability to prepare and eat foods. A low-sodium diet, weight management, and alcohol restriction are typically advocated for heart failure patients, but we know little about the effects of such therapies on outcomes, especially the higher-order HRQL concepts (ie, health perceptions, overall quality of life). Further, compliance with dietary recommendations is low; prior investigators have documented that although 80% of heart failure patients recognize the need to limit salt intake, only one-third reported always doing so.[19] No data are available on compliance with weight loss recommendations or alcohol restriction, but one can imagine that it may be similar to salt restriction because "comfort" foods and drink may be particularly desired when one is ill.

In Chapter 8, Wilson and colleagues discussed the burgeoning yet still inconclusive evidence about exercise in heart failure. Exercise training can improve symptoms, functional status, mood, health perceptions, and overall quality of life, although few investigators have considered quality of life as an outcome; thus, the database remains small with regard to the effect of exercise on overall quality of life. Although no investigator has found exercise training to decrease quality of life, some have found that exercise fails to improve it, especially in older, "sicker" patients. This finding is of concern and underscores the importance of continuing this line of research because elders and patients with the worst heart failure consume the greatest proportion of health care resources and are increasingly the targets of intervention studies. The impact of exercise training on survival is unknown, although it is currently being examined in major randomized clinical trials. Moreover, little is known about how to counsel patients best to maximize their ability to perform activities that are important to them, such as daily personal and household activities, leisure domestic and social activities, and sexual activity. Enhancing patients' ability to perform these activities without symptoms or distress will be a major step in improving patients' quality of life.

Primary prevention of heart failure and secondary prevention of progression of existing heart failure should be major strategies embraced by all health care providers and systems of care. However, despite the obvious importance of such preventive strategies to combating the rising incidence, prevalence, and costs of heart failure, they have not received the attention from clinicians or researchers that is warranted. Secondary prevention, in particular, receives little attention. Possibly discouraged by negative prognosis and poor quality of life, many clinicians seem reluctant to suggest risk factor modification for their patients with heart failure. In Chapter 9, Doering and colleagues presented evidence that following several secondary preventative avenues may improve outcomes for patients with heart failure. Although little research has been conducted on secondary prevention in heart failure, risk factor modification that addresses hypertension, hyperlipidemia, diabetes, smoking, alcohol consumption, sedentary lifestyle, and obesity may prevent progression of heart failure and may improve ventricular function. What is completely unknown is the influence of lifestyle changes required for risk factor modification on the quality of life of patients with heart failure. On the one hand, if ventricular function is improved and symptoms lessened, quality of life might improve. On the other hand, patients already beleaguered by living with a chronic illness might view any further imposed lifestyle changes as onerous, and their quality of life might decrease. This question is among the many that researchers need to answer regarding primary and secondary prevention in heart failure.

The small but promising pool of literature on biobehavioral therapy in the management of patients with heart failure was discussed in Chapter 10. This unique approach to patient management included the specific interventions of relaxation, biofeedback, stress reduction, and cognitive therapy. These therapies are promising because they can influence positively both physiologic and psychologic manifestations of heart failure while increasing patients' sense of control. These therapies appear to reduce rehospitalizations and improve symptoms, mood, and overall quality of life, and their impact appears to compare favorably with other nonpharmacologic therapies, such as exercise and heart failure disease management.

A fundamental requirement for the success of any therapy—pharmacologic, surgical, or nonpharmacologic/noninvasive—is patient compliance with the prescribed components of the therapy. However, as Hill pointed out in Chapter 11, several investigators have documented poor compliance among patients with heart failure. At least 50% of hospital heart failure admissions are thought to be preventable, and noncompliance plays a major role in most preventable cases. Clinicians, however, have been slow to recognize the importance of emphasizing compliance in their interactions with patients. The clinician's role does not end with transmitting information about heart failure and its management but must include strategies to support patient adherence, as well. Moreover, clinicians should examine the system by which care is delivered to see whether organizational factors support compliance. Evidence from other cardiovascular conditions suggests that if patients, providers, and health care delivery systems attended better to compliance, outcomes could be improved but data to support this are lacking in heart failure.

Patient and family education is the cornerstone of nonpharmacologic therapy but is an aspect of care that is poorly standardized and rarely based on research. Knox and colleagues, in Chapter 12, noted that most heart failure hospitalizations are due to failure to comply with a sodium-restricted diet, medications prescribed, exercise and activity guidelines, daily weight monitoring, the need to notify health care personnel regarding symptom changes, and timely follow-up. They argued that knowledge attainment is only one goal; strategies that address problem solving, social, and emotional factors and that promote behavioral change and improve compliance must also be employed by clinicians. The problem is that, too often, patient education involves giving advice, rather than true counseling, and this may be why patients and families remain unsatisfied with the education received. They point out that problems in the current system, such as premature hospital discharge, trying to teach stressed patients during a short hospital stay, and inadequate communication among providers adds to the inadequacies of patient education efforts.

Social support has been shown to have a potent influence on outcomes such as compliance, mood, hospitalizations, recurrent events, and survival.[20–22] We are just beginning to understand the importance of this variable in heart failure, although the small database available suggests that it has the same influence.[23,24] Baas and colleagues, in Chapter 13, suggested that numerous internal and external factors beyond social support provide supportive resources that are vital for patients with heart failure as they strive to maintain their quality of life, assume responsibility for their own care, and attain personal goals. They further argue that a major goal of clinicians caring for patients with heart failure is to facilitate supportive internal and external resources and that heart failure disease management approaches may be successful, in part, because they do facilitate a number of these resources. Possibly some of the greatest gains to be made in improving outcomes in heart failure will be made as clinicians come to understand the role of internal and external supportive resources and become more adept at promoting them.

Potentially one of the most powerful external supportive resources is the patient's family. Yet, as O'Connor discussed in Chapter 14, although clinicians may recognize this, traditionally they have done little to formally acknowledge or promote the family's integral role in the improvement of patient outcomes. The reality of acute care is that responsibility for heart failure patients must be transferred to the family after discharge. However, families rarely have the clinical expertise to assume care and, even if they do, they always have the emotional overlay that makes the provision of care difficult. More attention to the process of families assuming care is needed.

ARE WE FOCUSING ON THE BEST OUTCOMES?

At the current time, event-free survival remains the primary outcome in federally funded clinical trials. Cost-effectiveness and associated variables (eg, resource use indicators, such as rehospitalization) are becoming recognized as increasingly important to include in research. We believe that the time is coming when HRQL will be recognized as essential because informed consumers are increasingly involved in their health care. With involvement comes choice and, given a choice about outcomes, many patients will choose quality over quantity of life.[25]

A decade ago, quality of life seemed to be hopelessly mired in vagueness. Recently, investigators have proposed conceptual models of the essential components and theoretical models of the manner in which these concepts relate. Sophisticated statistical analyses of quality of life databases have been used to explore patients' perceptions of this construct. For example, in a recent meta-analysis of quality of life research, Smith and colleagues[26] found that patients emphasize mental health when defining overall quality of life but that physical functioning is emphasized over mental health when formulating health perceptions (one component of HRQL). Specifically, health perceptions are influenced by physical functioning, which is influenced by symptoms (Figure 21–2). Analyses such as these help us to improve our understanding of HRQL.

Valid, reliable, and sensitive generic and disease-specific measures of quality of life and HRQL increasingly are available. Access to such instruments has encouraged heart failure investigators to include HRQL as an outcome in many, if not most, of the important clinical trials. Further, many investigators are using the same instruments (eg, Minnesota Living with Heart Failure Questionnaire and Medical Outcomes Study SF-36), which has allowed comparisons across populations and data aggregation for sophisticated analyses in large samples. Such techniques facilitate our understanding of the impact of heart failure on HRQL.

Not only are we beginning to understand that heart failure is a diagnosis with a significant influence on HRQL, but we are also just beginning to understand the interventions that truly influence HRQL. Pharmaceutical therapy alone is not powerful enough to improve HRQL significantly. Surgical therapy may be sufficient but it is not available to the majority of heart failure patients. Many of the therapies in general use (eg, dietary sodium restriction) are sufficient to influence symptoms if patients can be counseled sufficiently to comply with therapy. However, symptom improvement is not sufficient to improve overall quality of life in patients with heart failure. Exercise, biobehavioral approaches, and perhaps social support may improve HRQL, at least in some heart failure patients, but the database is not sufficient as yet for sweeping conclusions. We must, therefore, conclude at this point that, once diagnosed with heart failure, a combination of therapies is the best approach to improving the quality of life of these patients.

We are also just beginning to understand the patient characteristics that predispose to successful heart failure management and better HRQL. A recent study demonstrated that a patient's educational level and functional status were significant predictors of self-care management ability, when measured as the importance that heart failure patients place on various symptoms.[27] However, only 10% of the variance in self-care management was explained by these two variables. Specifically, individuals with higher education may master self-care easier than may those with lower education. Interestingly, those with poorer functional status may be better at self-care, perhaps because of experience with the illness. Once we understand more about the predictors of self-care and success in heart failure management, we may be able to turn our collective attention to those individuals who need more assistance (eg, the homeless or those with intermittent cognitive impairment).

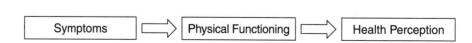

Figure 21–2 The relationships between symptoms, physical functioning, and health perceptions.

Interdisciplinary Collaboration

Disease management models appear to hold promise for a collaborative approach to improving outcomes in heart failure patients. Chapter 16 argued that disease management could be differentiated into (1) multidisciplinary, (2) case management by telephone or community outreach, and (3) heart failure clinic models. Each of these models was described in detail in Chapters 17 through 20. Despite the arbitrary distinction among the models, it should be noted that there are endless variations on the theme and that each of the programs tested seems to work to some degree. Patients enrolled in any of the different health care delivery models experience improved outcomes in terms of rehospitalization rates, costs, and quality of life. The few studies in which mortality was examined suggest a survival advantage for those enrolled in a heart failure disease management program, compared with those receiving usual care. The consistency of findings might be because, regardless of the model used, disease management always involves some level of interdisciplinary collaborative care.

Perhaps the message that is clearest from the explosion of disease management programs nationwide is that individuals from a single discipline cannot sufficiently meet the needs of the complex heart failure patient population. To achieve the desired outcomes (lower morbidity, higher survival, better HRQL) in a cost-effective manner, a comprehensive, interdisciplinary team is needed.

Interdisciplinary collaborative care is care provided by a team whose members are comprised of more than one discipline and who jointly share responsibility for planning care that is aimed at improving outcomes.[28] Interdisciplinary care is characterized by formation of a partnership among members of the individual disciplines. This partnership emphasizes coordination of care, effective communication, shared responsibility and authority, and joint decision-making that includes decisions about desired outcomes. Effective interdisciplinary collaborations recognize and optimize each of these factors while working to minimize situations where care is simply handed from discipline to discipline.

Heart failure patient and family care is too complex to be effectively delivered by a single discipline. It requires a comprehensive approach that is best delivered in an interdisciplinary collaborative environment. Failure of disciplines to collaborate has been linked to patient dissatisfaction and negative markers of quality care. Benefits of effective interdisciplinary collaboration include improved continuity of care and increased efficiency and quality of care, with the ultimate benefit of improved patient outcomes.[29,30] The best evidence in heart failure care indicates that interdisciplinary collaboration integrated into health care delivery models results in the best heart failure outcomes.

One major barrier to effective interdisciplinary collaborative care is the fear held by various professionals in different disciplines regarding maintenance of professional integrity within the interdisciplinary collaboration. Because nurses historically have struggled with issues of authority, power, and recognition related to their relationship with physicians, they may be tempted to leave physicians out of their collaborative ventures. Physicians often are not socialized to understand the unique contributions that other disciplines can make, and they often fail to consider the possibility of including others in their collaborative ventures or fail to consider them as equal partners. However, the various disciplines are equally vital to ensuring the success of ventures that aim to improve patient outcomes.

As disciplines work to maintain professional integrity within an interdisciplinary collaboration, they must overcome several potential problems.[28] First, communication among members of an interdisciplinary team must reflect partnerships in decision-making and shared needs, demands, values, goals, and outcomes. On the simplest level, this means that, for example, members should speak with each other about health care, not about medical or nursing care. Second, members of interdisciplinary teams need to consider carefully issues of power and authority. Effective collaboration demands negotiation and sharing of power and authority.

We need to move beyond historical issues and games (remember the "doctor–nurse game"?). Another factor that members of interdisciplinary teams need to contend with is professionalism that divides members. Each discipline has different expertise and professional expectations that, of course, are the basic reason for the collaboration. However, this professionalism also can set up boundaries that are difficult for members of other disciplines to cross if we do not take care to communicate so that no team members are excluded. Coming to an understanding of the issues important to each discipline's professional integrity can be enlightening and invigorating. Finally, each member of the team needs to feel free to communicate her or his discipline's values and to feel that these values are respected. Although optimally effective interdisciplinary teams have shared values, it is a mistake for any one discipline's values to be completely submerged by those of another. The essence of maintaining professional integrity is respecting the unique perspective of other disciplines and joining values for the good of patient care.

WHAT DOES THE FUTURE HOLD?

In the coming decade, the heart failure problem is expected to assume the same magnitude worldwide that it does now in the United States, and the problem will continue to grow in the United States. As such, heart failure prevention must become a priority for clinicians and researchers. Widespread adoption of primary preventive strategies to combat the seemingly inexorable rise in heart failure incidence and prevalence is vital. Research for addressing techniques for prevention of progression from cardiovascular disease to heart failure needs to be done. For example, does heart failure develop less frequently in acute myocardial infarction patients who exercise regularly after the event? Equally important is promotion of secondary prevention efforts, such as prevention of heart failure after acute myocardial infarction with widespread use of β-blockers and ACE inhibitors. More research is needed in this area to define how effective secondary prevention might

be in prevention of progression and promotion of regression of heart failure. In addition, it is important to determine how best to encourage clinicians to endorse and prescribe risk factor modification, and how to persuade patients to adopt prescribed lifestyle changes. Research also is needed to determine whether adoption of lifestyle changes adversely affects patients' quality of life and, if so, how to ameliorate negative affects.

As a group, most preventive strategies fit under the umbrella of nonpharmacologic and noninvasive interventions (referred to as *nonpharmacologic* for simplicity). The lack of work done in the area of prevention and risk factor modification is indicative of the lack of work done in the entire area of nonpharmacologic intervention. Pharmacologic therapy receives the most interest from researchers and clinicians, yet, at this stage of heart failure care, it may be advances in nonpharmacologic therapy that offer the most potential for improving outcomes. Because pharmacologic therapy operates in the background of nonpharmacologic therapy, advances in nonpharmacologic therapy also improve the effectiveness of drug therapy.

Nonpharmacologic therapy includes a wide range of therapies, including, at the macro level, heart failure disease management. At the micro level, nonpharmacologic therapy consists of components that fit within many comprehensive disease management programs and includes exercise, biobehavioral therapy, diet and nutrition, education and counseling, and behavioral strategies to enhance adherence. Many questions remain regarding optimal use of these therapies, particularly the umbrella therapy—disease management.

Despite the great promise of heart failure disease management to improve patient and health care resource use outcomes, the area of disease management research is mired in uncertainty and possibly has become a victim of its own success. Clinicians, seeing the success of a few heart failure programs, quickly adapted these programs, enrolled patients, and published outcomes from their programs. Consequently, the literature on heart failure disease management has mushroomed in the past 5 years, with the result that there has been little opportunity for clinicians and researchers to build on the work of each other. The end result is a literature with more questions than answers. For example, what components (eg, comprehensive education and counseling, optimization of medical therapy, flexible diuretic regimen, exercise training, vigilant follow-up) are essential to produce the positive results seen in most heart failure disease management programs? Of the major models of heart failure disease management (ie, multidisciplinary care, community care management, telephonic case management, and heart failure clinic models), is one more effective than another? How can we maximize interdisciplinary collaboration? Is the disease management approach appropriate for all patients with heart failure? Recent evidence indicates that, although all heart failure patients may need intensive education and counseling, some patients with less severe disease may suffer worse outcomes when they participate in disease management.[31] Given this information, it is important to determine which patients may be best served by which programs. Ultimately, to untangle many of these issues, we need progress in research and statistical methodology that will allow us to test patient, provider, system, and intervention variables simultaneously.

Similar questions about which patient groups are best served by a given therapy remain for other nonpharmacologic therapies. For example, which patient groups should be targeted for exercise training and at what intensities? Is home training as effective as supervised training in a rehabilitation or other health care setting? How do we identify which patients are best served by which levels of sodium restriction? For many patients, relatively rigid sodium restriction is associated with improved outcomes. On the other hand, given that sodium restriction has some negative effects, including activation of the renin-angiotensin system and volume depletion in some patients, is a rigid sodium restriction necessary for all patients, or are some patients harmed by such therapy? Is alcohol restriction necessary for all heart failure patients or only those with alcoholic cardiomyopathy? Will specific mi-

cronutrients (eg, Coenzyme 10, Hawthorne) be useful and in which patients? When any such therapy is prescribed, what is the best strategy or combination of strategies to promote its acceptance and adherence by the patient?

Largely unexplored are therapies that address specifically psychosocial factors that place patients at risk for poor quality of life, rehospitalization, and higher mortality. These include social isolation, depression, and anxiety. These are the risk factors of the future that clinicians and researchers need to consider in depth.

Perhaps the most important goal for the future is promoting application of existing research in practice. Over and over, investigators have documented the failure of clinicians to apply the results of clinical trials in their practices or to take advantage of the many published evidence-based guidelines to improve the management of their patients with heart failure.[32-37] Certainly clinicians' efforts to individualize care and to take patients' unique physical, psychologic, and social situations into account when planning and prescribing therapy might explain some of the discrepancy between "ideal" care and that seen in routine clinical practice. However, other factors also are operating in most cases, and these include failure of clinicians to remain current when faced with rapid advances in research related to patient management, difficulty applying results of clinical trials and guideline recommendations to individual patients, and fear of change. Innovative research that addresses these issues is sorely needed if we are to achieve the goal of promoting evidence-based care for all patients with heart failure.

To conclude, we are currently in an exciting time of continued rapid growth and change in clinical practice and research related to heart failure care. The increasing incidence and prevalence of heart failure, combined with the cost of caring for these patients in the future, provide us with an opportunity to address many of the difficult issues that will confront society as our population ages. Currently, the greatest efforts are concentrated in investigations of pharmacologic therapy. Achievement of improved morbidity, mortality, and quality of life outcomes for a greater number of patients with heart failure might best be realized by a more systematic, balanced, collaborative approach to practice and research that equally considers nonpharmacologic/noninvasive, surgical, and pharmacologic therapies and their interactions.

REFERENCES

1. Gillum RF. Trends in acute myocardial infraction and coronary heart disease death in the United States. *J Am Coll Cardiol.* 1994;23:1273–1277.

2. Gifford RW. A missed opportunity: Our failure to control hypertension optimally. *J Clin Hypertens.* 2000;2:21–24.

3. Mokdad AH, Serdula MK, Dietz WH, et al. The spread of the obesity epidemic in the United States, 1991–1998. *JAMA.* 1999;282:1519.

4. Hollander P. Confronting obesity: Toward prevention of diabetes and cardiovascular disease. *Cardiol Rev.* 2000;17:41–48.

5. Senni M, Tribouilloy CM, Rodeheffer RJ, et al. Congestive heart failure in the community: A study of all incident cases in Olmsted County, Minnesota, in 1991. *Circulation.* 1998;98:2282–2289.

6. Konstam MA, Dracup K, Baker DW, et al. Heart failure: Evaluation and care of patients with left-ventricular systolic dysfunction. Rockville, MD: Agency for Health Care Policy and Research, Public Health Services, U.S. Department of Health and Human Services; 1994.

7. Cardiology Preeminence Roundtable. *Beyond Four Walls.* Washington, DC: The Advisory Board Company; 1994.

8. Rich MW, Beckham V, Wittenberg C, Leven CL, Freedland KE, Carney RM. A multidisciplinary intervention to prevent the readmission of elderly patients with congestive heart failure. *N Engl J Med.* 1995;333:1190–1195.

9. Packer M, Bristow MR, Cohn JN, et al. The effect of carvedilol on morbidity and mortality in patients with chronic heart failure. *N Engl J Med.* 1996;334:1349–1355.

10. RALES Investigators. Effectiveness of spironolactone added to an angiotensin-converting enzyme inhibitor and a loop diuretic for severe chronic congestive heart failure (the Randomized Aldactone Evaluation Study [RALES]). *Am J Cardiol.* 1996;78:902–907.

11. Pitt B, Zannad F, Remme WJ, et al. The effect of spironolactone on morbidity and mortality in patients with severe heart failure. *N Engl J Med.* 1999;341:709–717.

12. Dracup K, Walden JA, Stevenson LW, Brecht ML. Quality of life in patients with advanced heart failure. *J Heart Lung Transplant.* 1992;11:273–279.

13. Rector TS, Johnson G, Dunkman WB, et al. Evaluation by patients with heart failure of the effects of enalapril compared with hydralazine plus isosorbide dinitrate on quality of life. V-HeFT II. *Circulation.* 1993;87:V171–VI77.

14. Gorkin L, Norvell NK, Rosen RC, et al. Assessment of quality of life as observed from the baseline data of the Studies of Left Ventricular Dysfunction (SOLVD) trial quality-of-life substudy. *Am J Cardiol.* 1993;71.

15. Carlson B, Riegel B, Moser D. Barriers and challenges to self-care in heart failure patients. Manuscript in process.

16. Monane M, Bohn RL, Gurwitz JH, Glynn RJ, Avorn J. Noncompliance with congestive heart failure therapy in the elderly. *Arch Intern Med.* 1994;154:433–437.

17. Stewart S, Pearson S. Uncovering a multitude of sins: Medication management in the home post acute hospitalization among the chronically ill. *Aust NZ J Med.* 1999;29:220–227.

18. Bennett SJ, Huster GA, Baker SL, et al. Characterization of the precipitants of hospitalization for heart failure decompensation. *Am J Crit Care.* 1998;7:168–174.

19. Ni H, Nauman D, Burgess D, Wise K, Crispell K, Hershberger RE. Factors influencing knowledge of and adherence to self-care among patients with heart failure. *Arch Intern Med.* 1999;159:1613–1619.

20. Hatchett L, Friend R, Symister P, Wadhwa N. Interpersonal expectations, social support, and adjustment to chronic illness. *J Pers Soc Psychol.* 1997;73:560–573.

21. Schreurs KM, de Ridder DT. Integration of coping and social support perspectives: implications for the study of adaptation to chronic diseases. *Clin Psychol Rev.* 1997;17:89–112.

22. Shumaker SA, Brownell A. Toward a theory of social support: Closing conceptual gaps. *J Soc Issues.* 1984;40:11–36.

23. Krumholz HM, Butler J, Miller J, et al. Prognostic importance of emotional support for elderly patients hospitalized with heart failure. *Circulation.* 1998;97:958–964.

24. Struthers AD, Anderson G, Donnan PT, MacDonald T. Social deprivation increases cardiac hospitalizations in chronic heart failure independent of disease severity and diuretic non-adherence. *Heart.* 2000;83:12–16.

25. Rector TS, Tschumperlin LK, Kubo SH, et al. Use of the Living with Heart Failure Questionnaire to ascertain patients' perspectives on improvement in quality of life versus risk of drug-induced death. *J Cardiac Failure.* 1995;1:201–206.

26. Smith KW, Avis NE, Assmann SF. Distinguishing between quality of life and health status in quality of life research: A meta-analysis. *Quality Life Res.* 1999;8:447–459.

27. Rockwell J, Riegel B. Predictors of self-care in persons with heart failure. *Heart Lung.* 2000; in press.

28. Lindeke LL, Block DE. Maintaining professional integrity in the midst of interdisciplinary collaboration. *Nurs Outlook.* 1998;46:213–218.

29. Knaus WA, Draper EA, Wagner DP, Zimmerman JE. An evaluation of outcomes from intensive care in major medical centers. *Ann Intern Med.* 1986;104:410–418.

30. Zimmerman JE, Shortell SM, Rousseau DM, et al. Improving intensive care: Observations based on organizational case studies in nine intensive care units: A prospective, multicenter study. *Crit Care Med.* 1993;21:1443–1451.

31. Riegel B, Carlson B, Glaser D, Hoagland P. Which heart failure patients respond best to a multidisciplinary disease management approach? *J Cardiac Failure,* in press.

32. Clinical Quality Improvement Network Investigators. Mortality risk and patterns of practice in 4606 acute care patients with congestive heart failure. The relative importance of age, sex, and medical therapy. *Arch Intern Med.* 1996;56:1669–1673.

33. Nohria A, Chen Y, Morton DJ, Walsh R, Vlases PH, Krumholz HM. Quality of care for patients hospitalized with heart failure at academic medical centers. *Am Heart J.* 1999;137:1028–1034.

34. Stafford RS, Saglam D, Blumenthal D. National patterns of angiotensin-converting enzyme inhibitor use in congestive heart failure. *Arch Intern Med.* 1997;157:2460–2464.

35. Sueta CA, Chowdhury M, Boccuzzi SJ, et al. Analysis of the degree of undertreatment of hyperlipidemia and congestive heart failure secondary to coronary artery disease. *Am J Cardiol.* 1999;83:1303–1307.

36. McDermott MM, Feinglass J, Lee P, et al. Heart failure between 1986 and 1994: Temporal trends in drug-prescribing practices, hospital admissions, and survival at an academic medical center. *Am Heart J.* 1997;134:901–909.

37. Ashton CM, Bozkurt B, Colucci WB, et al. Veteran Affairs Quality Enhancement Research Initiative in chronic heart failure. *Med Care.* 2000;38:126–137.

List of Sources

CHAPTER 1

Exhibit 1–1 *Source:* Adapted with permission from P.A. McKee, et al., The Natural History of Congestive Heart Failure: The Framingham Study, *The New England Journal of Medicine*, Vol. 285, pp. 1441–1446, Copyright © 1971 Massachusetts Medical Society. All rights reserved.

Figure 1–1 *Source:* Reprinted from *Morbidity and Mortality: 1998 Chartbook on Cardiovascular, Lung and Blood Diseases*, 1998, National Heart, Lung and Blood Institute, U.S. Department of Health and Human Services.

Figure 1–2 *Source:* Reprinted from Changes in Mortality From Heart Failure - United States, 1980–1995, *Mortality and Morbidity Weekly Report*, Vol. 47, pp. 633–637, 1998, the Centers for Disease Control and Prevention.

Table 1–1 *Source:* Adapted with permission from W.B. Kannel, K. Ho, and T. Thom, Changing Epidemiological Features of Cardiac Failure, *British Heart Journal*, Vol. 72, pp. S3-S9, © 1994, BMJ Publishing Group.

Table 1–2 *Source:* Adapted with permission from M. Senni, et al., Congestive Heart Failure in the Community: Trends in Incidence and Survival in a 10-year Period, *Archives of Internal Medicine*, Vol. 159, pp. 29–34, © 1999, American Medical Association.

Table 1–3 *Source:* Data from References 9–10, 26–28.

CHAPTER 2

Figure 2–1 *Source:* Reprinted with permission from I.B. Wilson and P.D. Cleary, Linking Clinical Variables with Health-Related Quality of Life: A Conceptual Model of Patient Outcomes, *Journal of the American Medical Association*, Vol. 273, No. 1, p. 60, Copyright 1995, American Medical Association.

CHAPTER 5

Figure 5–1 *Source:* Reprinted with permission from *The American Heart Journal*, Vol. 129, No. 6, p. 1167, © 1995, Mosby, Inc.

Figure 5–2 *Source:* Reprinted with permission from *Journal of Thoracic and Cardiovascular Surgery*, Vol. 115, No. 2, p. 384, © 1998, Mosby, Inc.

Figure 5–3 Courtesy of Thermo Cardiosystems, Woburn, MA.

Figure 5–4 Courtesy of Baxter Healthcare, Oakland, CA.

Figure 5–5 *Source:* Reprinted from *The Journal of Heart and Lung Transplantation*, Vol. 18, No. 7, p. 614, Copyright 1999, with permission from Elsevier Science.

Figure 5–6 *Source:* Reprinted from *The Journal of Heart and Lung Transplantation*, Vol. 18, No. 7, p. 612, Copyright 1999, with permission from Elsevier Science.

CHAPTER 6

Table 6–1 *Source:* Adapted from D.K. Moser and P.L. Worster, Impact of Psychosocial Factors on Physiologic Outcomes in Failure, *Journal of Cardiovascular Nursing*, Vol. 14, pp. 106–115, © 2000, Aspen Publishers, Inc.

CHAPTER 7

Figure 7–1 Courtesy of Baxter Healthcare, Oakland, CA.

Figure 7–2 Courtesy of Baxter Healthcare, Oakland, CA.

Figure 7–3 Courtesy of Baxter Healthcare, Oakland, CA.

Figure 7–4 Courtesy of Baxter Healthcare, Oakland, CA.

Figure 7–5 Courtesy of Baxter Healthcare, Oakland, CA.

Table 7–1 *Source:* Data from National Cholesterol Education Panel, Second Report of the Expert Panel on Detection, Evaluation, and Treatment of High Blood Cholesterol in Adults, Circulation, Vol. 89, pp. 1329–1445, © 1994, American Heart Association and S.M. Grundy, et al., Guide to Primary Prevention of Cardiovascular Diseases, *Circulation*, Vol. 95, pp. 2329–2331, © 1997, American Heart Association.

Table 7–2 *Source:* Data from J.L. Kee, *Laboratory and Diagnostic Tests*, 4th Edition, © 1995, Appleton & Lange.

CHAPTER 8

Figure 8–1 *Source:* Reprinted from *American Journal of Cardiology*, Vol. 69, C. Liang, et al., Characteristics of Peak Aerobic Capacity in Symptomatic and Asymptomatic Subjects with Left Ventricular Dysfunction, pp. 1207–1211, Copyright 1992 with permission from Excerpta Medica Inc.

Figure 8–3 *Source:* Reprinted with permission from D.M. Mancini, et al., Contribution of Skeletal Muscle Atrophy to Exercise Intolerance and Altered Muscle Metabolism in Heart Failure, *Circulation*, Vol. 85, pp. 1364–1373, © 1992, Lippincott, Williams & Wilkins.

Figure 8–4 *Source:* Reprinted with permission from H. Drexler, Alterations of Skeletal Muscle in Chronic Heart Failure, *Circulation*, Vol. 85, pp. 1751–1759, © 1992, Lippincott, William & Wilkins.

Figure 8–6 *Source:* Reprinted with permission from M.J. Sullivan, et al., Exercise Training in Patients with Severe Left Ventricular Dysfunction, Hemodynamic and Metabolic Effects, *Circulation*, Vol. 78, pp. 506–515, © 1988, Lippincott Williams & Wilkins.

Figure 8–7 *Source:* Reprinted with permission from A.J.S. Coats, et al., Controlled Trial of Physical Training in Chronic Heart Failure, *Circulation*, Vol. 85, pp. 2119–2131, © 1992, Lippincott, Williams & Wilkins.

Figure 8–8 *Source:* Reprinted with permission from R. Belardinelli, et al., Randomized, Controlled Trail of Long-Term Moderate Exercise Training in Chronic Heart Failure, *Circulation*, Vol. 99, pp. 1173–1182, © 1999, Lippincott Williams & Wilkins.

CHAPTER 9

Table 9–3 *Source:* Adapted from *The Sixth Report of the Joint National Committee on Prevention, Detection, Evaluation and Treatment of High Blood Pressure*, 1997, National High Blood Pressure Education Program, National Heart, Lung, and Blood Institute, U.S. Department of Health and Human Services.

CHAPTER 10

Table 10–1 *Source:* Reprinted with permission from *Alternative Therapies in Health and*

Medicine, American Association of Critical Care Nurses.

CHAPTER 11

Table 11–1 *Source:* Reprinted with permission from The Multilevel Compliance Challenge: Recommendations for a Call to Action, *Circulation*, Vol. 35, pp. 1085–1090, © 1997, Lippincott Williams & Wilkins.

CHAPTER 12

Appendix 12–A Courtesy of Evanston Northwestern Healthcare, Evanston, IL.

Exhibit 12–1 *Source:* Adapted from M. Konstam, et al., *Heart Failure: Evaluation and Care of Patients with Left Ventricular Systolic Dysfunction*, 1994, Agency for Health Care Policy and Research, Public Health Service, U.S. Department of Health and Human Services.

Exhibit 12–2 *Source:* Adapted with permission from M.W. Rich, Heart Failure Disease Management, *Journal of Cardiac Failure*, Vol. 5, pp. 64–75, © 1999, W.B. Saunders.

Exhibit 12–3 Courtesy of Disease Management Systems.

Exhibit 12–4 Courtesy of Evanston Northwestern Healthcare, Evanston, IL.

Figure 12–1 Courtesy of Evanston Northwestern Healthcare, Evanston, IL.

Figure 12–2 Courtesy of Evanston Northwestern Healthcare, Evanston, IL.

Table 12–1 *Source:* Reprinted with permission from S.B. Dunbar, et al., Heart Failure: Strategies to Enhance Patient Self-Management, *AACN Clinical Issues*, Vol. 9, pp. 244–256, © 1998, Lippincott Williams & Wilkins.

Table 12–2 *Source:* Data from J.O. Prochaska, et al., Stages of Change and Decision Balance for 12 Problem Behaviors, *Health Psychology*, Vol. 13, pp. 39–46, © 1994.

CHAPTER 14

Figure 14–1 *Source:* Data from R.D. Kerns, in *Family Assessment and Intervention in Managing Chronic Illness, A Biopsychosocial Perspective*, P.M. Nicassio and T.W. Smith, eds., pp. 207–244, © 1995, American Psychological Association.

CHAPTER 15

Figure 15–1 *Source:* Data from I.B. Wilson and P.D. Cleary, Linking Clinical Variables with Health-Related Quality of Life. A Conceptual Model of Patient Outcomes, *Journal of the American Medical Association*, Vol. 27, pp. 59–65, © 1995, American Medical Association.

CHAPTER 16

Figure 16–1 *Source:* Reprinted with permission from Changing Climate in Heart Failure: Towards a New Era, *Cardiovascular Research and Reports*, Vol. 19, No. 5, pp. 15–22, © 1998, Le Jacq Communications, Inc.

Figure 16–2 *Source:* Reprinted with permission from Changing Climate in Heart Failure: Towards a New Era, *Cardiovascular Research and Reports*, Vol. 19, No. 5, pp. 15–22, © 1998, Le Jacq Communications, Inc.

CHAPTER 17

Table 17–1 *Source:* Data from References 6–9 and 11.

CHAPTER 19

Appendix 19–A Courtesy of Stanford Cardiac Rehabilitation Program, Palo Alto, CA.

Figure 19–3 *Source:* Reprinted from *American Journal of Cardiology*, Vol. 79, J.A. West, et al., A Comprehensive Management System for Heart Failure Improves Clinical Outcomes and Reduces Medical Resource Utilization, pp. 58–63, Copyright 1997, with permission from Excerpta Medica, Inc.

Table 19–2 *Source:* Reprinted from *American Journal of Cardiology*, Vol. 79, J.A. West, et al., A Comprehensive Management System for Heart Failure Improves Clinical Outcomes and Reduces Medical Resource Utilization, pp. 58–63, Copyright 1997, with permission from Excerpta Medica, Inc.

CHAPTER 20

Table 20–1 *Source:* Data from References 1, 2, 4, and 6.

Table 20–2 *Source:* Reprinted with permission from *Journal of Cardiac Failure.*

CHAPTER 21

Figure 21–1 *Source:* Data from I.B. Wilson and P.D. Cleary, Linking Clinical Variables with Health-Related Quality of Life. A Conceptual Model of Patient Outcomes, *Journal of the American Medical Association*, Vol. 27, pp. 59–65, © 1995, American Medical Association.

Index

A

Acquired valve disease, 5
Adaptive potential assessment model
  affiliation-individuation, theoretical linkages, 205, 206
  self-care, theoretical linkages, 205, 206
  supportive resources, 204–205
Adult day care, 225, 226
Adult learning, principles, 186
Affiliation, defined, 202
Affiliation-individuation
  adaptive potential assessment model, theoretical linkages, 205, 206
  developmental residual, theoretical linkages, 205, 206
  self-care, theoretical linkages, 205, 206
  supportive resources, 202–203
Age-adjusted mortality rate, 14
Aging
  cardiovascular system, 5
  caregiver, 222
  heart failure, 5
    incidence, 8
    mortality, 12
  patient education, 186
Albumin, 101
Alcohol, 146, 310
  compliance, 146
Alcoholic cardiomyopathy, 146
Alternative models of care
  economic outcomes, 35–38
  randomized clinical trial, 35–38

Angiotensin-converting enzyme inhibitor, 15, 33, 139–140, 344
  Digoxin Investigators Group (DIG) trial, 45, 47
  noncompliance, 169
    physician factors, 171–172
Anthropometric measurement, 100–101
Anxiety, 85
  family, 221
Appraisal of Caregiving Scale, 256
Area Agency on Aging, 225, 226
Attributable risk, defined, 4
Autocorrelation, 53
Autonomy, 202

B

Behavior, outcomes measurement, 255
Behavior modification program, exercise training, 147–148
Behavioral health assessment, 136–138
β blocker, 139, 140, 344
  noncompliance, physician factors, 171–172
Biceps, 104, 108
Biobehavioral therapy, 85–86, 152–160, 346
  cardiovascular disease, 153–155
    cost-effectiveness, 156
    maintenance of effects, 154–155
    physiologic outcomes, 153–154
    psychologic outcomes, 154
  heart failure, 155–159
  potential mechanisms of action, 86
Biochemical serum marker, 101–102

Biofeedback
    cardiovascular disease, 153–155
        cost-effectiveness, 156
        maintenance of effects, 154–155
        physiologic outcomes, 153–154
        psychologic outcomes, 154
    defined, 153
    heart failure, 155–159
Biofeedback-relaxation training, 85–86
Biologic functioning, 250–251
Bisoprolol, 171
Blood pressure, control of, 168
Blood urea nitrogen creatinine, 103–104
Body mass index, 101
Burden Interview, 256

C

Cachexia
    catecholamine, 113
    cytokine, 112–113
    defined, 112
    management, 112–117
    sample menus, 114–116
    sodium restriction, 117
Canadian Cardiovascular Society Functional
    Classification, 246–247
Captopril, 27, 129, 140
Cardiac cachexia, 112
Cardiac rehabilitation program, 131–133
    components, 132–133
    patient selection, 133
Cardiac transplantation, 54, 65–71
    actuarial survival, 65, 66
    donor shortage, 66–67
    immunosuppression, 65
    quality of life
        age, 69–70
        complications, 69–70
        gender, 69–70
        long-term studies of outcomes, 69
        racial/ethnic background, 69–70
        research methodologic issues, 70–71
    technique, 65–66
Cardiomyopathy, quality of life, 59

Cardiopulmonary exercise testing, exercise
    training, 129, 130
Cardiovascular disease
    biobehavioral therapy, 153–155
        cost-effectiveness, 156
        maintenance of effects, 154–155
        physiologic outcomes, 153–154
        psychologic outcomes, 154
    biofeeback, 153–155
        cost-effectiveness, 156
        maintenance of effects, 154–155
        physiologic outcomes, 153–154
        psychologic outcomes, 154
    relaxation, 153–155
        cost-effectiveness, 156
        maintenance of effects, 154–155
        physiologic outcomes, 153–154
        psychologic outcomes, 154
    risk factor signs, 104–105
    social support research, 208–210
Cardiovascular Heart Study, 9, 11
Cardiovascular system, aging, 5
Caregiver, 255–257. See also Family
    aging, 222
    benefits, 223–224
    caregiver burden, 223, 256
    caring for, 222–229
    characterized, 222
    developmental burden, 223
    economic value, 222–223
    effects of caregiving, 222–224
    emotional burden, 223
    hardiness, 225–227
    health care workers, 225
    internal resources, 224–225, 225–227
    interventions to support, 225–227
    mitigating negative effects, 224–225
    outcomes measurement
        caregiver burden, 256
        caregiver symptoms, 256–257
        caregiving appraisal, 256
    physical burden, 223
    reciprocity, 223
    social support, 224
Caregiver Strain Index, 256

Carvedilol, 34
  clinical trial, 45, 46–47
  cost-effectiveness, 34
  Prospective Randomized Evaluation of
    Carvedilol in Symptoms and Exercise
    (PRECISE) trial, 45, 46–47
Case management
  defined, 282
  disease management, 271–272
  models, overview, 318–322
  telephone, 322–326
Catecholamine, cachexia, 113
Cause, defined, 4
Change, 184–186
  action stage, 184–185
  contemplation stage, 184–185
  maintenance stage, 184–185
  precontemplation stage, 184–185
  preparation stage, 184–185
Cholesterol, 7, 101–102
Chronic Heart Failure Questionnaire, 23, 25, 250
Chronic illness
  family, 220
    affective response, 221
    amount of disability, 221
    disease process, 220–221
    symptomology, 221
  health-related quality of life, 19–20
Chronic pain, family, 220, 221
Cigarette smoking, 7
Clinical practice guidelines, heart failure, 131
Clinical trial
  carvedilol, 45, 46–47
  digoxin, 45, 47
  enalapril, 44–46
  isosorbide dinitrate, 44–46
  metoprolol, 45, 48–49
  vesnarinone, 45, 47–48
Clock Drawing Test, 248–249
Cognitive functioning, 248–249
Cognitive-behavioral intervention, 85
Cognitive-behavioral transactional model of
  family functioning, 219
Communication, ineffective communication
  patterns, 180–181

Community case management, 282–298
  defined, 282
  Mount Carmel Health
    components, 291–295
    costs, 296–297
    critique, 296
    home health care, 297–298
    implementation, 290–291
    outcomes, 295
    patient independence, 297
    patient referral, 297
    pitfalls, 296–298
    program development, 290–291
  patient education, 292–293
  program, 284–290
    components, 285–288
    outcomes, 285–288
    patients, 285–288
    results, 284–290
    study design, 285–288
  rationale, 282–284
Comorbidity, xvi
Compliance, xiii, 165–175, 346–347. *See also*
  Noncompliance
  actions to increase
    by health care organizations, 166–167
    by patients, 166
    by providers, 166
  alcohol, 146
  challenge of, 165
  defined, 165
  exercise training, 147
  hospital readmisison, 169
  importance, 165
  medical nutrition recommendations, 120–121
  medication
    counseling, 172
    multidisciplinary treatment approach, 172
  mortality, 169
  nutritional management, 120–121
  pharmacologic therapy, 171–172
  research recommendations, 173–175
    patient level, 174
    provider level, 174–175
    systems level, 175–176

Compound symmetry, dependent variable, 53
Comprehensive clinical intervention, 37
Comprehensive discharge planning and home
    follow-up protocol, hospitalization,
    readmissions, 36–37
Computer telephony, telemanagement, 188
Congenital heart disease, 5
Constant covariance, dependent variable, 53
Control, 202, 213
Coronary artery bypass grafting, 54, 56
Coronary artery disease, 54
Coronary heart disease, 5
    heart failure, relationship, 3
    risk factors, 5, 6
Cost-effectiveness
    behavioral therapy, 155
    biofeedback, 155
    carvedilol, 34
    pharmacologic therapy, 33–35
    relaxation, 155
Creatinine, 13
Critical pathway guidelines
    heart failure, 181, 182
    patient education, 181, 182
Custodial home care, 225, 226
Cytokine, 26
    cachexia, 112–113

D

Dehydration, signs, 104
Dependent variable
    compound symmetry, 53
    constant covariance, 53
    normality transformation, 53
    repeated measures, 53
Depression, 85
    family, 221
Developmental residual
    affiliation-individuation, theoretical linkages,
        205, 206
    supportive resources, 204
Diabetes, 6, 143
Diet, 310
Diet history, 107–110
    current dietary intake evaluation, 107–108
    diminished cognitive function, 109
    dyspnea, 109, 110
    fatigue, 109, 110

medical history, 108
    medication, 110
    social and cultural factors, 110
    symptoms of heart failure, 108–110
Dietary sodium restriction, 140
Digitalis Investigation Group study, 33
Digoxin
    clinical trial, 45, 47
    Digoxin Investigators Group (DIG) trial, 45,
        47
    economic impact, 33
Digoxin Investigators Group (DIG) trial
    angiotensin-converting enzyme inhibitor, 45,
        47
    digoxin, 45, 47
    diuretic, 45, 47
Direct cost, heart failure, 31–32
Disease management, 184, 267–279, 350
    case management models, 271–272
    classification, 279
    clinic models, 272
    criteria, 268
    critique of published research, 272–275
    definition, 267–268
    differences in models of care, 272–273
    differences in patients studied, 273–274
    differences in study methods, 274–275
    evolution, 268–275
    models, 268–272
    multidisciplinary approach, 270–271
    program design, 275–279
        steps, 275–279
Diuretic, 139, 140, 141, 309, 311
    Digoxin Investigators Group (DIG) trial, 45,
        47
Donor shortage, quality of life, 67–71
    short-term studies on outcomes, 67–69
Duke Activity Status Instrument, 247–248
Dysfunctional myocardium, surgical
    revascularization, 55
Dyslipidemia, 7
Dyspnea, 124
    diet history, 109, 110

E

Edema, self-monitoring skills teaching, 120
Educational materials, patient education, 186,
    188–189

e-Health, 188
Electrolyte, 102–104
Enalapril, 140
　clinical trial, 44–46
　left ventricular dysfunction, 45, 46
　veterans Administration Heart Failure Trials,
　　44–46
Evans County study, 9, 10
Exercise, 146–148, 311, 346
　Prospective Randomized Evaluation of
　　Carvedilol in Symptoms and Exercise
　　(PRECISE) trial, 45, 46–47
　standards, consensus American Heart
　　Association statement, 131–132
　systolic dysfunction, 26
Exercise intolerance
　hemodynamic factors, 125
　pathophysiology, 124–128
　traditional explanation, 124–125
Exercise training, 86–92, 124–133, 128–131, 147
　behavior modification program, 147–148
　cardiopulmonary exercise testing, 129, 130
　compliance, 147
　exercise prescriptions in clinical practice,
　　131–133
　hemodynamic monitoring, 129, 130
　impact on quality of life, 87–90
　intervention, 87–90
　maximal exercise test, 133
　patient selection, 133
　patients, 87–90
　potential mechanisms of action, 91–92
　quality of life measurement, 87–90
　study design, 87–90
　variable response, 129, 131
Exertional dyspnea, pulmonary artery wedge
　pressure, 124
Exertional fatigue, 124
Eye, 104, 107

F

Family, 206–208, 347. *See also* Caregiver
　anxiety, 221
　chronic illness, 220
　　affective response, 221
　　amount of disability, 221
　　disease process, 220–221
　　symptomology, 221
　chronic pain, 220, 221
　depression, 221
　patient education, 181
　transitioning care, 219–230
Family theory, 219–222
Fatigue
　diet history, 109, 110
　skeletal muscle flow, 124
Fluid, 102–104
Fluid overload, 140–141
Fluid restriction, 310
Food Guide Pyramid, 107
Framingham Study, 3, 4, 6
　hypertension, 6
　left ventricular hypertrophy, 6
Functional health pattern
　general assessment, 137
　specific assessment, 137
Functional Status Questionnaire, 247
Functioning, 246–249
Fy-antigen, 7

G

Group-based cognitive-behavioral intervention,
　85
Guidelines, heart failure, 258
*Guidelines for the Evaluation and Management
　of Heart Failure,* 131

H

Hardiness, 225–227
Health Perceptions Questionnaire, 246
Health resource utilization, multidisciplinary
　approach, 38
Health-related quality of life, 347–348
　causal model, 19
　chronic illness, 19–20
　Comprehensive Health, Well-Being, and
　　Quality of Life Framework, 19
　concepts, 243, 345
　conceptual model, 18–19, 18–28
　　for clinicians, 20–25
　defined, 18
　dimensions, 19
　multidimensional construct, 18–19
　outcomes measurement, 241–251
　　biologic functioning, 250–251

Canadian Cardiovascular Society
Functional Classification, 246–247
Chronic Heart Failure questionnaire, 250
Clock Drawing Test, 248–249
cognitive functioning, 248–249
Duke Activity Status Instrument, 247–248
Functional Status Questionnaire, 247
functioning, 246–249
generic measures, 242–243
health perception, 245–246
Health Perceptions Questionnaire, 246
Heart Condition Assessment, 248
Medical Outcomes Short Form-36 Item
Questionnaire (SF-36), 244–245
Mini-Mental State Examination, 248
Minnesota Living with Heart Failure
questionnaire, 243–244
New York Heart Association (NYHA)
Functional Classification, 246
overall well-being, 243–245
physical functioning, 246–248
physiologic functioning, 250–251
Quality of Life Index, 245
Quality of Life Questionnaire in Severe
Heart Failure, 244
Sickness Impact Profile, 245
Specific Activity Scale, 247
symptoms, 249–250
Yale scale, 249–250
pharmacologic therapy
clinical trials, 44–49
impact, 43–49
Wilson and Cleary model, 20–27
biologic factors, 21, 25–27
empirical data, 25–27
functioning, 21–22, 26–27
general health perceptions, 22
levels, 20–22
measuring variables, 23–25
outcome measure, 23
physiologic factors, 21, 25–27
quality of life, 22
symptoms, 21, 25–26
Heart Condition Assessment, 248
Heart failure
aging, 5
incidence, 8
mortality, 12
biobehavioral therapy, 155–159

biofeedback, 155–159
causes, 5–7
clinical manifestations, 3
clinical practice guidelines, 131
coronary heart disease, relationship, 3
critical pathway guidelines, 181, 182
cycle of dependence, 179
defined, 3
diagnosis, criteria, 3, 4
direct cost, 31–32
economic impact, 31–38
key concepts, 31–32
emerging model, 270
epidemic, causes, 3
epidemiology, 3–15
future, 350–352
guidelines, 258
home management, 227–229
hospitalization, 12
cost, 31–32
length of stay, 12
readmission, 12
improving outcomes, 344–348
incidence, xv, 7–8
economic impact, 32
Framingham Study, 7, 8
indirect cost, 31–32
intangible cost, 31–32
model of traditional care, 269
morbidity, 12
mortality, 12–15
race, 12–13
sex, 12–13
multidisciplinary care, xiii
norm-based data, 24
nutritional management, management of
symptoms, 117–118
pathophysiology, 43
premature discharge, 180
prevalence, xv, 8–11
age, 11
race, 11
sex, 11
prognosis, 12–15
age-adjusted mortality rate, 14
factors, 13
functional classification, 13
type of underlying heart disease, 13
as public health problem, 3

relaxation, 155–159
research, xv
  methodological limitations, 3–4
risk factors, 5–7
  multiple, 7
severity, economic impact, 32
social support research, 208–210
standards, 258
summary, 343–350
telemanagement, 187–188
  high risk for rehospitalization, 187
trends, 8
Heart failure clinic, 301–315
  components, 302
  patient evaluation, 307
  patient management, 307–308
  studies, 302, 303–306
  University of California, Los Angeles
    (UCLA) Medical Center, 308–315
    alcohol, 310
    cost, 315
    diet, 310
    diuretic, 309, 311
    exercise, 311
    fluid restriction, 310
    medication compliance, 311–312
    outcomes, 312–313
    outcomes measurement, 314–315
    outcomes variables, 313–314
    patient education, 310–312
    smoking, 310
    weight, 310–311
Heart failure disease management program,
  78–85
  impact on quality of life, 80–83
  intervention, 80–83
  lessons from negative studies, 85
  mechanisms of action, 84–85
  patients, 80–83
  quality of life measurement, 80–83
  study design, 80–83
Heart transplant. *See* Cardiac transplantation
HeartMate implantable left ventricular assist
  device, 60–61
Height, 100
Hematocrit, 102
Hemodynamic monitoring, exercise training,
  129, 130
Hemoglobin, 102

Hibernating myocardium, surgical
  revascularization, 55
Hierarchical linear model, quality of life
  research, 53–54
Home assessment, 228
Home health care, 227–229, 297–298
  patient education, 227–228
Home-based intervention
  hospitalization, readmission, 36
  randomized clinical trial, 36–37
Hope, 212–213
Hospice, 225, 226
Hospital cost, heart failure, 31–32
Hospital readmisison, compliance, 169
Hospitalization, 12, 173
  length of stay, 12
  premature discharge, 180
  readmission, 12
    causes, 178
    comprehensive discharge planning and
      home follow-up protocol, 36–37
    home visit, 36–37
    home-based intervention, 36
    noncompliance, 178
  social support, 209
Hydralazine, 33
Hydralazine-isosorbide dinitrate, Veterans
  Administration Heart Failure Trials, 44–46
Hyperlipidemia, 142–143
Hypertension, 5–6, 138–142, 168
  Framingham Study, 6
  lifestyle modification, 138–139, 140
  management, 138–141
    outcomes, 141–142
  pharmacotherapy, 139–141
  population-attributable risk, 6
  Studies of Left Ventricular Dysfunction
    (SOLVD) registry, 138
Hypervolemia
  altered laboratory values, 103
  management, 118–119, 120
  signs, 104
Hypovolemia, altered laboratory values, 103

I

Immunosuppression, cardiac transplantation, 65
Implantable left ventricular assist device, 60–65
  benefits, 62

as bridge to heart transplantation, 60, 62
complications, 62–63
de-airing, 61–62
as destination therapy, 63
implantation, 61
quality of life, 63–65
    research methodologic issues, 64–65
    Randomized Evaluation of Mechanical
      Assistance for the Treatment of
      Congestive Heart Failure, 63
Inactivity, 146–148
Incidence, defined, 4
Indirect cost, heart failure, 31–32
Individuation, defined, 202
Insulin resistance, 143
Intangible cost, heart failure, 31–32
Interactive voice response, telemanagement,
    188
Interdisciplinary collaboration, 349–350
Ischemic left ventricular dysfunction, surgical
    revascularization, 55
Isolated systolic hypertension, 6
Isosorbide dinitrate, 33
    clinical trial, 44–46

K

Knowledge, outcomes measurement, 255

L

Left ventricular dysfunction
    enalapril, 45, 46
    Studies of Left Ventricular Dysfunction, 45,
      46
Left ventricular hypertrophy, 5
    Framingham Study, 6
Length of stay, outcomes measurement, 253
Lipid
    level guidelines, 101–102
    management, 142–143
    targets, 142
Longitudinal analysis, quality of life research,
    52–53
    attrition, 53

M

Malnutrition
    management, 112–117
    sample menus, 114–116
Maximal exercise test, exercise training, 133
Medical Outcomes Short Form-36 Item
    Questionnaire (SF-36), 244–245
Medical Outcomes Study, 23, 24
Medication
    compliance, 311–312
      counseling, 172
      multidisciplinary treatment approach, 172
    diet history, 110
Metoprolol, 34
    clinical trial, 45, 48–49
    Metoprolol CR/XL Randomised Intervention
      Trial in Congestive Heart Failure, 45,
      48–49
Mini-Mental State Examination, 248
Minnesota Living with Heart Failure
    questionnaire, 23, 24–25, 243–244
Mitral regurgitation, 56–58
Mitral valve repair, 56–58
    quality of life, 58–60
      research methodologic issues, 59–60
Mixed model, quality of life research, 53–54
Modeling and Role Modeling theory, 201, 202–
    205, 214, 215
    goals, 215–216
Monitoring and Educating Using Disease
    Management to Improve Compliance
    Instrument, patient education, 186, 192–196
Morbidity
    pharmacologic therapy, 43–44
    quality of life, association, 77–78
Mortality
    compliance, 169
    pharmacologic therapy, 43–44
    quality of life, association, 77–78
Multidisciplinary disease management model,
    331–339
    analysis, 337–339
    existing programs, 331–337
    future research, 337–339

Jewish Hospital of St. Louis Model, 331–334
Sharp HealthCare Multidisciplinary Disease Management Program, 334–336
summary of published reports, 332
Multidisciplinary treatment approach, 172
health resource utilization, 38
MULTIFIT, 322–326
Multilevel model, quality of life research, 53–54
Multivitamin supplement, 117
Myocardial infarction, population-attributable risk, 6

N

National Health and Nutrition Examination Survey, 9–11
New York Heart Association (NYHA) Functional Classification, 246
Nicotine replacement treatment, 145
Noncompliance, 165–175, 178, 311–312. *See also* Compliance
angiotensin-converting enzyme inhibitor, 169
physician factors, 171–172
beta blocker, physician factors, 171–172
defined, 165
desired treatment outcomes, 184
extent, 169–170
family factors contributing to, 168–170
impact, 165–168
issues, 184
patient factors, 168–170, 183, 184
provider factors, 171–172, 183, 184
readmission, 178
system factors, 172–173
Nonpharmacologic therapy, 345, 350–351
quality of life, 77–93
integrated theory to explain mechanism, 92
recommendations for research and practice, 92–93
Normality transformation, dependent variable, 53
Novacor left ventricular assist device, 60–61, 62
Nutrition, 345–346

Nutrition supplementation, 117
Nutritional assessment
components, 139
Subjective Global Assessment, 110–112
Nutritional cardiac disease, 5
Nutritional management, 99–121
compliance, 120–121
heart failure, management of symptoms, 117–118
nutrition assessment, 99–112, 139

O

Obesity, 7, 143–144
management, 144
Osmolality, 103
Outcome measure, 23
Outcomes evaluation
defined, 236
examples, 238
outcomes management, comparison, 237
outcomes research, comparison, 237
Outcomes management
defined, 236
examples, 238
outcomes evaluation, comparison, 237
outcomes research, comparison, 237
Outcomes measurement, 235–260, 314–315
behavior, 255
caregiver, 255–257
caregiver burden, 256
caregiver symptoms, 256–257
caregiving appraisal, 256
conceptual considerations, 235–236
data management, 239
defining goals and objectives, 236
determining approach, 236
developing conceptual framework, 236
future research, 258–260
health-related quality of life, 241–251
biologic functioning, 250–251
Canadian Cardiovascular Society Functional Classification, 246–247
Chronic Heart Failure questionnaire, 250
Clock Drawing Test, 248–249

cognitive functioning, 248–249
Duke Activity Status Instrument, 247–248
Functional Status Questionnaire, 247
functioning, 246–249
generic measures, 242–243
health perception, 245–246
Health Perceptions Questionnaire, 246
Heart Condition Assessment, 248
Medical Outcomes Short Form-36 Item
    Questionnaire (SF-36), 244–245
Mini-Mental State Examination, 248
Minnesota Living with Heart Failure
    questionnaire, 243–244
New York Heart Association (NYHA)
    Functional Classification, 246
overall well-being, 243–245
physical functioning, 246–248
physiologic functioning, 250–251
Quality of Life Index, 245
Quality of Life Questionnaire in Severe
    Heart Failure, 244
Sickness Impact Profile, 245
Specific Activity Scale, 247
symptoms, 249–250
Yale scale, 249–250
initial considerations, 235–239
instrument reliability, 240
instrument selection, 23, 239–241, 242
instrument validity, 240
knowledge, 255
length of stay, 253
managing expectations, 239
measuring financial outcomes, 251–254
    charges/costs, 252
measuring processes influencing outcomes,
    254–258
operational issues, 239
practical issues, 240–241
purpose clarification, 235–236
quality of care, 257–258
resource use, 251–252
resources to support, 259
risk adjustment, 252
self-care, 255
unplanned resource utilization, 253–254
Outcomes research
defined, 236
examples, 238

outcomes evaluation, comparison, 237
outcomes management, comparison, 237
Outpatient education seminar, 188

P

Patient education, 178–190, 310–312, 347
aging, 186
community case management, 292–293
consumer information, 197
critical pathway guidelines, 181, 182
deficit of knowledge, 183
educational materials, 186, 188–189
environmental barriers, 186–187
failure to include supporters, 181
family, 181
follow-up, 183
home health care, 227–228
improving health care systems, 184
individualized, 186
ineffective communication patterns, 180–181
Monitoring and Educating Using Disease
    Management to Improve Compliance
    Instrument, 186, 192–196
new models, 181–183
outpatient education seminar, 188
principles, 186
promoting behavior change, 184–186
strategies, 186–187
teaching in stressful environment, 180
telemanagement, 187–188
    high risk for rehospitalization, 187
traditional, 179–181
Patient independence, 297
Patient referral, 297
Performance-based measure, 24
Perfusion scintigraphy, surgical
    revascularization, 55
Pharmacologic therapy, 344–345
compliance, 171–172
cost-effectiveness, 33–35
health-related quality of life
    clinical trials, 44–49
    impact, 43–49
hypertension, 139–141
impact on physiologic parameters, 43–44
limitations, 152–153

morbidity, 43–44
mortality, 43–44
Philadelphia Geriatric Center Caregiving
Appraisal Scale, 256
Physical examination, 104–107
Physical functioning, 246–248
Physiologic functioning, 250–251
Population-attributable risk
hypertension, 6
myocardial infarction, 6
Positron emission tomography, surgical
revascularization, 55
Potassium, 103
Prazosin, 33
Prealbumin, 101
Prevalence, defined, 4
Prevention, 346
Progressive pump failure, 13
Prospective Randomized Evaluation of
Carvedilol in Symptoms and Exercise
(PRECISE) trial
carvedilol, 45, 46–47
exercise tolerance, 45, 46–47
PROVED trial, 33
Pulmonary artery wedge pressure, exertional
dyspnea, 124
Pulse pressure, 6

Q

Quality of care, outcomes measurement, 257–258
Quality of life, xiii, xv
cardiac transplantation
age, 69–70
complications, 69–70
gender, 69–70
long-term studies of outcomes, 69
racial/ethnic background, 69–70
cardiomyopathy, 59
defined, 18
donor shortage, 67–71
short-term studies on outcomes, 67–69
implantable left ventricular assist device,
63–65
interventions to improve, 78–93
mitral valve repair, 58–60
morbidity, association, 77–78
mortality, association, 77–78

nonpharmacologic therapy
integrated theory to explain mechanism,
92
recommendations for research and
practice, 92–93
surgical revascularization, 58–60
surgical therapy, impact, 52–71
Quality of Life Index, 245
Quality of life research
cardiac transplantation, methodologic issues,
70–71
hierarchical linear model, 53–54
implantable left ventricular assist device,
methodologic issues, 64–65
longitudinal analysis, 52–53
attrition, 53
methodologic issues, 52–54
mitral valve repair, methodologic issues, 59–
60
mixed model, 53–54
multilevel model, 53–54
random regression model, 53–54
recommendations for future research, 71
study sample, 53
surgical revascularization, methodologic
issues, 59–60

R

RADIANCE trial, 33
Random regression model, quality of life
research, 53–54
Randomized clinical trial
alternative models of care, 35–38
home-based intervention, 36–37
Randomized Evaluation of Mechanical
Assistance for the Treatment of Congestive
Heart Failure, implantable left ventricular
assist device, 63
Reciprocity
caregiver, 223
social network, 207
Regurgitant mitral valve, 56–58
Relative risk, defined, 4
Relaxation
cardiovascular disease, 153–155
cost-effectiveness, 156
maintenance of effects, 154–155

physiologic outcomes, 153–154
    psychologic outcomes, 154
  defined, 153
  heart failure, 155–159
Relaxation training, 85–86
Respiratory muscle, abnormalities, 127
Respite care, 225, 226
Rheumatic valve disease, 5
Rib, 104, 106
Risk adjustment, outcomes measurement, 252
Risk factor
  defined, 4
  modification, 136–151
Risk ratio, defined, 4

S

Scapula, 104, 106
Secondary prevention, 346
Self-care model
  adaptive potential assessment model,
    theoretical linkages, 205, 206
  affiliation-individuation, theoretical linkages,
    205, 206
  outcomes measurement, 255
  supportive resources, 203–204
    self-care actions, 203–204
    self-care knowledge, 203
    self-care resources, 203
Self-Care Resource Inventory, supportive
  resources, 204
Self-efficacy, 213–214
Serum cholesterol, 101–102
Serum creatinine, 103–104
Serum glucose, 102
Serum osmolality, 103
Serum potassium, 103
Serum sodium, 102–103
Sharp HealthCare Multidisciplinary Disease
  Management Program, multidisciplinary
  disease management model, 334–336
Short Form-12 Health Survey, 24
Short Form-20, 23, 24
Short Form-36 Health Survey, 23–24
Sickness Impact Profile, 245
Six-minute walk test, 24
Skeletal muscle
  abnormalities in heart failure, 124–128

  fatigue, 124
  inactivity, 128
Skilled home health care, 225, 226
Smoking, 144–146, 310
  hemodynamic data, 144–145
  mechanism of action, 144
Smoking cessation, 145
Social network
  quality, 207
  reciprocity, 207
  size, 207
Social support, 347
  caregiver, 224
  health
    relationships, 208
    theoretical explanations, 208
  hospitalization, 209
  multifaceted construct, 207
Social support research
  cardiovascular disease, 208–210
  heart failure, 208–210
  supportive resources
    overview, 206
    theory development, 206–208
Sodium, 102–103, 345–346
Sodium restriction
  cachexia, 117
  Kaiser/Stanford Heart Failure Program
    Sodium Progress Report #2, 329–330
Sodium retention, 140–141
  management, 118–119, 120
  signs, 104
Specific Activity Scale, 247
Spironolactone, 344
Spouse, 206–207
Standards, heart failure, 258
Stanford cardiac rehabilitation program
  experience, 322–326
Strength training, 147
Studies of Left Ventricular Dysfunction
  (SOLVD) registry
  hypertension, 138
  left ventricular dysfunction, 45, 46
Study sample, quality of life research, 53
Subjective Global Assessment, nutrition
  assessment, 110–112
Sudden death, 13
Supplement, 117

Support group, 210
Supportive resources, 201–216
  Adaptive Potential Assessment Model,
    204–205
  affiliated-individuation, 202–203
  developmental residual, 204
  external resources, 205–212
  health care providers, 211–212, 214–215
  information as, 210–211
  internal resources, 212–214
  interrelationships of component theories of
    modeling and role modeling, 205, 206
  overview, 201–202
  self-care model, 203–204
    self-care actions, 203–204
    self-care knowledge, 203
    self-care resources, 203
  Self-Care Resource Inventory, 204
  social support research
    overview, 206
    theory development, 206–208
  theoretical approach to, 202–205
Surgical revascularization, 54–56
  assessing contractile reserve, 55
  dysfunctional myocardium, 55
  hibernating myocardium, 55
  ischemic left ventricular dysfunction, 55
  perfusion scintigraphy, 55
  positron emission tomography, 55
  procedure, 55–56
  quality of life, 58–60
  quality of life research, methodologic issues,
    59–60
  results, 56
Surgical therapy, quality of life, impact, 52–71
Systolic dysfunction, exercise capacity, 26
Systolic Hypertension in the Elderly Program,
  141–142, 168
Systolic pressure, 6

T

Telemanagement
  computer telephony, 188
  heart failure, 187–188
    high risk for rehospitalization, 187
  interactive voice response, 188

patient education, 187–188
    high risk for rehospitalization, 187
Telephone, case management, 322–326
Temple, 104, 105
Triceps, 104, 108
Triglyceride, 101–102
  management, 142–143
Tumor necrosis factor-alpha, 26

U

University of California, Los Angeles (UCLA)
  Medical Center, heart failure clinic, 308–315
  alcohol, 310
  cost, 315
  diet, 310
  diuretic, 309, 311
  exercise, 311
  fluid restriction, 310
  medication compliance, 311–312
  outcomes, 312–313
  outcomes measurement, 314–315
  outcomes variables, 313–314
  patient education, 310–312
  smoking, 310
  weight, 310–311
Urine osmolality, 103
Urine sodium, 103

V

Valve disease, 5
Vasodilator, 33
Vesnarinone, clinical trial, 45, 47–48
Vesnarinone Trial, 45, 47–48
Veterans Administration Heart Failure Trials
  enalapril, 44–46
  hydralazine-isosorbide dinitrate, 44–46
Vigor, 214

W

Weight, 100–101, 310–311
  self-monitoring skills teaching, 120

Y

Yale scale, 249–250